C. Simon, W. Stille, P. J. Wilkinson
Antibiotic Therapy in Clinical Practice

Antibiotic Therapy

in Clinical Practice

By

Prof. Dr. C. Simon

University Children's Hospital, Kiel, W. Germany

and

Prof. Dr. W. Stille

University Centre for Internal Medicine, Frankfurt am Main,
W. Germany

and

Dr. P. J. Wilkinson

Microbiology and Public Health Laboratory, Plymouth, England

With 36 Figures and 72 Tables

19 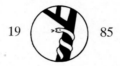 85

F. K. SCHATTAUER VERLAG · STUTTGART – NEW YORK

The reproduction of general descriptive names, trade names, trade marks etc. in this publication, even when there is no special identification mark, is not to be taken as a sign that such names, as understood by the Trade Marks and Merchandise Marks Law, may be freely used.

For various reasons, the lists of antibiotics and chemotherapeutic agents in this book may not be complete. The omission of a commercially available preparation does not necessarily imply that it is less suitable for therapy than the alternatives described.

Notice

Not all of the drugs mentioned in this book have been approved by FDA for use in infants or in children under age 6 or age 12. Such drugs should not be used if effective alternatives are available; they may be used if no effective alternatives are available or if the known risk of toxicity of alternative drugs or the risk of nontreatment is outweighed by the probable advantages of treatment.

Because of the possibility of an error in the article or book from which a particular drug dosage is obtained, or an error appearing in the text of this book, our readers are urged to consult appropriate references, including the manufacturer's package insert, especially when prescribing new drugs or those with which they are not adequate familiar.   – The AUTHORS

CIP-Kurztitelaufnahme der Deutschen Bibliothek

Simon, Claus: Antibiotic therapy in clinical practice / by
C. Simon and W. Stille and P. J. Wilkinson. –
Stuttgart ; New York : Schattauer, 1985
    Einheitssacht.: Antibiotika-Therapie in Klinik und Praxis ‹engl.›
    ISBN 3-7945-0936-6

NE: Stille, Wolfgang ; Wilkinson, Peter J.:

Authorized English edition.
Translated by Dr. F. MIELKE, Hamburg.
Original German edition: C. SIMON, W. STILLE: Antibiotika-Therapie in Klinik und Praxis.
5th edition. Schattauer, Stuttgart – New York 1982.

Composing, printing and binding: Mayr Miesbach Druckerei und Verlag GmbH, Am Windfeld 15, D-8160 Miesbach, Germany

ISBN 3-7945-0936-6

Foreword

This book attempts to give a clear, systematic presentation of the pharmacology and mode of action of antimicrobial agents, together with practical guidance in their use in the treatment of infectious disease. We hope it will be of value not only to the clinician but also to medical students, pharmacists and pharmacologists, microbiologists and any concerned with the diagnosis and management of infection.

Any rational choice of antimicrobial agent must be based on a firm clinical and microbiological diagnosis; how this should be made is discussed in the clinical sections of the text. Severe and life-threatening infections need antibiotics before laboratory results are available and clear guidance is given for such cases. The indications and contraindications for each agent are detailed, together with examples of inappropriate use.

Effective treatment requires the antimicrobial to be given at optimal dosage in relation to the age and general condition of the patient and the route of administration. Our recommendations are based on controlled studies, where available, and on the clinical experience of ourselves and others.

Despite the current range of antibiotics, both new and old, the treatment of most important infections is largely standard. Certain differences in practice between Britain, other European countries and the USA are mentioned. Prescribing habits and trade names vary from country to country and this book is intended for an international readership; generic names are therefore used throughout, but as comprehensive a list of proprietary names as practicable is given for each antibiotic.

In Germany, this book has achieved five editions and a sixth is in preparation. The British coauthor of the first English edition has contributed to a thorough revision of the text which should enable its use as a handy, up to date reference work by a wider readership.

We are very grateful to the Schattauer Verlag, and particularly to Prof. Dr. Dr. P. Matis, for their help and support in the production of this book.

Autumn 1984   C. Simon, W. Stille, P. J. Wilkinson

Authors' Addresses:

Prof. Dr. C. SIMON
   Universitäts-Kinderklinik
   Schwanenweg 20, 2300 Kiel, F.R.G.

Prof. Dr. W. STILLE
   Zentrum der Inneren Medizin der Universität
   Theodor-Stern-Kai 7, 6000 Frankfurt/M., F.R.G.

Dr. P. J. WILKINSON MRC Path.
   Public Health Laboratory, Derriford Hospital
   Derriford Road, Plymouth PL8 8DH, U.K.

Contents

A. Basic Concepts of Chemotherapy

1. Classification of Antibiotics

Antibiotics are substances produced by fungi and bacteria, which in small quantities can inhibit the growth of microorganisms or even kill them. *Chemotherapeutic agents* are artificial substances with antimicrobial activity and are not found in nature. There are no fundamental differences between antibiotics and chemotherapeutic agents. Synthetic antibiotics (e. g. chloramphenicol) and chemically modified (semisynthetic) antibiotics (e. g. ampicillin) occupy an intermediate position.

Table 1. Classification of the β-lactam antibiotics.

Group	Subgroup	Important derivatives
Penicillins (Penams)	Benzyl penicillin	Benzyl penicillin sodium Procaine benzyl penicillin Benzathine benzyl penicillin
	Phenoxypenicillins (acid-stable)	Phenoxymethyl penicillin Propicillin Azidocillin
	Aminobenzyl penicillins	Ampicillin Amoxycillin Bacampicillin Pivampicillin Talampicillin
	Acylamino-(ureido-) penicillins	Azlocillin Mezlocillin Piperacillin Apalcillin
	Carboxy- penicillins	Carbenicillin Carfecillin Carindacillin Ticarcillin Temocillin
	Penicillinase- stable penicillins	Oxacillin Cloxacillin Dicloxacillin Flucloxacillin Methicillin Nafcillin

Table 1. (continued).

Group	Subgroup	Important derivatives
Penicillins	Other penicillins	Mecillinam Pivmecillinam
Cephalosporins (Cephems)	Cephalothin group	Cephalothin Cephaloridine and others
	Cefazolin group	Cefazolin Cefazedone
	Cefuroxime group	Cefuroxime Cefamandole Cefotiam
	Cefoxitin group	Cefoxitin Cefotetan Cefmetazole Latamoxef
	Cefotaxime group	Cefotaxime Ceftriaxone Ceftizoxime Cefmenoxime Ceftazidime
	Oral cephalosporins	Cephalexin Cefaclor Cefadroxil Cephradine Cefroxadine
	Other cephalosporins	Cefsulodin Cefoperazone
Carbapenems	–	Thienamycin Olivanic acid
Monolactams	–	Aztreonam Nocardicin
β-Lactamase inhibitors	–	Clavulanic acid Sulbactam

There are several classifications of the important antibiotics and chemotherapeutic agents based on their chemical structure, their biological origin and their therapeutic use (Tables 1–3). Antibiotics of the same class have similar modes of action and spectra of activity; they generally share resistance and are similar in their toxicity.

Table 2. Classification of antibiotics other than the β-lactams.

Group	Subgroup	Important derivatives
Aminoglycosides	Older aminoglycosides	Streptomycin Neomycin Paromomycin Kanamycin
	Newer aminoglycosides	Gentamicin Sisomicin Tobramycin Netilmicin Amikacin
Other broad-spectrum antibiotics	Tetracyclines	Tetracycline Oxytetracycline Doxycycline Minocycline
	Chloramphenicol group	Chloramphenicol Thiamphenicol
Narrow-spectrum antibiotics	Macrolides	Erythromycin Josamycin Oleando-, Spiramycin
	Polymyxins	Polymyxin B Colistin
	Others	Clindamycin Fusidic acid Spectinomycin
Cell wall antagonists (not β-lactams)	–	Vancomycin Fosfomycin Cycloserine

Table 3. Classification of the antibacterial chemotherapeutic agents.

Group	Derivatives
Sulphonamides	Short-acting sulphonamides Medium-acting sulphonamides Long-acting sulphonamides Ultra-long-acting sulphonamides Poorly absorbed sulphonamides
Sulphonamide-diaminopyrimidine combinations	Co-trimoxazole Co-trimoxole Co-trimetrole Co-trimazine Co-tetroxazine

Table 3. (continued).

Group	Derivatives
Nitrofurans	Nitrofurantoin Nitrofurazone Nifuratel
Older gyrase inhibitors	Nalidixic acid Oxolinic acid Pipemidic acid Piromidic acid Cinoxacin
Newer gyrase inhibitors	Norfloxacin Ciprofloxacin Ofloxacin Pefloxacin Enoxacin
Nitroimidazoles	Metronidazole Tinidazole Ornidazole

A few antibiotics, which act selectively on certain pathogens (e. g. staphylococci, Pseudomonas or Mycobacterium tuberculosis) are called *narrow-spectrum antibiotics*. *Broad-spectrum antibiotics* are effective against a wider range of pathogens. A complete spectrum of activity cannot yet be achieved by a single drug, however, and a combination is always required for this purpose. Because of their toxicity, some antibiotics are restricted to local use (e. g. neomycin, paromomycin, bacitracin) and may be grouped as *topical antibiotics*.

2. Antibacterial Activity

Mode of action: The antibacterial activity of an antibiotic may be measured in vitro by determining the minimal inhibitory concentration (MIC). While some antibiotics merely inhibit the multiplication of bacteria *(bacteriostasis)*, others actively kill microorganisms *(bactericidal activity)*. The most important bactericidal antibiotics are the penicillins, the cephalosporins and the aminoglycosides.

Whether or not an antibiotic is bactericidal depends not only on the type of antibiotic, its mode of action and concentration at the site of action, but also on the bacterial species, the numbers of bacteria present (i. e. the inoculum size *in vitro*), the duration of action and the phase of growth of the organism. Thus penicillins and cephalosporins are bactericidal only on actively proliferating organisms; polymyxin and the aminoglycosides, on the other hand, also act on bacteria in the resting phase.

The bactericidal effect is of greatest importance during the first 4–8 hours, and is only clinically relevant if a high percentage of the bacteria (>99%) are killed during this period. Bacteria can also die as part of their own aging process while under the influence of bacteriostatic drugs. A bactericidal effect is valuable in certain diseases in which the causative agent can only be eradicated with difficulty (e. g. bacterial endocarditis). Many aspects of the clinical importance of bactericidal activity are obscure. The existing bactericidal antibiotics are by no means instantly bactericidal; the bacteria generally die after a latent period. The example of chloramphenicol in typhoid fever shows that a bacteriostatic antibiotic is not necessarily inferior to a bactericidal one in every disease.

Some **pathogenic organisms may persist** when β-lactam antibiotics act on resting bacteria, that is, small numbers of dormant, sensitive bacteria survive. The explanation is that autolytic bacterial enzymes necessary for cell division are inhibited by the antibiotic. These *persisters* are thus morphologically normal bacteria which have survived lethal concentrations of penicillin. The daughter cells, produced subsequently, remain fully sensitive when the effect of the antibiotic ceases. Because of this phenomenon, antibacterials may fail to sterilise the lesion in many infections, which explains in part the failures of treatment encountered in immune deficiency diseases and bone marrow suppression. In other words, despite satisfactory tissue concentrations, the bactericidal antibiotics, currently available, may be unable to eradicate the pathogens of infection without the aid of the body's defence mechanisms.

Penicillins and cephalosporins can give rise in a hypertonic medium (e. g. urine) to forms of gram-negative organisms whose cell walls are deficient. These *spheroplasts* (with defective cell walls) or *protoplasts* (with absent cell walls) survive and no longer react to the antibiotic; in some cases, they revert to their normal bacterial form after the end of therapy. Their clinical relevance is doubtful. Spheroplasts can be cultivated in the presence of subinhibitory concentrations of antibiotics. With penicillins and cephalosporins, this leads to the appearance of filamentous and other morphologically changed forms. At subinhibitory concentrations, different antibiotics show differing partial activities. The "minimal antibacterial concentration" is a measure of the subinhibitory activity of an antibiotic, i. e. that concentration which can still lead to a measurable inhibition of bacterial growth.

The **mechanism of action** of most antibiotics is well known, and is generally similar in drugs of the same group, giving rise to a pattern of complete cross-resistance. Antibiotics act by inhibiting bacterial cell wall synthesis, inhibiting the synthesis of cytoplasmic components, damaging the cytoplasmic membrane or disrupting nucleic acid synthesis (Table 4). A knowledge of these mechanisms is important in understanding the basis of the combined action of antibiotics, since a synergistic (potentiated) effect only occurs when the partners in the combination have different sites of action.

Table 4. Sites of action of antibiotics.

Cell wall synthesis	Cytoplasmic membrane (permeability)	Synthesis of cytoplasmic components	Nucleic acid synthesis
β-Lactam antibiotics Vancomycin Fosfomycin Cycloserine	Colistin Polymyxin B Amphotericin B Nystatin	Chloramphenicol Tetracycline Erythromycin Lincomycin Aminoglycosides	Rifampicin Griseofulvin Fusidic acid Gyrase inhibitors

References

HELM, E. B.: Antibakterielle Aktivität von Antibiotika in Körperflüssigkeiten. Beecham, Neuss 1977.
SHAH, P. M., W. JUNGHANNS, W. STILLE: Dosis-Wirkung-Beziehung der Bakterizidie bei E. coli, K. pneumoniae und Staphylococcus aureus. Dtsch. med. Wschr. *101:* 325 (1976).

3. Bacterial Resistance

Sensitivity to antibiotics varies between different species of bacteria, between different strains of the same species and even within the same bacterial population. The antibiotic sensitivity pattern of some bacterial species, such as pneumococci, gonococci, meningococci and Haemophilus influenzae is largely predictable; other species such as staphylococci, enterococci, Escherichia coli, Klebsiella, Pseudomonas aeruginosa, Proteus and Mycobacterium tuberculosis show considerable variations. The sensitivities of these species should therefore be tested in vitro before starting antibiotic treatment.

Bacterial resistance is present when the bacteria multiply at an antibiotic concentration which can be achieved in the tissues. Resistance is due either to inherent insensitivity to the antibiotic, or to inactivation by bacterial enzymes (Table 5).

Table 5. Examples of chromosomal and plasmid-mediated antibiotic resistance.

| Mechanisms of antibiotic resistance ||
Chromosomal mutation	Plasmid transfer (extrachromosomal)
Increased formation of an inactivating enzyme (e. g. by Escherichia coli against *ampicillin*).	Enzymatic hydrolysis of the β-lactam ring (by *penicillin* and *cephalosporin* β-lactamases).
Decreased permeability (e. g. to *benzyl penicillin* in gonococci).	Acetylation by bacterial acetyltransferases (e. g. of *chloramphenicol* by Haemophilus).
Reduced binding to bacterial ribosomes (e. g. of *streptomycin* in enterococci).	Enzymatic changes by phosphorylases (e. g. of *gentamicin* by gram-positive bacteria).
	Disruption of transport across the cell membrane *(tetracyclines)*.
	Metabolic by-pass by the formation of a new bacterial enzyme (e. g. of dihydrofolate reductase, which confers resistance to *trimethoprim*).

Certain penicillins and cephalosporins are inactivated by species-specific β-lactamases which hydrolyse the β-lactam ring of the antibiotic. The β-lactamases of gram-positive bacteria are secreted outside the cell, while those of gram-negative bacteria remain within the periplasmic space (Fig. 1). There are also β-lactamase inhibitors (e. g. clavulanic acid) which increase the resistance of

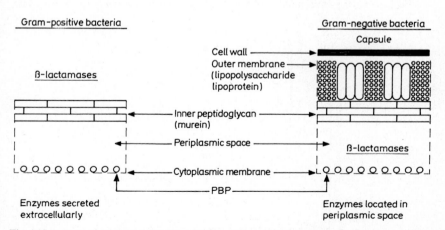

Fig. 1. Structure of capsule, cell wall and cell membrane of gram-positive and gram-negative bacteria. PBP = penicillin binding protein.

certain bacteria against the penicillins. Aminoglycosides are also modified by bacterial enzymes (acetylase, phosphorylase, adenylase), which explains differences in the spectrum of activity of different members of this group. Chloramphenicol can be acetylated by the action of a bacterial acetyltransferase on the two free hydroxyl groups, which destroys its antibacterial activity. Other factors determining resistance to penicillins and cephalosporins are the ability of the antibiotic to penetrate the outer layers of the bacterial cell wall, and changes in the cell wall structure which can lead to antibiotic tolerance.

Resistance may be classified as follows:

1. **Natural resistance,** where the sensitivity of a bacterial species is permanent and genetically determined (e. g. the ineffectiveness of benzyl penicillin against Pseudomonas aeruginosa). Such resistance is chromosomally mediated.

2. **Mutational resistance:** This is unrelated to previous antibiotic therapy. Individual members of a bacterial population which have become resistant through mutation do not multiply disproportionately until selected by treatment with that antibiotic.

3. **Secondary resistance** does not develop until therapy has begun. Exposure to the antibiotic selects for resistant variants which appear in small numbers in larger bacterial populations and arise through mutation. Secondary resistance can develop at varying speeds according to the rate of mutation and the transfer quota for high frequency resistance. Resistance develops rapidly with streptomycin *(one-step resistance),* within a few days with erythromycin and fusidic

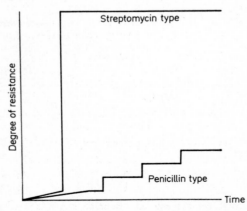

Fig. 2. One-step resistance (streptomycin type) and multiple-step resistance (penicillin type).

acid, and much more slowly with polypeptide antibiotics and others *(multiple-step resistance)* (Fig. 2). This is why antibiotics to which resistance develops rapidly have a higher clinical failure rate. In such cases regular bacteriological cultures are recommended to detect any relapse or change in infecting organism promptly.

4. **Transferable resistance,** plasmid-mediated (or infectious drug resistance) occurs predominantly in gram-negative bacilli (Escherichia coli, Klebsiella, Salmonella, Shigella, Pseudomonas aeruginosa, Serratia, Proteus, Vibrio and Yersinia). During the process of conjugation, plasmids (extrachromosomal genetic material) are transferred from one bacterial species to another; this process requires the mediation of a "resistance transfer factor". The multiple resistance of salmonellae or shigellae against sulphonamides, tetracycline, chloramphenicol or streptomycin can thus be transferred to a sensitive strain of Escherichia coli. Other examples of transferable resistance include that to ampicillin and carbenicillin, kanamycin and gentamicin or trimethoprim. Resistance can also be transferred between bacteria of the same species. Extra-chromosomal resistance transfer by plasmids has also been observed in staphylococci, in which it is mediated by bacteriophages. The transfer of multiple resistance occurs not only *in vitro* but also *in vivo*; it has been demonstrated in the human intestine, on other mucous membranes and on the skin. This is often lost spontaneously later. Antibiotic supplements in animal feedstuffs, which could play a part, are not nowadays permitted.

Genetics of antibiotic resistance: Bacteria can acquire resistance to antimicrobials either through chromosomal mutation or by plasmid transfer. Plasmids are extrachromosomal elements of bacterial DNA (including *R-factors*) which can, like the chromosome, carry genetic information about antibiotic resistance. Mutations mediating antibiotic resistance arise spontaneously with a frequency which is not affected by exposure to antibiotics. Plasmid-mediated resistance is generally of greater clinical importance than chromosomal, since bacteria which have undergone chromosomal mutation are metabolically impaired and less well able to multiply than non-mutant members of the population.

Plasmid-mediated resistance is usually based on the synthesis of proteins which either act as enzymes or change the cell wall in such a way that the antibiotics can no longer penetrate. R-(Resistance-)plasmids can be transferred from one bacterial cell to another by conjugation, transduction mediated by bacteriophages or by transformation (direct DNA transfer after the destruction of a cell). Conjugation is the main method of transfer for gram-negative organisms and bacteriophage transduction for gram-positive (e. g. staphylococci).

Another means of resistance transfer is by means of minute mobile elements of DNA (*transposons*) which are often found on plasmids and can move from plasmid to plasmid or to the chromosome. A transposon can mediate single or multiple resistance and can, after entering a bacterial cell, become incorporated in its plasmid or chromosome.

Chromosomal and plasmid-mediated resistance involve different mechanisms (Table 5). It is not uncommon for more than one resistance mechanism to be present in a single bacterial strain.

Clinical importance of resistance: Necessary antibiotics should not be withheld because of the fear of resistance, although patients at particular risk (e. g. with severe burns or leukaemia) should be carefully monitored for the development of secondary infections with resistant organisms during and after antibiotic treatment. The danger of resistance is reduced by the use of combinations (e. g. in tuberculosis or agranulocytosis); the use of rifampicin or fusidic acid as single agents should be avoided since both can give rise to one-step mutational resistance.

When an antibiotic becomes ineffective against a proportion of cases of a given infection in a hospital (e. g. benzyl penicillin against staphylococci), an alternative, usually effective antibiotic (e. g. flucloxacillin) should be used for the initial, "blind" therapy of severe infections such as osteomyelitis which are likely to be caused by those organisms.

In large hospitals it is sometimes worth monitoring the resistance situation systematically as a basis for general recommendations for antibiotic use. Broad-spectrum antibiotics which favour the selection of resistant organisms in patients should then only be used for clear indications such as infections with many possible bacterial causes. In such situations, antibiotics which have been found to exert only a slight selection pressure, e. g. piperacillin, should be preferred to agents such as ampicillin which select strongly. The uncritical use of antibiotics for general prophylaxis or in viral infections should always be avoided because of the risk of spread of resistant strains. Careful measures to minimise the risk of cross-infection will also help to control the dissemination of such bacteria in hospitals.

Cross-resistance (more precisely: *parallel resistance*) is the simultaneous resistance in a given bacterial strain to several antibiotics of the same group, that is, with generally similar chemical structures and the same or related modes of action. Two-way cross-resistance involving a single antibiotic is always related to resistance to another antibiotic of the same group; examples occur amongst the tetracyclines, between neomycin and kanamycin, and between polymyxin B and colistin. Cross-resistance can also be one-way where, for example, resistance to antibiotic A is linked with resistance to antibiotic B, but resistance primarily to antibiotic B may be associated with sensitivity to antibiotic A. An example of this is kanamycin resistance in mycobacteria which is linked with resistance to streptomycin; streptomycin-resistant strains are mostly sensitive to kanamycin, however. Differentiation between one-way and two-way cross-resistance is important in therapy because giving a closely related antibiotic will be unsuccessful where cross-resistance is two-way. There is no point in giving amoxycillin when ampicillin has failed. When antibiotics with one-way cross-resistance are used, it is best to give first that antibiotic which allows the alternative drug to be given, should resistance to the first agent arise.

References

BRADLEY, H. E., J. G. WETMIER, D. S. HODES: Tolerance in Staphylococcus aureus. Evidence for bacteriophage role. J. infect. Dis. *141:* 233 (1980).

BRITZ, M. L., R. G. WILKINSON: Chloramphenicol acetyltransferase of Bacteroides fragilis. Antimicrob. Ag. Chemother. *14:* 105 (1978).

CURTIS, N. A. C., D. ORR, G. W. ROSS et al.: Affinities of penicillins and cephalosporins for the penillin-binding proteins of Escherichia coli K-12 and their antibacterial activity. Antimicrob. Ag. Chemother. *16:* 533 (1979).

CURTIS, N. A., D. ORR, G. W. ROSS et al.: Competition of β-lactam antibiotics for the penicillin-binding proteins. Antimicrob. Ag. Chemother. *16:* 325 (1979).

DAVIES, J.: Aminoglycosides-aminocyclitol antibiotics and their modifying enzymes. In: LORIAN, V. (ed.): Antibiotics in Laboratory Medicine. p. 474. Williams and Wilkins, Baltimore 1980.

GALE, E. F. E., E. CUNLITTE, P. E. REYNOLDS et al.: The Molecular Basis of Antibiotic Action XXX. Wiley, New York 1972.

GEORGE, R. H., D. E. HEALING: Thymidine-requiring Haemophilus influenzae and Staphylococcus aureus. Lancet *2:* 1081 (1977).

GRIECO, M. H.: Antibiotic resistance. Med. Clin. North Amer. *66:* 25 (1982).

HAKENBECK, R., M. TARPAS, A. TOMASZ: Multiple changes of penicillin-binding proteins in penicillin-resistant clinical isolates of Streptococcus pneumoniae. Antimicrob. Ag. Chemother. *17:* 364 (1980).

FOSTER, T. J., T. G. B. HOWE, K. U. V. RICHMOND: Translocation of the tetracycline resistance determinant from R-100-1 to E. coli chromosome. J. Bacteriol. *124:* 1153 (1975).

PERCHESON, P. B., I. E. BRYAN: Penicillin-binding components of penicillinase-susceptible and resistant strains of Streptococcus pneumoniae. Antimicrob. Ag. Chemother. *12:* 390 (1980).

WEINSTEIN, R. A., C. NATHAN, R. GRUENSFELDER et al.: Endemic aminoglycoside resistance in gram-negative bacilli: Epidemiology and mechanisms. J. infect. Dis. *141:* 338 (1980).

4. Pharmacokinetics

Pharmacology must be taken into account when planning antibiotic treatment, particularly the choice of agent, route of administration and dosage. Antibiotics vary greatly in their absorption, blood concentrations, tissue diffusion, distribution in the body, metabolism, accumulation and excretion. Antibiotic pharmacokinetics also vary with the patient's age, disease and organ function. Another important factor is the galenic form of the preparation, which may differ considerably with different preparations of the same antibiotic.

The **absorption rate** after oral administration affects the blood concentration-time curve. Some antibiotics are well absorbed by mouth, whereas others require parenteral administration. Rapid oral absorption leads to higher tissue levels than slow absorption in drugs which diffuse well and whose half-life is not too short. The rate of absorption after i. m. injection also varies, as between benzyl penicillin and procaine penicillin, and this is shown as variation in peak blood levels and the duration of adequate therapeutic concentrations, both of which are important for bactericidal activity at the site of infection. Bacteriostatic antibiotics need prolonged concentration at the site of infection in order to exceed the minimal inhibitory concentration of the infecting organism.

Tissue diffusion is very important in therapy, although the tissue concentration is unfortunately difficult to determine. Studies with radioactively labelled antibiotics in animals are also difficult to evaluate, since they fail to distinguish between the active agent and labelled metabolites. The concentration of free antibiotic in the plasma (i. e. the part which is not bound to plasma proteins) is an important factor in determining tissue concentrations in the healthy patient. Intracellular antibiotic concentrations of agents such as rifampicin, chloramphenicol and tetracyclines are extremely difficult to measure. The extent to which an antibiotic penetrates tissues is reflected by its concentrations in lymph, synovial fluid, cerebrospinal fluid, saliva, tears and in artificially produced blisters; in animals it may be measured in subcutaneous fibrin implants or perforated synthetic capsules.

There is a general tendency towards an equilibrium between blood and tissue concentrations which requires a variable time to achieve since it depends on the capacity for diffusion of the antibiotic concerned. Maximal tissue concentrations therefore occur later than maximal blood concentrations and they also decline more slowly. The concentration in inflamed tissues is particularly important. Since this concentration is difficult to measure, it may be estimated as the serum concentration at the mid-point of the interval between two consecutive doses. Median concentrations are just as important as the serum peak and trough concentrations. The *trough* (or valley) *concentration* is the residual concentration just before the next dose.

Comparison of single tissue concentrations should be based on measurements made in the steady state only, i.e. during constant i.v. infusion. The different composition and metabolism of different tissues can easily explain the variability of tissue kinetics in different organs. Glomerular filtration, tubular secretion and tubular reabsorption affect the concentration in the renal parenchyma, so blood and urine concentrations are both unsuitable indices of antibiotic concentrations in the kidney itself. The concentration in renal lymph, moreover, which is regarded as an indicator of the interstitial antibiotic content, is the result of both tubular reabsorption and plasma transudation, and so it is not identical with the renal parenchymal concentration. Antibiotic concentrations in well perfused organs, e.g. the lungs and liver, are usually higher than in the eyes or bones.

The **antibiotic concentrations in body fluids** (cerebrospinal fluid, bile, urine, amniotic fluid etc.) are important in the treatment of certain infections such as meningitis, cholangitis, urinary infections and chorioamnionitis. Note that the pharmacokinetics of an antibiotic in inflamed tissue or in systemic disease may differ greatly from the conditions found in the healthy person. Thus cerebrospinal fluid concentrations of penicillin are higher in meningitis than when the meninges are not inflamed, showing an increased permeability of the blood-brain barrier. Antibiotic concentrations in the bile, on the other hand, can be lower in obstructive jaundice. The concentration in bronchial secretions is relevant to bronchiectasis, that in pleural effusion or empyema pus to pleurisy, and that in wound secretions to wound infection. The tissue diffusion, total clearance and renal clearance of antibiotics with a short half-life, such as the penicillins and cephalosporins, are impaired or delayed in geriatric patients, who generally have higher blood and lower tissue concentrations than young adults.

Protein binding: It is generally agreed that only the unbound portion has antibacterial activity. The proportions of bound to unbound antibiotic depend on the plasma and tissue concentrations and are kept in an equilibrium defined by the adsorption isotherms (steady state). The degree of protein binding varies with different antibiotics and depends not only on the concentration but also on the pH, the protein content of the blood and inflamed tissue, the simultaneous administration of other drugs which can displace the first antibiotic, and the age (protein binding is less in the newborn). Many drugs are much less bound in chronic renal failure. There are also different physico-chemical mechanisms of protein binding and different types of protein (human, animal). Blood and tissue concentrations in animals are not generally applicable to man.

The variation in published information about protein binding *in vitro* is partly due to differences of method and partly to the dependence of protein binding on drug concentration. Theoretical calculations of tissue levels ("free concentrations"), based on the percentage protein binding, do not relate to the true situation *in vivo*. Many questions about the clinical relevance of protein binding are still unanswered. An important function is the transport of substances in the blood and their deposition in inflamed, protein-rich tissue. Free and bound antibiotics are concentrated in infected organs and tissues in relation to their degree of protein binding. Highly protein-bound drugs are less bound in inflamed tissue with a low protein content than in the blood, and their antibacterial activity at these sites is correspondingly greater. Highly protein-bound antibiotics can also achieve high total concentrations in inflamed tissues by virtue of their normal properties of diffusion, which depend on molecular size, lipophilia, ionic dissociation etc. Increased vascular permeability also increases the concentration of antibiotics at sites of inflammation. Protein binding cannot therefore be considered in isolation; it must always be related to the other properties of the antibiotic such as solubility, tissue penetration, metabolism and excretion rate.

Most antibiotics are **metabolised** to varying extents and at different rates. The products of oxidation, reduction, hydrolysis and conjugation are usually antibacterially inactive or at least less active than the parent compound, and appear in the blood, urine, bile or faeces. This inactivation is usually associated with detoxication of the antibiotic, as happens to chloramphenicol through its conjugation with glucuronic acid. Occasionally, however, metabolic products can have enhanced toxicity, as in the acetylation of sulphonamides.

Most antibiotics are **eliminated** predominantly through the kidneys, by glomerular filtration and also, in some cases, by tubular secretion. A few antibiotics (e. g. rifampicin, fusidic acid, cefoperazone, ceftriaxone) are mainly excreted in the bile and faeces. Intestinal reabsorption may occur and is sometimes useful in treatment. Renal insufficiency leads to the accumulation of antibiotics whose primary route of elimination is through the kidneys, and this may cause toxic side-effects. The plasma half-life of the agent is one index of its rate of elimination and is used to determine the optimal dose interval. The plasma half-life in premature babies, in the full-term neonate and in infants of up to one month may be prolonged because of immaturity of renal function. Antibiotics in this group of patients should usually be given at lower dosage or at extended dose intervals.

References

Dost, F. H.: Grundlagen der Pharmakokinetik. Thieme, Stuttgart 1968.

Gibaldi, M.: Biopharmaceutics and clinical pharmacokinetics. Lea & Febiger, Philadelphia 1977.

Gladtke, E., H. M. v. Hattingberg, W. Kübler: Einführung in die Pharmakokinetik. 2nd Ed. Springer, Berlin 1977.

Notari, R. E.: Biopharmaceutics and pharmacokinetics. Marcel Decker Inc., New York 1977.

Ritschel, W. A.: Handbook of Basic Pharmacokinetics. 1st ed. Drug Intelligence Publ., Hamilton 1976.

Schönfeld, H. (ed.): Pharmacokinetics. Karger, Basel 1978.

Simon, C., D. Kiosz, V. Malerczyk: Die Plasmaeiweißbindung von Clindamycin, Cephazolin und Cephradin bei Neugeborenen und Erwachsenen. Klin. Päd. *187:* 71 (1975).

Swarbrick, J. (ed.): Dosage Form Design and Bioavailability. Lea & Febiger, Philadelphia 1973.

Wagner, J. G.: Biopharmaceutics and relevant pharmacokinetics. 2nd Ed. Drug Intelligence Publ., Hamilton Ill. 1977.

B. Properties of Antibiotics and Chemotherapeutic Agents

1. Penicillins

β-Lactam antibiotics: The penicillins and cephalosporins are the most important β-lactam antibiotics. They have a similar mechanism of action which is to inhibit peptidoglycan synthesis within the bacterial cell wall. The differences of activity between penicillins and cephalosporins are due to variations in their affinity for the binding proteins of the bacteria, their ability to penetrate the bacterial cell membrane *(crypticity)* and their stability to β-lactamase.

A number of new β-lactam antibiotics have been discovered in recent years, including ring-substituted cephalosporins such as latamoxef, and others which are neither penicillins nor cephalosporins (see Fig. 3). New possibilities for treatment are provided by the clavulanic acid derivatives, carbapenems and monolactams (monocyclic β-lactams).

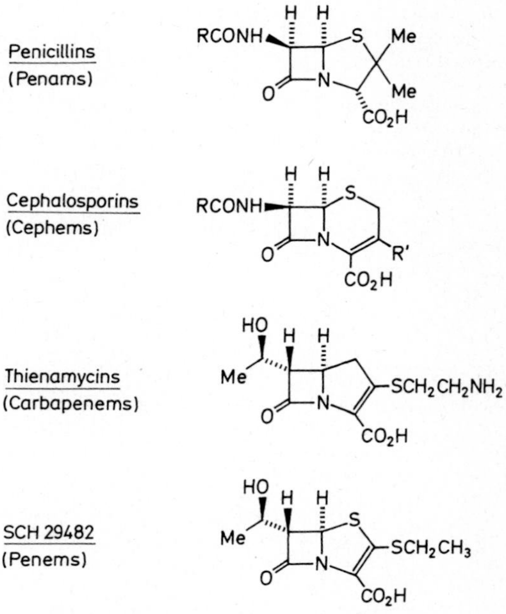

Fig. 3. Structural formulae of the β-lactam antibiotics (penicillins, cephalosporins, thienamycins and penems).

Most β-lactam antibiotics in current use are semi-synthetic. The 6-amino-penicillanic acid or the 7-aminocephalosporanic acid rings can be substituted in a number of different ways. The apparently random nature of derivatives is in fact subject to fixed rules which have become clear as understanding of the structure-activity relationships of the β-lactam antibiotics has increased (Fig. 4). Thus acylamino derivatives are generally active against Pseudomonas and the Enterobacteriaceae, and are concentrated well in the bile. Aminothiazol-oxime derivatives have particularly good antibacterial activity and are very stable to the β-lactamases of members of the Enterobacteriaceae. Oxymethyl derivatives are also very stable to the β-lactamase of Bacteroides fragilis. Because the oxymethyl derivatives penetrate the bacterial cell poorly, they are generally less active. Tetrazolium derivatives have good pharmacokinetic qualities but cause intolerance to alcohol. There may be problems of inactivation with acetyl derivatives.

β-Lactam antibiotics can nowadays be synthesised readily and assembled almost as required like a system of building blocks. Relatively few derivatives combine a good profile of activity with suitable biological qualities, however. Although some

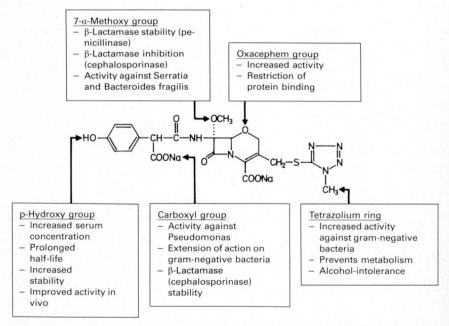

Fig. 4. Structure-activity relationships in the β-lactam antibiotics, exemplified by latamoxef.

derivatives seem to be the final product of medical development, the following three qualities have not yet been successfully combined in a single penicillin or cephalosporin:
– strong anti-pseudomonas activity,
– strong anti-bacteroides activity,
– strong anti-staphylococcal activity.
These three qualities are best represented at present in thienamycin and its derivatives, i. e. the carbapenems.

Properties of the penicillins: Derivatives of 6-aminopenicillanic acid. Bactericidal action on proliferating bacteria, but no effect in the resting phase (inhibition of bacterial cell wall synthesis). The following penicillins are important therapeutically: benzyl penicillin, phenoxymethyl penicillin, propicillin and azidocillin, the penicillinase-stable penicillins (oxacillin, cloxacillin, dicloxacillin, flucloxacillin, nafcillin), ampicillin and its derivatives (bacampicillin, pivampicillin, talampicillin), amoxycillin, the carboxy penicillins (ticarcillin, carfecillin, carindacillin), and the acylamino penicillins (azlocillin, mezlocillin, and piperacillin). These drugs differ from each other not only in their chemical structure (Fig. 5) but also in their range of action.

The **main indications** for the different penicillins are listed in Table 6. Benzyl penicillin is the drug of choice for streptococcal and pneumococcal infections as well as for infections with sensitive strains of staphylococci. Ampicillin is the first choice for infections with enterococci, Haemophilus and Proteus mirabilis. Because of their stability to staphylococcal penicillinase, oxacillin, cloxacillin, dicloxacillin, flucloxacillin and nafcillin are used as penicillinase-resistant anti-staphylococcal penicillins. Azlocillin, ticarcillin and piperacillin are effective agents in infections with sensitive strains of Pseudomonas, although they are not stable to penicillinase.

Parenteral penicillins are given at intervals corresponding to their pharmacokinetics. Treatment should be started with a loading dose. In acute and serious infections, benzyl penicillin is given parenterally as a short i. v. infusion or i. v. injection in a medium or high dosage (4–20 megaunits of benzyl penicillin, or 6–15 g of another penicillin daily).

After clinical signs of improvement, treatment may be continued with high doses of an oral penicillin (3 g), usually either phenoxymethyl penicillin or amoxycillin. Mild infections may be treated with oral penicillins from the outset. Depot penicillins give relatively low serum levels and are therefore only recommended for infections with very sensitive bacteria (streptococci, pneumococci, treponemes), as prophylaxis for rheumatic fever, and for patients who cannot take oral penicillins because of vomiting etc. Topical and rectal

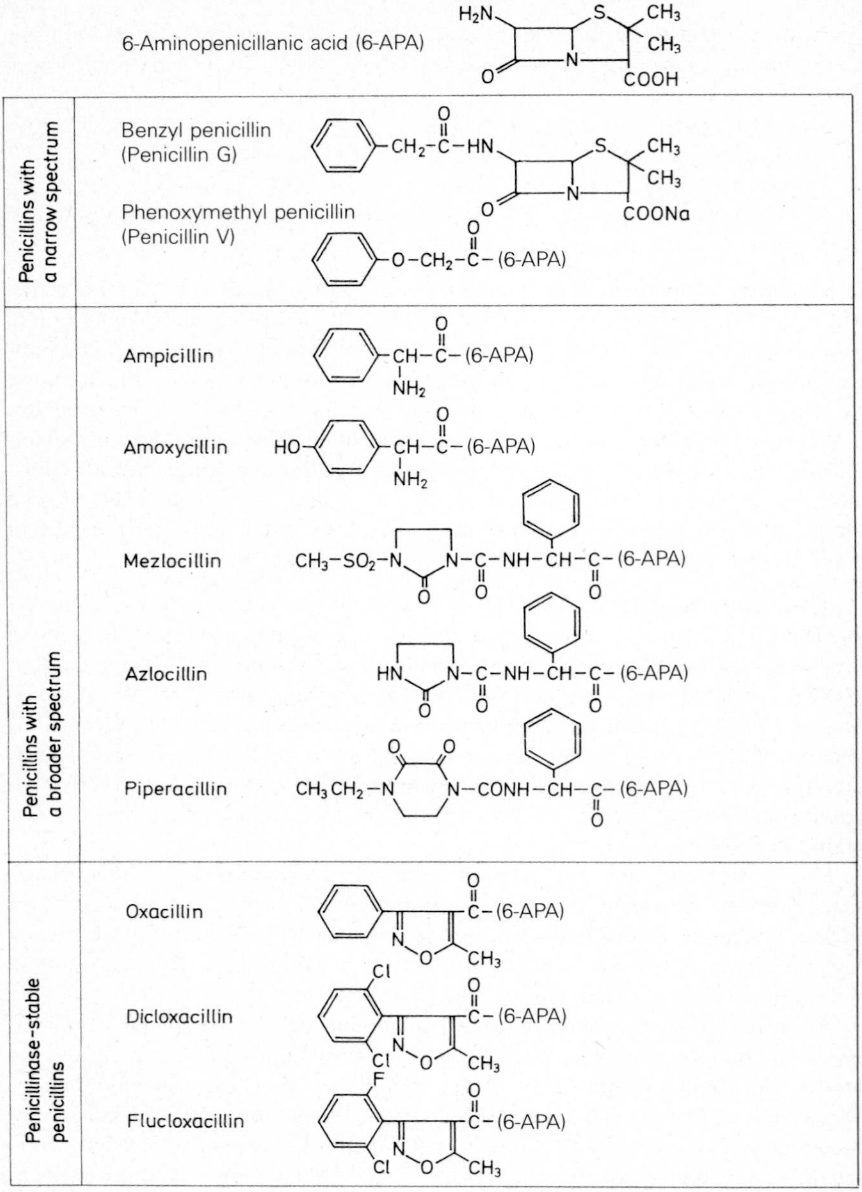

Fig. 5. Chemical structure of the important penicillins.

Table 6. Clinical efficacy of penicillins (principal indications shown thus: [+ + +] or [+]).

Drug	Staphylococci (without production of penicillinase)	Staphylococci (with production of penicillinase)	Str. pneumoniae, Str. pyogenes, gono-, meningococci, Treponema pallidum	Enterococci	Esch. coli	Klebsiella	Proteus mirabilis	Proteus vulgaris	Pseudomonas aeruginosa	Haemophilus	Serratia marcescens
Benzyl penicillin, phenoxymethyl penicillin	[+ + +]	∅	[+ + +]	+	∅	∅	∅	∅	∅	∅	∅
Ampicillin	+ +	∅	+ +	[+ +]	+ +	∅	[+ +]	+	∅	[+ +]	∅
Mezlocillin	+	∅	+ +	[+ +]	[+ +]	+ +	+ +	[+ +]	+ +	+ +	+ +
Piperacillin	+	∅	+ +	+ +	[+ +]	[+ +]	+ +	[+ +]	[+ +]	+ +	+ +
Azlocillin	+	∅	+	+ +	+ +	∅	+ +	∅	[+ +]	+ +	∅
Penicillinase-resistant penicillins	+ +	[+ +]	+ +	∅	∅	∅	∅	∅	∅	∅	∅

administration of penicillins are not recommended because they are often ineffective and carry a considerable risk of allergy.

General evaluation *of the penicillins:*
Advantages: Bactericidal, well tolerated, large dose range, no or only slow development of resistance during therapy.
Disadvantages: Relatively narrow spectrum of activity (except piperacillin and mezlocillin), risk of allergy, rapid excretion.

a) Benzyl Penicillin (Penicillin G)

Properties: Benzyl penicillin is used as its readily soluble sodium or potassium salt or as a poorly soluble depot penicillin (procaine penicillin, benzathine penicillin, clemizole penicillin). It is unstable in acid solution. One international unit of sodium or potassium penicillin is equivalent to 0.6 μg (1 μg = 1.67 units). One megaunit is therefore 600 mg. One megaunit of procaine penicillin corresponds to 1 g, and 1 megaunit of benzathine penicillin corresponds to 750 mg of the pure substance.

Mode of action: Bactericidal on proliferating bacteria, by inhibition of cell wall synthesis by blocking bacterial transpeptidase. A few "persister" organisms may survive; they are morphologically normal bacteria which are not actively multiplying and whose cell wall synthesis is complete. They can survive lethal concentrations of penicillin and resume growth once the penicillin has been removed.

Spectrum of activity:
Good or moderate sensitivity (minimal inhibitory concentration 0.001 to 0.5 units/ml) is shown by Streptococcus pyogenes, Lancefield group B streptococci, pneumococci, viridans streptococci, anaerobic streptococci, gonococci, meningococci, diphtheria bacilli, spirochaetes (treponemes, Borrelia), Actinomyces israeli and Pasteurella multocida. Many gram-negative anaerobes (e. g. Bacteroides melaninogenicus, Fusobacteria) are highly sensitive.
Variable sensitivity is shown by Staphylococcus aureus and epidermidis, Listeria, Clostridia, Bacillus anthracis, and Campylobacter species. Most staphylococcal strains are resistant, but benzyl penicillin is very active against sensitive strains.
Weak sensitivity (or resistance) shown by enterococci (Streptococcus faecalis, Streptococcus faecium), Proteus mirabilis, Brucella, Haemophilus influenzae and Bordetella pertussis.

Resistance[1] (minimal inhibitory concentration greater than 5 units/ml) is shown by the coliforms, salmonellae, Bacteroides fragilis, Nocardia asteroides and vibrios.

Resistance: The frequency of *primary resistance* amongst staphylococci differs from place to place (30–90%), and amongst pneumococci and gonococci is low but increasing. Multi-resistant pneumococci are resistant not only to benzyl penicillin but also to tetracycline, chloramphenicol, erythromycin and clindamycin. Some strains are also resistant to rifampicin. Penicillin-resistant gonococci from East Asia are also mostly resistant to tetracycline, erythromycin and spectinomycin.

Secondary resistance is uncommon and develops slowly (multiple step resistance) through mutation, the selection of resistant variants, or the induction of penicillinase in potential penicillinase producers under the prolonged influence of penicillin. The β-lactam ring of the penicillin is split hydrolytically by bacterial penicillinase, giving rise to antibacterially inactive penicilloyl compounds. *Penicillin-tolerant* strains of Staphylococcus aureus and Streptococcus sanguis are inhibited bacteriostatically, but they are only very slowly destroyed, if at all. Penicillin-tolerant strains of Staphylococcus aureus can have simultaneous tolerance to cephalosporins and vancomycin, but not to gentamicin.

Cross-sensitivity to acylamino penicillins is found in bacteria sensitive to benzyl penicillin.

Pharmacokinetics:
Oral administration is ineffective because the drug is not stable to gastric acid.
Absorption is rapid and complete after i.m. injection of the water-soluble benzyl penicillin, but is retarded with depot penicillins.
Serum concentrations after i.m. or i.v. administration depend on the dose and dose-interval, and differ between benzyl penicillin and the depot penicillins (Fig. 6).
The maximum serum level is 75 units/ml *after an i.v. bolus injection* of 1 megaunit of benzyl penicillin; after an *i.v. infusion over one hour* it is 24 units/ml. The corresponding mean peak concentrations after 5 megaunits are 394 units/ml and 134 units/ml. *Constant infusion* of 0.165 and 0.833 megaunits/hour (equivalent to a daily dose of 4 and 20 megaunits) gives rise to mean serum concentrations of 5.8 and 22.2 units/ml respectively. Thus, as a rule of thumb, the mean serum concentrations in units/ml achieved with constant i.v. infusion correspond approximately to the number of megaunits administered per day.

---

[1] Limit of sensitivity at moderate dosage of up to 5 megaunits daily.

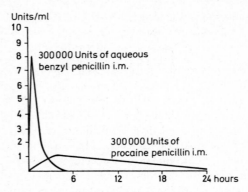

Fig. 6. Serum concentrations with different penicillins.

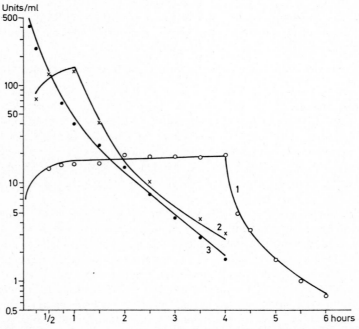

Fig. 7. Measured serum concentrations of benzyl penicillin (sodium salt) and curves calculated from them, after 4 hours of continuous infusion (0.5 megaunits/h = 12 megaunits/day, curve 1), after a short infusion of one hour (5 megaunits, curve 2), and after a bolus intravenous injection (5 megaunits, curve 3).

Because excretion is so rapid, the serum concentrations after i. v. bolus injection fall below those achieved through constant i. v. infusion within 1¼ hours; concentrations after a short (1 hour) i. v. infusions fall below those of constant infusion within 1¾ hours (Fig. 7). In order to maintain a minimum serum level of 0.1 units/ml, a further i. v. injection or short infusion of 5 megaunits is required after 8 hours.

A 1-hour i. v. infusion of 10 megaunits of benzyl penicillin gives rise to a maximum serum concentration of 400 units/ml, which falls to 2.2 units/ml in the absence of probenecid and to 9.6 units/ml when given at the same time as 1 g of probenecid, 5 h after the infusion has finished. Mean serum concentrations of 2.8, 8, 20 and 70 units/ml are found 1 hour after the *i. m. injection of* 0.2, 0.5, 1, and 5 megaunits of sodium benzyl penicillin (Table 7). Depot penicillins give a slower rise and fall with relatively low serum concentrations. The serum concentrations after 0.4 megaunits of procaine penicillin are

0.6 units/ml at 1 and 2 h, 0.5 units/ml at 6 h and 0.1 units/ml at 12 h;

after 0.6 megaunits of procaine penicillin they are

1.0 units/ml at 1 and 2 h, 0.9 units/ml at 6 h and 0.6 units/ml at 12 h.

The advantage of giving higher doses of sodium benzyl penicillin by the i. m. route is that serum concentrations decline more slowly because of the more prolonged absorption of the higher dose. Combined preparations of sodium

Table 7. Mean serum concentrations in adults after the i. m. injection of various preparations of penicillin.

Time (h)	Mean serum concentrations (units/ml) after the injection of	
	Benzyl penicillin sodium (5 megaunits)	Benzyl penicillin sodium (0.25 megaunits) + Procaine penicillin (0.75 megaunits)
¼	54.6 ± 8.3	6.0 ± 2.0
½	76.0 ± 21.0	6.1 ± 2.1
¾	78.0 ± 9.8	6.2 ± 1.8
1	69.0 ± 11.4	4.7 ± 2.4
1½	46.0 ± 9.6	3.6 ± 1.3
2	33.8 ± 3.8	2.1 ± 1.0
2½	23.4 ± 6.7	2.0 ± 1.1
3	16.1 ± 9.4	1.9 ± 0.8
3½	9.1 ± 0.9	1.8 ± 0.8
4	8.1 ± 3.4	1.6 ± 0.5
6	2.8 ± 2.2	1.2 ± 0.3
8	0.9 ± 1.1	1.0 ± 0.4
10	0.3 ± 0.5	0.8 ± 0.3
12	<0.1	0.6 ± 0.3

benzyl penicillin and procaine penicillin are generally preferred for i. m. use in clinical practice, since they combine high initial concentrations with a prolonged period of effect (Table 7).

Low serum concentrations of at least 0.03 units/ml for 3–4 weeks, which are useful in the long-term prophylaxis of rheumatic fever, are maintained *after benzathine penicillin* (1.2 megaunits i. m.). 0.2 units/ml persist in the serum 2 weeks after 2.4 megaunits of this preparation.

Half-life after parenteral benzyl penicillin: 40 min.

Plasma protein binding: ca. 50%.

CSF penetration is poor, but improved in the presence of meningeal inflammation. In purulent meningitis, large single doses of benzyl penicillin give cerebrospinal concentrations which are high enough to kill pneumococci and meningococci (0.08–0.3 units/ml 1 h after 4 megaunits i. v.).

Tissue concentrations: Good penetration of kidneys, lungs, liver, prostate, skin and mucous membranes.

Poor diffusion into muscle, bone, nervous tissue, brain and aqueous humor.

Concentrations in inflammatory, pleural, pericardial, peritoneal and synovial effusions reach 25–75% of the serum concentrations. About ¼ of the maternal serum concentration is found in the fetal circulation. High concentrations in amniotic fluid. 5–10% of serum concentration in breast milk.

Excretion: 85–95% excreted in the urine after parenteral administration with very high urinary concentrations of several times the serum value. Urinary recovery is reduced in the newborn, in renal insufficiency and with the simultaneous administration of probenecid. There is no spontaneous reduction in clearance with single doses of up to 5 megaunits.

Low biliary excretion; the concentrations in hepatic bile are of the same order as those of the blood.

Side effects:

1. *Penicillin hypersensitivity:* The most frequent complication of penicillin therapy (0.5–2.0%). The allergens are the intact penicillin molecule and also antibacterially inactive metabolites of 6-amino-penicillanic acid, e. g. penicilloic acid. Since all penicillins are derived from 6-amino-penicillanic acid, they can all produce an allergic response in the hypersensitive individual.

   Cross-allergy between the penicillins and cephalosporins is rare, so cephalosporins may still be considered as alternative agents in cases of penicillin allergy, though the patient should be carefully observed during therapy.

   The occurrence of penicillin allergy depends on *several factors,* e. g.

   a) the type of penicillin: Skin reactions are commoner after ampicillin than after benzyl or phenoxymethyl penicillin;

b) the functional state of the reticuloendothelial system: patients with infectious mononucleosis often develop allergy after ampicillin;

c) the route of administration: the topical application of penicillin on the skin or mucous membranes has a high association with penicillin allergy.

If hypersensitivity has been present for some time, the allergic response may occur immediately after the first dose or develop within 8–14 days during treatment. A mild reaction may consist only of a morbilliform or scarlatiniform rash on the trunk and extremities which can disappear spontaneously during treatment. Urticarial or oedematous skin rashes with or without fever and sometimes accompanied by joint swelling, laryngeal oedema, cerebral oedema, conjunctivitis or other symptoms should be taken more seriously. The development of urticaria is a clear contraindication to any further penicillin therapy. *Anaphylactic shock* is fortunately rare but may be extremely serious and lethal in 10% of cases. Affected patients suffer sudden vasomotor collapse, loss of consciousness, muscle cramps and respiratory distress. Rapid and intensive therapy (see below) may be lifesaving. Drug fever, neutropenia, thrombocytopenia and haemolytic anemia are rarely seen.

True penicillin allergy may be confused with the rare *allergy to procaine* and may be due to degradation products. The Hoigné syndrome, which follows the accidental intravascular injection of depot penicillin, is accompanied by severe general reactions, fear of imminent death, loss of consciousness without circulatory collapse, hallucinations, double vision, tinnitus, vertigo, paraesthesiae and tachycardia. These symptoms are not due to allergy and disappear completely within 15–30 min. They are caused by microemboli of the depot penicillin in capillaries.

Tests: No satisfactory method of testing for the presence of penicillin allergy has so far been developed. Specific serum IgE can be demonstrated in individuals who have never shown signs of allergy. A negative IgE, on the other hand, does not exclude the presence of allergy. When a patient gives a history, or for other reasons is suspected of penicillin allergy, the following *preliminary tests* may be useful if there is a need for further penicillin therapy:

Scratch test: A drop of penicillin solution (1000–5000 units/ml) is applied to a fresh skin scratch. An immediate reaction with erythema and pruritus occurs within 15 min in allergic individuals.

Intradermal test with 0.02 ml of a solution of 1000 units/ml. This test is dangerous and serious, occasionally fatal reactions have occurred. Positive results occur more frequently with penicilloyl polylysin (Pre-Pen, Kremers-Urban, Milwaukee, Wisc., USA). A wheal and flare reaction with erythema generally occurs within 30 min in allergic individuals, though it can be delayed. The frequency of positive reactions is increased when benzyl penicillin and penicilloyl-polylysin are tested simultaneously. False positive and false negative reactions have been reported. The value of skin testing, for which the scratch test is the best, is the recognition of patients in whom an immediate and severe reaction is likely to follow a further dose of a penicillin.

When the scratch and intradermal tests are negative, a careful *exposure test* may be performed. A solution of 200000 units of benzyl penicillin in 500 ml of fluid is infused very slowly and stopped immediately at the first sign of any possible allergic reaction. Depot penicillins must never be given when there is any suspicion of penicillin allergy, because of the danger of a protracted allergic response.

Treatment of penicillin allergy:
When rashes occur during treatment, discontinue penicillin. For allergic shock, which is often associated with pulmonary, laryngeal and cerebral oedema, inject 0.5 mg adrenaline i. m. or subcutaneously, followed, if necessary, by 0.5 mg slowly i. v.; repeat up to 3 times at intervals of 5–10 min if necessary. Continuous infusion of vasoconstrictors such as noradrenaline 5 mg or angiotensin 2.5 mg in 500 ml is recommended to maintain the blood pressure, together with 50–100 mg of prednisone and calcium i. v. For laryngeal oedema, intubate or perform a tracheotomy and give artificial respiration. Injections of penicillinase and antihistamines are ineffective. The patient should be observed carefully for a few hours after clinical improvement has been established, since symptoms can recur. When severe, protracted shock follows the injection of depot penicillins, particularly clemizole and benzathine penicillin, the site of injection must be excised.

2. *Neurotoxicity* with convulsions is reported after intrathecal instillation and also in meningitis, epilepsy and uraemia after very high systemic doses of benzyl penicillin, in excess of 20 megaunits. The potassium salt of benzyl penicillin can give rise to hyperkalaemia, muscle spasm, coma and cardiac arrest when given in excess and the sodium salt is preferable. 1 megaunit of potassium benzyl penicillin contains 1.5 milliequivalents of potassium. In some high dose penicillin preparations, the sodium and potassium salts are mixed in a ratio intended to avoid electrolyte disturbances. A maximum daily dosage of 20–30 megaunits of benzyl penicillin in adults, or of 12 megaunits in children, should not generally be exceeded. Patients in severe renal failure (decompensated retention or uraemia) require only 50% of the normal dose of penicillin.

3. *The Herxheimer reaction* at the beginning of treatment of syphilis, particularly congenital and secondary syphilis, with penicillin: fever, chills, systemic and focal reactions. *Treatment:* 50–100 mg prednisone i. v.

Main indications: Infections caused by streptococci, pneumococci, meningococci, penicillin-sensitive staphylococci; syphilis, gonorrhoea, diphtheria, scarlet fever, follicular tonsillitis, peridontitis, erysipelas, rheumatic fever, subacute bacterial endocarditis, prophylaxis of infective endocarditis, erysipeloid, lobar pneumonia, meningitis due to sensitive pathogens, anthrax, animal bites infected with Pasteurella multocida, leptospirosis, actinomycosis, tetanus, gas gangrene, wound infections developed outside hospital.

Depot penicillin gives lower blood concentrations than benzyl penicillin, which is rapidly absorbed after i. m. injection. Depot penicillins are indicated in patients who cannot take penicillin by mouth because of vomiting, and also in infections with very sensitive bacteria such as spirochaetes and gonococci, where quite low concentrations are effective. Severe infections should be treated with aqueous preparations in high dosage, either as an i. v. infusion or as a large intramuscular injection.

Inappropriate use: Benzyl penicillin *should not be used alone* in
severe sepsis where the causative organism is unknown, since it is ineffective against penicillinase-producing strains;
urinary infections;
atypical pneumonia (pathogens commonly insensitive to penicillin).

Contra-indication: Penicillin allergy. Caution with too high a dose (greater than 10 megaunits) in renal failure and epilepsy (risk of neurotoxicity). Do not give the potassium salt in severe renal failure.

Route: Use a 5–10% solution for i. m. injection of sodium benzyl penicillin, and up to 20% for i. v. injection. Give frequently, either every 4–6 h in small doses, or by short i. v. infusion over ½–1 h for higher doses and in severe illness. In some cases, benzyl penicillin infusion can be given by day and i. m. depot penicillin at night. A depot injection of penicillin can be given at the start of outpatient therapy of infections with very sensitive organisms, followed by oral penicillin. The oral, rectal and topical administration of benzyl penicillin is not recommended.

Intrathecal benzyl penicillin is not generally necessary, and intralumbar injection of a depot penicillin must be avoided.

Dosage:
Adults: 1 megaunit daily for sensitive pathogens, and 20 megaunits i. m. and/or i. v. for less sensitive bacteria.
Small children: 0.04–0.06 megaunits/kg daily or 0.2–0.5 megaunits/kg i. m. or i. v.

Infants: 0.04–0.1 megaunits/kg daily or 0.2–0.5 (–1) megaunits/kg i. m. or i. v. Do not exceed a daily dose of 10 megaunits of benzyl penicillin (adults) in *severe renal failure,* or 50% of the normal daily dose; depot penicillin should only be given every 2 (–6) days.

Dose interval: Every 4–6 hours with sodium and potassium benzyl penicillin and every 8 hours in the newborn and infants (delayed excretion because of renal immaturity); depot penicillins vary according to preparation and dose (generally every 12–24 hours).

The administration of **probenecid** can inhibit the tubular secretion of benzyl penicillin, resulting in higher serum levels. Adults are given 0.5 g orally 4 times a day and children (2 years and above) 10 mg/kg 4 times a day. Contra-indicated in blood dyscrasia, renal failure, uric acid calculus, gout. Probenecid used to be particularly recommended in severe sepsis and endocarditis in order to achieve higher blood and tissue concentrations. Probenecid is also used in the USA in the single dose treatment of gonorrhoea with benzyl penicillin or ampicillin.

Instillation of benzyl penicillin is possible but has only a brief effect because of its rapid absorption. Dosage:
Intrapleural: 100000–200000 units for adults, half that for children (in a solution with 2000–5000 units/ml).
Intraarticular: 50000–100000 units in 2–5 ml.
Intrathecal (lumbar route): 5000–10000 units for adults, 8000 units for children of school age, 5000 units for small children, 2500 units for infants. All these doses are of sodium benzyl penicillin in a solution containing 1000 units/ml. Depot penicillin should not be given. The injection volume should be at least 10 ml, warmed to 37° C, and with the same quantity of CSF drawn off. The penicillin solution may be further diluted with CSF. Give by slow injection (1 ml/min) and only 30–50% of the intralumbar dose for suboccipital and intraventricular instillation.

Preparations:
Benzyl penicillin, ampoules of 0.4, 1, 10 and 20 megaunits (Crystapen).
Clemizole penicillin, ampoules of 1 megaunit (Clemipen, Megacillin, Preve-cillin).
Procaine penicillin, ampoules of 0.6; 1.2; 2.4 megaunits (Wycillin).
Benzathine penicillin, ampoules of 1.2 megaunit (Bicillin, Penadur 6-3-3, Penduran, Penidural, Permapen, Retarpen, Tardocillin 1200).
Benethamine penicillin 475 mg + procaine penicillin 250 mg + benzyl penicillin sodium 300 mg (Triplopen).

Benzathine penicillin (20%) + procaine penicillin (80%) in ampoules of 1 megaunit (Depotpen).

Benzathine penicillin (75%) + procaine penicillin (25%) in ampoules of 1.2 megaunit (Bicillin C-R 900/300).

Combinations of high or low dose benzyl penicillin and depot penicillin are widely used in many countries.

Compound preparations with streptomycin are no longer acceptable because of the unnecessary risk of side effects with streptomycin, the inadequate spectrum and the possibility of underdosage of benzyl penicillin.

Summary:

Advantages: Wide therapeutic range, maximum concentrations achieved by injection, relatively low serum protein binding (50%), more active against sensitive strains than other penicillins, depot effect with procaine, clemizole, and benzathine penicillins.

Disadvantages: Inactivation by penicillinase-producing bacteria, oral administration not possible because of instability to acid and poor oral absorption. Hypersensitivity reactions complicating parenteral administration (particularly of depot preparations) are more dangerous than with the oral route.

References

APPELBAUM, P. C., J. N. SCRAGG, A. J. BOWEN, A. BHAMJEE, A. F. HALLET, R. C. COOPER: Streptococcus pneumoniae resistant to penicillin and chloramphenicol. Lancet 2: 995 (1977).

BLOG, F. B., A. CHANG, G. A. J. DEKONING, A. P. ORANJE, E. STOLZ, G. BOSSCHER-KOETSIER, M. P. E. DE-JONGE-SUY, M. F. MICHEL, E. O'NEIL, S. DE WEERDT-VAN AMEYDEN, L. GAASTRA: Penicillinase-producing strains of Neisseria gonorrhoeae isolated in Rotterdam, Brit. J. vener. Dis. 53: 98 (1977).

COOKSEY, R. C., R. R. FACKLAM, C. THORNSBERRY: Antimicrobial susceptibility patterns of Streptococcus pneumoniae. Antimicrob. Ag. Chemother. 13: 645 (1978).

DIXON, J. M. S., A. E. LIPINSKI, M. E. P. GRAHAM: Detection and prevalence of pneumococci with increased resistance to penicillin. Canad. med. Assoc. J. 117: 1159 (1977).

HALDANE, E. V., S. AFFLAS: Penicillin-tolerant staphylococcus aureus. Lancet 2: 39 (1977).

HANSMAN, D.: Penicillin-insensitive pneumococci and pneumococcal infections. Med. J. Aust. 1: 132 (1976).

HOROWITZ, L.: Atopy as factor in penicillin reactions. New Engl. J. Med. 292: 1243 (1975).

KRAFT, D., A. ROTH, P. MISCHER, H. PICHLER, H. EBNER: Specific and total serum IgE measurements in the diagnosis of penicillin allergy. A long term follow-up study. Clinical Allergy 7: 21 (1977).

LACKNER, F., W. HAIDER, D. KRAFT, G. KRYSTOF, H. PICHLER, S. FITZAL: Zur Wertung von Exanthemen nach hochdosierten intravenösen Penicillinkombinationen in der Intensivpflege. Int. J. clin. Pharmacol. 13: 90 (1976).

MEERS, P. D., R. B. MATTHEWS: Multiple resistant pneumococcus. Lancet 2: 219 (1978).
RAICHLE, M. E., H. KUTT, S. LOUIS, F. McDOWELL: Neurotoxicity of intravenously administered penicillin G. Arch. Neurol. 25: 232 (1971).
SABATH, L. D., N. WHEELER, M. LAVERDIERE, D. BLAZEVIC, B. J. WILKINSON: A new type of penicillin resistance of Staphylococcus aureus. Lancet 1: 443 (1977).
SIMON, C., J. VOCK, V. MALERCZYK: Zur Blutspiegelkinetik bei hochdosierter parenteraler Penicillin G-Therapie. Dtsch. med. Wschr. 96: 1393 (1971).

b) Phenoxy Penicillins

Common proprietary names:
Phenoxymethyl penicillin: Apsin VK, Beromycin, Cliacil, Co-Caps, Crystapen V, Distaquaine VK, Econocil VK, Fenoxypen, Icipen, Isocillin, Megacillin oral, Pencompren, Penicillin VK, Ospen, Stabillin V-K, Star-Pen, Ticillin V-K, V-Tablopen, V-Cil-K.
Propicillin: Baycillin, Oricillin. Not available in Britain.
Phenethicillin: Broxil.
Azidocillin: Longatren, Nalpen, Syncillin. Not available in Britain.

Synonyms: Acid-resistant penicillins, oral penicillins.

Properties: Phenoxymethyl penicillin (Penicillin V) is a biosynthetic product; propicillin (phenoxypropyl penicillin) and phenethicillin (phenoxyethyl penicillin) and azidocillin (α-azidobenzyl penicillin) are semi-synthetic products (see Fig. 4 for chemical structure). The potassium salts of phenoxymethyl penicillin, phenethicillin, propicillin and azidocillin are readily soluble in water, while the phenoxymethyl penicillin free acid is only poorly water-soluble. Acid-stability is quite good with all the acid-resistant penicillins. In some countries (e. g. Germany), phenoxy penicillins are still dosed in units. 1 megaunit of phenoxymethyl penicillin, phenethicillin and azidocillin correspond approximately to 600 mg (1 g contains approx. 1.6 megaunits). For propicillin, 1 megaunit corresponds to 700 mg (1 g = 1.42 megaunits).

Mechanism and spectrum of action: All the acid-resistant penicillins act like benzyl penicillin. Only propicillin has a slighter improved penicillinase stability, but it is quite inadequate in infections caused by penicillinase-producing staphylococci.

Antibacterial activity: Propicillin and phenethicillin are 2–4 times less active than benzyl penicillin, phenoxymethyl penicillin and azidocillin against sensitive gram-positive bacteria. The last three agents are very similar in their activity. Like ampicillin, azidocillin has comparable activity against Haemophilus influenzae and Bordetella pertussis, and is, like ampicillin, also active against enterococci.

Resistance: Uncommon and slow to develop (like benzyl penicillin). Cross-resistance amongst penicillinase-forming bacteria is found between the acid-resistant penicillins, benzyl penicillin and ampicillin.

Pharmacokinetics:

Maximal serum concentrations in mg/l (Fig. 8) after oral administration of

propicillin (700 mg)	7.1 (after 2.50 h),
phenoxymethyl penicillin potassium (600 mg)	3.8 (after 0.75 h),
phenethicillin (600 mg)	3.4 (after 0.75 h),
azidocillin (600 mg)	5.3 (after 0.50 h).

In the elderly (60–80 years) without cardiac or renal disease, the serum concentrations after oral intake of 1 megaunit of propicillin (700 mg) are twice as high and the area under the blood concentration-time curve twice as large as in young, healthy adults. Since absorption of the antibiotic is not reduced and the rate of elimination is similar to that in young adults, it must be assumed that propicillin is less well distributed in the tissues of the older patient.

The rates of absorption of propicillin and phenoxymethyl penicillin are about the same (approx. 50%), as shown by comparisons of the areas under the blood concentration-time curves for intravenous and oral administration. The blood

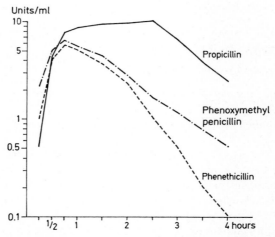

Fig. 8. Mean serum concentration-time curves in healthy adults after oral administration of 1 megaunit of propicillin (700 mg) and 1 megaunit phenoxymethyl penicillin and phenethicillin (600 mg), respectively.

concentration of propicillin is twice as high as that of phenoxymethyl penicillin, which is primarily explained by the fact that propicillin is metabolised more slowly than phenoxymethyl penicillin. With azidocillin, at least 75% of the oral dose is absorbed and blood levels after oral administration are comparable with those which would be expected from the i.m. route. Phenoxymethyl penicillin and phenethicillin are not absorbed as well after meals as in the fasting state. Half-life of phenoxymethyl penicillin, propicillin and azidocillin: 30 min; of phenethicillin: 20 min.

Plasma protein binding: Phenoxymethyl penicillin: 60%, propicillin: 80–85%, phenethicillin: 80%, and azidocillin: 84%.

Tissue diffusion and *CSF penetration* are similar to benzyl penicillin.

Excretion: Phenoxymethyl penicillin is 30–50% excreted in the urine, propicillin 50%, phenethicillin 20–30% and azidocillin 60% of the oral dose. More inactive metabolites (penicilloic acid) are excreted with phenoxymethyl penicillin than with propicillin. 5% of the dose of azidocillin is excreted in the urine as ampicillin, which is formed from azidocillin in the body.

Side effects: The risk of sensitisation is smaller than with benzyl penicillin, which is given parenterally. Neurotoxicity does not occur.

Main indications: Mild infections caused by penicillin-sensitive bacteria, e.g. sore throat, erysipelas, scarlet fever, prophylaxis against recurrence of rheumatic fever, prophylaxis against scarlet fever.

Inappropriate use: Meningitis, septicaemia, endocarditis, infections caused by less sensitive bacteria which require large i.v. doses.

Contra-indication: Penicillin allergy.

Administration and dosage: Can only be given by mouth. The minimum recommended doses are:

Adults and children of school age: 500,000 units (0.5 megaunit) 3 times a day (or 500 mg t.i.d.);

Younger children (aged 1–6 years): 300,000 units (0.3 megaunit) 3 times a day (or 250 mg t.i.d.);

Infants: 150,000 units (0.15 megaunit) 3 times a day (or 125 mg t.i.d.);

Newborn: 100,000 units (0.1 megaunit) 2–3 times a day (or 62.5 mg t.i.d.).

Azidocillin: 1.5–2 g a day for adults, 750 mg a day for children (2–10 years); 60 mg/kg a day for children under 2 years. Give in 3 divided doses in each case.

Preparations: *Phenoxymethyl penicillin:* Tablets of 200,000, 400,000, 500,000, 600,000, 800,000 units and 1, 1.2 and 1.5 megaunits (capsules or tablets of 125 mg,

250 mg and 500 mg); syrup with 1 ml = 50,000 units, 1 ml = 60,000 units and 1 ml = 80,000 units (syrup with 125 mg or 250 mg in 5 ml).
Propicillin: Tablets or coated tablets of 200,000, 400,000, 600,000 and 1 million units; syrup.
Phenethicillin: Tablets of 250 mg.
Azidocillin: Capsules of 500 mg, tablets of 750 mg, granules in sachets of 250 mg.

Summary: Despite differences in their antibacterial activity and pharmacokinetics, the different acid-resistant penicillins have similar clinical activity when given for the correct indications and at sufficient dosage. Azidocillin has additional activity against Haemophilus influenzae and Bordetella and is therefore particularly suitable for the treatment of respiratory infections and otitis media.

References

COLE, M., M. D. KENIG, V. A. HEWITT: Metabolism of penicillins to penicilloic acids and 6-amino-penicillanic acid in man. Antimicrob. Ag. Chemother. *3:* 463 (1973).
MICHEL, M. F., J. P. VAN WAARDHUIZEN, K. F. KERREBIJN: A comparison of serum concentrations after oral administration of acidocillin and ampicillin. Chemotherapy (Basle) *18:* 77 (1973).
SIMON, C., V. MALERCZYK, U. MÜLLER, G. MÜLLER: Zur Pharmakokinetik von Propicillin bei geriatrischen Patienten im Vergleich zu jüngeren Erwachsenen. Dtsch. med. Wschr. *97:* 1999 (1972).
SIMON, C., V. MALERCZYK, C. G. V. WULFFEN: In-vitro-Aktivität und Pharmakokinetik von Propicillin, Penicillin V und Phenethicillin. Med. Welt *27* (N. F.): 2476 (1976).
SIMON, C., W. JUNK, V. MALERCZYK: Azidocillin (In-vitro-Aktivität, Pharmakokinetik und Behandlungsergebnisse bei Keuchhusten). Arzneimittel-Forsch. *26:* 424 (1975).

c) Penicillinase-Stable Penicillins (Anti-Staphylococcal Penicillins)

Common proprietary names:
Dicloxacillin: Dichlor-Stapenor, Diclocil, Dycill, Dynapen, Pathocil. Not sold in Great Britain.
Flucloxacillin: Floxapen, Staphylex.
Oxacillin: Bactocill, Cryptocillin, Stapenor, Oxacillin, Prostaphlin. Not sold in Great Britain.
Cloxacillin: Cloxapen, Orbenin. No longer sold in Germany.
Methicillin: Celbenin, Staphcillin. No longer sold in Britain or Germany.
Nafcillin: Nafcil, Unipen. Not sold in Britain or Germany.

Properties: Methicillin was the first penicillinase-resistant penicillin to be used in therapy. Since it can only be given parenterally, is relatively toxic and has a low *in vitro* activity on penicillinase-producing staphylococci, it has been superceded by the penicillinase-stable isoxazolyl penicillins oxacillin, nafcillin, cloxacillin, dicloxacillin and flucloxacillin, which have been developed since. These penicillins are water-soluble and acid-stable and so can be given by mouth. They differ from each other in pharmacokinetic properties only, and not in their antibacterial activity.

Mode of action: Like benzyl penicillin.

Spectrum of activity: Effective against penicillinase-producing staphylococci. Methicillin has only $\frac{1}{50}$ of the activity of benzyl penicillin against penicillin sensitive staphylococci, streptococci, pneumococci and other gram-positive bacteria; the other penicillinase-stable penicillins have $\frac{1}{10}$ of the activity of benzyl penicillin against these organisms. Penicillin-tolerant staphylococcal strains are also tolerant to penicillinase-resistant penicillins.

Resistance: Methicillin-resistant staphylococci are unevenly distributed, occur more frequently in hospitals, and are generally sensitive to fusidic acid, gentamicin and vancomycin. Methicillin resistance may be overlooked if special laboratory techniques are not used. Methicillin resistance is best detected *in vitro* either in culture media containing 5% NaCl or after overnight incubation at 30° C. Secondary resistance has not been observed during therapy. There is complete cross-resistance in staphylococci between all the penicillinase-stable penicillins and the cephalosporins (except cefamandole). Methicillin is traditionally used in the laboratory to test for resistance to the penicillinase-stable penicillins. Penicillin-sensitive staphylococci are always sensitive to methicillin and the isoxazolyl penicillins.

Pharmacokinetics:
Oral absorption is best with dicloxacillin and flucloxacillin. Cloxacillin and oxacillin, which are less acid-stable than dicloxacillin, are less well absorbed. Absorption of nafcillin is incomplete and irregular. Absorption is better on an empty stomach (1 h before or 2–4 h after meals). Maximal blood concentrations occur after 1–2 h. Methicillin is not acid-stable and is virtually not absorbed after oral administration.
Serum concentrations (mg/l) after 500 mg by mouth 1 h after a meal (Fig. 9): flucloxacillin 7.6 and 2.3 (after 1½ or 4 h), dicloxacillin 5.9 and 2.0 (after 1½ and 4 h). Oral dicloxacillin produces serum levels twice as high as cloxacillin and four times as high as oxacillin.

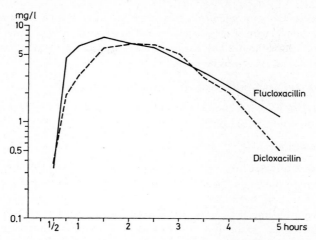

Fig. 9. Mean serum concentration-time curve in 10 healthy adults after a single oral dose of 500 mg of flucloxacillin or dicloxacillin, 1 h after a standard breakfast.

Serum concentrations (mg/l) after i. v. injection of 500 mg: flucloxacillin 15.7 and 2.0 (after 1 and 4 h), oxacillin 1.7 and less than 0.1 (after 1 and 4 h); nafcillin serum levels are much lower than those of oxacillin because of stronger inactivation in the liver.

Half-life of dicloxacillin and flucloxacillin: 45 min; oxacillin: 25 min; nafcillin 60 min.

Plasma protein binding: 97% with dicloxacillin, 95% with flucloxacillin and cloxacillin, 93% with oxacillin, 87% with nafcillin, 38% with methicillin.

CSF penetration is poor, up to 10% of the serum concentration in meningitis. Passes into the fetal circulation.

Excretion in the urine after parenteral administration: 65% with dicloxacillin, 35% with flucloxacillin, 30% with cloxacillin, 25% with oxacillin, 15–30% with nafcillin. Oxacillin is more rapidly excreted than dicloxacillin, and is more extensively metabolised than either dicloxacillin or flucloxacillin. Excretion of inactive metabolites (penicilloic acid) is highest with nafcillin and oxacillin, less with cloxacillin and flucloxacillin, and least with dicloxacillin. In contrast to the other drugs, 8% of an intramuscular dose of nafcillin is eliminated via the bile.

Side effects: Similar to benzyl penicillin. Methicillin, which is very little used today, has caused allergic bone marrow depression (granulocytopenia) and kidney damage. Nafcillin may also lead to neutropenia (reversible). Increased serum transaminases and neutropenia have been reported after oxacillin. Local irritation is frequently found with dicloxacillin, both i. m. (pain) and i. v. (phlebitis); it is less frequent with oxacillin and flucloxacillin. The parenteral administration of dicloxacillin should therefore be avoided.

Indication: Infection with penicillin-resistant staphylococci.

Inappropriate use: Infections with penicillin-sensitive or methicillin-resistant staphylococci, streptococci, pneumococci, gonococci, meningococci etc.

Contra-indication: Allergy to penicillin.

Administration: For oral administration (before meals), dicloxacillin and flucloxacillin are preferable because of their better absorption and higher, more persistent serum concentrations.

When given by injection, oxacillin, cloxacillin and flucloxacillin have better local tolerance than dicloxacillin. Oxacillin (1% solution) is preferable for local instillation. Intravenous injection should be given slowly to avoid irritation of the vein; short i. v. infusions over 30 min are preferable.

Dosage: Daily doses lower than those given here are not advised.
Oral administration of dicloxacillin and flucloxacillin (fasting):
    Adults and older children: 2–4 g daily,
    smaller children: 1–2 g daily,
    newborn: 0.5–1 g daily,
in 4 (−6) divided doses.
I. m. or i. v. administration of flucloxacillin or cloxacillin (more severe infections):
    Adults and children of school age: 3–4 (−10) g daily,
    smaller children: 2–3 (−6) g,
    infants: 1–2 (−4) g,
    newborn: 40 mg/kg daily,
in 4–6 hourly injections or short infusions.
Probenecid may be given in addition (500 mg 4 times a day for adults), which delays the renal excretion of the penicillinase-resistant penicillins and thus increases the serum concentrations. It should not be given to children under 2 years.
Intralumbar instillation of oxacillin: 10–20 g (adults) and 5–10 mg (children).

Preparations:
Dicloxacillin: Capsules of 250 mg.
Flucloxacillin: Capsules of 250 and 500 mg, ampoules of 250, 500 mg and 1 g.
Cloxacillin: Capsules of 250 mg.

Oxacillin: Capsules of 250 mg, ampoules of 500 mg and 1 g.
Methicillin: Ampoules of 1 g, 4 g, and 6 g.
Nafcillin: Ampoules of 500 mg, 1 g, and 2 g.

Summary: Effective in infections with penicillinase-producing staphylococci. Less effective than benzyl penicillin against other gram-positive bacteria. Prefer dicloxacillin or flucloxacillin for oral use, and flucloxacillin by injection.

References

BRUCKSTEIN, A. H., A. A. ATTIA: Oxacillin hepatitis. Two patients with liver biopsy, and review of the literature. Amer. J. Med. *64:* 519 (1978).

CHU, J. Y., D. M. O'CONNOT, R. R. SCHMIDT: The mechanisms of oxacillin induced neutropenia. J. Ped. *90:* 668 (1977).

COLE, M., M. D. KENIG, V. A. HEWITT: Metabolism of penicillins to penicilloic acid and 6-aminopenicillanic acid in man and its significance in assessing penicillin absorption. Antimicrob. Ag. Chemother. *3:* 463 (1973).

COGAN, M. C., A. I. ARIEL: Sodium wasting, acidosis and hyperkalemia induced by methicillin interstitial nephritis. Evidence for selective distal tubular dysfunction. Amer. J. Med. *64:* 500 (1978).

DISMUKES, W. E.: Oxacillin-induced hepatic dysfunction. JAMA *226:* 861 (1973).

GALLAGHER, P. J., D. J. WAYNE: Haematuria during methicillin therapy. Postgrad. med. J. *47:* 511 (1971).

JENSEN, H. A., A. B. HALVEG, K. I. SAUNAMÄKI: Permanent impairment of renal function after methicillin nephropathy. Brit. med. J. *4:* 406 (1971).

LEVENTHAL, J. M., A. B. SILKEN: Oxacillin-induced neutropenia in children. J. Ped. *89:* 769 (1976).

MALONE, A. J. jr., S. FIELD, J. ROSMAN, W. P. SHEMERDIAK: Neurotoxic reaction to oxacillin. New Engl. J. Med. *296:* 453 (1977).

OLANS, R. N., L. B. WEINER: Reversible oxacillin hepatotoxity. J. Pediat. *89:* 835 (1976).

SANJAD, S., G. G. HADDAD, V. H. NASSAR: Nephropathy, an underestimated complications of methicillin therapy. J. Pediat. *84:* 873 (1974).

SCHIFFER, C. A., H. J. WEINSTEIN, P. H. WIERNIK: Methicillin associated thrombocytopenia. Ann. intern. Med. *85:* 338 (1976).

SIMON, C., V. MALERCZYK, B. HODGSON: Flucloxacillin, ein neues Staphylokokken-Antibiotikum. Dtsch. med. Wschr. *98:* 1502 (1972).

SUTHERLAND, R., E. A. P. CROYDON, G. N. ROLINSON: Flucloxacillin, a new isoxazolyl penicillin compared with oxacillin, cloxacillin and dicloxacillin. Brit. med. J. *4:* 455 (1970).

ULLMAN, U.: The binding of isoxazolyl penicillins to human serum proteins. Arzneimittel-Forsch. *27:* 2136 (1977).

WESTERMAN, E. L., M. W. BRADSHAW, T. W. WILLIAMS Jr.: Agranulocytosis during therapy with orally administered cloxacillin. Amer. J. clin. Path. *69:* 559 (1978).

WOODROFF, A. J., N. M. THOMSON, R. MESDOWS, J. R. LAWRENCE: Nephropathy associated with methicillin administration. Aust. N. Z. J. Med. *4:* 256 (1974).

YOW, M. D., L. H. TABLER, F. F. BARRETT, A. A. MINTZ, G. R. BLANKINSHIP, G. E. CLARK, D. J. CLARK: A ten-year assessment of methicillin-associated side-effects. Pediatrics *58:* 329 (1976).

d) Ampicillin

Common proprietary names: Amblosin, Amfigen, Binotal, Britcin, Penbritin, Penbrock, Pen trexyl, Vidopen etc.

Description: A semisynthetic penicillin derivative (α-aminobenzyl penicillin) with an extended spectrum.

Mode of action: Bactericidal, by inhibition of peptidoglycan synthesis in the cell wall. Not stable to penicillinase from staphylococci or enterobacteria.

Spectrum of action: As benzyl penicillin, but with additional moderate or good activity (inhibitory concentration up to 5 mg/l) against enterococci, Listeria, Haemophilus influenzae and Campylobacter. Benzyl penicillin is 2–4 times more active against gram-positive bacteria. The frequency of ampicillin-resistant strains of Haemophilus is increasing, but these are still reliably sensitive to cefuroxime, cefamandole, cefotaxime and cefaclor. Simultaneous resistance of Haemophilus to ampicillin and chloramphenicol is rare.

Variable activity against salmonellae, shigellae, Escherichia coli (resistance rate 20–50%) and Proteus mirabilis (non-penicillinase-producing strains). The following bacteria are resistant: Klebsiella, Enterobacter, Citrobacter, Yersinia enterocolitica, Serratia marcescens, Bacteroides fragilis, Pseudomonas aeruginosa, and generally also Proteus vulgaris, Proteus rettgeri and Proteus morganii. When combined with a β-lactamase inhibitor such as clavulanic acid, there is synergistic action on β-lactamase-producing strains of Escherichia coli, Klebsiella, Bacteroides fragilis and Staphylococcus aureus.

Resistance: Complete cross-resistance with amoxycillin. Penicillin-resistant strains of gonococci are also resistant to ampicillin. Some cross-resistance of aerobic gram-negative bacilli with azlocillin, mezlocillin, piperacillin and the cephalosporins. Resistance rarely develops during therapy and has not been observed with Haemophilus either.

Pharmacokinetics:
Absorption by mouth (30–40%) is markedly less than after parenteral administration.
Maximum serum concentrations after 500 mg by mouth (after meals): mean of 2 mg/l after 1½ hours; after 500 mg i. m.: 10 mg/l after ½ hour (Fig. 10). *Half-life:* 1 hour. *Plasma protein binding:* 18%.
Good *tissue diffusion; CSF penetration* poor, as with benzyl penicillin, but sufficient to treat meningitis when a large dose is given i. v. Concentrations in

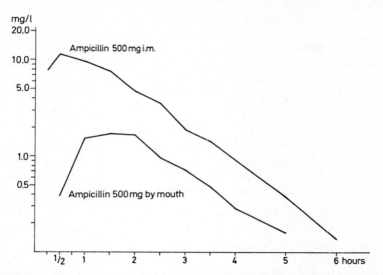

Fig. 10. Blood concentration after 500 mg of ampicillin i. m. and orally (1 h after a meal).

hepatic bile are as high as in serum, and higher in gall-bladder bile. Ampicillin crosses the placenta and passes into the fetal circulation and amniotic fluid.

20–30% of the oral dose and 60% of the i. v. dose are *excreted* in the urine after 24 hours; high urine concentrations (1000–2000 mg/l are found after 0.5–1 g i. m.). Eliminated also in the bile and faeces. Biliary recovery after i. v. administration: 0.1%.

Side effects: Toxicity is as low as benzyl penicillin. Typical allergy, as shown in urticaria or anaphylactic shock is no more frequent than with benzyl penicillin. Macular rashes occur in 5–20% of patients during or after 8–14 days of treatment. The cause of the rash seems in part to be toxic, since it is more frequent at higher dosage and with degradation of ampicillin in the infusion. Treatment may be continued in life-threatening situations, provided there is very careful observation. Other penicillins should only be used subsequently with great care, since cross-allergy may occur. 5–20% of cases have gastrointestinal reactions (nausea, vomiting, diarrhoea) due in part to disturbance of the normal intestinal flora. Like clindamycin, ampicillin can cause pseudomembranous enterocolitis, which may become chronic and is related to the presence of toxin-producing strains of Clostridium difficile in the large bowel. This serious complication may be effectively treated with oral vancomycin (see p. 363). Urinary infection is often followed by a reinfection with resistant bacteria (Klebsiella or Enterobacter).

Main indications: Haemophilus meningitis and other haemophilus infections (where shown to be sensitive), enterococcal endocarditis and other severe enterococcal infections, salmonella endocarditis, osteomyelitis and meningitis, listeriosis, prolonged salmonella excretion after gastroenteritis (some dispute this last indication).

Other indications: Acute and chronic urinary infections with sensitive pathogens, long-term treatment of chronic bronchitis, cholecystitis and cholangitis, gynaecological infections, pertussis. For oral treatment, amoxycillin or the ampicillin esters, which are better absorbed, are preferable.

Inappropriate use: Typical or proven staphylococcal, streptococcal and pneumococcal infections, sore throat, fever of unknown origin, primary pneumonia, wound infections, topical or local application.

Contra-indications: Penicillin allergy, infectious mononucleosis (50–100% of patients develop a rash).

Administration: In severe infections and in patients who are unable to swallow, give as a 10–20% solution i.m., slowly i.v., or if in large doses, by short i.v. infusion. Prepare a fresh solution every 6–8 hours if given by slow i.v. infusion because of progressive inactivation in vitro at room temperature; do not give other additives in the same infusion. Ampicillin is poorly absorbed by the oral route, so bacampicillin, pivampicillin, talampicillin or amoxycillin are preferable by mouth.

Dosage: Standard daily dosage in *adults* of 2–4 g by mouth and 1.5–2 g parenterally; this dosage may be increased to 10–20 g. Reduce dosage in renal failure giving the normal single dose every 12 hours when the creatinine clearance is 10–50 ml/min, and every 24 hours at creatinine clearances below 10 ml/min. In *children:* 100–150 (–200) mg/kg (orally) and 100–400 mg/kg (parenterally); 200–400 mg/kg in meningitis. Divide daily dose into 3–4 single doses. For *intrathecal* use in adults, give 10–20 mg once a day only, and in children 5–10 mg.

Preparations: Capsules and tablets of 250 mg and 500 mg, tablets of 1 g, ampoules of 500 mg, 1, 2, and 5 g, syrup of 50 mg/ml; and powder of 250 mg.

Summary:
Advantages: Broader spectrum of activity than benzyl penicillin; good tissue diffusion.

Disadvantages: High rate of resistance among gram-negative rods, poor absorption by mouth, frequent rashes. In many cases, better replaced by piperacillin or mezlocillin for parenteral use, and by an ampicillin ester (bacampicillin, talampicillin) or amoxycillin for oral use.

References

BASS, J. W., D. M. CROWLEY, R. W. STEELE, F. S. H. YOUNG, L. B. HARDEN: Adverse effects of orally administered ampicillin. J. Pediatr. *83:* 106 (1973).

BELL, S. M., D. D. SMITH: Ampicillin-resistant Haemophilus influenzae, type b. Med. J. Aust. *1:* 517 (1975).

BIÖRKLUND, A., E. DAHLQUIST, C. KAMME, N. I. NILSSON: Ampicillin-resistant Haemophilus influenzae in otitis media. Lancet *1:* 1135 (1975).

BYSJÖ, E., K. DORNBUSCH: Occurrence and transfer of ampicillin resistance associated with ampicillin-resistant. Haemophilus influenzae isolated from a case at a day-care centre. Scand. J. infect. Dis. *9:* 293 (1977).

DELAGE, G., Y. DECLERCK, J. LESCOP, P. DERY, F. SHARECK: Haemophilus influenzae type b infections: Recurrent disease due to ampicillin-resistant strains. J. Pediatrics *90:* 319 (1977).

GURWITH, M. J., H. R. RABIN, K. LOVE and the Co-operative Antibiotic Diarrhea Study Group: Diarrhea associated with clindamycin and ampicillin therapy: preliminary results of a co-operative study. J. infect. Dis. (Suppl.) *135:* 104 (1977).

HOWARD, A. J., C. J. HINCE, J. D. WILLIAMS: Antibiotic resistance in Streptococcus pneumoniae and Haemophilus influenzae. Report of a study group on bacterial resistance. Brit. med. J. *1:* 1657 (1978).

KEATING, J. P., A. L. FRANK, L. L. BARTON, F. J. TEDESCO: Pseudomembranous colitis associated with ampicillin therapy. Amer. J. Dis. Child. *128:* 369 (1974).

LUSK, R. H., F. R. FEKETY Jr., J. SILVA Jr., T. BODENDORFER, B. J. DEVINE, H. KAWANISHI, L. KORFF, D. NAKAUCHI, S. ROGERS, S. B. SISKIN: Gastrointestinal side effects of clindamycin and ampicillin therapy. J. infect. Dis. (Suppl.) *135:* 111 (1977).

MALMVALL, B.-E., P. BRANEFORS-HELANDER: R-factor involvement in a local outbreak of ampicillin-resistant Haemophilus influenzae infections. Scand. J. infect. Dis. *10:* 53 (1978).

PHILLIPS, J. A., F. H. LOVEJOY Jr., Y. MATSUMIYA: Ampicillin-associated diarrhoea: Effect of dosage and route of administration. Pediatrics *58:* 869 (1976).

READ, L., J. R. COVE-SMITH: Pseudomembranous enterocolitis complicating ampicillin therapy. Postgrad. med. J. *53:* 324 (1977).

ROBERTSON, M. B., K. J. BREEN, P. V. DESMOND, M. L. MASHFORD, A. M. McHUGH: Incidence of antibiotic-related diarrhoea and pseudomembranous colitis: A prospective study of lincomycin, clindamycin and ampicillin. Med. J. Aust. *1:* 243 (1977).

SCHWARTZ, R., W. RODRIGUEZ, W. KHAN, S. ROSS: The increasing incidence of ampicillin-resistant Haemophilus influenzae. A cause of otitis media. JAMA. *239:* 320 (1978).

SIMON, C., V. MALERCZYK, G. ZIEROTT, K. LEHMANN, U. THIESEN: Blut-, Harn- und Gallenspiegel von Ampicillin bei intravenöser Dauerinfusion. Arzneimittel-Forsch. *25:* 654 (1975).

e) Ampicillin Derivatives

The ampicillin derivatives in current use are amoxycillin, bacampicillin, pivampicillin, and talampicillin. The older derivatives hetacillin, epicillin and ciclacillin are now little used if at all. They differ from ampicillin in their pharmacokinetic properties but not in their antibacterial activity (except for the weaker ciclacillin).

α) Amoxycillin

Proprietary names: Amoxil, Amoxypen, Clamoxyl, Infectomycin, Larotid, Polymox, Trimox, Wymox.

Properties: Chemically α-amino-p-hydroxybenzyl penicillin (Fig. 5, p. 24) as the trihydrate, which is poorly soluble in water but dissolves better in phosphate buffer (pH 8.0). Relatively acid-stable, like ampicillin. Monosodium salt for injection is very water-soluble.

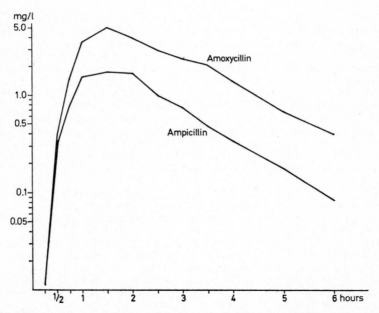

Fig. 11. Mean serum concentrations after the oral administration of 500 mg of amoxycillin and ampicillin.

Antibacterial activity: Spectrum and *in vitro* activity similar to ampicillin. Rapidly bactericidal to gram-negative bacilli.

Pharmacokinetics: *Absorption* is almost complete after oral administration. Maximum blood concentrations after 2 hours are more than twice as high as after the same dose of ampicillin by mouth (Fig. 11). Absorption is unaffected by food intake. Mean serum concentrations of 20 mg/l (1 h) and 2 mg/l (4 h) follow the i. v. injection of 1 g. *Plasma protein binding:* 17%. *Urinary recovery* 60–70% in 6 hours after oral intake, and 70–80% after i. v. administration.

Indications: As ampicillin, with the addition of typhoid fever, particularly with chloramphenicol resistance or when chloramphenicol is contra-indicated.

Side effects: As with ampicillin. Intestinal upset is less frequent because of the almost complete absorption after oral administration.

Administration and dosage: 1–1.5 (–3) g daily according to bacterial sensitivity; 50 (–100) mg/kg in small children, in 3 (–4) divided doses.
Larger doses may be given i. v. in severe infections. Intravenous injection or short infusion (1 g every 6–8 h) may also be given at the beginning of treatment and in patients with vomiting or unconsciousness. Do not mix with lignocaine when injecting i. m., because of inactivation.

Preparations: Capsules of 375 mg and 500 mg, tablets of 500 mg, 750 mg and 1 g, syrup containing 50 mg/ml, drops containing 100 mg/dl, and ampoules containing 500 mg, 1 g, 2 g, and 5 g.

Summary: Almost complete absorption after oral administration, hence smaller dosage possible than with ampicillin, with a lower risk of intestinal upset. Because of the high rate of resistance in gram-negative rods, amoxycillin, like ampicillin, cannot be recommended as a single agent in the initial treatment of severe infections.

References

COMBER, K. R., R. J. BOON, R. SUTHERLAND: Comparative effects of amoxycillin and ampicillin on the morphology of Escherichia coli in vitro and correlation with activity. Antimicrob. Ag. Chemother. *12:* 736 (1977).
FANG, L. S. T., N. E. TOLKOFF-RUBIN, R. H. RUBIN: Efficacy of single-dose and conventional amoxicillin therapy in urinary-tract infection localized by the antibody-coated bacteria technique. New Engl. J. Med. *298:* 413 (1978).
FARID, Z., S. BASSILY, I. A. MIKHAIL, D. C. EDMAN, A. HASSAN, W. F. MINER: Treatment of chronic enteric fever with amoxicillin. J. Infect. Dis. *132:* 698 (1975).

PILLAY, N., E. B. ADAMS, D. NORTH-COOMBES: Comparative trial of amoxycillin and chloramphenicol in treatment of typhoid fever in adults. Lancet 2: 333 (1975).
ROLINSON, G. N., A. C. McDONALD, D. A. WILSON: Antibacterial action of β-lactam antibiotics on Escherichia coli with particular reference to ampicillin and amoxycillin. J. Antimicrob. Chemother. 3: 541 (1977).
RONALD, A. R., F. A. JAGDIS, G. K. M. HARDING, S. A. HOBAN, P. L. MUIR, M. J. GURWITH: Amoxicillin therapy of acute urinary tract infections in adults. Antimicrob. Ag. Chemother. 11: 780 (1977).
SIMILÄ, S., K. KOUVALAINEN, P. MÄKELÄ: Pseudomembranous colitis after amoxycillin. Lancet 2: 317 (1976).
SIMON, C., W. TOELLER: Amoxycillin, ein neues Aminobenzylpenicillin. Arzneimittel-Forsch. 24: 181 (1974).
SPYKER, D. A., R. J. RUGLOSKI, R. L. VANN, W. M. O'BRIEN: Pharmacokinetics of amoxicillin: dose dependence after intravenous, oral and intramuscular administration. Antimicrob. Ag. Chemother. 11: 132 (1977).

β) Pivampicillin

Proprietary names: Maxifen, Pivatil, Pondocillin.

Properties: Pivaloyl oxymethyl ester of ampicillin, marketed as the hydrochloride. Readily soluble in water, odourless, with a bitter taste. When taken by mouth, pivampicillin is rapidly and almost completely (99%) transformed by non-specific esterases in the serum and intestinal wall into pivalinic acid (20%) and ampicillin-hydroxymethyl ester. The latter then breaks down spontaneously into ampicillin (70%) and formaldehyde (6%). 50% of the pivalinic acid (trimethyl acetic acid) produced in this way is excreted as the glucuronide in the urine. Formaldehyde breaks down rapidly in the body, particularly in the erythrocytes and the liver, into formic acid and then into CO_2 and H_2O.

Antibacterial action: Pivampicillin itself is almost completely inactive. The ampicillin released by its metabolism in the body has the characteristic spectrum and normal activity of ampicillin (see p. 44).

Pharmacokinetics: Rapid and almost complete (90%) *absorption* after oral administration. Maximal blood concentrations after 1–1½ h are proportional to the dose, with single doses of 170, 350 and 700 mg. The maximal *blood concentrations* (Fig. 12) are at least twice as high as those found after oral ampicillin, and of the same order as those found after i. m. ampicillin. The *urine recovery* is 65–75% (20–30% with ampicillin). The simultaneous intake of food considerably impairs the absorption of ampicillin but improves absorption and gastric tolerance of pivampicillin. Thus a much smaller dose of pivampicillin is needed to achieve the same blood concentration as oral ampicillin. The *half-life,*

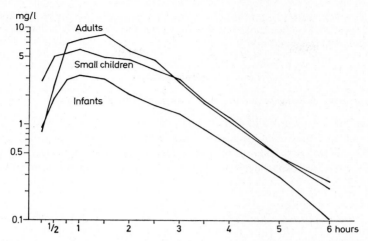

Fig. 12. Mean serum concentrations after a single oral dose of 700 mg pivampicillin hydrochloride (in adults) and of 15 mg pivampicillin base per kg body weight in small children aged 2–3 years and infants aged 5–8 months.

plasma protein binding and excretion are similar to those of ampicillin (p. 44). *Tissue concentrations* are related to blood concentrations.

Side effects: As for oral ampicillin. Ingestion when fasting occasionally leads to heartburn, a sensation of epigastric distension, and vomiting; intestinal upset is less frequent than with ampicillin because the intestinal flora is less disturbed on account of the better absorption. Pivalinic acid shows very little toxicity in animals (mean LD_{50} in mice after i. v. administration is 451 mg/kg). No side effects related to pivalinic acid have been observed in man so far.

Indications: As for ampicillin.

Administration and dosage: 1.4–2.8 g a day for *adults,* 50–100 mg/kg for *small children* in 3 or 4 divided doses (preferably after meals).

Preparations: Capsules and tablets of 350 and 700 mg; syrup of 32.5 mg/dl.

References

MARGET, W., F. DASCHNER, K. UNERTL: Investigations on pivampicillin treatment in newborns and infants. Infection *1:* 41 (1973).

PEDERSEN-BJIERGAARD, L., K. E. PETERSON: Oral absorption of pivampicillin and ampicillin in young children: Cross-over-study using equimolar doses of a suspension. Clin. Pharmacokinetics 2: 451 (1977).

γ) Bacampicillin

Proprietary names: Ambaxin, Ambocamp, Bacacil, Penglobe.

Properties: An ampicillin ester (aminopenicillin) for oral use, which is almost completely absorbed from the gastrointestinal tract and very rapidly hydrolysed to ampicillin in the body. 800 mg of the ester correspond to 556 mg of free ampicillin. Bacampicillin hydrochloride is readily soluble in water and chloroform, and is acid-stable.

Structural formula:

Mode and spectrum of activity: As ampicillin.

Pharmacokinetics: *Rapid absorption* of about 95% of the oral dose; maximal serum concentrations after 1 h (but after 2½ h with ampicillin).

Maximal serum concentrations after 800 mg orally are generally much higher than those after the equimolar dose of ampicillin (556 mg) (Fig. 13), with a mean individual maximum concentration of 15.9 mg/l, which has declined after 4 h to 2.0 mg/l, and after 6 h to 0.5 mg/l. After oral bacampicillin, the concentrations in blister fluid are four times higher, and in saliva and tears three times higher than those found after oral ampicillin at equimolar dosage. There is a dose-related increase in serum concentrations when the dose is doubled from 400 to 800 mg. Food intake does not impair absorption.

Urine recoveries over the first 6 h with oral bacampicillin: 57%, with i.v. ampicillin: 60%, with oral ampicillin: 30%.

Side effects as with oral ampicillin though loose stools and diarrhoea are less frequent because of the almost complete gastrointestinal absorption. Well tolerated by mouth.

Main indications: Respiratory and urinary infection by sensitive pathogens.

Contra-indications: As with benzyl penicillin.

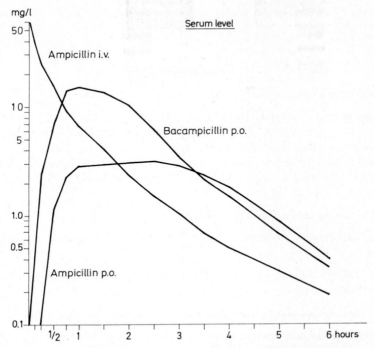

Fig. 13. Mean serum concentrations after 800 mg of bacampicillin by mouth, compared with 556 mg of ampicillin by mouth and i. v.

Administration and dosage: 800 mg 3 times a day in tablet form (20 mg/kg 3 times a day for children).

Preparations: Film tablets of 400 and 800 mg.

Summary: Better than oral ampicillin because of its complete absorption and good gastrointestinal tolerance.

References

EKSTRÖM, B., U. FORSGREN, L. MAGNI, B. SJÖBERG, J. SJÖVALL, R. TOLF: Bacampicillin, a well-absorbed pro-drug of ampicillin. J. Drug. Res. 2: 39 (1977).
MAGNI, L., B. SJÖBERG, J. SJÖVALL, J. WESSMAN: Clinical pharmacological studies with bacampicillin. Chemotherapy 5: 109 (1976).

SIMON, C., V. MALERCZYK, M. KLAUS: Absorption of bacampicillin and ampicillin and penetration into body fluids (skin blister fluid, saliva, tears) in healthy volunteers. Scand. J. infect. Dis. *Suppl. 211* (1978).

δ) Talampicillin

Proprietary name: Talpen.

Properties: The phthalidyl thiazolidine carboxylic ester of ampicillin which, like bacampicillin and pivampicillin, is rapidly and completely absorbed from the gastro-intestinal tract after oral dosage. Mucosal and erythrocytic esterases release free ampicillin into the circulation and the inactivated ester moiety is excreted through the liver and kidneys. 500 mg of the ester corresponds to 338 mg of free ampicillin.

Mode and spectrum of activity: As ampicillin.

Pharmacokinetics: Identical behaviour to that of pivampicillin and bacampicillin.

Side effects: As with oral ampicillin, except that, as with pivampicillin and bacampicillin, gastro-intestinal intolerance is much reduced.

Main indications and contra-indication: As with the other ampicillin esters.

Administration and dosage: 500 mg 3–4 times a day in tablet form (10 mg/kg 3–4 times a day for children).

Summary: This was the first of the ampicillin esters to be marketed in Great Britain, where it is frequently used. A good form of delivery of ampicillin by the oral route.

References

LEIGH, D. A., D. S. REEVES, K. SIMMONS, A. L. THOMAS, P. J. WILKINSON: Talampicillin: a new derivative of ampicillin. Brit. med. J. *1:* 1378 (1976).

f) Carboxypenicillins

α) Carbenicillin

The first carboxybenzyl penicillin, which is still commercially available for the treatment of infections with Pseudomonas and Proteus but, because of its weak activity, has now been largely superceded by ticarcillin, azlocillin and piperacillin.

β) Carbenicillin Esters

Proprietary names: For *carindacillin:* Carindapen, Geocillin.
For *carfecillin:* Uticillin, Vexyl.

Description: Carindacillin is the indanyl ester and carfecillin the phenyl ester of carbenicillin. Both esters are acid-stable and absorbed after oral administration, by being rapidly hydrolysed into carbenicillin which passes into the bloodstream. The indanol or phenol released by hydrolysis is bound to glucuronic acid and excreted predominantly in the urine.

Structural formulae of carbenicillin and its esters:

Generic Name	R
Carbenicillin	
Carindacillin	
Carfecillin	

Spectrum of activity: Sufficient carbenicillin for effective treatment of Pseudomonas aeruginosa and Proteus species is only present in the urine. Infections with Pseudomonas at other sites must be treated with the parenteral form or an alternative antibiotic.

Pharmacokinetics: Maximal serum concentrations average 10 mg/l after 1 g of carindacillin by mouth, and 8 mg/l after the same dose of carfecillin. *Urinary concentration* of carindacillin: 300–2000 mg/l; of carfecillin: 200–1000 mg/l. *Uri-*

nary recovery: 30% and 20–25% respectively. The indanol released through the hydrolysis of carindacillin in the body is excreted in the urine as a glucuronide-sulphate conjugate, and the same occurs with the phenol released from carfecillin. The urinary concentrations are not sufficient for treatment in patients with *renal failure* (creatine clearance less than 10 ml/min).

Side effects: Relatively frequent diarrhoea, vomiting, nausea, disagreeable taste, all of which occur more frequently with carindacillin.

Indications: Oral continuation of the treatment of persistent or recurrent urinary infection with Pseudomonas aeruginosa, Proteus vulgaris and other indole-positive species (Proteus morganii and Proteus rettgeri), for which no other oral antibiotic treatment is available.

Administration and dosage: 1 g 3–4 times a day by mouth as film tablets for 1–2 weeks; 20 mg/kg 3–4 times a day for children. Longer treatment is possible. 500 mg 3 times a day is often sufficient with carfecillin.

Preparations: Tablets of 500 mg.

Summary: When tolerated by the patient, a possible antibiotic treatment of chronic and recurrent urinary infections caused by Pseudomonas aeruginosa, Proteus vulgaris and related indole-positive species.

References

BAILEY, R. R., J. B. EASTWOOD, I. B. VAUGHAN: The pharmacokinetics of an oral form of carbenicillin in patients with renal failure. Postgrad. med. J. *48:* 422 (1972).
BAKER, D. A., V. T. ANDRIOLE: The treatment of difficult urinary-tract infections with carbenicillin indanyl sodium. J. infect. Dis. *(Suppl.) 127:* 136 (1973).
BOROWSKI, J., A. MUSIEROWICZ, J. CZERNIAWSKI, D. DZIERZANOWSKA, M. ZAREBSKI, Z. GINGEL: Laboratory and clinical studies on carfecillin. J. Antimicrob. Chemother. *2:* 175 (1976).
HODGENS, G. R., R. L. PERKINS: Carbenicillin indanyl sodium oral therapy of urinary tract infections. Arch. intern. Med. *131:* 679 (1973).
HOLLOWAY, W. J., W. A. TAYLOR: Long term oral carbenicillin therapy in complicated urinary tract infections. J. infect. Dis. (Suppl) *127:* 143 (1973).
KNIRSCH, A. K., D. C. HOBBS, J. KORST: Pharmacokinetics toleration, and safety of indanyl carbenicillin in man. J. infect. Dis. (Suppl.) *127:* 105 (1973).
LEIGH, D. A., K. SIMMONS: The treatment of simple and complicated urinary tract infections with carfecillin, a new oral ester of carbenicillin. J. Antimicrob. Chemother. *2:* 293 (1976).
WILKINSON, P. J., D. S. REEVES, R. J. WISE, J. T. ALLEN: Volunteer and clinical studies with carfecillin: a new orally administered ester of carbenicillin. Brit. med. J. *2:* 250 (1975).
WISE, R.: Editorial. For and against carfecillin – a matter of resistance? J. Antimicrob. Chemother. *1:* 4 (1975).

γ) Ticarcillin

Proprietary names: Aerugipen, Ticar, Ticarpen.

Properties: A carbenicillin derivative, α-carboxy-3-thienylmethyl penicillin, commercially available as the disodium salt, containing 5.2–6.5 milliequivalents/g of sodium. It is water-soluble and the solution is colourless or slightly yellow. Solutions stored at 4° C should be discarded after 3 days.

Structural formula:

Spectrum of activity: Identical with that of carbenicillin, but with 2–3 times the *in vitro* activity on Pseudomonas aeruginosa. Strains of Pseudomonas are considered resistant at minimal inhibitory concentrations of 100 mg/l or more, so less than 5% of clinically encountered strains are currently resistant. There is no difference in activity from carbenicillin on Escherichia coli and Proteus species (particularly the indole-positive strains). Most strains of Mima, Herellea, Klebsiella, Citrobacter and Serratia are resistant as are all strains of Enterobacter species and the enterococci. Synergy with the aminoglycosides (tobramycin, gentamicin, amikacin) is found against Pseudomonas aeruginosa.

Pharmacokinetics:
Rapid *absorption* after intramuscular injection (maximal serum concentration after 30–45 min). Not absorbed by mouth.
Mean serum concentrations: 107 and 175 mg/l respectively, 1 h after i.v. injection of 3 g and 5 g, and 14 and 28 mg/l respectively after 4 h. 740 ± 56 mg/l after short i.v. infusion of 5 g over 30 min; 981 ± 53 mg/l after i.v. infusion of 10 g over 60 min. Serum concentration of 260 mg/l found with constant i.v. infusion of 1 g/h. *Half-life* 70 min. *Plasma protein binding* 45%.
Excretion almost entirely through the kidneys. *Urinary recovery* greater than 95%. Urinary concentration during the first 6 h after i.v. infusion of 5 g is greater than 10,000 mg/l.

Side effects: As for benzyl penicillin (allergy, neurotoxicity etc.). Hypernatraemia, hypokalaemia and thrombophlebitis are less frequent than with carbenicillin due to the smaller dose. Daily sodium load 94 milliequivalents with

18 g of ticarcillin daily. Bleeding disorders with prolongation of bleeding time are caused by impaired platelet function and depend on the dose given.

Indications: Pseudomonas infections (septicaemia or meningitis, skin, soft tissue or urinary infections, pneumonia, bronchiectasis, purulent otitis media). Septicaemia and meningitis caused by Pseudomonas aeruginosa should always be treated in combination with an aminoglycoside such as tobramycin, amikacin or netilmicin.

Contra-indication: Penicillin allergy. Take care in patients receiving anticoagulants because of the possibility of an increased bleeding tendency.

Administration: Adequate dilution is necessary with the i. v. route (1 g in 10 or preferably 20 ml of distilled water for injection to avoid local venous irritation). Short i. v. infusion is preferable. Dissolve in 1% lignocaine for i. m. injection (1 g in 2 ml) and do not exceed 2 g per injection. Do not mix with aminoglycosides (gentamicin, tobramycin, netilmicin or amikacin) in the same solution for injection or infusion, because inactivation has been reported *in vitro,* though not *in vivo.*

Dosage: 18–20 g a day for *adults;* 300 mg/kg for *children* and *neonates,* in 4 (–6) i. v. injections or short infusions daily and preferably in combination with tobramycin or gentamicin (for dosage, see p. 136). 2 g every 8 h are sufficient in severe renal failure (creatinine clearance 10–30 ml/min), or 2 g every 12 h (creatinine clearance less than 10 ml/min).

For *Pseudomonas meningitis:* intrathecal instillation (intraventricular in the newborn) of 40 mg (adults), 10–20 mg (children older than 2 years) or 5–10 mg (children under 2 years) may be given.

Preparations: Ampoules of 1 g, 2 g, 5 g and 10 g.

Summary: Less active than azlocillin and piperacillin in Pseudomonas infections. Dose-dependent side effects.

References

NELSON, J. D., S. SHELTON, H. KUSMIESZ: Clinical pharmacology of ticarcillin in the newborn infant: Relation to age, gestational age, and weight. J. Pediat. *87:* 474 (1975).
PARRY, M. F., H. C. NEU: Pharmacokinetics of ticarcillin in patients with abnormal renal function. J. infect. Dis. *133:* 46 (1976).
PARRY, M. F., H. C. NEU: Ticarcillin for treatment of serious infections with Gram-negativ bacteria. J. infect. Dis. *134:* 476 (1976).

Schimpff, S. C., S. Landesman, D. M. Hahn, H. C. Standiford, C. L. Fortner, V. M. Young, P. H. Wiernik: Ticarcillin in combination with cephalothin or gentamicin as empiric antibiotic therapy in granulocytopenic cancer patients. Antimicrob. Ag. Chemother. *10:* 837 (1976).
Simon, C., M. Leuth, V. Malercyk: Ticarcillin, In-vitro-Aktivität und Pharmakokinetik. Dtsch. med. Wschr. *99:* 2460 (1974).
Ullmann, U.: The protein binding of ticarcillin and tobramycin. J. Antimicrob. Chemother. *2:* 213 (1976).
Wise, R., D. S. Reeves, A. S. Parker: Administration of ticarcillin, a new antipseudomonal antibiotic, in patients undergoing dialysis. Antimicrob. Ag. Chemother. *5:* 119 (1974).

δ) Temocillin

Proprietary name: Temopen.

Properties: Temocillin is the first 6-methoxy-penicillin with an unusually high stability to β-lactamases produced by gram-negative bacteria. The methoxy group was introduced at the 6α-position in the nucleus. Temocillin has a free carboxylic acid group and a thienyl group similar to ticarcillin. It is available as disodium salt. The structural formula is:

Spectrum of activity: Temocillin is active against the majority of gram-negative bacteria including β-lactamase-producing strains of Haemophilus influenzae and Neisseria gonorrhoeae. Gram-positive bacteria, Pseudomonas aeruginosa, Acinetobacter species, Campylobacter jejuni and Bacteroides fragilis are resistant. Against sensitive bacteria the in vitro activity is generally superior to that of other penicillins and cephalosporins. Some strains of Enterobacter cloacae, Serratia marcescens and Providencia stuartii are resistant. There is a partial cross-resistance with other penicillins and cephalosporins.

Pharmacokinetics: *Mean serum concentrations* 90 mg/l at 1 h after i. v. injection of 1 g; 35 mg/l at 4 h and 10 mg/l at 12 h. Not absorbed by mouth. *Plasma protein binding:* 85%. *Half-life:* 4.5 h. *Urinary recovery:* 80%, mostly filtered by the glomeruli.

Side effects: Similar to ticarcillin (see p. 57).

Indications: Urinary and gynaecological infections with known sensitive gram-negative rods.

Administration and dosage: Preferably as i. v. injection or short i. v. infusion. 2–4 g a day in 2 or 3 divided doses are usually adequate because of the relatively long half-life.

Preparations: Ampoules of 1 g and 2 g.

Summary: Highly active against enterobacteria, but inactive against Pseudomonas species, Bacteroides fragilis and gram-positive bacteria. Should only be used for infections with known sensitive microorganisms.

References

BOLIVAR, R., S. S. WEAVER, G. P. BODEY: Comparative in vitro study of temocillin (BRL 17421), a new penicillin. Antimicrob. Ag. Chemother. *21:* 641 (1982).

BROWN, R. M., R. WISE, J. M. ANDREWS: Temocillin, in vitro activity and the pharmacokinetics and tissue penetration in healthy volunteers. J. Antimicrob. Chemother. *10:* 295 (1982).

CHEN, H. Y., J. D. WILLIAMS: Temocillin compared to ampicillin against Haemophilus influenzae and with other penicillins against intestinal aerobic gram-negative rods. J. Antimicrob. Chemother. *10:* 279 (1982).

CLARKE, A. M., S. J. V. ZEMCOV: Comparative in vitro activity of temocillin (BRL 17421), a new penicillin. J. Antimicrob. Chemother. *11:* 319 (1983).

GREENWOOD, D., A. COWLISHAW, A. ELEY: In vitro activity of temocillin, a new β-lactamase-stable penicillin active against enterobacteria. Antimicrob. Ag. Chemother. *22:* 198 (1982).

JULES, K., H. C. NEU: Antibacterial activity and β-lactamase stability of temocillin. Antimicrob. Ag. Chemother. *22:* 453 (1982).

VAN LANDUYT, H. W., M. PYCKAVET, A. LAMBERT, J. BOELAERT: In vitro activity of temocillin (BRL 17421), a novel β-lactam antibiotic. Antimicrob. Ag. Chemother. *22:* 535 (1982).

MALOTTKE, R., J. POTEL: Mikrobiologische Untersuchungen mit dem neuen Penicillin BRL 17421 (Temocillin). Infection *11:* 47 (1983).

PIOT, P., E. VAN DYCK: In vitro activity of BRL 17421 against Haemophilus influenzae, Neisseria gonorrhoeae, and Branhamella catarrhalis. Antimicrob. Ag. Chemother. *21:* 166 (1982).

SLOCOMBE, B., M. J. MASKER, P. H. BENTLEY: BRL 17421, a novel β-lactam antibiotic, highly resistant to β-lactamases, giving high and prolonged serum levels in humans. Antimicrob. Ag. Chemother. *20:* 38 (1981).

VERBIST, L.: In vitro activity of temocillin (BRL 17421), a novel β-lactamase-stable penicillin. Antimicrob. Ag. Chemother. *22:* 157 (1982).

YOURASSOWSKY, E., M. P. VAN DER LINDEN, M. J. LISMONT, F. CROKAERT: Growth curve patterns and bacterial morphology of Escherichia coli subjected to different temocillin (BRL 17421) concentrations. J. Antimicrob. Chemother. *10:* 289 (1982).

g) Acylamino Penicillins

The group contains derivatives of ampicillins. The amino group was first substituted by ureido side-chains, so the name ureido penicillins is also used for this group. The actual derivatives contain more complicated rings and are better classified as acylamino penicillins. All derivatives are more or less active against Pseudomonas aeruginosa, enterobacteria and enterococci. They penetrate rapidly into the bacterial cell wall (good crypticity), but are not stable against β-lactamases from staphylococci or resistant strains of Enterobacter, Serratia and Klebsiella.

α) Azlocillin

Proprietary names: Azlin, Securopen.

Properties: An acylureido penicillin (an ampicillin derivative, in which the amino group of the side-chain has been substituted). The monosodium salt is about 40% soluble in water. The 10% solution can be stored at room temperature for at least 6 h without loss of activity. 5 g azlocillin contain 11 milliequivalents of sodium.

Spectrum of activity: Broader than carbenicillin because of its much greater activity against Pseudomonas aeruginosa (4–8-fold), enterococci (10-fold) and Bacteroides fragilis (2-fold). Mean MIC (minimal inhibitory concentration) of azlocillin against Pseudomonas is 8 mg/l, against enterococci 1–2 mg/l and against Bacteroides fragilis 16 mg/l. Ticarcillin and mezlocillin are only ⅓ as active as azlocillin against Pseudomonas (Table 35, p. 285). Mezlocillin is more active than azlocillin against other gram-negative bacilli such as Escherichia coli, Proteus species, Klebsiella, Enterobacter, Serratia etc. All penicillinase-producing staphylococci are resistant, as are the majority of enterobacters and serratias. There is synergy with the aminoglycosides against Pseudomonas, Klebsiella, Serratia, Proteus and enterococci.

Resistance: Incomplete cross-resistance with piperacillin, ticarcillin, mezlocillin and ampicillin. Some strains of Pseudomonas are resistant to ticarcillin but sensitive to azlocillin. Azlocillin-resistant gram-negative rods are sometimes sensitive to mezlocillin and piperacillin (e. g. Escherichia coli, Klebsiella, Serratia). Complete cross-resistance with benzyl penicillin against staphylococci, mycoplasmas etc., and with ampicillin against Haemophilus influenzae.

Pharmacokinetics:
Not absorbed by mouth.

Mean serum concentrations after i. v. injection of 2 g: 60 mg/l at 1 h, and 6 mg/l at 4 h; after i. v. infusion of 5 g over 30 min 430 mg/l at end of infusion and 35 mg/l at 4 h afterwards.

Half-life: 1¼ h. *Plasma protein binding:* 30%.

Urinary excretion 60% at 6 h in the active form. An unknown amount is transformed by the body into inactive metabolites.

Side effects: As with benzyl penicillin. False-positive non-enzymatic tests for urinary sugar and urobilinogen may occur during therapy. Skin rashes are less common than with ampicillin. Reversible leucopenia occurs rarely.

Indications: Pseudomonas infections such as ecthyma gangrenosum, pneumonia in patients on ventilation, infected burns, septicaemia in leukaemics, aspiration pneumonia etc. Best given in combination with an aminoglycoside. When the causative organism is unknown, azlocillin may be combined with one of the β-lactamase-stable cephalosporins.

Inappropriate use: Infections against which other penicillins such as benzyl penicillin, mezlocillin or piperacillin would be more active. Infections by penicillin-resistant staphylococci.

Contra-indication: Penicillin allergy.

Administration and dosage: Preferably as i. v. injection or short i. v. infusion. Intramuscular injection is possible but sometimes painful. In severe or fulminating infections, give 5 g 3 times a day as a short i. v. infusion to adults and 80 mg/kg 3 times a day to children; otherwise give 2 g 3 times a day to adults and 30 mg/kg 3 times a day to children. In renal failure (creatinine clearance less than 30 ml/min) the usual single dose should be given every 12, instead of every 8 h. The 1% aqueous solution may be used for local irrigation.

Preparation: Ampoules of 500 mg, 1 g, 2 g and 10 g.

Summary: An effective anti-pseudomonal penicillin which has completely supplanted carbenicillin. An important partner in combination with the β-lactamase-stable cephalosporins in initial therapy.

References

DASCHNER, F.: In vitro-Kombinationswirkung von Carbenicillin, Mezlocillin und Azlocillin mit Gentamicin und Sisomicin auf Pseudomonas aeruginosa, Serratia marcescens, Klebsiella pneumonia und indolpositive Proteus-Stämme. Infection *4, Suppl. 4:* 331 (1976).

HELM, E. B., W. RISTOW, P. M. SHAH, P. SCHACHT, W. STILLE: Behandlung von Pseudomonas-Infektionen mit dem neuen Ureidopenicillin Azlocillin. Dtsch. med. Wschr. *102:* 1211 (1977).

KÖNIG, B., K. METZGER, P. MÜRMANN, H. OFFE, W. SCHRÖCK: Azlocillin: Ein neues Penicillin gegen Pseudomonas aeruginosa und andere gramnegative Bakterien. Infection *5:* 60 (1977).

LODE, H., U. NIESTRATH, P. KOEPPE, H. LANGMAACK: Azlocillin und Mezlocillin: Zwei neue semisynthetische Acylureidopenicilline. Infection *5:* 163 (1977).

STEWART, D., G. P. BODEY: Azlocillin: In vitro studies of a new semisynthetic penicillin. Antimicrob. Ag. Chemother. *11:* 865 (1977).

SUTTER, V. L., S. M. FINEGOLD: Susceptibility of anaerobic bacteria to 23 antimicrobial agents. Antimicrob. Ag. Chemother. *10:* 736 (1976).

VENT, J., H. LATURNUS: Bestimmung der Knochenkonzentration von Azlocillin. Arch. orthop. Unfall-Chir. *90:* 259 (1977).

WIRTH, K., M. SCHOMERUS, J. H. HENGSTMANN: Zur Pharmakokinetik von Azlocillin, einem neuen halbsynthetischen Breitspektrum-Antibiotikum. Infection *4:* 25 (1976).

β) Mezlocillin

Proprietary names: Baypen, Mezlin.

Properties: An acylureido penicillin. The sodium monohydrate is readily soluble in water. The 10% aqueous solution for i.v. injection is colourless or slightly yellow and remains stable for up to 24 h at room temperature. Approx. 9.3 milliequivalents of sodium are contained in 5 g.

Spectrum of activity: Broader than ampicillin, to include some of the indole-positive strains of Proteus (Proteus vulgaris), Providencia, Serratia, Klebsiella, Enterobacter and Pseudomonas aeruginosa. Mezlocillin is 2–3 times more active than azlocillin against the Enterobacteriaceae, with the exception of Pseudomonas aeruginosa (mean MIC of mezlocillin 32 mg/l, and of azlocillin 8 mg/l). A variable number of strains are resistant to mezlocillin at concentrations of 64 mg/l or more, however, including Providencia (60%), Klebsiella aerogenes (40%), Serratia marcescens (40%), Enterobacter (20–40%), Pseudomonas aeruginosa (10–40%) and Escherichia coli (10–30%). At concentrations of 32 mg/l or more, mezlocillin is active against most of the non-sporing anaerobes (Bacteroides species, including Bacteroides fragilis). All penicillinase-producing staphylococci are resistant, as are ampicillin-resistant strains of Haemophilus. Synergy is found in combination with the aminoglycosides against Pseudomonas, Klebsiella, Serratia and Proteus.

Pharmacokinetics:
Not absorbed by mouth.
Mean serum concentrations: 140 mg/l at ½ h and 13 mg/l at 4 h after an i.v. injection of 2 g. Mean concentrations after i.v. infusion of 5 g over 30 min were

426 mg/l at the end of the infusion, 178 mg/l 1 h later and 33 mg/l 4 h after the end of the infusion. *Half-life:* 50 min; *plasma protein binding:* 30%.

Excretion: 55–60% in active form in the urine, and relatively high biliary excretion also. An unknown amount is decomposed into antibacterially inactive metabolites.

Side effects: As with benzyl penicillin. The urinary excretion of metabolites can lead to false positive non-enzymatic urinary tests for sugar and urobilinogen.

Rashes are no more frequent than with benzyl penicillin. As with other β-lactam antibiotics, a transient neutropenia sometimes occurs.

Indications: Infections of the genitourinary and biliary tract with sensitive gram-negative bacilli including Bacteroides species. Metronidazole still remains the best first-line antibacterial agent in Bacteroides fragilis infections, however. Severe systemic infections (septicaemia, endocarditis, meningitis etc.) in combination with an aminoglycoside or with a penicillinase-stable penicillin (e.g. flucloxacillin).

Inappropriate uses: Infections with organisms sensitive to benzyl penicillin. Staphylococcal infections.

Contra-indication: Penicillin allergy.

Administration and dosage: Preferably as i.v. injection or short i.v. infusion over 30 to 60 min. Do not mix with other drugs in the syringe or infusion solution, particularly aminoglycosides. Dosage for severe systemic infections: 5 g 3 times a day or 10 g twice a day (200–300 mg/kg/day for children); for urinary infections and non-life-threatening infections with sensitive bacteria: 2 g 3 times a day (80–100 mg/kg/day for children).

Preparations: Ampoules of 500 mg, 1 g, 2 g, 5 g and 10 g.

Summary: A bactericidal broad-spectrum penicillin which is superior to ampicillin in both activity and breadth of spectrum. It is recommended for infections with sensitive gram-negative bacilli, particularly biliary and abdominal infections.

References

BODEY, G. P., T. PAN: Mezlocillin: In vitro studies of a new broad-spectrum penicillin. Antimicrob. Ag. Chemother. *11:* 74 (1977).

FU, K., H. C. NEU: The comparative synergistic activity of amikacin, gentamicin, netilmicin and azlocillin, mezlocillin, carbenicillin and ticarcillin against Serratia marcescens. J. Antibiot. *31:* 135 (1978).

ISELL, B. F., G. P. BODEY, S. WEAVER: Clinical pharmacology of mezlocillin. Antimicrob. Ag. Chemother *13:* 180 (1978).
METZGER, K.: Dosisfindung in der antibakteriellen Chemotherapie. Arzneimittel-Forsch. *27:* 286 (1977).
WERNER, H., C. KRASEMANN, J. UNGERECHTS, H. J. SCHMITZ: Die in-vitro-Aktivität von Mezlocillin, Azlocillin und Carbenicillin gegen Bacteroidaceae unter besonderer Berücksichtigung der Fragilis-Gruppe. Infection *5:* 17 (1977).
WISE, R., A. P. GILLETT, J. M. ANDREWS, K. A. BEDFORD: Activity of azlocillin and mezlocillin against gramnegative organisms. Antimicrob. Ag. Chemother. *13:* 559 (1978).

γ) Piperacillin

Proprietary names: Pipracil, Pipril.

Properties: An acylamino penicillin related to azlocillin and mezlocillin. The monosodium salt is readily soluble in water and is relatively stable (10% loss of action after 24 hours at 25° C in a buffered solution). The 10% aqueous solution is isotonic with blood. 1 g of piperacillin sodium contains 2 milliequivalents of sodium.

Mode of action: Bactericidal in the log phase of bacterial growth.

Spectrum of activity: Piperacillin combines the spectra of azlocillin and mezlocillin; because of its greater intrinsic activity, there are generally fewer strains with reduced sensitivity or resistance to piperacillin than with azlocillin or mezlocillin. Against Pseudomonas aeruginosa, piperacillin is generally one dilution step more active than azlocillin and 3–4 dilution steps more active than mezlocillin (see Table 35, p. 285).

Against Escherichia coli and Klebsiella pneumoniae, piperacillin is generally 1–2 dilution steps more active than mezlocillin in ⅔ of the strains encountered. Piperacillin is 1–2 dilutions more active than mezlocillin against almost all strains of Proteus mirabilis, Proteus vulgaris, Enterobacter aerogenes, Citrobacter freundii and salmonellae. Mezlocillin is slightly more active against enterococci. There are no essential differences between piperacillin and azlo- or mezlocillin against Haemophilus or anaerobes (including Bacteroides fragilis). Piperacillin has no activity on penicillinase-producing staphylococci. There is synergy with aminoglycosides against gram-negative bacilli and enterococci.

Resistance: Incomplete cross-resistance with ticarcillin, azlo-, mezlo-, and ampicillin. Complete cross-resistance with benzyl penicillin against staphylococci and with ampicillin against Haemophilus. Piperacillin is inactivated by β-lactamases produced by staphylococci and Bacteroides fragilis.

Pharmacokinetics: *Mean concentrations:* 40 mg/l (1 h), 3.6 mg/l (4 h) and 1 mg/l (6 h) after i. v. injection of 2 g. After an i. v. infusion of 4 g serum concentrations are 60 mg/l 1 h after end of infusion, 8 mg/l (4 h) and 2.5 µg/ml (6 h). Constant serum concentration of 15 mg/l is maintained during continuous i. v. infusion (0.33 g/h = 8 g/24 h). *Half-life:* 1 h. *Plasma protein binding:* 20%. *Urinary excretion* in active form: 60–70%. *Urinary concentrations* after 2 g i. v.: 4000–10000 mg/l during the first 3 hours. Biliary concentrations (hepatic bile): 200–2400 mg/l. A proportion is metabolised in the body. *Tissue diffusion* good but *CSF concentration* relatively low.

Side effects: As with benzyl penicillin. Skin rashes are less frequent than with ampicillin. As with other β-lactam antibiotics, transient neutropenia occasionally occurs.

Indications: Urinary, genital and biliary infections caused by sensitive gram-negative bacilli, and proven or suspected Pseudomonas infections (preferably in combination with tobramycin), as well as severe systemic infections (septicaemia, meningitis, pneumonia etc.) in combination with an aminoglycoside or cephalosporin.

Inappropriate use: Use as a single agent in life-threatening systemic bacterial infections of unknown origin, particularly where resistant organisms such as Staphylococcus aureus, Enterobacter or Bacteroides fragilis are possible pathogens.

Contra-indication: Penicillin allergy.

Administration and dosage: Preferably as an i. v. injection or short i. v. infusion. Do not mix in the syringe or the infusion solution with other drugs or with an aminoglycoside.
Normal dosage: 2 g 3–4 times a day (30 mg/kg 3–4 times a day in children). The dose can be doubled in severe or life-threatening infections (4 g 3–4 times a day). In renal failure (serum creatine greater than 5 mg/dl), do not exceed a daily dose of 6 g. I. m. injection is only recommended for single doses of up to 2 g, and the substance may be dissolved in 0.5% lignocaine solution if necessary.

Preparations: Ampoules of 1 g, 2 g, 4 g and 6 g.

Summary: The most active broad-spectrum penicillin to date, especially in the gram-negative range including Pseudomonas and the non-sporing anaerobes. Not active against many staphylococci. In the initial treatment of life-threatening infections, give only in combination with an aminoglycoside or cephalosporin.

References

BODEY, G. P., B. LeBLANC: Piperacillin: In vitro evaluation. Antimicrob. Ag. Chemother. *14* (1): 78 (1978).

BRAVENY, I., K. MACHKA: Antibakterielle Wirkung von Piperacillin in der Kombination mit Cefotiam und Cefotaxim. Fortschr. antimikrob. Chemother. *3-1:* 33 (1984).

FU, K. P., H. C. NEU: Piperacillin, a new penicillin active against many bacteria resistant to other penicillins. Antimicrob. Ag. Chemother. *13* (3): 358 (1978).

GENTRY, L. O., J. G. JEMSEK, E. A. NATELSON: Effects of sodium piperacillin on platelet function in normal volunteers. Antimicrob. Ag. Chemother. *19:* 532 (1981).

KUCK, N. A., G. S. REDIN: In vitro and in vivo activity of piperacillin, a new broad-spectrum semisynthetic penicillin. J. Antibiot. *31* (11): 1175 (1978).

STASZEWSKI, S., A. RESTLE, W. STILLE: Piperacillin in Kombination mit modernen Cephalosporinen – eine In-vitro-Untersuchung. FAC *3-1:* 7 (1984).

VERBIST, L.: In vitro activity of piperacillin, a new semisynthetic penicillin with an unusually broad spectrum of activity. Antimicrob. Ag. Chemother. *13* (3): 349 (1978).

VOGEL, F., J. HARTLAPP, N. SPANNBRUCKER, K. KRACK: Kombinationstherapie mit Cefotiam und Piperacillin bei immunsupprimierten Patienten. FAC *3-1:* 43 (1984).

WHITE, G. W., J. B. MALOW, V. M. ZIMELIS, H. PAHLAVANZADEH, A. P. PANWALKER, G. G. JACKSON: Comparative in vitro activity of azlocillin, ampicillin, mezlocillin, piperacillin and ticarcillin, alone and in combination with an aminoglycoside. Antimicrob. Ag. Chemother. *15:* 540 (1979).

δ) Apalcillin

Proprietary name: Lumota.

Description: An acylamino penicillin developed in Japan with a similar spectrum and activity to piperacillin (see p. 65).

Structural formula of apalcillin:

Spectrum of activity: Apparently slightly greater activity against Pseudomonas, but little or no action on Bacteroides fragilis, Serratia marcescens or penicillin-resistant staphylococci. Primarily resistant strains of Escherichia coli, Klebsiella pneumoniae and Proteus species occur.

Pharmacokinetics: *Maximal serum concentrations* of 140 and 190 mg/l are found 2 hours after an i. v. infusion of 2 g and 3 g respectively. *Plasma protein binding:* 96%. *Half-life:* 80 min. *Urinary recovery:* 20%. High *excretion* in the bile and some metabolism in the body. Pharmacokinetic properties are not, therefore, as favourable as with piperacillin.

Side effects: Relatively frequent increase in serum transaminases and (in animals) histamine release and reduction in blood pressure. Diarrhoea in 5–10%.

Dosage: 2–3 g 3 times a day, as i.v. infusion.

Summary: No advantages in comparison to piperacillin, inferior pharmacokinetics and more side effects.

References

NOGUCHI, H.: Antibacterial activity of Apalcillin against gram-negative bacilli. Antimicrob. Ag. Chemother. *13:* 745 (1978).

h) Mecillinam

Proprietary name: Selexid, Selexidin (Pivmecillinam).

Synonyms: Amdinocillin, amidino penicillin.

Spectrum of activity: A broad-spectrum penicillin developed in Denmark by Leo (the amidino derivative of 6-aminopenicillanic acid) with strong activity against gram-negative bacilli such as Escherichia coli, Proteus mirabilis, Proteus vulgaris, Klebsiella pneumoniae, Enterobacter cloacae, Yersinia, Citrobacter, salmonellae and shigellae (minimum inhibitory concentrations generally 0.1–0.5 mg/l). Less active against gram-positive bacilli such as streptococci, pneumococci or penicillin-sensitive staphylococci. No activity against Pseudomonas aeruginosa, enterococci or penicillinase-producing staphylococci, or against most strains of Serratia marcescens or Haemophilus influenzae. Intense synergy with ampicillin against most strains of Escherichia coli and Klebsiella pneumoniae, as well as with cephalosporins, aminoglycosides and tetracyclines against other bacteria. The mode of action of mecillinam differs from that of other penicillins because it is active on only one binding protein, leading to a marked production of spheroblasts and a slower bacteriolysis. The synergistic combination with pivampicillin (Miraxid) is currently undergoing clinical trials.

Pharmacokinetics: Poorly absorbed by mouth, but well absorbed as the ester (pivmecillinam or bacmecillinam). Mean *serum concentrations* 1 h after the oral administration of 200 mg and 400 mg of pivmecillinam are 3 and 5 mg/l respectively. *Half-life:* 1 h. *Plasma protein binding:* 10%. *Urinary recovery:* 50% (after oral administration). Good tolerance except for allergic reactions and occasional nausea and vomiting after oral administration.

Indications: Mecillinam is suitable for the treatment of infections with gram-negative bacilli (e. g. in urine) and may be given parenterally as well as orally (as pivmecillinam or bacmecillinam). May be used in salmonella infections.

Dosage: 200–400 mg of pivmecillinam orally 3 times a day, 5–15 mg/kg (as tablets) 3 times a day for children below the age of 6. In salmonella infections, 1.2–2.4 g a day.

References

AARASS, I., K. W. SKARSTEN, H. C. NEES: Pivmecillinam in the treatment of post-operative bacteriuria in gynecological patients. A double-blind comparison with pivmecillinam and pivampicillin. J. Antimicrob. Chemother *3:* 227 (1977).
BRESKY, B.: Controlled randomized study comparing amoxycillin and pivmecillinam in adult out-patients presenting with symptoms of acute urinary tract infection. J. Antimicrob. Chemother. *3* (Suppl. *B*): 121 (1977).
GEDDES, A. M., P. D. CLARKE: The treatment of enteric fever with mecillinam. J. Antimicrob. Chemother. *3* (Suppl. *B*): 1011 (1977).
Leading Article: Mecillinam. Lancet *1:* 252 (1978).
MITCHARD, M., J. ANDREWS, M. J. KENDALL, R. WISE: Mecillinam serum levels following intravenous injection: A comparison with pivmecillinam. J. Antimicrob. Chemother. *3* (Suppl. *B*): 83 (1977).
REEVES, D. S.: Antibacterial activity of mecillinam. J. Antimicrob. Chemother. *3* (Suppl. *B*): 5 (1977).
ROHOLT, K.: Pharmacokinetic studies with mecillinam and pivmecillinam. J. Antimicrob. Chemother. *3* (Suppl. B): 71 (1977).
SPRATT, B. G.: The mechanism of action of mecillinam. J. Antimicrob. Chemother. *3* (Suppl. *B*): 13 (1977).
STILLE, W., E. BISCHOF LÉGER, E. B. HELM: Kombinationseffekte von Mecillinam mit Ampicillin bzw. Cephazolin. Arzneimittel-Forsch. *28:* 1661 (1978).

i) Penicillin Combinations

A number of fixed combinations are commercially available, in which ampicillin, carbenicillin or mezlocillin are combined with penicillinase-stable penicillins, such as oxa-, cloxa-, and dicloxacillin. Because of the high proportion of bacteria resistant to ampicillin, carbenicillin and mezlocillin, they are now becoming obsolete. Free combinations of anti-pseudomonal penicillins such as azlocillin or piperacillin with other β-lactam antibiotics (e. g. of the cefotaxime group), which would considerably extend the spectrum and increase the activity, are potentially much more useful nowadays. Combinations of antibiotics at various doses are available in many countries.

2. Cephalosporins

Classification: Cephalosporins can be classified according to their chemical structure, clinical uses and historical factors. Because of their great variety, it is difficult to classify the cephalosporins on the basis of their chemical properties alone, and this is not therefore helpful in clinical practice. A classification according to their activity and spectrum would be useful for clinical usage but is complicated by the degree of overlap and duplication. Subdivision of the cephalosporins into 1–4 generations in the approximate order of their historical discovery is arbitrary and of no great practical value, although such a classification is widely used and accepted. We believe the most useful classification of the cephalosporins to be in groups based on a compound representative of that group, namely:

1. *Cephalothin-cefazolin group.*
2. *Cefuroxime group* (with cefuroxime, cefamandole and cefotiam).
3. *Cefoxitin group* (the 7-methoxy cephalosporins).
4. *Cefotaxime group* (with cefotaxime, ceftriaxone, ceftizoxime, cefmenoxime, ceftazidime).
5. *Other cephalosporins* (cefsulodin, cefoperazone).
6. *Oral cephalosporins* (with cephalexin, cefadroxil, cefaclor, cephradine, and cefroxadine).

There are well established representatives of each group which should be considered for particular indications because of their spectrum of action and pharmacokinetic properties. The reasons for these preferences are dealt with below as well as in the chapter "Choice of the antibiotic" (p. 249) and the chapters concerned with therapy.

a) Cephalothin-Cefazolin Group

Proprietary names:

for *cephalothin:*	Cephalothin, Cepovenin, Keflin;
for *cephaloridine:*	Cephaloridin, Ceporin, Glaxoridin, Loridine;
for *cefazolin:*	Ancef, Cefacidal, Gramaxin, Kefzol;
for *cefazedone:*	Refosporin;
for *cephacetrile:*	Celospor;
for *cephapirin:*	Cefadyl.

Mode of action: Like the penicillins, the cephalosporins inhibit bacterial cell wall synthesis and are bactericidal only during bacterial growth.

Table 8. Structural formula of the cephalosporins.

$$R_1-NH-CH-CH \quad \overset{S}{\diagdown} CH_2$$

Compound	R_1	R_2
7-Aminocephalo-sporinic acid	H–	
Cephalothin		
Cephaloridine		
Cefazolin		
Cefamandole		
Cefuroxime		
Cefsulodin		
Cefotiam		2HCl

Spectrum of activity: *Very sensitive* strains include gram-positive bacteria such as pneumococci, streptococci, staphylococci, gonococci, meningococci, diphtheria bacilli and Bacillus anthracis. Certain staphylococci are designated penicillin-tolerant, and although they are inhibited by cephalosporins at low concentrations, they are only killed in high concentrations. The sensitivity of gram-negative bacteria *in vitro* is variable amongst species such as Escherichia coli, Klebsiella pneumoniae, Proteus mirabilis and others. Cefazolin and cefazedone are more active *in vitro* against gram-negative bacilli, particularly Escherichia coli and Klebsiella, than cephaloridine and cephalothin. The following bacteria are *resistant:* Pseudomonas aeruginosa, Proteus morganii and rettgeri, enterococci (Streptococcus faecalis), most strains of Proteus vulgaris and Haemophilus influenzae, as well as Providencia, Serratia, Citrobacter, Edwardsiella, Arizona, Acinetobacter, Bacteroides fragilis, Campylobacter, Nocardia, Mycoplasma, Moraxella, Brucella and most of the Enterobacter species.

Resistance: *Primary* resistance is common in gram-negative bacteria but quite rare with gram-positive organisms. *Secondary* resistance during therapy is rare and arises slowly. *Cross-resistance* occurs with Staphylococcus aureus between cephalosporins and penicillinase-stable penicillins (oxacillin, cloxacillin, di- and flucloxacillin) but not with Staphylococcus epidermidis (i. e. methicillin-resistant strains of Staphylococcus epidermidis can be sensitive to cephalothin). Partial cross-resistance is found with ampicillin, the acylamino penicillins and ticarcillin. No cross-resistance with benzyl penicillin.

Pharmacokinetics:
Not absorbed after oral administration. *Rapid* absorption after i. m. injection. *Serum concentrations* of cefazolin and cefazedone are much higher, dose for dose, than those found with cephaloridine, cephalothin, cephacetrile and cephapirin. The mean serum concentrations after 1 g of *cefazolin* i. v. are 52 mg/l after 1 h, 33 mg/l after 2 h and 5.6 mg/l after 6 h; at the corresponding times after the same dose of cephalothin, they are only 2.9, 0.6 and less than 0.1 mg/l. The mean serum concentrations after 1 g of *cefazedone* i. v. are 65 mg/l (1 h), 34 mg/l (2 h) and 6.4 mg/l (6 h). The serum concentrations 1 hour after the *i. m. injection* of 0.5 g are highest with cefazolin and cefazedone, about half as high with cephaloridine, and much lower with cephacetrile, cephalothin and cephapirin.

Half-life of cephalothin: 27 min; cephacetrile: 60 min; cephapirin: 36 min; cefazolin: 94 min; cefazedone: 140 min; cephaloridine: 90 min. *Protein binding* in the blood: cephalothin: 70%; cefacetrile: 24–28%; cephapirin: 50%; cefazolin: 84%; cefazedone: 93%; cephaloridine: 20%. *Tissue diffusion* is similar to that of the penicillins. Poor *CSF penetration,* though slightly improved in meningitis.

Concentrations in the *pleura, peritoneal* and *synovial* fluid: approx. 50–100% of the serum value. Approximately 50% of the maternal concentration may be measured in the cord blood. Relatively high concentrations in the amniotic fluid. *Excretion* primarily through the *kidneys;* the proportions recoverable in active form are: cephalothin 64%, cephacetrile 75%, cephapirin 70%, cefazolin 92%, cefazedone 97% and cephaloridine 85%. Cephaloridine is predominantly filtered by the glomeruli, whereas cephalothin and cephacetrile are mostly secreted by the tubules. A greater proportion of cefazolin and cefazedone is filtered by the glomeruli than of cephalothin. 20–30% of cephalothin, cephacetrile and cephapirin are metabolised in the body and excreted in the urine as desacetyl compounds which have weak antibacterial activity. High concentrations are found in the urine. Therapeutically adequate biliary concentrations are achieved with cefazolin, and cefazedone.

Side effects:
1. *Allergic reactions* (fever, rashes, urticaria etc.) in 1–4%. Anaphylactic shock is possible, but less common than with the penicillins. Although in some series up to 10% of penicillin-allergic patients have experienced similar, though usually milder reactions with the cephalosporins, such cross-allergy is seldom of critical importance. The great majority of patients with penicillin allergy tolerate cephalosporins because they do not release any penicilloyl compounds in the body.
2. *Allergic leukocytopenia,* rapidly reversible after cessation of therapy. Blood count should be checked after prolonged therapy or if allergic symptoms or fever occur during treatment.
3. *Local reactions* such as induration or pain after i. m. injection (especially with cephalothin) and thrombophlebitis (after more than 6 g of cephalothin by slow i. v. infusion).
4. *Risk of impaired renal function* with cephaloridine overdosage; the initial signs are proteinuria and casts in the urine. The daily dose of cephaloridine should not therefore exceed 4 g. This dose restriction does not apply to the other cephalosporins. Since high doses have produced renal damage in animals, no cephalosporin should be given at unnecessarily high dosage. Suggested daily maxima for cephalothin and cephacetrile are 8 g and for cefazolin and cefazedone 6 g. When there is pre-existing renal impairment, excessive doses of cephalothin (12–24 g a day) can cause further damage to the kidneys. Renal damage has also been reported with the combination of cephalothin or cephaloridine with gentamicin. Prior damage through shock (acute tubular necrosis), haemolysis, frusemide etc. are probably as important as the overdosage itself. When renal function is otherwise good, the combination of

cephaloridine or cephalothin with gentamicin or other aminoglycosides probably carries little risk.

5. The *direct Coombs test* can become *positive* during therapy with cephalosporins, particularly with cephalothin. The cephalosporins are assumed either to damage the surface of the red cells, allowing normal serum globulin to accumulate at this site, or to facilitate the deposition of a cephalosporin-globulin complex on the red cell surface which reacts with anti-human globulin. For all that, haemolytic anaemia is extremely rare during cephalosporin therapy.

Indications have become fewer with the introduction of the new β-lactamase-stable cephalosporins. Cefazolin and cefazedone (the best drugs in this group) are still useful in:

1. Primary pneumonia (community-acquired).
2. Wound infections (community-acquired).
3. Indications for benzyl penicillin in the presence of penicillin allergy (cross allergy with penicillin is 10% or less).

Cephaloridine should no longer be used on account of its potential nephrotoxicity.

Incorrect use: Trivial infections or those which should respond to antibiotics which are easier to give. Methicillin-resistant staphylococcal infections (cross-resistance). Severe systemic infections (sepsis), where multi-resistant enterobacteria may be involved.

Contra-indications: Cephalosporin allergy and cephaloridine-induced renal failure (oliguria, anuria). Do not exceed the recommended dose, and do not combine with frusemide.

Administration: I.m. injection (0.5 g) is possible with cefazolin, cefazedone, cephacetrile and cephapirin. Slow i.v. injection, short infusion or even constant infusion are preferable with cephalothin and higher doses of cefazolin and cefazedone. Intrathecal instillation of cephaloridine is available.

Dosage:
Cephalothin, cephacetrile, cephapirin: 3–8 g a day for adults, 50–100 (–200) mg/kg for children, in 3–4 divided doses (according to dosage). In renal failure, give 1 g every 6 hours where the creatinine clearance is 10–25 ml/min and 0.5 g when the creatinine clearance is 2–10 ml/min.

Cefazolin, cefazedone: 3–4 (–6) g a day for adults, 60 (–100) mg/kg for children, in 3 (–4) divided doses. In renal failure, reduce normal daily dose to 60% where creatinine clearance is 40–60 ml/min, to 25% where creatinine clearance is 20–40 ml/min and to 10% where creatinine clearance is 5–20 ml/min.

Preparations: Ampoules of 250 mg, 500 mg, 1 g, 2 g, and 4 g. Lignocaine solution is provided for i.m. injection only.

Summary: Because of their better antibacterial activity and pharmacokinetic properties, cefazolin and cefazedone are the only two recommended antibiotics in this group. Both these drugs also act on penicillinase-producing staphylococci. They have a fairly broad spectrum of action, low toxicity and give rise to high urine concentrations. Nevertheless, they have generally poor activity against gram-negative bacilli and are not active against Pseudomonas aeruginosa.

References

BARZA, M.: The nephrotoxicity of cephalosporins: An overview. J. infect. Dis. (Suppl.) *137:* 60 (1978).

BERGAN, T., E. K. BRODWALL, O. ØRJAVIK: Pharmacokinetics of cefazolin in patients with normal and impaired renal function. J. Antimicrob. Chemother. *3:* 435 (1977).

BERNARD, B., L. BARTON, M. ABATE, C. A. BALLARD: Maternal-fetal transfer of cefazolin in the first twenty weeks of pregnancy. J. infect. Dis. *136:* 377 (1977).

BRODWALL, E. K., T. BERGAN, O. ØRJAVIK: Kidney transport of cefazolin in normal and impaired renal function. J. Antimicrob. Chemother. *3:* 585 (1977).

BROGARD, J. M., F. KUNTZMANN, J. LAVILLAUREIX: Blood levels, renal and biliary excretions of a new cephalosporin, cephacetrile (Ciba 36278 Ba). Schweiz. med. Wschr. *103:* 110 (1973).

BROGARD, J. M., M. DORNER, M. PINGET, M. ADLOFF, J. LAVILLAUREIX: The biliary excretion of cefazolin. J. infect. Dis. *131:* 625 (1975).

COLE, D. R., J. PUNG: Penetration of cefazolin into pleural fluid. Antimicrob. Ag. Chemother. *11:* 1033 (1977).

DASH, C. H.: Penicillin allergy and the cephalosporins. J. Antimicrob. Chemother. *1 (Suppl.):* 107 (1975).

DELLINGER, P., T. MURPHY, V. PINN, M. BARZA, L. WEINSTEIN: Protective effect of cephalothin against gentamicin-induced nephrotoxicity in rats. Antimicrob. Ag. Chemother. *9:* 192 (1976).

FILLASTRE, J. P., R. LAUMONIER, G. HUMBERT, D. DUBOIS, J. METAYER, A. DELPECH, J. LEROY, M. ROBERT: Acute renal failure associated with combined gentamicin and cephalothin therapy. Brit. med. J. *2:* 396 (1973).

KIOSZ, D., C. SIMON, V. MALERCZYK: Die Plasmaeiweißbindung von Clindamycin, Cephazolin und Cephradin bei Neugeborenen und Erwachsenen. Klin. Pädiat. *187:* 71 (1975).

KLEINKNECHT, D., D. GANEVAL, D. DROZ: Acute renal failure after high doses of gentamicin and cephalothin. Lancet *1:* 1129 (1973).

RAM, M. D., S. WATANATITTAN: Levels of cefazolin in human bile: J. Infect. Dis. (Suppl.) *128:* 361 (1973).

SABATH, L. D., N. WHEELER, M. LAVERDIERE, D. BLAZEVIC, B. J. WILKINSON: A new type of penicillin resistance of Staphylococcus aureus. Lancet *1:* 443 (1977).

SIMON, C., V. MALERCZYK, E. BRAHMSTAEDT, W. TOELLER: Cephazolin, ein neues Breitspektrumantibiotikum. Dtsch. med. Wschr. *98:* 2448 (1973).

SIMON, C., V. MALERCZYK, B. TENSCHERT, F. MÖHLENBECK: Concentrations de cefazoline et de céfradine dans les éspaces intra et extravasculaires. Rev. Méd. (Paris) *37:* 1885 (1977).
SIMON, C., V. MALERCZYK, B. TENSCHERT, F. MÖHLENBECK: Die geriatrische Pharmakologie von Cefazolin, Cefradin und Sulfisomidin. Arzneimittel-Forsch. *26:* 1377 (1976).
TURES, J. F., W. F. TOWNSEND, H. D. ROSE: Cephalosporin-associated pseudomembranous colitis. JAMA *236:* 948 (1976).

b) Cefuroxime Group

Proprietary names: For *cefamandole:* Kefadol, Mandokef, Mandol; for *cefuroxime:* Curocef, Zinacef; for *cefotiam:* Halospor, Spizef.

Properties: Cefamandole is a heterocyclic cephalosporin and is given as cefamandole nafate for reasons of stability. It is rapidly and almost completely hydrolysed into cefamandole in the body. Like cefamandole, cefuroxime is a second generation cephalosporin with improved antibacterial activity (structural formula p. 71). Cefotiam is a 7-aminothiazolacetamido cephalosporin. The sodium salts of cefamandole nafate and cefuroxime are readily soluble in water as is the dihydrochloride of cefotiam. Cefamandole nafate contains 0.27 mg of sodium carbonate per mole. When dissolved in water, 30% of the ester is rapidly hydrolysed; 70% is hydrolysed in the body.

Spectrum of activity: Cefamandole, cefuroxime and cefotiam are largely stable to β-lactamases. β-lactamase resistance in these cephalosporins and in cefoxitin is due to the molecular grouping around the β-lactam ring which comprises mandelamido and tetrazole groups for cefamandole and the methyloxime group for cefuroxime. This group has much better activity than cephalothin against almost all gram-negative bacilli, and, to a lesser extent, against the gram-positive

Table 9. Activity against 499 clinical bacterial isolates tested *in vitro* with cephalothin (CT), cefuroxime (CU), cefamandole (CM), cefotiam (CI) and cefoxitin (CX). n = number of strains examined.
MIC$_{50\%}$ = minimal inhibitory concentration in 50% of the strains.

Species	n	MIC$_{50\%}$ (mg/l) CT	CU	CM	CI	CX
Escherichia coli	102	3.1	3.1	3.1	0.1	3.1
Proteus mirabilis	105	25.0	12.5	12.5	3.1	3.1
Proteus vulgaris	60	>200.0	200.0	200.0	25.0	6.2
Klebsiella pneumoniae	65	6.2	3.1	6.2	0.2	3.1
Enterobacter aerogenes	102	>200.0	12.5	0.8	0.4	50.0
Citrobacter freundii	15	50.0	12.5	25.0	25.0	50.0

cocci. Only cefamandole and cefotiam have reasonably good activity against staphylococci, with minimal inhibitory concentrations between 0.4 and 0.8 mg/l. Cefuroxime and cefotiam are particularly active against streptococci of Lancefield groups A and B, gonococci including penicillinase-producing strains and meningococci. Cefamandole is active particularly against Enterobacter species, salmonellae and staphylococci (including these resistant to methicillin and cephalothin). Cefamandole, cefuroxime and cefotiam are all active against Haemophilus influenzae, mostly at concentrations of 0.4–1.6 mg/l as well as against ampicillin-resistant strains. Table 9 shows the variations in activity of cefamandole, cefuroxime and cefotiam against different enterobacteria in 50% of the strains tested. The following organisms are completely resistant: Pseudomonas aeruginosa, enterococci, Mycoplasma, Chlamydia and mycobacteria. Cefamandole, cefuroxime and cefotiam have little or no activity against Bacteroides fragilis, while cefuroxime and cefotiam have little or no activity against cephalothin-resistant staphylococci.

Resistance: A variable proportion of Enterobacteriaceae are resistant to cefamandole, cefuroxime and/or cefotiam (according to the organism involved, see Table 34, p. 281). There is incomplete cross-resistance between the old and the new (β-lactamase-stable) cephalosporins and incomplete cross-resistance between cefoxitin, cefuroxime, cefamandole and cefotiam, which should be taken into account in sensitivity testing.

Pharmacokinetics:
Not absorbed by mouth. *Serum concentrations* after i. v. injection of 1 g (Fig. 14): 16.5 mg/l (1 h) and 1.1 mg/l (4 h) with cefamandole; 24.1 mg/l (1 h) and 3.7 mg/l (4 h) with cefuroxime; 19 mg/l (1 h) and 1.1 mg/l (4 h) with cefotiam. With a continuous i. v. infusion of 0.166 g/h (= 4 g/24 h), the *mean serum concentrations* are 8.1 mg/l with cefamandole and 12.0 mg/l with cefuroxime. *Half-life* of cefamandole: 50 min, cefuroxime: 70 min and cefotiam: 45 min. All penetrate tissues well but CSF poorly. Skin blister concentrations at equilibrium with cefamandole are 3 times as high and with cefuroxime 8 times as high as with cephalothin. *Plasma protein binding* of cefamandole: 67%, cefuroxime: 20%, cefotiam: 40%.
Urinary excretion of 90% of cefamandole and cefuroxime in active form within the first 6 h by glomerular filtration and active tubular secretion, and of 70% with cefotiam. A small amount is excreted with the bile. Little or no metabolism (except for cefotiam at approx. 20%). Probenecid retards renal excretion and doubles the half-life. Cefamandole is partially removed by haemodialysis, while cefuroxime is almost completely removed. Cefamandole and cefuroxime are only partially removed by peritoneal dialysis.

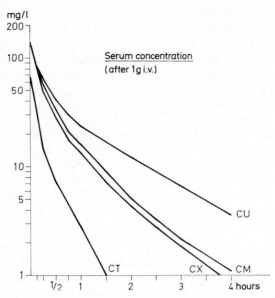

Fig. 14. Mean serum concentrations of cefuroxime (CU), cefamandole (CM), cefoxitin (CX) and cephalothin (CT) after i. v. injection of 1 g of each into 10 healthy adults, as a cross-over study.

Side effects: Similar to the older cephalosporins, but without the nephrotoxicity of cephaloridine. Cefamandole may cause alcohol intolerance (compare latamoxef and cefoperazone, pp. 86, 100) and hypoprothrombinaemia.

Indications: Initial therapy before culture and sensitivities are available of severe bacterial infections which could be due to staphylococci or also to resistant gram-negative rods. Indications of this sort are septicaemia, secondary pneumonia, postoperative urinary infections and severe wound and tissue infections. The gaps in the spectrum due to Pseudomonas and enterococci can be covered by giving azlocillin or piperacillin at the same time. Combination with an aminoglycoside (gentamicin, tobramycin, amikacin or netilmicin) to enhance the antibacterial effect continues to be indicated in severe infections with Enterobacteriaceae (septicaemia, pneumonia or endocarditis). Cefamandole, cefuroxime and cefotiam are also specifically indicated in infections with ampicillin-resistant strains of Haemophilus and with otherwise resistant bacilli. Cefamandole and cefotiam are often more effective against infections with Enterobacter aerogenes and staphylococci, whereas cefuroxime and cefotiam are better in infections with Klebsiella pneumoniae and penicillin-resistant gonococci.

Contra-indications: Similar to the other cephalosporins.

Administration: Either by i. v. injection, short i. v. infusion (30 min) or continuous i. v. infusion. Cefamandole must not be added to solutions containing calcium or magnesium. Do not mix with other drugs (e. g. aminoglycosides) in the same solution. The i. m. injection of cefamandole can be painful and is better dissolved therefore in 0.5% lignocaine.

Dosage: In *severe* (life-threatening) *systemic infections,* 2 g 3 times a day for adults (50 mg/kg 3 times a day for children).

For *local infections* (without severe systemic features): 1 g 3 times a day for adults (25 mg/kg 3 times a day for children).

For *gonorrhoea:* Single dose of 1.5 g of cefuroxime i. m. divided between 2 separate injection sites and preferably combined with a single oral dose of 1 g probenecid.

The dosage interval should be prolonged in patients with *chronic renal failure* to 8 h when the creatinine clearance is 30–50 ml/min, to 12 h at 10–29 ml/min, to 24 h at 5–9 ml/min and to 48 h for less than 5 ml/min. The normal single dose, according to the severity of the infection is then given at longer intervals. Do not give more than 0.75–1 g as a single dose when the creatinine clearance is less than 10 ml/min.

Preparations: *Cefamandole:* Ampoules of 500 mg, 1 g, 2 g; *Cefuroxime:* Ampoules of 250 mg, 750 mg, 1.5 g; *Cefotiam:* 500 mg, 1 g and 2 g.

Summary: These agents are important compounds because of their considerably improved activity against gram-negative bacilli. The gaps which still remain in the spectrum of activity (Pseudomonas, enterococci) can be covered by combination with other antibiotics.

References

Azimi, P. H.: Clinical and laboratory investigation of cefamandole therapy of infections in infants and children. J. infect. Dis. (Suppl.) *137:* 155 (1978).

Eykyn, S., C. Jenkins, A. King, I. Phillips: Antibacterial activity of cefuroxime, a new cephalosporin antibiotic, compared with that of cephaloridine, cephalothin, and cephamandole. Antimicrob. Ag. Chemother. *9:* 690 (1976).

Foord, R. D.: Cefuroxime: Human pharmacokinetics. Antimicrob. Ag. Chemother. *9:* 741 (1976).

Goodwin, C. S.: Cefuroxime: pharmacokinetics after a short infusion, and in vitro activity against hospital pathogens. J. Antimicrob. Chemother. *3:* 253 (1977).

GREENWOOD, D., N. J. PAARSON, F. O'GRADY: Cefuroxime: a new cephalosporin antibiotic with enhanced stability to enterobacterial β-lactamases. J. Antimicrob. Chemother. *2:* 337 (1976).

LEVINE, L. R., E. McCAIN: Clinical experience with cefamandole for treatment of serious bone and joint infections. J. infect. Dis. (Suppl.) *137:* 119 (1978).

MEYERS, B. R., B. LENG, S. Z. HIRSCHMANN: Cefamandole: Antimicrobial activity in vitro of a new cephalosporin. Antimicrob. Ag. Chemother. *8:* 737 (1975).

NORRBY, R., R. D. FOORD, P. HEDLUND: Clinical and pharmacokinetic studies on cefuroxime. J. Antimicrob. Chemother. *3:* 355 (1977).

PHILLIPS, I., A. KING, C. WARREN: The activity of penicillin and eight cephalosporins on Neisseria gonorrhoeae. J. Antimicrob. Chemother. *2:* 31 (1976).

RICHMOND, M. H., S. WOTTON: Comparative study of seven cephalosporins: Susceptibility to beta-lactamase and ability to penetrate the surface layers of Escherichia coli. Antimicrob. Ag. Chemother. *10:* 219 (1976).

SACK, K., U. KAISER, B. ZÜLLICH: Experimentelle Untersuchungen zur Nierenverträglichkeit von Cefuroxim. Infection *5:* 92 (1977).

SIMON, C.: Cefuroxim, ein neues β-Lactamase-stabiles Cephalosporin. Schweiz. med. Wschr. *108:* 1398 (1978).

SIMON, C., MALERCZYK, F. NIXDORF: In vitro activity and clinical pharmacology of cefamandole in comparison to cephalothin. J. Antimicrob. Chemother. *4:* 85 (1978).

SIMON, C.: Pharmacokinetics of cefuroxime in comparison to cefalothin. Proc. roy. Soc. Med. *70: (Suppl. 9):* 19 (1977).

SIMON, C.: D-Streptokokken (Enterokokken und Non-Enterokokken) und Cephalosporinempfindlichkeit. Med. Welt *34:* 1353 (1983).

SYKES, R. A. GRIFFITHS, D. M. RYAN: Comparative activity of ampicillin and cefuroxime against three types of Haemophilus influenzae. Antimicrob. Ag. Chemother. *11:* 599 (1977).

WOLD, J. S., R. R. JOOST, H. R. BLACK, R. S. GRIFFITH: Hydrolysis of cefamandole nafate to cefamandole in vivo. J. infect. Dis. *(Suppl.) 137:* 17 (1978).

c) 7-Methoxy Cephalosporins

The 7-methoxy cephalosporins (or cephamycins) differ from the other cephalosporins by possessing a 3 cepham nucleus with a methoxy group in the 7-α position. This class includes cefoxitin, cefotetan, cefmetazole and latamoxef. They are all very stable to β-lactamases, including those produced by Bacteroides fragilis. They are not active against Pseudomonas, however, except for latamoxef, in which a sulphur atom is replaced by an oxygen atom in the ring (Table 10).

α) Cefoxitin

Proprietary names: Mefoxin, Mefoxitin.

Mode of action: Highly resistant to almost all bacterial β-lactamases. Relatively poor penetration of the outer membrane of gram-negative bacteria.

Table 10. Structural formula of the 7-methoxy cephalosporins.

Generic Name	R_1	R_2	X
Cefoxitin		$-OCONH_2$	S
Cefmetazole	$NC-CH_2-S-CH_2-$		S
Cefotetan			S
Latamoxef			O

Spectrum of activity: Cefoxitin is more active than cefazolin against gram-negative bacilli such as Escherichia coli and Proteus mirabilis by 1–2 or more dilution stages. Moreover, cefoxitin inhibits the majority of cefazolin-resistant organisms (Proteus vulgaris, Proteus rettgeri, Proteus morganii, Klebsiella pneumoniae, Serratia marcescens, Providencia and others). Cefoxitin is generally more active against Bacteroides species and is also stable to the β-lactamase of Bacteroides fragilis. Activity against staphylococci and streptococci of Lancefield groups A and B is less than with cefazolin, and the activity against Haemophilus is less than that of cefamandole, cefuroxime, cefotiam and the cephalosporins of the cefotaxime group. The following bacteria are resistant: Pseudomonas aeruginosa, enterococci, some Enterobacteriaceae, all mycoplasmas, chlamydiae and mycobacteria.

Resistance: Primary resistance is rare amongst the Enterobacteriaceae with the exceptions of Citrobacter freundii and Enterobacter cloacae. Resistance does not arise during therapy. Some cross-resistance is found with the cephalosporins of the cephalothin group and incomplete cross-resistance with cefamandole, cefuroxime, cefotiam and members of the cefotaxime group, so bacterial sensitivity to these agents should always be specifically tested.

Pharmacokinetics: *Not absorbed* by mouth.

Serum concentrations after *injection* of 1 g i. v.: 13.2 mg/l (1 h) and 0.9 mg/l (4 h). During continuous i. v. *infusion* of 0.166 g/h (= 4 g/24 h), the mean serum concentrations are 7.5 mg/l (3 times higher than with cephalothin).

Concentrations in blister fluid are also 3 times higher (80% of serum level). Penetrates *tissues* well but CSF poorly.

Half-life: 45 min. *Plasma protein binding:* 50%.

Excretion is predominantly renal, with 90% appearing in active form in the urine within 6 h. A small amount is secreted in the bile and some is also metabolised and excreted in the urine as decarbamyl cefoxitin. Probenecid delays renal excretion and doubles the serum concentrations and half-life.

Side effects: Similar to the older cephalosporins. Usually no cross-allergy with penicillins and administration in penicillin allergy is justifiable if the patient is under careful observation. Cefoxitin should only be given in life-threatening situations and under frequent haematological control when there have been any previous signs of hypersensitivity to other cephalosporins. Cefoxitin may induce β-lactamase of Pseudomonas aeruginosa in vitro but there is no evidence that this is of clinical relevance.

Indications:
1. *Initial therapy* of severe bacterial infections which may be caused by gram-positive cocci, resistant gram-negative rods and Bacteroides fragilis. Indications of this nature are sepsis of uncertain cause, secondary pneumonia (p. 352), postoperative urinary infections and severe wound and tissue infections. Because of its effectiveness against anaerobes, cefoxitin may be used in the treatment of mixed infections with anaerobes such as gangrene, tonsillar abscess, lung abscess and peritonitis.
2. Therapy of infections with *known sensitive organisms,* particularly where otherwise resistant pathogens are sensitive to cefoxitin (e. g. Klebsiella, Serratia, Proteus rettgeri).
3. *Combined therapy* of bacterial infections. Combination with azlocillin covers the gaps in the spectrum of cefoxitin due to Pseudomonas and enterococci. Combination with an aminoglycoside (gentamicin, amikacin or netilmicin) may enhance the antibacterial effect in severe infections which may involve resistant Enterobacteriaceae (pneumonia, septicaemia, endocarditis).

Contra-indications: Allergy to cephalosporins.

Administration: Preferably by i. v. injection or short i. v. infusion (30 min). Continuous i. v. infusion and i. m. injection are also possible but, because i. m. injection is painful, dissolve in 0.5% lignocaine. Do not mix with other drugs, particularly aminoglycosides (risk of precipitation).

Dosage: For *severe (life-threatening) systemic infections:* 2 g 3–4 times a day (50 mg/kg 3–4 times a day for children).

For *local infections* in the absence of severe systemic infection: 1 g 3 times a day (25 mg/kg 3 times a day for children).

Prolong the dose-interval for patients with *chronic renal failure* to 8 h when the creatinine clearance is 30–50 ml/min, to 12 h when 10–29 ml/min, to 24 h when 5–9 ml/min and to 48 h when less than 5 ml/min. The normal single dose is then given at extended intervals, according to the severity of the infection. Only when the creatinine clearance is less than 10 ml/min should the single dose of 750 mg not be exceeded.

Cefoxitin is dialysable. Give 2 g at the end of each haemodialysis.

Preparations: Injection bottles of 1 g and 2 g; infusion bottles of 2 g.

Summary: A β-lactamase-stable, broad-spectrum antibiotic with good activity against anaerobes. The Pseudomonas and enterococcal gap can be covered in initial therapy by combination with other antibiotics.

References

BUSH, R. P., T. E. MAXIM, N. ALLEN, T. A. JACOB, F. J. WOLF: Analysis of cefoxitin, cephalothin and their deacylated metabolites in human urine by high-performance liquid chromatography. J. Chromatography *99:* 609 (1974).

DARLAND, G., J. BIRNBAUM: Cefoxitin resistance to beta-lactamase: a major factor for susceptibility of Bacteroides fragilis to the antibiotic. Antimicrob. Ag. Chemother. *11:* 725 (1977).

DASCHNER, F. D., E. E. PETERSEN et al.: Antibiotic prophylaxis in gynecology: Cefoxitin concentrations in serum, myometrium, endometrium and salpinges. Infection *10:* 341 (1982).

GEDDES, A. M., L. P. SCHNURR, A. P. BALL, D. McGHIE, G. R. BROOKES, R. WISE, J. ANDREWS: Cefoxitin: a hospital study. Brit. med. J. *1:* 1126 (1977).

RICHMOND, M. H., S. WOTTON: Comparative study of seven cephalosporins: Susceptibility to beta-lactamases and ability to penetrate the surface layers of Escherichia coli. Antimicrob. Ag. Chemother. *10:* 219 (1976).

SHAH, P. M., E. B. HELM, W. STILLE: Behandlung von Cephalothin- und Cefazolin-resistenten Infektionen mit Cefoxitin. Münch. med. Wschr. *120:* 375 (1978).

SIMON, C., E. MEYER, V. MALERCZYK: Cefoxitin, ein neues β-Lactamase-stabiles Antibiotikum. Arzneimittel-Forsch. *28:* 1541 (1978).

WERNER, H., R. FIRSCHING, C. KRASEMANN: In-vitro-Empfindlichkeit von Bacteroidaceae gegen Cefoxitin und Cephalothin. Infection *5:* 13 (1977).

β) Cefotetan

Spectrum of activity: Currently the most active 7-methoxy cephalosporin against gram-negative rods (considerably more effective than cefoxitin and cefmetazole); however, it is less effective against staphylococci and streptococci, for which 2–4 times higher concentrations are required. Activity against Bacteroides fragilis and other anaerobes is about the same as cefoxitin. A percentage of strains are resistant: with Staphylococcus aureus, 25%; with Enterobacter cloacae, Serratia marcescens and Citrobacter freundii, 35% each; with Bacteroides fragilis, 20%. Pseudomonas aeruginosa and the enterococci (Streptococcus faecalis) are always resistant; Clostridium difficile and Bacteroides thetaiotaomicron are slightly sensitive. Very stable against bacterial β-lactamase *in vitro* and *in vivo*. Given as the disodium salt.

Pharmacokinetics: *Half-life* 3 hours after i. v. administration. *Plasma protein binding:* 90%. 70% *excreted* unchanged in the urine, 15% in a tautomeric form with similar antibacterial activity. Partially excreted through the bile. Present information suggests that the clinical examination of cefotetan is worthwhile because of the improved activity and longer half-life. Because of the tetrazole sidechain alcohol intolerance must be expected (see p. 22).

References

ADAM, H. K., H. L. HOUGHTON, R. A. YATES, J. YOUNG, R. J. DONNELLY: Pharmacokinetics and tolerance of a 24-h infusion of cefotetan disodium (with and without loading dose) in normal Caucasian volunteers. J. Antimicrob. Chemother. *11:* 193 (1983).

COX, C. E., S. J. CHILDS, W. G. WELLS, S. MIRELMANT, W. C. LESKY: Preliminary report on a comparative trial of cefotetan and cefoxitin in the treatment of urinary tract infections. J. Antimicrob. Chemother. *11:* 227 (1983).

GUIBERT, J., M. D. KITZIS, C. YVELIN, J. F. ACAR: Pharmacokinetics of single intravenous and intramuscular doses of cefotetan in normal human volunteers. J. Antimicrob. Chemother. *11:* 201 (1983).

HART, C. A., A. PERCIVAL: Susceptibilities of gentamicin-resistant Gram-negative aerobic bacilli to cefotetan and other β-lactams. J. Antimicrob. Chemother. *11:* 95 (1983).

HAUTMANN, R., F. PRANADA, Zs. PUSZTAI-MARKOS: Cefotetan in complicated urinary tract infections – clinical experience. J. Antimicrob. Chemother. *11:* 223 (1983).

LEIGH, D. A., J. MARRINER: In-vitro activity of cefotetan and other cephalosporins against multiresistant strains of Enterobacteriaceae. J. Antimicrob. Chemother. *11:* 103 (1983).

MOOSDEEN, F., J. MASKELL, J. PHILPOTT-HOWARD, J. D. WILLIAMS: Cefotetan activity against gram-negative aerobes and anaerobes. J. Antimicrob. Chemother. *11:* 59 (1983).

NOLEN, T. M., H. L. PHILLIPS, H. J. HALL: Clinical evaluation of cefotetan in the treatment of lower respiratory tract infections. J. Antimicrob. Chemother. *11:* 233 (1983).

RUCKDESCHEL, G.: Activity of cefotetan against non sporing anaerobes: a comparative study. J. Antimicrob. Chemother. *II Suppl. A:* 117 (1983).

WERNER, H.: Inhibitory activity of cefotetan and other β-lactams against anaerobes. J. Antimicrob. Chemother. *11:* 107 (1983).

WRIGHT, N., R. WISE, T. HEGARTY: Cefotetan elimination in patients with varying degrees of renal dysfunction. J. Antimicrob. Chemother. *11:* 213 (1983).

YATES, R. A., H. K. ADAM, R. J. DONNELLY, H. L. HOUGHTON, E. A. CHARLESWORTH, E. A. LAWS: Pharmacokinetics and tolerance of single intravenous doses of cefotetan disodium in male Caucasian volunteers. J. Antimicrob. Chemother. *11:* 185 (1983).

γ) Cefmetazole

Spectrum of activity: A newly developed 7-methoxy cephalosporin with better activity than cefoxitin. Activity against staphylococci is greater than that of other cephalosporins of the cefoxitin and cefotaxime groups. More active than cefoxitin against Enterobacteriaceae by 1–2 dilution steps. Similar in activity against Bacteroides fragilis. Pseudomonas and enterococci are resistant. Cefmetazole is very stable to bacterial β-lactamases.

Pharmacokinetics: *Half-life:* 45–60 min after i. v. administration. *Plasma protein binding:* 85%. Almost completely excreted in the active form in the urine. Relatively high biliary concentrations.

Evaluation: Cefmetazole is a further development of cefoxitin and is of interest because of its good anti-staphylococcal activity. It has been widely used in Japan since 1980.

δ) Latamoxef

Proprietary names: Moxalactam, Moxam.

Synonym: Lamoxactam.

Chemically, latamoxef belongs to the oxa-β-lactam group (a sulphur atom has been substituted by a hydrogen atom in the 7-aminocephalosporanic acid). Certain characteristics of latamoxef can be explained by different functional groups (Fig. 4, p. 22).

Spectrum of activity is similar to cefotaxime. Latamoxef is more active than cefotaxime against Bacteroides fragilis, Enterobacter cloacae and Citrobacter freundii, but less active against Staphylococcus aureus, Staphylococcus epidermidis and Streptococcus viridans (Table 12, p. 89). Some strains of Pseudomonas aeruginosa are resistant to latamoxef but nearly all strains are sensitive to ceftazidime.

Pharmacokinetics: *Serum concentrations* (after 1 g i. v.): Table 14, p. 90. *Half-life:* 130 min. *Plasma protein binding:* 40%. *Urinary recovery:* 75%. The amount of latamoxef excreted in the bile is not known exactly but high concentrations of microbiologically active drug appear in the faeces and cause major changes in the stool concentration of certain bacteria (Escherichia coli, other enterobacteria and anaerobes).

Side effects: As with other cephalosporins but bleeding diatheses (caused by hypoprothrombinaemia and/or disorders of platelet function) are not uncommon. Prophylactic administration of vitamin K (10 mg per week) is recommended. The prothrombin time should be measured every second day during therapy. The risk of bleeding disorders is increased in patients with renal insufficiency, disturbed liver function, gastrointestinal disorders or during total parenteral nutrition. In such cases, other tests should also be performed (bleeding time, platelet count and platelet aggregation). When bleeding occurs, treatment with latamoxef should be discontinued and fresh frozen plasma, prothrombin complex or platelet concentrate may be given. Latamoxef may cause alcohol intolerance (see also p. 92).

Indications: Use should be restricted to severe infections due to agents resistant to other, better tolerated antibiotics. Suitable for intra-abdominal and gynaecological bacterial infections of unknown origin, lung abscesses and aspiration pneumonia, which are often mixed infections with gram-positive or gram-negative bacteria, including fusobacteria and bacteroides. Latamoxef has been used in clinical trials for the treatment of meningitis caused by gram-negative bacilli (enterobacteria).

Daily dose: 2–4 g for adults, 50–100 mg/kg for children.

Preparations: Ampoules of 1 g and 2 g.

Summary: Because of its good activity against anaerobes and most enterobacteria latamoxef is a useful antibiotic in a few clinical situations but bleeding disorders (a relatively frequent side effect) are the reason for prophylactic administration of vitamin K and careful monitoring of bleeding time, prothrombin time and other tests.

References

DELGADO, D. G., C. J. BRAU, C. G. COBBS, W. E. DISMUKES: In vitro activity of LY 127935, a new 1-oxa cephalosporin, against aerobic gram-negative bacilli. Antimicrob. Ag. Chemother. *16:* 864 (1979).
DEMARIA, A. JR., S. ALVAREZ, J. O. KLEIN, W. R. McCABE: In vitro studies of moxalactam (LY 127935), a new beta-lactam antibiotic with significant activity against gram-negative bacteria. Infection *8:* 261 (1980).

FLOURNOY, D. J., F. A. PERRYMAN: LY 127935, a new beta-lactam antibiotic versus proteus, Klebsiella, Serratia, and Pseudomonas. Antimicrob. Ag. Chemother. *16:* 641 (1979).

GIBBS, R. S., et al.: Therapy of obstetrical infections with moxalactam. Antimicrob. Ag. Chemother. *17 (6):* 1004 (1980).

HALL, W. H., B. J. OPFER, D. N. GERDING: Comparative activities of the oxa-β-lactam LY 127935, cefotaxime, cefoperazone, cefamandole, and ticarcillin against multiply resistant gram-negative bacilli. Antimicrob. Ag. Chemother. *17:* 273 (1980).

JORGENSEN, J. H., S. A. CRAWFORD, G. A. ALEXANDER: In vitro activities of cefotaxime and moxalactam (LY 127935) against Haemophilus influenzae. Antimicrob. Ag. Chemother. *17:* 516 (1980).

KAPLAN, S. L., E. O. MASON jr., H. GARCIA, S. J. KVERNLAND, E. M. LOISELLE, D. C. ANDERSON, A. A. MINTZ, R. D. FEIGIN: Pharmacokinetics and cerebrospinal fluid penetration of moxalactam® in children with bacterial meningitis, J. Pediat. *98:* 152 (1981).

LANDESMAN, S. H., M. L. CORRADO, C. C. CHERUBIN, M. GOMBERT, D. CLERI: Diffusion of a new beta-lactam (LY 127935) into cerebrospinal fluid. Amer. J. Med. *69:* 92 (1980).

NEU, H. C., N. ASWAPOKEE, K. P. FU, P. ASWAPOKEE: Antibacterial activity of a new 1-oxa-cephalosporin compared with that of other β-lactam compounds. Antimicrob. Ag. Chemother. *16:* 141 (1979).

OARSONS, J. N., J. M. ROMANO, M. E. LEVISON: Pharmacology of a new 1-oxa-β-lactam (LY 127935) in normal volunteers. Antimicrob. Ag. Chemother. *17:* 226 (1980).

PARSONS, J. N., J. M. ROMANO, M. E. LEVISON: Pharmacology of a new 1-oxa-β-lactam (LY 127935) in normal volunteers. Antimicrob. Ag. Chemother. *17:* 226 (1980).

SCHAAD, U. B., G. H. MCCRACKEN jr., N. THRELKELD, M. L. THOMAS: Clinical evaluation of a new broad-spectrum oxa-beta-lactam antibiotic, moxalactam®, in neonates and infants. J. Pediatr. *98:* 129 (1981).

SCHAAD, U. B., G. H. MCCRACKEN, CH. A. LOOCK, M. L. THOMAS: Pharmacokinetics and bacteriological efficacy of moxalactam (LY 127935), netilmicin, and ampicillin in experimental gram-negative enteric bacillary meningitis. Antibicrob. Ag. Chemother. *17:* 406 (1980).

SRINIVASAN, S., K. P. EU, H. C. NEU: The pharmacokinetics of moxalactam® in normals compared with the pharmacokinetics of cefazolin. Antimicrob. Ag. Chemother. *19:* 302 (1981).

WERNER, H., C. KRASEMANN: In-vitro-Aktivität des Oxa-Beta-Laktams LY 127935 gegenüber Bacteroides fragilis und anderen anaeroben gramnegativen Stäbchen. Infection *8, Suppl. 3:* 342 (1980).

WISE, R., S. BAKER, N. WRIGHT, R. LIVINGSTON: The pharmacokinetics of LY 127935, a broad spectrum oxa-β-lactam. J. Antimicrob. Chemother. *6:* 319 (1980).

d) Cefotaxime Group

Proprietary names:

for *cefotaxime:*   Claforan;
for *ceftriaxone:*   Rocephin;
for *ceftizoxime:*   Cefizox, Ceftiz;
for *cefmenoxime:*   Bestcall, Tacef;
for *ceftazidime:*   Fortum (see below).

Table 11. Structural formula of the cephalosporins of the cefotaxime group.

R_1—CO—NH—[7]—S—[3]—R_2, O=—N, COOH

Generic Name	R_1	R_2
Cefotaxime		$-CH_2-OCOCH_3$
Ceftizoxime		$-H$
Cefmenoxime		
Ceftriaxone		
Ceftazidime		
Cefoperazone		
Latamoxef		

Properties: Cefotaxime derivatives have an extended spectrum, very high activity against enterobacteria and some activity against Pseudomonas aeruginosa. This improvement has been achieved by coupling the aminothiazol side-chain of cefotiam with the oxime side-chain of cefuroxime. The aminothiazol-oxime derivative *cefotaxime* is the parent substance of the group.

Ceftriaxone, ceftizoxime and *cefmenoxime* are chemical analogues of cefotaxime with substitution only at position R_2 (Table 11) which gives different pharmacokinetics but the same activity. Ceftizoxime is the non-substituted derivative of cefotaxime. Cefmenoxime has the same methyltetrazole side-chain as cefamandole, cefoperozone etc. *Ceftazidime* is substituted at the oxime side-chain as well and therefore has a separate position within the group, and is described separately below.

Mode of action: There are differences in β-lactamase stability, in their ability to penetrate the bacterial cell wall and their affinity for the so-called penicillin binding proteins (PBP).

Spectrum of activity: Very similar within the cefotaxime group and considerably extended and more active than the older cephalosporins. Unlike the older cephalosporins, the agents in the cefotaxime group are effective at very low concentrations against Haemophilus influenzae (ampicillin-sensitive and -resistant strains).

Table 12. Differences of *in vitro* activity in newer cephalosporins. E. = Enterobacter, Staph. = Staphylococcus, Strept. = Streptococcus.

Agent	*In vitro* activity	
	relatively good	relatively poor
Cefotaxime Ceftriaxone Ceftizoxime Cefmenoxime	Klebsiella Proteus vulgaris	Pseudomonas Acinetobacter
Cefoperazone	Pseudomonas	Acinetobacter E. cloacae
Latamoxef	Bacteroides fragilis E. cloacae Citrobacter	Pseudomonas Staph. aureus Strept. viridans
Ceftazidime	Pseudomonas Acinetobacter E. cloacae Proteus vulgaris	Staph. aureus

Table 13. Activity against Staphylococcus aureus of newer cephalosporins in comparison with cephalothin. GM = geometrical mean of minimal inhibitory concentrations (mg/l), $MIC_{50\%}$ and $MIC_{90\%}$ = minimal inhibitory concentrations at 50% or 90% of the strains examined.

Antibiotic	GM	$MIC_{50\%}$	$MIC_{90\%}$
Cefotaxime	2.0	1.6	3.1
Ceftriaxone	4.1	3.1	6.2
Ceftizoxime	4.0	1.6	3.1
Cefmenoxime	2.0	1.6	3.1
Latamoxef	10.0	8.0	16.0
Cefoperazone	3.8	3.1	6.2
Ceftazidime	6.8	4.0	8.0
Cephalothin	0.2	0.1	0.4

Activity differs against different species of bacteria (Table 12). Among the newer cephalosporins cefotaxime and analogous antibiotics are most active against Klebsiella pneumoniae and Proteus vulgaris. Ceftazidime is also relatively more active against Enterobacter cloacae. All cefotaxime derivatives are less active than cephalothin against staphylococci (Table 13). Ceftizoxime is only slightly active against Pseudomonas. Ceftazidime (p. 96) is the most active against Pseudomonas aeruginosa and Acinetobacter. The differences of clinical relevance are also listed in Tables 33 and 34 (p. 280 and 281), which include the minimal inhibitory concentrations for 50% and 90% of the strains examined. As the percentage of resistant strains for each drug is continually changing, a combination should be used to cover gaps in the spectrum.

The following bacteria are resistant: enterococci, Clostridium difficile, Legionella pneumophila, Mycoplasma and Chlamydia species.

Combinations with an aminoglycoside (gentamicin, tobramycin) are often synergistic against sensitive bacteria. There may also be synergy or at least an additive effect in combination with an acylamino penicillin.

Table 14. Mean serum concentrations of newer cephalosporins after i. v. injection of 1 g.

Antibiotic	Serum concentration (mg/l) after			
	1 h	4 h	6 h	12 h
Cefotaxime	12	1.1	0.3	0
Ceftriaxone	120	65	50	30
Ceftizoxime	30	5	2	0
Cefmenoxime	25	4	1	0
Latamoxef	65	16	9	0.9
Cefoperazone	58	14	7	1.0
Ceftazidime	40	10	5	0.6

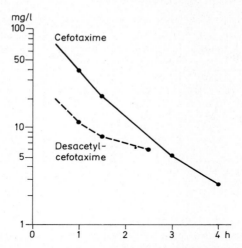

Fig. 15. Mean serum level of cefotaxime and desacetyl-cefotaxime after i. v. injection of 2 g in 10 healthy adult volunteers.

Resistance: Secondary resistance is rare. Partial cross-resistance in gram-negative strains with cephalosporins of the cephalothin group. Complete cross-resistance with methicillin-resistant strains of Staphylococcus aureus. Ampicillin-resistant strains of Haemophilus and penicillin-resistant gonococci are sensitive to all the cephalosporins of the cefotaxime group.

Pharmacokinetics: *Not absorbed* by mouth. After i. v. injection of 1 g (Table 14 and Fig. 15), the *serum levels* after 1 h are highest with ceftriaxone and lower with ceftizoxime, cefmenoxime and cefotaxime. The *concentrations* are still relatively high after 6 h with ceftriaxone, while they have declined to 2 mg/l, 1 mg/l and 0.3 mg/l with ceftizoxime, cefmenoxime and cefotaxime, respectively. There are corresponding differences in concentration between the individual antibiotics in short i. v. infusion, continuous i. v. infusion and i. m. injection. The *half-life* is longest with ceftriaxone (7–8 h), shorter with ceftizoxime and cefmenoxime (70 min), shortest with cefotaxime (60 min), and 2 h with the other derivatives (Table 15). *Plasma protein binding* is 97% with ceftriaxone (in concentrations up to 150 mg/l), 60% with cefmenoxine and less than 50% with the other newer cephalosporins. All members diffuse quite well into tissues, but poorly into the CSF when the meninges are not inflamed. Therapeutically effective CSF concentrations for purulent meningitis can be achieved particularly with cefotaxime.

Table 15. Pharmacokinetic data for newer cephalosporins.

Antibiotic	Half-life (min)	Plasma protein binding (%)	Urinary recovery	Tubular secretion	Biliary excretion
Cefotaxime	60	40	50	+	(+)
Ceftriaxone	385 – 480	97	40 – 60	Ø	+
Ceftizoxime	70	30	80	Ø	(+)
Cefmenoxime	70	60	80	Ø	(+)
Latamoxef	130	40	75	Ø	(+)
Cefoperazone	110	90	25	(?)	++
Ceftazidime	110	10	70	Ø	(+)

Urinary output of active agent in the first 24 h: 50% with cefotaxime, 40–60% with ceftriaxone and 70–80% with ceftizoxime and cefmenoxime. The biliary concentrations are generally higher than the serum levels. Ceftriaxone is excreted to a much greater extent in the bile than the other members of the group. Approximately ⅓ of the dose of cefotaxime is metabolised in the body, which explains the relatively low serum concentrations (Table 14). The metabolites detected have been desacetyl cefotaxime, which has reduced antibacterial activity, and 2 inactive lactones. Small quantities of metabolites have also been detected with ceftriaxone and ceftizoxime (in animals). The renal excretion of cefotaxime is also by tubular secretion, so probenecid increases the serum concentrations. Excretion is predominantly by glomerular filtration with the other antibiotics. In *renal failure,* the half-life of ceftriaxone and cefotaxime is less prolonged than with the other antibiotics of this group.

Side effects: Similar to the other parenteral cephalosporins. Good renal tolerance. Allergic side effects seem to occur more frequently with ceftriaxone. The alcohol intolerance with cefmenoxime is related to the blockage of acetaldehyde dehydrogenase (caused by the tetrazole side-chain). The acetaldehyde concentration increases after consumption of alcoholic beverages and the following symptoms can occur: erythema, sweating, hypotension, tachycardia, vomiting, headache and dizziness. There may be a delayed reaction up to 72 h after administration of the antibiotic. In order to avoid this antabuse-(disulfiram-)like effect, no alcohol should be consumed within 2–4 days of stopping therapy. Caution with infusions which contain alcohol. There is no particular risk of bleeding disorders with cefotaxime but bleeding during therapy has been observed with ceftriaxone.

Indications:
1. *Initial therapy* of severe, life-threatening infections (sepsis, pneumonia, osteomyelitis, wound and tissue infections), particularly if – because of severe underlying disease – the body's defences are impaired and multi-resistant gram-negative bacilli may be present. Also recommended for the initial therapy of urinary infections in urological surgery, where multi-resistant bacteria occur more often. If Bacteroides fragilis is suspected, combine with metronidazole. Always combine these agents in severe systemic infections, either with an aminoglycoside or with an acylamino penicillin.
2. Treatment of severe generalised or local infections (pneumonia, pyelonephritis, cholangitis) *due to cefazolin-resistant bacteria,* which are also insensitive to the acylamino penicillins.
3. Severe infections in patients with *penicillin allergy* (cross-sensitivity should be excluded prior to therapy).

Inappropriate uses: Less severe bacterial infections and those which would be expected to respond to benzyl penicillin, amoxycillin, cefazolin or cefazedone. Safety of newer derivatives in pregnancy is not yet established.

Contra-indication: Allergy to cephalosporins. Reduce dose in renal and hepatic failure.

Administration and dosage: Preferably 2–3 times a day as a short i.v. infusion (20–30 min) or slow i.v. injection (5 min). Continuous i.v. infusion also possible. I.m. injection may be painful; if necessary, dissolve in 0.5% lignocaine solution and do not exceed a dose of 1 g. Daily dose according to severity of infection: 2–4 g (50–100 mg/kg for children). Highest dose (e.g. for meningitis): 6 g a day for adults, 200 mg/kg for children.

Preparations: Ampoules of 500 mg, 1 g and 2 g.

Summary: The cephalosporins of the cefotaxime group have been a major advance in therapy because of their considerably improved activity and extension of their spectrum.

Anti-pseudomonal activity is incomplete with most members of this group and the activity against staphylococci is generally less than with cephalothin. Because clinical experience has been the longest with cefotaxime, this drug seems to be the most appropriate representative of the group for use at present.

References

ADAM, D., R. TIMMLER: Pharmakokinetik von Ceftizoxim mit und ohne Probenecid. Arzneim.-Forsch./Drug. Res. *32 (I):* 416 (1982).

ANGEHRN, P., P. J. PROBST, R. REINER, R. W. THEN: Ro 13-9904, a long-acting broad-spectrum cephalosporin: in vitro and in vivo studies. Antimicrob. Ag. Chemother. *18:* 913 (1980).

BAUMGARTNER, J. D., M. P. GLAUSER: Pharmacokinetic and microbial susceptibility studies of ceftriaxone. Eur. J. clin. Microbiol. *2:* 501 (1983).

BECHARD, D. L.: The efficacy of ceftizoxime in the therapy of bacteraemia. J. Antimicrob. Chemother. *10, Suppl. C:* 175 (1982).

BELOHRADSKY, B. H., K. BRUCH, D. GEISS, D. KAFETZIS, W. MARGET, G. PETERS: Intravenous cefotaxime in children with bacterial meningitis. Lancet *I:* 61 (1980).

BERGAN, T., T. KALAGERT, K. BLOCK HELLUM, C. O. SOLBERG: Penetration of cefotaxime and desacetylcefotaxime into skin blister fluid. J. Antimicrob. Chemother. *10:* 193 (1982).

BESKID, G., J. G. CHRISTENSON, R. CLEELAND, W. DELORENZO et al.: In vivo activity of Ceftriaxone (Ro 13-9904), a new broad spectrum semicynthetic cephalosporin. Antimicrob. Ag. Chemother. *20:* 159 (1981).

DASCHNER, F., H. M. JUST, CH. BECKER: In-vitro-Kombinationswirkung von Cefmenoxim mit Aminoglykosiden bei gramnegativen Erregern krankenhauserworbener Infektionen. Fortschr. antimikrob. antineoplast. Chemother. *2-2:* 233 (1983).

FUCHS, P. C., R. N. JONES, C. THORNSBERRY, A. L. BARRY et al.: Cefmenoxime (SCE 1365), a new cephalosporin: In vitro activity, comparison with other antimicrobial agents, beta-lactamase stability, and disk diffusion testing with tentative interpretive criteria. Antimicrob. Ag. Chemother. *20:* 747 (1981).

GERDING, D. N., L. R. PETERSON: Comparative tissue and extravascular fluid concentrations of ceftizoxime. J. Antimicrob. Chemother. *10 Suppl. C:* 105 (1982).

GRANNEMAN, G. R., L. SENELLO, F. J. STEINBERG, R. C. SONDERS: Intramuscular and intravenous pharmacokinetics of Cefmenoxim, a new broad-spectrum cephalosporin, in healthy subjects. Antimicrob. Ag. Chemother. *21:* 141 (1982).

HEIMANN, G., M. EICKSCHEN, K. SEEGER: Pharmakokinetik von Cefotaxim im Kindesalter. Infection *8:* 454 (1980).

HELM, E. B., D. WURBS, R. HAAG, D. BENTELE, P. M. SHAH: Elimination of bacteria in biliary tract infections during ceftizoxime therapy. Infection *10:* 67 (1982).

HINKLE, A. M., G. P. BODEY: In vitro evaluation of Ro 13-9904. Antimicrob. Ag. Chemother. *18:* 574 (1980).

HITZENBERGER, G.: Pharmakokinetik von Ceftizoxim. Wien. med. Wschr. *131:* 391 (1981).

HÖFFKEN, G., H. LODE, P. KOEPPE, M. RUHNKE, K. BORNER: Pharmacokinetics of Cefotaxime and Desacetyl-Cefotaxime in Cirrhosis of the Liver. Chemotherapy *30:* 7 (1984).

KAFETZIS, D. A., D. CRAIG BRATER, J. E. FANOURAGAKIS: Ceftriaxone distribution between maternal blood and fetal blood and tissues at parturition and between blood and milk post partum. Antimicrob. Ag. Chemother. *23:* 870 (1983).

KAMINMURA, T.: Laboratory evaluation of ceftizoxime, a new parenteral cephalosporin. Arzneimittel-Forsch. *30*/II: 1662 (1980).

KOJO, H.: Antibacterial activity of ceftizoxime (FK 749), a new cephalosporin, against cephalosporin-resistant bacteria, and its stability to β-lactamase. Antimicrob. Ag. Chemother. *16:* 549 (1979).

v. LOEWENICH, V., R. MIETHING, M. UIHLEIN, H. KNOTHE, M. GREIPEL-ZAMORSKI: Cefotaxim- und Desazetyl-Cefotaxim-Spiegel im Liquor cerebrospinalis von Neu- und Frühgeborenen. Pädiat. Pädol. *18:* 361 (1983).

DE LOUVOIS, J., A. MULHALL, R. HURLEY: The safety and pharmacokinetics of cefotaxime in the treatment of neonates. Pediat. Pharmacol. *2:* 275 (1982).

LÜTHY, R., R. MÜNCH, J. BLASER, W. BHEND, W. SIEGENTHALER: Human pharmacology of cefotaxime (HR 756), a new cephalosporin. Antimicrob. Ag. Chemother. *16:* 127–133 (1979).

MÜHLBERG, W., D. PLATT: Elimination von Desacetylcefotaxim bei geriatrischen Patienten mit Multimorbidität. Klin. Wschr. *60:* 1497 (1982).

MULLANEY, D. T., J. F. JOHN: Cefotaxime therapy: evaluation of its effect on bacterial meningitis, CSF drug levels, and bactericidal activity. Arch. intern. Med. *143:* 1705 (1983).

NABER, K., D. ADAM, F. KEES, W. LINTZ, H. GROBECKER: Cefmenoxim: Pharmakokinetik bei jüngeren Probanden gegenüber älteren Patienten und Gewebekonzentrationen im Urogenitaltrakt. Fortschr. antimikrob. antineoplast. Chemother. *2-2:* 297 (1983).

NEU, H. C., P. ASWAPOKEE, K. P. FU, I. HO, C. MATTHIJSSEN: Cefotaxime kinetics after intravenous and intramuscular injection of single and multiple doses. Clin. Pharmacol. Ther. *27:* 677 (1980).

NISHIDA, M., T. KAMIMURA, N. OKADA, Y. MATSUMOTO, Y. MINE, T. MURAKAWA: Comparison of antibacterial activity of a new cephalosporin, ceftizoxime (FK 749) with other cephalosporin antibiotics. J. Antibiotics *32:* 1319 (1979).

NODA, K.: Metabolic fate of (^{14}C)-ceftizoxime, a parenteral cephalosporin antibiotic, in rats and dogs. Arzneimittel-Forsch. *30/II:* 1665 (1980).

OKONOGI, K.: β-Lactamase stability and antibacterial activity of Cefmenoxime (SCE-1365), a novel cephalosporin. Antimicrob. Ag. Chemother. *20:* 171 (1981).

QUENTIN, C. D., R. ANSORG: Penetration of cefotaxime into the aqueous humor of the human eye after intravenous application. Graefe's Arch. klin exp. Ophthalmol. *220:* 245 (1983).

ROOS, R., W. MARGET, H. TRUJILLO, D. A. KAFETZIS, C. J. PAPADATOS, H. M. VON HATTINGBERG, B. H. BELOHRADSKY, K. BRUCH: Multizentrische Studie über Cefotaxim bei Meningitis und Sepsis im Kindesalter. Klinische Ergebnisse, Serum-Pharmakokinetik und Liquorspiegel. Infection *8:* 501 (1980).

SCHAAD, U. B., K. STOECKEL: Single-dose pharmacokinetics of ceftriaxone in infants and young children. *21:* 248 (1982).

SEDDON, M., R. WISE, A. P. GILLET, R. LIVINGSTON: Pharmacokinetics of Ro 13-9904, a broad-spectrum cephalosporin. Antimicrob. Ag. Chemother. *18:* 240–242 (1980).

SHANNON, K., A. KING, C. WARREN, I. PHILLIPS: In vitro antibacterial activity and susceptibility of the cephalosporin Ro 13-9904 to beta-lactamases. Antimicrob. Ag. Chemother. *18:* 292 (1980).

WISE, R., N. WRIGHT, P. J. WILLS: Cefotaxime: pharmacology of cefotaxime and its desacetyl metabolite in renal and hepatic disease. Antimicrob. Ag. Chemother. *19:* 526 (1981).

WISE, R., J. M. ANDREWS: A comparison of the pharmacokinetics and tissue penetration of ceftriaxone, moxalactam and cefotaxime. Eur. J. clin. Microbiol. *2:* 505 (1983).

WISE, R., S. BAKER, R. LIVINGSTON: Comparison of cefotaxime and moxalactam pharmacokinetics and tissue levels. Antimicrob. Ag. Chemother. *18:* 369 (1980).

e) Ceftazidime

Proprietary name: Fortum.

Properties and in vitro activity: The pentahydrate (with sodium carbonate) is highly soluble in water (releasing carbon dioxide). 1 g of ceftazidime contains 2.3 milliequivalents of sodium. Ceftazidime has almost the same antibacterial spectrum as cefotaxime but it is 10 times as active as cefotaxime and 2–3 times as cefsulodin against Pseudomonas aeruginosa (Table 35, p. 285). Resistant strains of Pseudomonas aeruginosa are rare. Ceftazidime is better than most other cephalosporins against Proteus vulgaris, Serratia marcescens, Acinetobacter species and Enterobacter cloacae (Table 12, p. 89). On the other hand, the in vitro activity of ceftazidime against staphylococci is only one third that of cefotaxime (Table 13, p. 90) and one fifteenth that of latamoxef against Bacteroides fragilis. With other anaerobes there is less differences in activity. Ceftazidime is, like other cephalosporins, not active against methicillin- and cephalothin-resistant staphylococci, Streptococcus faecalis, Listeria monocytogenes, Campylobacter species or Clostridium difficile.

Pharmacokinetics (Tables 14, 15): Mean *serum concentrations* after i. v. injection of 1 g are 40 mg/l (1 h), 10 mg/l (4 h) and 0.6 mg/l (12 h). Serum *half-life* 2 hours. Serum *protein binding* 10%. Relatively good *tissue penetration*. The *CSF levels* are low in the absence of inflammation.

Urinary excretion unchanged in the active form by glomerular filtration (80–90% in the first 24 h). *Biliary excretion* <1%. Metabolites have not been found in urine and bile.

Side effects similar to cefotaxime. No intolerance of alcohol. Bleeding disorders have not been observed in clinical trials, due to the absence of a carboxyl and a tetrazole groups.

Indications: As for cefotaxime (p. 93). Ceftazidime may be used for infections caused by organisms resistant to other antibiotics including aminoglycosides and other cephalosporins. When appropriate it may be used safely in combination with an aminoglycoside or another β-lactam antibiotic, for example in the presence of severe neutropenia, or with an antibiotic active against anaerobes when the presence of Bacteroides fragilis is suspected.

Contra-indications: Hypersensitivity to cephalosporins. Ceftazidime should be given with caution to patients with immediate hypersensitivity reactions to penicillins.

Table 16. Recommended maintenance doses of ceftazidime in renal insufficiency.

Creatinine clearance ml/min	Approx. serum creatinine μmol/l (mg/dl)	Recommended unit dose of ceftazidime (g)	Frequency of dosing (hourly)
50 – 31	150 – 200 (1.7 – 2.3)	1.0	12
30 – 16	200 – 350 (2.3 – 4.0)	1.0	24
15 – 6	350 – 500 (4.0 – 5.6)	0.5	24
<5	>500 (>5.6)	0.5	48

Administration and dosage: Ceftazidime may be given intravenously or by deep intramuscular injection. For intramuscular use it should be reconstituted with 0.5% or 1% lignocaine hydrochloride. The dosage depends on the severity, sensitivity and type of infection and on the age, weight and renal function of the patient.

Adults: The adult dosage range for ceftazidime is 1 to 6 g per day: for instance, 500 mg, 1 g or 2 g given 8- or 12-hourly by i. v. or i. m. injection. In urinary tract infections and in many less serious infections, 500 mg or 1 g 12-hourly is usually adequate. In the majority of infections, 1 g 8-hourly or 2 g 12-hourly should be given. In very severe infections, especially in immunocompromised patients including those with neutropenia, 2 g 8- or 12-hourly should be administered. Cystic fibrosis: In patients with normal renal function who have pseudomonal lung infections, high doses of 100 to 150 mg/kg/day as three divided doses should be used. In adults with normal renal function 9 g/day has been used safely.

Infants and children: The usual dosage range for children aged over two months is 30 to 100 mg/kg/day, given as two or three divided doses; for children aged over two months but under 1 year it is generally 25 to 50 mg/kg twice daily. Doses up to 50 mg/kg three times per day, to a maximum of 6 g daily, may be given to infected immunocompromised or fibrocystic children.

Neonates and children up to 2 months of age: Whilst clinical experience is limited, a dose of 25 to 60 mg/kg/day given as two divided doses has proved to be effective. In the neonate the serum half-life of ceftazidime can be three to four times that in adults.

Dosage in impaired renal function: After a loading dose of 1 g the recommended maintenance doses of ceftazidime are shown in Table 16. During haemodialysis the serum half-life ranges from 2 to 5 hours. The appropriate maintenance dose should be repeated following each haemodialysis period.

Preparations: Ampoules of 500 mg, 1 g, 2 g.

Summary: Ceftazidime is one of the most active cephalosporins for severe bacterial infections, especially these caused by Pseudomonas aeruginosa or other gram-negative bacilli resistant to other antibiotics. In immunocompromised patients, for instance in the treatment of febrile neutropenic patients, ceftazidime should be combined with an aminoglycoside or another β-lactam antibiotic.

References

BLASER, J., A. BAUERNFEIND, M. VOGT, R. LÜTHY: Monotherapie von systemischen Pseudomonas-aeruginosa-Infektionen mit Ceftazidim. Dtsch. med. Wschr. *108, 35:* 1312 (1983).

O'CALLAGHAN, P., P. B. ACRED, D. M. HARPER: Glaxo GR-20263, a new broad-spectrum cephalosporin with anti-pseudomonal activity. Antimicrob. Ag. Chemother. *17:* 876 (1980).

HARRIS, A. M., S. J. PLESTED, P. B. HARPER: A comparison of the in-vitro properties of ceftazidime with those of new broad-spectrum cephalosporins and gentamicin. J. Antimicrob. Chemother. *8, Suppl. B:* 43 (1981).

SIMPSON, I. N., S. J. PLESTED, P. B. HARPER: Investigation of the β-lactamase stability of ceftazidime and eight other new cephalosporin antibiotics. J. Antimicrob. Chemother. *9:* 357 (1982).

VERBIST, L., J. VERHAEGEN: GR-20263: a new aminothiazolyl cephalosporin with high activity against pseudomonas and enterobacteriaceae. Antimicrob. Ag. Chemother. *17:* 807 (1980).

WISE, R., J. M. ANDREWS, K. A. BEDFORD: Comparison of in vitro activity of GR-20263, a novel cephalosporin derivative, with activities of other beta-lactam compounds. Antimicrob. Ag. Chemother. *17:* 884 (1980).

f) Cefsulodin

Proprietary names: Pseudocef, Monaspor.

Properties: A semi-synthetic cephalosporin with the following structural formula:

Readily water-soluble as the sodium salt.

Antibacterial activity: Greatest against Pseudomonas aeruginosa, where MIC's are relatively low. Generally active also against carbenicillin- and gentamicin-resistant strains of Pseudomonas. *Resistance* to Pseudomonas occurs in 1–3% only. Synergy in combination with aminoglycosides is frequently found, as is additive activity in combination with an anti-pseudomonal β-lactam antibiotic.

Staphylococci, pneumococci and gonococci are inhibited at concentrations between 0.5 and 4 mg/l but most gram-negative bacilli other than Pseudomonas are insensitive.

Pharmacokinetics: After i. v. injection of 500 mg, 1 g and 2 g, the mean serum concentrations are 20, 40 and 60 mg/l (1 h). *A serum concentration* of 100 mg/l is achieved after a short i. v. infusion of 2 g (30 min). *Half-life:* 1 ½ h. *Plasma protein binding:* 30%. *Urine recovery:* 90%. *Tissue diffusion* good.

Side effects: Similar to other parenteral cephalosporins. Renal function should be closely monitored, particularly when cefsulodin is combined with an aminoglycoside.

Indications: Proven Pseudomonas infections of the respiratory and urinary tracts, skin and bone, preferably in combination with an aminoglycoside. Combination with another cephalosporin or a penicillin without risk of antagonism is possible.

Administration and dosage: Preferably by short i. v. infusion over 30 min. Slow i. v. injection is also possible. Dissolve in 0.5% lignocaine solution for i. m. injection. 2–3(−6) g a day for *adults,* 50(−100) mg/kg for *children,* in 2–3 divided doses. Do not exceed a *maximum dose* of 6 g a day.

Preparations: Ampoules of 500 mg and 1 g.

Summary: A highly effective antibiotic for infections with Pseudomonas aeruginosa, but with no activity against other gram-negative bacilli; it can usually be given with safety in penicillin allergy.

References

GRIMM, H.: Bakteriologische In-vitro-Untersuchungen mit einem neuen gegen Pseudomonas wirksamen Cephalosporin: Cefsulodin. Arzneimittel-Forsch. *30 (II)* 1478 (1980).

SLACK, M. P. E., D. B. WHELDON, R. A. SWANN, E. PERKS: Cefsulodin, a cephalosporin with specific antipseudomonal activity, in vitro studies of the drug alone and in combination. J. Antimicrob. Chemother. *5:* 687 (1979).

ULLMANN, U.: Bacteriological studies with cefsudolin (CGP 7174/E), the first antipseudomonal cephalosporin. J. Antimicrob. Chemother. *5:* 563 (1979).

g) Cefoperazone

Proprietary names: Cefobid, Cefobis.

Activity: Ureido-cephalosporin with better activity against Pseudomonas aeruginosa in comparison to cefotaxime but less activity in comparison to ceftazidime. Spectrum of activity similar to cefotaxime. Cefoperazone is less active against Acinetobacter calcoaceticus and Enterobacter cloacae.

Pharmacokinetic data and tolerance are not so favourable as with cefotaxime and its derivatives: The bulk of cefoperazone is excreted with the bile into the intestines. Urinary excretion of active agent is only 20–25%.
Serum concentrations (after 1 g i. v.): Table 14, p. 90. *Half-life:* 110 min;· *plasma protein binding:* 90%.

When liver function is severely impaired, the half-life is prolonged threefold, the extrarenal clearance reduced to ⅛, and urinary excretion is three times as great.

Side effects: As with other cephalosporins but diarrhoea has been reported in 20–30% of cases and bleeding diatheses (caused by hypoprothrombinaemia and/or disorders of platelet function) are relatively frequent. Because of these side effects, use cefoperazone only in severe infections due to agents resistant to other antibiotics. May cause alcohol intolerance (see also p. 92).

Daily dose: 2–4 g for adults, 50–100 mg/kg for children.

Preparations: Ampoules of 500 mg, 1 g and 2 g.

References

ALLAZ, A.-F., P. DAYER, J. FABRE, M. RUDHARDT, I. BAFANT: Pharmacocinétique d'une nouvelle cephalosporine, la céfopérazone. Schweiz. med. Wschr. *109:* 1999 (1979).
CRAIG, W. A.: Single-dose pharmacokinetics of cefoperazone following intravenous administration. Clin. Ther. *3:* 46 (1980).
MATSUBARA, N., S. MINAMI, T. MURAOKA, I. SAIKAWA, S. MITSUHASHI: In vitro antibacterial activity of cefoperazone (T-1551), a new semisynthetic cephalosporin. Antimicrob. Ag. Chemother. *16:* 731 (1979).
NEU, H. C., N. ASWAPOKEE, K. P. FU, P. ASWAPOKEE: Antibacterial activity of a new 1-oxacephalosporin compared with that of other β-lactam compounds. Antimicrob. Ag. Chemother. *16:* 141 (1979).
SCHWIGON, C.-D., D. BARCKOW: Blutgerinnungsstörungen unter Cefoperazon und Lamoxactam. Diagnostik & Intensivtherapie *7:* 221 (1982).
SHIMIZU, K.: Cefoperazone: absorption, excretion, distribution and metabolism. Clin. Ther. *3:* 60 (1980).

h) Oral Cephalosporins

Proprietary names:

for *cephalexin:*	Cepexin, Ceporex, Ceporexin, Keflex, Oracef, Palitrex;
for *cefadroxil:*	Bidocef, Duracef, Ultracef;
for *cefaclor:*	Ceclor, Distaclor, Panoral;
for *cephradine:*	Anspor, Sefril, Velosef;
for *cefroxadine:*	Oraspor.

Properties: The chemical structure of cefadroxil differs from cephalexin solely by an additional para-hydroxyl group in the aromatic ring, and from cephradine by a double bond in the aromatic ring. Cefroxadine is the oxymethyl derivative of cephradine (Table 17). Cefaclor is also very similar to cephalexin, but a methyl group has been substituted by a chlorine group. All compounds are readily soluble in water and relatively stable; cefaclor is the only representative which is less stable than cephalexin in aqueous solution.

Table 17. Structural formula of the oral cephalosporins.

Generic Name	R_1	R_2
Cephalexin	C$_6$H$_5$–CH–NH$_2$	$-CH_3$
Cephradine	C$_6$H$_9$–CH–NH$_2$	$-CH_3$
Cefadroxil	HO–C$_6$H$_4$–CH–NH$_2$	$-CH_3$
Cefaclor	C$_6$H$_5$–CH–NH$_2$	$-Cl$
Cefroxadine	C$_6$H$_9$–CH–NH$_2$	$-OCH_3$

Spectrum of activity: Identical with cephalothin (see above), but less active against some organisms, particularly gram-negative rods. Some strains of Escherichia coli, Klebsiella and Proteus are resistant. Not active against Enterobacter aerogenes, Serratia marcescens, Pseudomonas aeruginosa, Bacteroides fragilis or enterococci. Little activity against Bordetella pertussis and Haemophilus influenzae. Cefaclor is 4–8 times as active as the other oral cephalosporins against streptococci, pneumococci and sensitive gram-negative bacilli (Escherichia coli, Klebsiella pneumoniae, Proteus mirabilis) and inhibits Haemophilus influenzae (ampicillin-sensitive) at concentrations of 1.6–3.2 mg/l and ampicillin-resistant strains at 3.2–6.4 mg/l. Resistance does not develop rapidly *in vitro* or *in vivo*.

Pharmacokinetics (Fig. 16): With *cephalexin* and *cephradine:* Absorption is largely complete after oral administration with maximal blood concentrations after 1½ hours (cephalexin) and 1 hour (cephradine). *Mean maximal serum concentration* after 1 g of cephalexin is 24.7 mg/l, and 7.5 mg/l after 4 h; after 1 g of cephradine orally, the maximum is 23 mg/l, and the concentration after 4 h

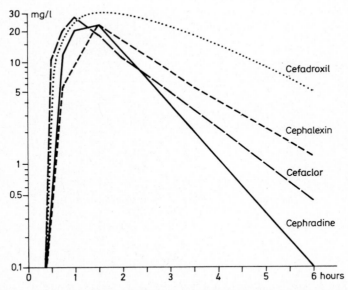

Fig. 16. Mean serum concentration in 10 healthy adults (volunteers) after an oral dose of 1 g cefadroxil (· · · ·), cephalexin (– – – –), cefaclor (————) and cephradine (——) each, given 1 h after a standardised breakfast.

1.5 mg/l. *Half-life* of cephalexin: 60 min; of cephradine: 32 min. *Plasma protein binding:* 12% with cephalexin, 13% with cephradine. *Penetration* of cephalexin and cephradine into purulent bronchial secretions and amniotic fluid is good. More than 90% is excreted unchanged *through the kidneys.* A small quantity of cephalexin is also excreted in the bile. The pharmacokinetics of *cefroxadine* are virtually identical with those of cephalexin.

Maximal serum concentrations after 1 g of *cefadroxil* by mouth are higher (28 mg/l) than after 1 g of cephalexin. Because of the longer half-life (1½ h), the serum concentrations decline more slowly than with cephalexin and the concentration is 4 times as high after 6 h. *Plasma protein binding:* 20%. *Urinary recovery:* 85%.

Mean serum concentrations of *cefaclor* are 17 mg/l (1 h) and 3.1 mg/l (3 h) after 500 mg, and 27 mg/l (1 h) and 5.1 mg/l (3 h) after 1 g. *Half-life:* 1 h. *Urinary recovery* (over 8 h): 60%. Partially metabolised in the body.

Side effects: As with parenteral cephalosporins, and also gastro-intestinal upset (vomiting, diarrhoea) in 1–3%.

Indications: Infections of the respiratory and urinary tracts and skin where caused by sensitive bacteria, particularly staphylococci, as well as many strains of Escherichia coli, Klebsiella and Proteus. Cefaclor is also useful in infections with Haemophilus. Prophylaxis of ascending urinary infections.

Inappropriate usage: Severe systemic infections where β-lactamase-stable cephalosporins would be more effective.

Contra-indications: Allergy to cephalosporins.

Administration and dosage: 0.5(−1) g 3 times a day, 50(−100) mg/kg for children; with cefadroxil: 1 g twice a day for adults, 50–100 mg/kg twice a day for children.

Preparations:

Cephalexin:	Capsules of 250 mg, tablets of 500 mg and 1 g, granules for 60 ml and 120 ml suspension (50 mg/ml), syrup (50 mg/ml) and 10 ml drops (100 mg/ml).
Cefadroxil:	Capsules of 500 mg, tablets of 1 g, powder for 60 ml syrup (50 mg/ml) and (forte) for 60 ml syrup (100 mg/ml).
Cefaclor:	Capsules of 250 mg and 500 mg, granules for 60 ml and 120 ml suspension (125 mg/5 ml and 250 mg/5 ml).
Cephradine:	Capsules of 500 mg, tablets of 1 g, granules for 60 ml suspension (50 mg/ml), ampoules of 1 g, 2 g and 4 g.
Cefroxadine:	Capsules of 250 mg.

Summary: Oral cephalosporins are frequently used and well tolerated in children but they are considerably less active than the newer parenteral cephalosporins. Cefaclor is distinguished from the other oral cephalosporins by its effectiveness against Haemophilus. Cefadroxil has the advantage of a longer half-life.

References

AHRENS, T., K. G. NABER: Activity of cefroxadine and cephalexin in urinary tract infections: A double-blind comparative study. Infection *11:* 31 (1983).

BACH, V. T., M. M. KHURANA, H. THADEPALLI: In vitro activity of cefaclor against aerobic and anerobic bacteria. Antimicrob. Ag. Chemother. *13:* 210 (1978).

BERGAN, T.: Pharmacokinetics of a new cephalosporin, CGP 9000 (cefroxadine), in healthy volunteers. Chemotherapy *26:* 225 (1980).

BILL, N. J., J. A. U. WASHINGTON: Comparison of in vitro activity of cephalexin, cephradine and cefaclor: Antimicrob. Ag. Chemother. *11:* 470 (1977).

BLOCH, R., J. J. SZWED, R. S. SLOAN, F. C. LUFT: Pharmacokinetics of *cefaclor* in normal subjects and patients with chronic renal failure. Antimicrob. Ag. Chemother. *12:* 730 (1977).

BUCK, R. E., K. E. PRICE: Cefadroxil, a new broad-spectrum cephalosporin: Antimicrob. Ag. Chemother. *11:* 324 (1977).

CUTLER, R. E., A. D. BLAIR, M. R. KELLY: Cefadroxil kinetics in patients with renal insufficiency. Infection *5:* 592 (1980).

DEGEN, J., L. RINGWELSKI, H. MAIER-LENZ: Konzentration von Cefadroxil im Nierengewebe und Serum nach oraler Applikation bei Patienten mit normaler und eingeschränkter Nierenfunktion. Arzneimittel-Forsch./Drug. Res. *33:* 1339 (1983).

GERARDIN, A., J. B. LECAILLON, J. P. SCHOELLER, G. HUMBERT, J. GUIBERT: Pharmacokinetics of cefroxadin (CGP-9000) in man. J. Pharmacokin. Biopharm. *10:* 15 (1982).

GINSBURG, C. M., G. H. McCRACKEN Jr., J. C. CLAHSEN, M. L. THOMAS: Clinical pharmacology of cefadroxil in infants and children: Antimicrob. Ag. Chemother. *13:* 845 (1978).

HALPRIN, G. M., S. M. McMAHON: Cephalexin concentrations in sputum during acute respiratory infections. Antimicrob. Ag. Chemother. *3:* 703 (1973).

HARHAUSEN, E., C. SIMON: Zum Nachweis von Cefaclor im Serum und Urin (einschließlich Stabilitätsprüfung) mit Hilfe der Hochdruckflüssigkeitschromatographie. Infection *7, Suppl. 6:* 603 (1979).

HARTSTEIN, A. I.: Comparison of pharmacological and antimicrobial properties of cefadroxil and cephalexin. Antimicrob. Ag. Chemother. *12:* 93 (1977).

HARVENGT, C., P. DE SCHEPPER, F. LAMY, J. HANSEN: Cephadrine absorption and excretion in fasting and nonfasting volunteers. J. clin. Pharmac. *13:* 36 (1973).

KAMMER, R. B., L. J. SHORT: Cefaclor: summary of clinical experience. Infection *7, Suppl. 6:* 631 (1979).

KNOTHE, H.: Die In-vitro-Aktivität von Cefaclor. Infection *7, Suppl. 6:* 518 (1979).

KORZENIOWSKI, O. M., W. M. SCHELD, M. A. SANDE: Comparative pharmacology of cefaclor and cephalexin. Antimicrob. Ag. Chemother. *12:* 157 (1977).

MÜLLER, O., U. RÜCKERT, K. FABRICIUS: Untersuchungen zur Exkretion von Cefaclor in menschlicher Galle. Infection 7, Suppl. 6: 624 (1979).
NABER, K., W. KALDEWEY: Vergleichsstudie Cefaclor versus Amoxicillin bei Harnwegsinfektionen. Infection 7, Suppl. 6: 617 (1979).
NEU, H. C., K. P. FU: Cefaclor: In vitro spectrum of activity and beta-lactamase stability: Antimicrob. Ag. Chemother. 13: 584 (1978).
NICHOLAS, P., B. R. MEYERS, S. Z. HIRSCHMAN: Cephalexin: Pharmacologic evaluation following oral and parenteral administration. J. clin. Pharmacol. 13: 463 (1973).
PFEFFER, M., A. JACKSON, J. XIMENES, J. P. DE MENEZES: Comparative human oral clinical pharmacology of cefadroxil, cephalexin, and cephradine: Antimicrob. Ag. Chemother. 11: 331 (1977).
PRESTON, D. A.: Summary of laboratory studies on the antibacterial activity of cefaclor. Infection 7, Suppl. 6: 557 (1979).
SANTORO, J., B. N. AGARWAL, R. MARTINELLI, N. WENGER, M. E. LEVISON: Pharmacology of cefaclor in normal volunteers and patients with renal failure. Antimicrob. Ag. Chemother. 13: 951 (1978).
SHADOMY, S., G. WAGNER, M. CARVER: In vitro activities of five oral cephalosporins against aerobic pathogenic bacteria. Antimicrob. Ag. Chemother. 12: 609 (1977).
SILVER, M. S., G. W. COUNTS, D. ZELEZNIK, M. TURCK: Comparison of in vitro antibacterial activity of three oral cephalosporins: Cefaclor, cephalexin, and cephradine. Antimicrob. Ag. Chemother. 12: 591 (1977).
SIMON, C.: Zur Pharmakokinetik von Cefadroxil, einem neuen Oral-Cephalosporin. Arzneimittel-Forsch. 30 (I): 502 (1980).
SINAI, R., S. HAMMBERG, M. I. MARKS, C. H. PAI: In vitro susceptibility of Haemophilus influenzae to sulfamethoxazole-trimethoprim and cefaclor, cephalexin, and cephradine. Antimicrob. Ag. Chemother. 13: 861 (1978).
YASUDA, K., S. KURASHIGE, S. MITSUHASHI: Cefroxadine (CGP-9000), an orally active cephalosporin. Antimicrob. Ag. Chemother. 18: 105 (1980).
ZAK, O., W. A. VISCHER, C. SCHENK, W. TOSCH, W. ZIMMERMANN, J. REGOS, E. R. SUTE, F. KRADOLFER, J. GELZER: CGP 9000: A new orally active, broad spectrum cephalosporin. J. Antibiot. 6: 653 (1976).

3. Other β-Lactam Antibiotics

a) Imipenem/Cilastatin

Proprietary name: Zienam.

Properties:

Imipenem (N-formimidoyl thienamycin) is a derivative of thienamycin and has been found to be 5–10 times more stable than thienamycin; its antibacterial activity is equal or slightly superior to that of thienamycin. Imipenem is a carbapenem and has the following structural formula:

The substitution of a methylene (CH_2) group for the sulphur atom makes imipenem more potent in its bactericidal effect. Attachment of the hydroxyethyl side-chain to the β-lactam ring in a trans orientation is responsible for its stability to bacterial β-lactamases.

Cilastatin is a competitive reversible inhibitor of dehydropeptidase-I, the renal enzyme which metabolises and inactivates imipenem. Cilastatin is a derivative of the heptene carbonic acid with the following structural formula:

Cilastatin has two functions. Firstly, it reduces hydrolysis of imipenem in the kidneys of the patient and increases urine concentrations of the active antibiotic; secondly, it inhibits nephrotoxicity of imipenem at a higher dosage (demonstrable in animal experiments). Imipenem has no effect on other human metallo-dipeptidases and is not active against bacteria. Imipenem and cilastatin sodium are present in Trademark (Zienam) in a 1:1 ratio.

Spectrum of activity: Imipenem inhibits cell wall synthesis and is highly bactericidal. It has a very broad spectrum of activity which embraces almost all the gram-positive organisms, including Streptococcus faecalis, Listeria monocytogenes, Mycobacterium avium-intracellulare, and gram-negative bacteria, including Pseudomonas aeruginosa, Citrobacter, Serratia, Acinetobacter and Enterobacter species. Imipenem also inhibits β-lactamase-producing strains of Haemophilus influenzae and Neisseria gonorrhoeae. It is more active than clindamycin and metronidazole against Bacteroides fragilis and most other anaerobes (Clostridia, Peptococcus, Peptostreptococcus, Actinomyces, Fusobacterium species etc.). The activity of imipenem against Proteus vulgaris and Proteus mirabilis is somewhat less than against the other enterobacteria. Imipenem is inactive against Pseudomonas cepacia and maltophilia, some strains of Streptococcus faecium and some methicillin-resistant staphylococci. There is very occasional partial cross-resistance with penicillins and cephalosporins.

Pharmacokinetics:

After i. v. infusion of 250 mg and 500 mg of *imipenem* over 20 min, *peak serum concentrations* range from 14–24 mg/l to 20–60 mg/l. *Half-life:* 60 min. *Protein binding:* 25%. *Urinary recovery:* 15–20%.

Cilastatin gives *peak serum levels* after i. v. infusion of 250 mg and 500 mg over 20 min between 15–25 mg/l and 30–50 mg/l. *Half-life:* 45 min. *Protein binding:* 25%. *Urinary recovery:* 55% as the parent drug and ca. 15% as the N-acetyl metabolite (with the same inhibitory activity against dehydropeptidase-I). Activity of dehydropeptidase-I in the kidneys returns to normal soon after the elimination of cilastatin from the bloodstream.

Concomitant administration of imipenem and cilastatin increases the serum levels of imipenem only slightly (Fig. 17); the half-life and protein binding are almost the same as when used singly but *urine concentrations* of imipenem are much higher and exceed 10 mg/l for up to 8 hours after 500 mg imipenem + 500 mg cilastatin i. v. *Urinary recovery* of imipenem (after combined treatment): 70% (the remainder is recovered as antibacterially inactive metabolites). Imipenem is not excreted in the faeces. No accumulation of imipenem in plasma or urine was found with the combination after repeated administration. Imipenem/cilastatin is dialysable.

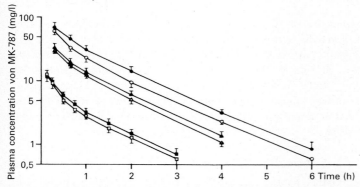

Fig. 17. Mean plasma concentration of *N*-formimidoyl thienamycin (MK-787) administered intravenously in doses of 150 mg (□), 500 mg (△), or 1,000 mg (○) alone (open symbols) or combined with equal doses of dehydro-peptidase inhibitors (filled symbols). The standard deviations are indicated by bars. After: S. R. NORRBY et al.: Antimicrob. Ag. Chemother. *23:* 300 (1983).

Side effects: Serious side effects are rare. In 5–10%, minor side effects were observed: gastrointestinal upset (nausea, vomiting and diarrhoea), local reactions (thrombophlebitis), allergic reactions (rashes) and haematological reactions (eosinophilia).

The direct Coombs test can become positive during therapy. A mild, transient change in prothrombin time was found in <2% of cases. No signs of nephrotoxicity or serious renal abnormality were observed.

Indications: Mixed infections and severe infections (prior to the identification of causative organisms), particularly septicaemia, intraabdominal, gynaecological, bone or joint infections. Failure of previous therapy with other broad-spectrum antibiotics.

Contra-indication: Hypersensitivity to any component of the drug. Use in pregnancy and in children not yet established. Reduce dosage in renal insufficiency.

Administration and dosage: The intravenous dosage form should be dissolved in an appropiate volume of compatible diluent (not in solvents containing lactate) and infused over 20 min. The daily dosage is 1.5–2 g administered in 3 or 4 divided doses. The maximum daily dose is 4 g. In patients with severe renal impairment (creatinine clearance <15 ml/min), reduce the normal daily dose to 50%. Patients on dialysis should be given an additional 500 mg after each haemodialysis.

Preparations: Ampoules containing 250 mg or 500 mg of imipenem +250 mg or 500 mg of cilastatin.

Summary: Imipenem is the first of a new class of β-lactam antibiotics with a very broad spectrum of activity against almost all aerobic and anaerobic bacteria and with a high potency. It may prove to be an alternative to a wide range of antibiotic combinations used previously for initial therapy in severe bacterial infections including mixed infections. To avoid metabolic degradation in the kidneys and to attain sufficient urinary concentrations, imipenem is combined with cilastatin which inhibits a renal dipeptidase that destroys imipenem and increases the renal tolerance of the drug.

References

AZNAR, J., M. C. GARCÍA IGLESIAS, E. J. PEREA: Comparative activity of imipenem (N-formimidoyl thienamycin) on enterococci and its interactions with aminoglycosides. J. Antimicrob. Chemother. *13:* 129 (1984).

BRAVENY, I., K. MACHKA, R. ELSSER: Antibacterial activity of N-formimidyl thienamycin in comparison with cefotaxime, lamoxactam, cefoperazone, piperacillin and gentamicin. Infection *10:* 45 (1982).

BROWN, J. E., V. E. DELBENE, C. D. COLLINS: In vitro activity of N-formimidoyl thienamycin, moxalactam and other new beta-lactam agents against Bacteroides fragilis: contribution of beta-lactamase to resistance. Antimicrob. Ag. Chemother. *19:* 248 (1981).

CULLMANN, W.: A comparison of antibacterial activities of N-formimidoyl thienamycin (MK 0787) with those of other recently developed β-lactam derivatives. Antimicrob. Ag. Chemother. *21:* 302 (1982).

ERON, L. J., D. L. HIXON, CH. H. PARK: Imipenem versus moxalactam in the treatment of serious infections. Antimicrob. Ag. Chemother. *24:* 841 (1983).

FAINSTEIN, V., B. LEBLANC, S. WEAVER, G. P. BODEY: Comparative in vitro study of thienamycin. Infection *10:* 50 (1981).

KESADO, T., K. WATANABE, Y. ASAHI, M. ISONO et al.: Susceptibilities of anaerobic bacteria to N-Formimidoyl-thienamycin (MKO 787) and to other antibiotics. Antimicrob. Ag. Chemother. *21:* 1016 (1982).

KROPP, H., J. G. SUNDELOF, J. S. KAHAN, F. M. KAHAN, J. BIRNBAUM: MK 0787 (N-formimidoyl thienamycin): Evaluation of in vitro and in vivo activities. Antimicrob. Ag. Chemother. *17:* 993 (1980).

KROPP, H., J. G. SUNDELOF, R. HAJDU, F. M. KAHAN: Metabolism of thienamycin and related carbapenem antibiotics by the renal dipeptidase dehydropeptidase-l. Antimicrob. Ag. Chemother. *22:* 62 (1982).

MARKOWITZ, N. et al.: In vitro susceptibility patterns of methicillin-resistant and -susceptible Staphylococcus aureus strains in a population of parenteral drug abusers from 1972 to 1981. Antimicrob. Ag. Chemother. *23:* 450 (1983).

NEU, H. C., P. LABTHAVIKUL: Comparative in vitro activity of N-formimidoyl thienamycin against gram-positive and gram-negative aerobic and anaerobic species and its β-lactamase stability. Antimicrob. Ag. Chemother. *21:* 180 (1982).

NORRBY, S. R., K. ALESTIG, B. BJÖRNEGARD, L. A. BURMAN, F. FERBER, J. L. HUBER, K. H. JONES, F. M. KAHAN, J. S. KAHAN, H. KROPP, M. A. P. MEISINGER, J. G. SUNDELOF: Urinary recovery of N-formimidyl thienamycin (MK 0787) as affected by coadministration of N-formimidyl thienamycin dehydropeptidase inhibitors. Antimicrob. Ag. Chemother. *23:* 300 (1983).

TISCHHAUSER, G.: The in vitro activity of N-formimidoyl thienamycin compared with other broad-spectrum cephalosporins and with clinidamycin and metronidazole. Infection *11:* 219 (1983).

WISE, R., J. M. ANDREWS, N. PATEL: N-Formimidoyl thienamycin a novel β-lactam: an in vitro comparison with other β-lactam antibiotics. J. Antimicrob. Chemother. *7:* 521 (1981).

WITTE, J. L., F. L. SAPICO, H. N. CANAWATI: In vitro susceptibility of methicillin-resistant and methicillin-susceptible Staphylococcus aureus strains to N-formimidoyl thienamycin. Antimicrob. Ag. Chemother. *22:* 906 (1982).

b) Aztreonam

The monolactams are a new group of naturally occuring monocyclic β-lactam antibiotics produced by bacteria, and the name monobactam is used for some derivatives. These compounds have a simple β-lactam ring but lack an attached thiazolidine ring. They are very stable to β-lactamases (with the exception of the chromosomally transmitted type IV enzyme). Squibb (USA) have developed the monobactam SQ 26180 which is produced from Chromobacterium violaceum. This was the starting point for the synthesis of 3-aminobactamic acid. Aztreonam (SQ 26776) is a derivative of this monobactam. Aztreonam has marked antibacterial activity and is therefore currently undergoing extensive clinical trials.

Spectrum of activity: It is active against almost all aerobic gram-negative bacilli including Pseudomonas aeruginosa, Serratia marcescens and Citrobacter freundii, but is not active against anaerobes (Bacteroides species etc.), Acinetobacter and Alcaligenes species, or against gram-positive bacteria. The anti-pseudomonal activity is approximately similar to that of cefsulodin. Aztreonam acts synergistically with gentamicin against aztreonam-resistant strains of Pseudomonas aeruginosa and Klebsiella pneumoniae. It has the following structural formula:

Clinical use: Aztreonam is widely used in clinical trials and apparently well tolerated. The value of a selective antibiotic only against gram-negative bacteria is limited. The main indications are known infections by sensitive enterobacteria or pseudomonas. Use without knowledge of the underlying pathogen is only justified in urinary infections. No cross-allergy with other β-lactams.

Proprietary name: Azactam.

Summary: First agent of a promising group of new β-lactams. More monobactams and monolactams are expected.

c) Clavulanic Acid

Proprietary names: Augmentan, Augmentin (in combination with amoxycillin), Synulox.

Properties: Clavulanic acid is obtained by the fermentation of Streptomyces clavuligerus and is structurally similar to the penicillin nucleus but has no acylamino side-chain and contains oxygen instead of sulphur at position 1. It has the following structural formula:

It has only weak antibacterial activity and would not be therapeutically effective if administered alone. Clavulanic acid is, however, a strong and irreversible β-lactamase inhibitor, especially of types II, III, IV and V. Clavulanic acid acts only against β-lactamases of type I if they are produced by Bacteroides fragilis. Amoxycillin-resistant (β-lactamase producing) strains of Staphylococcus aureus, Haemophilus influenzae, gonococci, Escherichia coli, Klebsiella pneumoniae, Proteus mirabilis, Proteus vulgaris and Bacteroides fragilis are generally as sensitive in the presence of clavulanic acid as amoxycillin-sensitive strains. Clavulanic acid does not protect amoxycillin from inactivation by the β-lactamases of Pseudomonas aeruginosa, Serratia marcescens, Enterobacter species, Proteus morganii or Proteus rettgeri. Some strains of Escherichia coli and Klebsiella do not become sensitive to amoxycillin through clavulanic acid because they produce a different type of β-lactamase. Enterobacteriaceae should therefore be tested *in vitro* for sensitivity to amoxycillin with clavulanic acid. Amoxycillin trihydrate for oral use and clavulanic acid as the potassium salt are combined in the ratio of 2:1 in Great Britain and 4:1 in Germany, because of the different dosage practices for amoxycillin in the two countries.

Large oral doses of clavulanic acid are not recommended because of poor tolerance. For parenteral use, the mixture is in the same ratio in Great Britain and Germany (5:1).

Pharmacokinetics: Clavulanic acid is well absorbed orally as the potassium salt. 125 mg of clavulanic acid by mouth give rise to a maximal serum concentration after 1.5 h (3 mg/l), and 0.6 mg/l after 4 h. 2.3 mg/l are detected one hour after 100 mg i. v., and 0.3 mg/l after 4 h. *Plasma protein binding: 20%. Half-life:* 75 min. *Urinary recovery: 35–40%* (with oral administration).

Amoxycillin has similar pharmacokinetics after oral and i. v. administration but the percentage urinary recovery is higher.

Side effects: 10% of patients suffer nausea, vomiting, and diarrhoea, predominantly due to the clavulanic acid. The recommended oral dose of clavulanic acid should not, therefore be exceeded.

Indications: Urinary infections with amoxycillin-resistant bacteria, the β-lactamases of which are inhibited by clavulanic acid (e. g. Escherichia coli and Klebsiella pneumoniae).

Administration and dosage: Orally: In Britain, 1–2 tablets of 375 mg (250 mg of amoxycillin and 125 mg of clavulanic acid) 3 times a day. In Germany, 1 tablet of 625 mg (500 mg amoxycillin and 125 mg clavulanic acid) 3 times a day. By i. v. injection: 600 mg (500 mg amoxycillin + 100 mg clavulanic acid) or 1.2 g (1 g amoxycillin + 0.2 g clavulanic acid), both 3 times a day.

Preparations: Tablets of 375 mg (Britain), 625 mg (Germany), suspension (31 mg/ml), ampoules of 600 mg and 1.2 g.

Summary: Clavulanic acid in combination with amoxycillin is a valuable addition to the range of oral antibiotics. It extends the spectrum of activity of amoxycillin against certain β-lactamase-producing bacteria (staphylococci, Haemophilus, gonococci, Escherichia coli, Klebsiella pneumoniae and Bacteroides fragilis). Clinical experience with this combination is still limited and its activity cannot be finally evaluated. Another combination is ticarcillin + clavulanic acid (Timentin) but the activity against Pseudomonas aeruginosa is not improved.

References

ADAM, D.: Pharmakokinetics of amoxicillin and clavulanic acid administered alone and in combination. Antimicrob. Ag. Chemother. 22: 353 (1982).

BALL, A. P., P. G. DAVEY, A. M. GEDDES, I. D. FARRELL, G. R. BROOKES: Clavulanic acid and amoxycillin: A clinical, bacteriological and pharmacological study. Lancet I: 620 (1980).

BALL, P., T. WATSON, S. MEHTAR: Amoxycillin and clavulanic acid in intra-abdominal and pelvic sepsis. J. Antimicrob. Chemother. 7: 441 (1981).

BEEUWKES, H., V. H. RÜTGERS: A combination of amoxicillin and clavulanic acid in the treatment of respiratory tract infections caused by amoxicillin-resistant Haemophilus influenzae. Infection 9: 244 (1981).

BROWN, A. G., D. BUTTERWORTH, M. COLE, G. HANSCOMB, G. D. HOOD, C. READING, G. N. ROLINSON: Naturally occuring β-lactamase inhibitors with antibacterial activity. J. Antibiot. 29: 668 (1976).

CHARNAS, R. L., J. FISHER, J. R. KNOWLES: Chemical studies on the inactivation of Escherichia coli RTEM β-lactamase by clavulanic acid. Biochemistry 17: 2185 (1978).

CLARKE, A. M., S. J. V. ZEMCOV: Clavulanic acid in combination with ticarcillin: an in-vitro comparison with other β-lactams. J. Antimicrob. Chemother. 13: 121 (1984).

FISHER, J., R. L. CHARNAS, J. R. KNOWLES: Kinetic studies on the inactivation of Escherichia coli RTEM β-lactamase by clavulanic acid. Biochemistry 17: 2180 (1978).

FUGLESANG, J. E., T. BERGAN: Antibacterial activity and kill kinetics of amoxicillin-clavulanic acid combinations against Escherichia coli and Klebsiella aerogenes. Infection *11:* 329 (1983).

GOLDSTEIN, F. W., M. D. KITZIS, J. F. ACAR: Effect of clavulanic acid and amoxycillin formulation against β-lactamase producing gram-negative bacteria in urinary tract infections. J. Antimicrob. Chemother. *5:* 705 (1979).

v. KLINGEREN, B., M. DESSENS-KROON: The influence of clavulanic acid on the susceptibility to amoxycillin of β-lactamase-producing strains of H. influenzae using different inoculum sizes. J. Antimicrob. Chemother. *5:* 322 (1979).

LEIGH, D. A., K. BRADNOCK, J. M. MARRINER: Augmentin (amoxicillin and clavulanic acid) therapy in complicated infections due to β-lactamase producing bacteria. J. Antimicrob. Chemother. *7:* 229 (1981).

MÜLLER, J. M., C. N. BAKER, C. THORNSBERRY: Inhibition of β-lactamase in Neisseria gonorrhoeae by sodium-clavulanate. Antimicrob. Ag. Chemother. *14:* 794 (1978).

NEU, H. C., K. P. FU: Clavulanic acid, a novel inhibitor of β-lactamases. Antimicrob. Ag. Chemother. *14:* 650 (1978).

NELSON, J. D., H. KUSMIESZ, S. SHELTON: Pharmacokinetics of potassium clavulanate in combination with amoxycillin in pediatric patients. Antimicrob. Ag. Chemother. *21:* 681 (1982).

NINANE, G., J. JOLY, M. KRAYTMAN, F. PIOT: Bronchopulmonary infection due to β-lactamase-producing Branhamella catarrhalis treated with amoxycillin/clavulanic acid. Lancet *II (8083):* 257 (1978).

PAISLEY, J. W., J. A. WASHINGTON: Combined activity of clavulanic acid and ticarcillin against ticarcillin-resistant gram-negative bacilli. Antimicrob. Ag. Chemother. *14:* 224 (1978).

PETERS, G., G. PULVERER, N. NEUGEBAUER: In vitro-activity of clavulanic acid and amoxycillin-resistant bacteria. Infection *8 (3):* 104 (1980).

PETERS, G., G. PULVERER, M. NEUGEBAUER: In vitro activity of clavulanic acid and amoxicillin combined against amoxicillin-resistant bacteria. Infection *8:* 104 (1980).

READING, G., M. COLE: Clavulanic acid: a β-lactamase-inhibiting β-lactam from Streptomyces clavuligerus. Antimicrob. Ag. Chemother. *11:* 852 (1977).

SCHAAD, U. B., P. A. CASEY, D. L. COOPER: Single-dose pharmacokinetics of intravenous clavulanic acid with amoxicillin in pediatric patients. Antimicrob. Ag. Chemother. *23:* 252 (1983).

WISE, R.: Clavulanic acid and susceptibility of Bacteroides fragilis to penicillin. Lancet *II:* 145 (1977).

WISE, R., J. M. ANDREWS, K. A. BEDFORD: In vitro study of clavulanic acid in combination with penicillin, amoxycillin and carbenicillin. Antimicrob. Ag. Chemother. *13:* 389 (1978).

WISE, R., I. A. DONOVAN, J. DRUMM, J. M. ANDREWS, P. STEPHENSON: The penetration of amoxycillin/clavulanic acid into peritoneal fluid. J. Antimicrob. Chemother. *11:* 57 (1983).

WITKOWSKI, G. et al.: Pharmakokinetic studies of amoxicillin, potassium clavulanate and their combination. Eur. J. clin. Microbiol. *1:* 233 (1982).

WUST, J., T. D. WILKINS: Effect of clavulanic acid on anaerobic bacteria resistant to β-lactam antibiotics. Antimicrob. Ag. Chemother. *13:* 130 (1978).

d) Sulbactam

A new β-lactam antibiotic (penicillanic acid sulfone) developed by Pfizer (USA) with weak antibacterial activity. Because of its capacity to inhibit β-lactamases, it can be used effectively in combination with penicillins (e. g. ampicillin). Synergy is thus achieved *in vitro* for certain otherwise resistant strains of bacteria and the spectrum of activity can thus be extended. The combination of piperacillin and sulbactam, for example, is active against penicillin-resistant strains of Staphylococcus aureus, Escherichia coli, Klebsiella pneumoniae and Bacteroides fragilis, but not against piperacillin-resistant strains of Pseudomonas. Because sulbactam is not absorbed by mouth, the pivaloyl oxymethyl ester (CP 47904) has been developed, which is hydrolysed in the intestinal mucosa to release sulbactam into the blood. Diarrhoea is a reported side effect. There is little clinical experience with this compound to date, but the combination of sulbactam with an amino penicillin may be useful in the future and a combination with bacampicillin is currently undergoing clinical evaluation.

Structural formula:

Reference

NEU, H. C., K. P. FU: Synergistic activity of piperacillin in combination with β-lactamase inhibitors. Antimicrob. Ag. Chemother. *18:* 582 (1980).

4. Tetracyclines

Common proprietary names:

Tetracycline: Achromycin, Economycin, Hostacyclin, Latycin, Mephacyclin, Supramycin, Tetrabid, Tetrachel, Tetralysal, Tetrex. Deteclo contains tetracycline, chlortetracycline and demeclocycline.

Oxytetracycline: Abbocin, Berkmycen, Chemocycline, Galenomycin, Imperacin, Oxymycin, Terramycin, Terravenös, Unimycin, Vendarcin.

Demeclocycline (formerly called demethylchlortetracycline): Declomycin, Ledermycin.

Rolitetracycline (N-pyrrolidinomethyltetracycline): Reverin, Syntetrin, Tetraverin, Velocycline.
Doxycycline: Dumoxin, Investin, Vibramycin and Vibravenös.
Minocycline: Klinomycin, Minocin.

Properties: A group of closely related broad-spectrum antibiotics with a naphthacene ring system. Tetracycline, oxytetracycline, rolitetracycline, minocycline and doxycycline differ from each other in the composition of their side-chains (Fig. 18), but they have an identical spectrum of action with the exception of minocycline, which retains activity against strains of staphylococci resistant to the other tetracyclines (Fig. 19). There are various differences in activity and pharmacokinetic properties (absorption, blood concentrations, plasma protein binding, excretion) between the different tetracyclines, on the basis of which doxycycline and minocycline, which have sustained activity, can be separated from the other tetracyclines, whose half-lives are shorter.

Mode of action: The bacteriostatic activity of the tetracyclines is based on the inhibition of protein synthesis in the bacterial cell by prevention of acylation of amino acids as they enter the ribosome on the growing peptide chain. This action affects both extracellular and intracellular bacteria. The activity of the tetracyclines is very dependent on the medium, and much activity is lost in certain body fluids (e. g. bile).

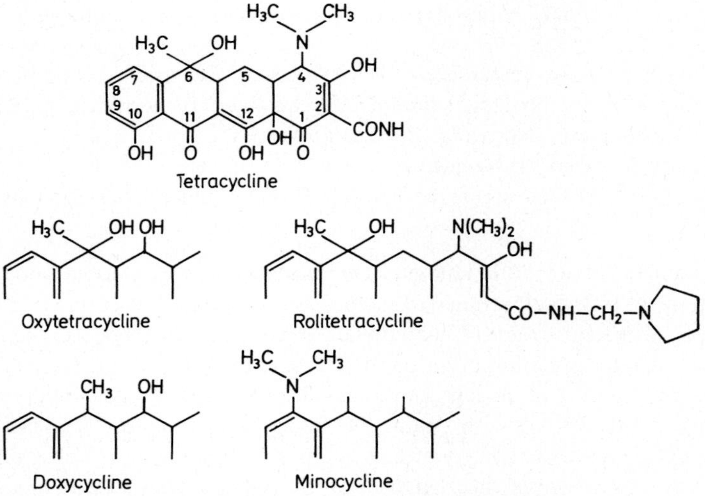

Fig. 18. Chemical structure of the tetracyclines.

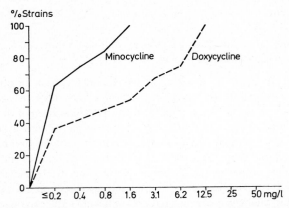

Fig. 19. Cumulative frequency of minimal inhibitory concentrations of minocycline and doxycycline in 52 tetracycline-resistant strains of Staphylococcus aureus.

Spectrum of activity:

Moderate or good sensitivity: Streptococci, pneumococci, gonococci, meningo-cocci, Listeria, actinomycetes, Pasteurella multocida, Yersinia, Haemophilus, Brucella, Pseudomonas mallei and pseudomallei, Vibrio cholerae and Vibrio parahaemolyticus, Campylobacter species, Leptospira, Francisella tularensis and Bordetella pertussis. Good activity also against mycoplasmas, chlamydiae (ornithosis, trachoma, lymphogranuloma inguinale) and rickettsiae (Q-fever, typhus).

Variable sensitivity: Enterococci, staphylococci, Escherichia coli, Klebsiella, Enterobacter, Acinetobacter, salmonellae, shigellae, Bacteroides species, clos-tridia, corynebacteria, Nocardia, Bacillus anthracis.

Little activity against mycobacteria.

Inactive against Pseudomonas aeruginosa, Proteus vulgaris, Serratia marcescens etc.

Resistance: There is little tendency for resistance to arise during therapy. The proportion of resistant strains of staphylococci varies from place to place (10–30%). Resistant strains of haemolytic streptococci, pneumococci, gonococci, clostridia and Haemophilus influenzae also occur (10–35% of Lancefield Group A streptococci, 2–30% of pneumococci and 3% of Haemophilus influenzae are resistant). Only 40–60% of strains of Bacteroides fragilis are sensitive to tetracyclines. Penicillin resistant strains are generally resistant to tetracyclines as well. There is cross-resistance between all the tetracyclines except minocycline against staphylococci, but no cross-resistance with other antibiotics.

Pharmacokinetics:

Absorption after oral administration is variable and depends on the individual preparation. Tetracycline and oxytetracycline are less completely absorbed than demeclocycline. Chlortetracycline is so poorly absorbed (at most 25%) that it should no longer be used. Comparative studies of i. v. and oral administration show doxycycline to be 75% and minocycline to be almost completely absorbed. The absorption of tetracycline is impaired by food, particularly milk and certain drugs (aluminium hydroxide, sodium bicarbonate, potassium and magnesium salts, ferrous sulphate). Increasing the oral dose of tetracycline beyond 250 mg, which achieves maximum absorption, does not usually increase the blood level proportionally, but simply results in greater loss in the faeces. Blood concentrations of doxycycline (Fig. 20) and minocycline, on the other hand, are doubled by increasing the dose from 100 to 200 mg, and doubled again from 200 to 400 mg. Maximal blood concentrations after oral administration are achieved after 2–3 hours.

Mean serum concentrations with regular oral administration of 250 mg tetracycline or oxytetracycline are between 1 and 3 mg/l. Maximal serum concentrations of 3 mg/l are found after a single daily dose of 100 mg of doxycycline or 200 mg of minocycline. Unlike minocycline, doxycycline shows some non-toxic accumulation, so a maintenance dose of 100 mg following an initial dose of 200 mg is sufficient. Minocycline requires a maintenance dose of 200 mg.

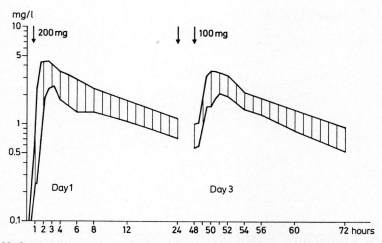

Fig. 20. Serum concentration in 8 adults after a single oral dose of 200 mg doxycycline (left) and after repeated oral doses of 100 mg doxycycline every 24 hours on day 3 (right).

Mean serum concentrations after a single i. v. injection of 250 mg of an injectable tetracycline: 3–5 mg/l after 3–4 h, 2–3 mg/l after 6 h and 1–2 mg/l after 12 h; of 200 mg doxycycline (see Fig. 21). 3.6 mg/l are achieved in the serum after an i. v. infusion of 200 mg of doxycycline for 1 hour, and 2.5 mg/l with 100 mg. After 200 mg of minocycline i. v. over 60 min, the serum concentration falls from 3.5 mg/l at the end of infusion to 1 mg/l after 12 h and 0.6 mg/l after 24 h. *Half-lives* of tetracycline, oxytetracycline and rolitetracycline: 8–9 hours; doxycycline and minocycline: 15 hours. The half-life of doxycycline is reduced to 7 hours when phenytoin or another barbiturate are given at the same time, due to enzyme induction in the liver.

Protein binding of tetracycline and oxytetracycline in the serum: 40%; rolitetracycline: 50%; doxycycline: 96%; minocycline: 75%.

Good *tissue diffusion* in the liver, kidneys, spleen, bones, lungs and genital tract. High biliary concentration. 50–75% of the maternal serum concentration is found in the cord blood, 20% in the amniotic fluid and 50–100% in the breast milk. Effective tetracycline concentrations are achieved in the pleural, pericardial, peritoneal and synovial fluids.

CSF penetration: Poor (at 1–10% of serum concentrations), but 20–40% with minocycline and improved penetration with meningeal inflammation.

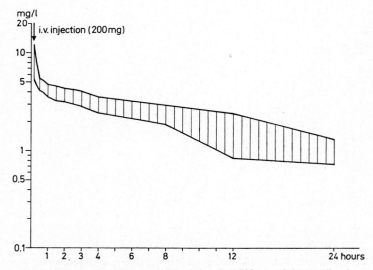

Fig. 21. Serum concentrations in 8 adults after 200 mg of doxycycline i. v.

Excretion of tetracycline and oxytetracycline is predominantly renal, mainly by glomerular filtration, at 10–25% after oral and 50–70% after i. v. administration. High urinary concentrations (50–300 mg/l). Delayed excretion of doxycycline and minocycline. *Urinary recovery* of doxycycline: 70% and 40% after i. v. and oral administration respectively; of minocycline: 5.9% and 5.5%. Urinary concentrations of doxycycline after 200 mg i. v. and orally: 60–200 mg/l; of minocycline after 200 mg orally: 4–25 mg/l. Because about 35% of absorbed minocycline is excreted into the intestines through the bile, more than 50% of the ingested antibiotic may be assumed to be metabolised in the body. The other tetracyclines are also excreted at high concentration in the bile when liver function is normal and the extrahepatic biliary tree is patent. They are then partly reabsorbed in the intestinal tract and partly metabolised in the body. After oral administration, the concentrations of tetracycline and oxytetracycline are particularly high in the faeces due to the incomplete absorption (200–2000 µg/g), while the better absorbed preparations (doxycycline and minocycline) are lost to a much lesser extent in the stools. Gastro-intestinal upset is therefore less common with these preparations, and they can be given in smaller doses.

Apart from doxycycline and minocycline, tetracyclines accumulate in *renal failure*. This can lead to liver damage and so require a reduction in dosage (see below). The half-life of doxycycline is prolonged to 15–24 hours according to the severity of renal failure, but repeated administration of the normal dose does not result in accumulation. The half-life of minocycline is prolonged in chronic renal failure.

Side effects:
1. *Gastrointestinal* upset with vomiting and diarrhoea due to irritation of the intestinal mucosa or disturbance of the gut flora. Stomatitis, glossitis, oesophagitis, proctitis, and vaginitis also occur. Pseudomembranous enterocolitis (caused by Clostridium difficile) is a rare but severe complication of tetracycline therapy and can develop after i. v. administration as well. It is doubtful whether the increased growth of candida in the intestines is the cause of gastrointestinal disturbances during tetracycline treatment. The prophylactic value of adding nystatin or amphotericin B to tetracycline preparations has not been established in comparative studies.
2. *Severe liver damage* can follow overdosage, particularly after parenteral administration in the third trimester of pregnancy or following the accumulation of tetracyclines in renal failure. The daily parenteral dose should not therefore exceed 750 mg (−1 g) of oxytetracycline or rolitetracycline, and 200 (−300) mg of doxycycline and minocycline. Special care is necessary during *pregnancy*. The combination of tetracyclines with other potentially

hepatotoxic drugs such as chlorpromazine, phenylhydantoin and phenyl-butazone derivatives should be avoided as far as possible.

3. *Photosensitivity* particularly occurs after demeclocycline which should there-fore not now be used. It may also occur with other tetracyclines but is rare with minocycline. Erythema and oedema are found on exposed areas of the body. Regression is slow, requiring 2–4 weeks, and residual pigmentation and detachment of the nails may persist. Exposure to the sun should therefore be avoided in patients receiving tetracycline therapy.

4. *Allergies* (rashes, anaphylactic shock) have only been observed rarely. There is cross-allergy between all the tetracyclines.

5. *Reversible leucocytopenia* due to allergic bone marrow depression is rare.

6. *The teeth of small children* can be stained yellow irreversibly, often with associated enamel defects and an increased tendency to caries. The tetra-cycline is deposited in the teeth, bones and nails as tetracycline calcium phosphate. Both deciduous and permanent teeth may be affected, depending on the phase of odontogenesis in which the tetracycline has been given between the 5th month of pregnancy and the end of the 6th year. Tetracycline should therefore be avoided between the 1st and 6th year and during pregnancy from the 5th month onward. Infants should only be given tetracycline where alternative drugs have failed and there are very clear indications for treatment. In such cases, the yellow discoloration of the teeth may have to be accepted. A temporary and completely reversible delay of bone growth in premature infants has only been observed when overdosage has been considerable.

7. Tetracycline therapy can give rise to a reversible increase in *intracranial pressure,* shown in the newborn as bulging of the fontanelle and as papilloedema in older children and adults, with visual disturbance and severe headache.

8. *Various types of renal damage* can occur, expressed either as deterioration of a pre-existing renal functional impairment and shown by an increase of serum creatinine and urea, or as renal damage associated with acute fatty change in the liver, also caused by tetracycline. A partially reversible *nephrogenic diabetes insipidus* which is resistant to vasopressin is occasionally caused by demeclocycline.

9. *Pseudoglycosuria:* Reduction tests (Fehling, Nylander) in the urine may be falsely positive at high tetracycline concentrations and, since polarisation analysis shows a substance which rotates to the right, may also simulate glycosuria.

10. Because of their magnesium content, some tetracycline derivatives for intravenous injection may cause cardiac arrhythmias in digitalised patients.

This can be avoided by injecting slowly over the recommended minimum period of 2 min. Injectable rolitetracycline, doxycycline and oxytetracycline are contra-indicated in myasthenia gravis on account of their magnesium content.

11. *Local irritation and phlebitis* sometimes complicate i. v. administration, and rapid injection can give rise to general symptoms such as dizziness, sweating, and circulatory collapse. Pain at the injection site commonly follows i. m. injection. *Ulceration of the oesophageal mucosa* has occasionally been reported after doxycycline and tetracycline capsules, but not tablets. This is mostly seen in patients with hiatus hernia.

12. Minocycline frequently causes *transient dizziness* at the onset of treatment, particularly in women, which is sometimes associated with drowsiness and nausea and may impair driving ability. It is probably due to central nervous system disturbance, and in some cases treatment has had to be stopped.

Main indications: Infections with sensitive gram-negative rods (Escherichia coli, Haemophilus influenzae, Bacteroides). Mixed infections originating in the mouth, throat or intestinal tract. Long-term treatment of chronic bronchitis, e. g. with one dose of doxycycline a day, which is well tolerated. Treatment of interstitial pneumonia with features suggestive of mycoplasma, ornithosis or Q-fever. Non-gonorrhoeal urethritis, due to Chlamydia trachomatis or Ureaplasma urealyticum. Infectious diseases such as brucellosis, tularaemia, plague, leptospirosis, lymphogranuloma inguinale, trachoma, cholera, rickettsiosis (typhus etc.), listeriosis, melioidosis (caused by Pseudomonas pseudomallei).

Other indications: Urinary infections, dysentery, enterococcal infections, syphilis and gonorrhoea in patients with penicillin allergy, acne and rosacea.

Inappropriate usage: Clinically typical or bacteriologically proven infections with staphylococci, streptococci, pneumococci or Pseudomonas aeruginosa, all of which are commonly resistant. Meningitis (poor CSF penetration). Typhoid fever (clinically ineffective although sensitive *in vitro*). Prophylactic administration in surgical operations (risk of staphylococcal or pseudomonas enterocolitis).

Caution is advised in pregnant women, particularly in the last trimester and in children up to 6 years because of the risk of yellow discoloration of the teeth. Caution also in patients with severe liver disease (risk of further hepatotoxicity), especially in acute hepatitis, as well as in renal failure.

Contra-indication: Myasthenia gravis (applies to all intravenous tetracyclines on account of their magnesium content).

Administration: Generally as coated tablets, film tablets or capsules after meals, and as syrup or drops in children. 3–4 divided doses are advised, except for demeclocycline and minocycline where 2 doses suffice, and doxycycline where one dose a day is enough. 1–2 single i. v. doses a day may be given to seriously ill patients and to those who cannot take the antibiotic by mouth. I. m. administration is possible but painful and has no particular advantage over the oral route. Continuous infusion of tetracycline hydrochloride is not recommended because of the high rate of phlebitis; it has been superceded by other injectable tetracyclines. Rolitetracycline can also be instilled intraperitoneally (150–500 mg in 5–20 ml) and intrapleurally (100–200 mg in 40–100 ml).

Dosage:
Oral: Doxycycline: 200 mg (4 mg/kg) on day 1, later reduced to 100 mg (2 mg/kg). Long-term treatment is also available in doses up to 200 mg a day (4 mg/kg) in severe infections. Minocycline 200 mg (4 mg/kg for children initially), then 100 mg every 12 h (or 2 mg/kg for children).

Tetracycline and oxytetracycline: 1–1.5 (−2) g, 20–30 mg/kg for children, in 2–4 divided doses 1 h before or 2 h after meals.

The possibility of intolerance means that the recommended dose should not be exceeded. It is not usually necessary to restrict treatment because of intolerance.

Intravenous: Doxycycline: 200 mg once a day initially followed by a maintenance dose of 100 (−200) mg as a slow i. v. injection; 2–4 mg/kg once a day for children. Minocycline: 200 mg a day for adults, 4 mg/kg for children, in 1 or 2 short i. v. infusions.

Rolitetracycline and oxytetracycline: 0.25–0.5 (−0.75) g a day in 2 (−3) divided doses, 10 mg/kg for children under 12 years (maximum single dose 100 mg). Because the preparations contain solubilisers and magnesium, injection must be slow (250 mg over at least 3 minutes). Do not mix with other drugs such as strophanthin.

Intramuscular: Rolitetracycline and oxytetracycline: 250–500 mg a day for adults, 10 mg/kg a day for children (maximum single dose 100 mg), given as 4 divided doses. Oxytetracycline depot injection: 250–500 mg in 1–2 (−4) divided doses (maximum single dose 250 mg), 10 mg/kg/per day for children.

Preparations:
Tetracycline: Coated tablets, capsules and tablets of 50 mg, 250 mg and 500 mg.
Oxytetracycline: Capsules and tablets of 50 mg, 250 mg and 500 mg.
Doxycycline and *minocycline:* Capsules and tablets of 50 mg and 100 mg.

For children: Drops or syrup. For i. v. injection: Ampoules of 100 mg, 250 mg and 275 mg. For i. v. infusion: Ampoules of 200 mg.

There are also many topical preparations which contain tetracycline.

Combined preparations: Tetracycline with oleandomycin (individual components underdosed), and combination of tetracyclines with other preparations, e. g. expectorants.

Summary:

Advantages: Broad spectrum of activity, resistance slow to develop during therapy, relatively favourable pharmacokinetics (good tissue diffusion), long-term therapy possible. Allergy very rare.

Disadvantages: Increasing resistance amongst the gram-negative bacilli, and only bacteriostatic at therapeutically attainable concentrations, so of no value as a single agent in the treatment of severe systemic infection before culture results are available. Should be avoided in late pregnancy and early childhood.

Doxycycline is preferred because it is well absorbed and tolerated and relatively little metabolised. If an intravenous tetracycline is necessary in severe infections or where oral administration is impossible, rolitetracycline, minocycline, or the i. v. forms of oxytetracycline and doxycycline are preferable to an oral tetracycline.

References

ALLEN, J. C.: Drugs five years later: Minocycline. Ann. intern. Med. *85:* 482 (1976).
ANDERSSON, K.-E., P. A. MARDH, M. ÅKERLUND: Passage of doxycycline into extracellular fluid. Scand. J. infect. Dis. *(Suppl.) 9:* 7 (1976).
ANDERSSON, H., K. ALESTIG: The penetration of doxycycline into CSF. Scand. J. infect. Dis. *(Suppl.) 9:* 17 (1976).
BROGAN, T. D., L. NEALE, H. C. RYLEY, B. H. DAVIES, J. CHARLES: The secretion of minocycline in sputum during therapy of bronchopulmonary infection in chronic chest diseases. J. Antimicrob. Chemother *3:* 247 (1977).
CAMMAN, U., W. STILLE: Tetracycline. Zuckschwerdt, Munich 1982.
CARRILHO, F., J. BOSCH, V. ARROYO, A. MAS, J. VIVER, J. RODES: Renal failure associated with demeclocycline in cirrhosis. Ann. intern. Med. *87:* 195 (1977).
CHOW, A. W., V. PATTERN, L. B. GUZE: Comparative susceptibility of anaerobic bacteria to minocycline, doxycycline, and tetracycline. Antimicrob. Ag. Chemother. *7:* 46 (1975).
DREW, T. M., R. ALTMAN, K. BLACK, M. GOLDFIELD: Minocycline for prophylaxis of infection with Neisseria meningitidis: High rate of side-effects in recipients. J. infect. Dis. *133:* 194 (1976).
FANNING, W. L., D. W. GUMP, R. A. SOFFERMAN: Side-effects of minocycline: A double blind study. Antimicrob. Ag. Chemother. *11:* 712 (1977).
GNARPE, H., K. DORNBUSCH, O. HÄGG: Doxycycline concentration levels in bone, soft tissue and serum after intravenous infusion of doxycycline. Scand. J. infect. Dis. *(Suppl.) 9:* 54 (1976).
GUMP, D. W., T. ASHIKAGA, T. J. FINK, A. M. RADIN: Side effects of minocycline: Different dosage regimens. Antimicrob. Ag. Chemother. *12:* 642 (1977).
HANSMAN, D.: Haemophilus influenzae typ b resistant to tetracycline. Lancet *2:* 893 (1975).
JACOBSON, J. A., B. DANIEL: Vestibular reactions associated with minocycline. Antimicrob. Ag. Chemother. *8:* 453 (1975).
NASH, P., L. SIDEMAN, V. PIDCOE, B. KLEGER: Minocycline in Legionnaires' disease. Lancet *1:* 45 (1978).
NEUVONEN, P. J., O. PENTTILÄ: Interaction between doxycycline and barbiturates. Brit. med. J. *1:* 535 (1974).

PENTTILÄ, O., P. J. NEUVONEN, K. AHO, R. LEHTOVAARA: Interaction between doxycycline and some antiepileptic drugs. Brit. med. J. *2:* 470 (1974).

PHILIPS, M. E., J. B. EASTWOOD, J. R. CURTIS, P. E. GOWER, H. E. DE WARDENER: Tetracycline poisoning in renal failure. Brit. med. J. *2:* 149 (1974).

SIMON, C., V. MALERCZYK, H. ENGELKE, I. PREUSS, H. GRAHMANN, K. SCHMIDT: Die Pharmakokinetik von Doxycyclin bei Niereninsuffizienz und geriatrischen Patienten im Vergleich zu jüngeren Erwachsenen. Schweiz. med. Wschr. *105:* 1615 (1975).

SIMON, C., V. MALERCZYK, J. PREUSS, K. SCHMIDT, H. GRAHMANN: In-vitro-Aktivität und Pharmakokinetik von Minocyclin. Arzneimittel-Forsch. *26:* 556 (1976).

SIMON, C., D. SOMMERWERCK, J. FRIEDHOFF: Der Wert von Doxycyclin bei Atemwegsinfektionen (Serum-, Speichel-, Sputum-, Lungen-, Pleuraexsudatspiegel). Praxis und Klinik der Pneumonologie *32:* 217 (1978).

SKLENAR, I., P. SPRING, L. DETTLI: One-dose and multiple-dose kinetics of minocycline in patients with renal disease. Ag. Act. *7/3:* 367 (1977).

SOMMERWERCK, D., C. SIMON, J. FRIEHOFF: Minocyclin zur Therapie von Atemwegsinfektionen (Sputum-, Pleuraexsudat- und Lungenspiegel). Dtsch. med. Wschr. *103:* 822 (1978).

STENBAEK, Ø., E. MYHRE, B. P. BERDAL: The effect of doxycycline on renal function in patients with advanced renal insufficiency. Scand. J. infect. Dis. *5:* 199 (1973).

WHELTON, A., M. SCHACH VON WITTENAU, T. M. TWOMEY, W. G. WALKER, J. R. BIANCHINE: Doxycycline pharmacokinetics in the absence of renal function. Kidney Int. *5:* 365 (1974).

WILLIAMS, D. N., L. W. LAUGHLIN, LEE YHU-HSIUMG: Minocycline: possible vestibular side-effects. Lancet *2:* 744 (1974).

5. Chloramphenicol Group

a) Chloramphenicol

Proprietary names: Chloromycetin, Paraxin.

Properties: p-Nitrophenyl-diochloracetyl-aminopropanediol. Unrelated to other antibiotics except thiamphenicol. Chloramphenicol is a very bitter, stable and poorly water-soluble compound. Chloramphenicol palmitate and stearoyl glycollate are insoluble in water and have no taste, so can be used in syrup. Chloramphenicol succinate is water-soluble and so suitable for parenteral administration. Phenylalanine in the culture medium antagonises the *in vitro* sensitivity of chloramphenicol and can therefore show false resistance.

Mode of action: Bacteriostatic on extra- and intracellular bacteria. Inhibits bacterial protein synthesis by blocking the transfer of soluble ribonucleic acid to ribosomes.

Spectrum of activity: Activity against most gram-positive and gram-negative bacteria as well as against rickettsiae (typhus), spirochaetes, chlamydiae, mycoplasmas, leptospiras, and Bacteroides (including B. fragilis). A variable number of strains of Staphylococcus aureus, Escherichia coli, Klebsiella, Enterobacter, Proteus, Salmonella, Shigella and Vibrio cholerae are chloramphenicol-resistant. Resistant strains have also been found occasionally in Haemophilus influenzae, pneumococci and meningococci. Mycobacteria, nocardia, fungi, protozoa and viruses are always resistant, as are most strains of Pseudomonas aeruginosa.

Resistance: Slight tendency for resistance to develop during therapy. Generally no cross-resistance with other antibiotics, except thiamphenicol.

Pharmacokinetics:
Rapid and almost complete *absorption* (90%) after oral administration which depends on particle size. Blood concentrations are 2–4 times higher with small particles. Maximal serum concentrations after 2–4 hours. Chloramphenicol is available as two antibacterially inactive esters, the palmitate (a suspension) and the stearoyl glycollate (a powder). They are hydrolysed in the gastrointestinal tract by esterases and lipases prior to absorption, and active chloramphenicol is released. Non-esterified chloramphenicol is preferable in patients with difficulties in digestion or enzyme deficiencies. Chloramphenicol monosuccinate sodium (antibacterially inactive) is rapidly absorbed after i. m. administration (maximum blood level after 1–2 h) and transformed into free chloramphenicol by hydrolysis in the liver.

Serum concentrations after repeated oral doses of 500 mg: 4–6 mg/l; after repeated doses of 1 g: 10–20 mg/l (Fig. 22). Values between 5–9 mg/l (after 1–2 h) are obtained after i. v. injection of 500 mg; 4–6 mg/l (after 3–4 h), 3–4 mg/l (after 5–7 h) and 3 mg/l (after 8—10 h). *Half-life:* 3 hours. *Binding* to *serum protein:* approx. 50%.

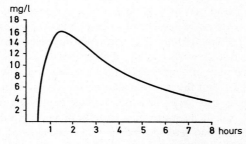

Fig. 22. Blood concentration curve after 1 g of chloramphenicol orally as a dispersible capsule.

Chloramphenicol is mostly present in the active form in the blood. It is partially inactivated in the body by binding to glucuronic acid (10% in serum, 90% in urine), and also by hydrolysis and reduction of the nitro compound to amine.

Good tissue diffusion in all organs. 50% of the serum concentrations are found in the CSF, also in the pleural, peritoneal and synovial fluids. In meningitis, the CSF concentration can increase to the level of the serum concentrations. Therapeutically effective concentrations are also found in the aqueous and vitreous humors. 30–80% of the maternal serum values are found in the cord blood and amniotic fluid, 0–50% in the breast milk.

Excretion: Predominantly through the kidneys (up to 90%) by glomerular filtration of free chloramphenicol (5–10%) and tubular secretion of the inactive glucuronides (about 90%). Urinary free chloramphenicol concentrations between 70 and 150 mg/l when 500 mg are given every 6 hours. Inactive metabolites accumulate in renal failure, but the serum concentrations of free chloramphenicol do not rise markedly. In patients with severe liver damage, the half-life of free chloramphenicol is prolonged up to 6 hours because of the reduced binding to glucuronic acid.

A small amount is excreted through the bile (concentrations of active chloramphenicol about 20–50% of serum concentrations); only very small amounts pass out with the faeces.

Side effects: *Aplastic blood dyscrasias* are the most dangerous side effects of chloramphenicol. They almost always occur as irreversible pancytopenia or aplastic anaemia, leukopenia or thrombocytopenia, or a combination of these disorders. They mostly occur after a later period of 2–8 weeks and are fatal in more than 50% of cases.

It is difficult to obtain reliable information about the frequency of aplastic chloramphenicol blood dyscrasias. An American survey of 1967 reviewed 408 cases from different countries over 11 years where bone marrow suppression was clearly associated with chloramphenicol. The published figures range between 1:5000–10000 and 1:40000–100000. The frequency increased with increasing total dosage, but blood disorders also followed short courses of treatment. Genetic factors (e. g. an inherited enzyme defect) may play a role in the development of these blood dyscrasias, but the precise cause has not so far been found.

Minor disturbances also occur, such as reversible depression of erythropoiesis, accompanied by a fall in haemoglobin, vacuolisation of pro-erythroblasts and granulocyte precursors and leukocytopenia. The reduced utilisation of iron in haemoglobin synthesis causes the serum iron to rise. The cause of these toxic disturbances is the inhibition of protein synthesis by the action of chloramphenicol on messenger RNA, and they appear regularly when serum concentrations exceed 25 mg/l.

Mild gastrointestinal symptoms such as flatulence and loose stools are quite common but not dangerous.

Allergies occur only rarely.

"Grey baby" syndrome. Newborn babies and premature infants treated with doses of more than 25 mg/kg may react with vomiting, meteorism, hypothermia, respiratory problems, grey skin coloration and uncontrolled circulatory collapse. These symptoms are often fatal within a few hours and result from the toxic accumulation of chloramphenicol which is not adequately conjugated to glucuronic acid in the immature liver for excretion in the urine. In such cases, the half-life is 6–7 times longer than usual.

Optic neuritis and peripheral neuritis: Very rare side effects, found particularly after long-term treatment of children with chloramphenicol for recurrent pulmonary infection in cystic fibrosis; vision sometimes returns after discontinuation of the antibiotic and treatment with large doses of vitamin B.

Indications: Typhoid and paratyphoid fevers (A and B), salmonella septicaemia and meningitis, haemophilus meningitis (particularly where ampicillin-resistant), Escherichia coli meningitis (when proved sensitive), purulent meningitis before culture results are available, peritonitis, intraocular infections, life-threatening infections with agents resistant to other antibiotics. Other former indications have been largely superceded by the new cephalosporins (e. g. cefotaxime). The position of the cheap and stable chloramphenicol is more important in many developing countries with restricted supply of other agents. Here it still belongs to the WHO list of essential drugs.

Inappropriate use: Infections against which other, less dangerous antibiotics are also effective; infections where bactericidal therapy is important (endocarditis, osteomyelitis, salmonella carriage); topical instillation of inactive chloramphenicol succinate which is only activated after i. v. administration when it is hydrolysed in the liver.

Contra-indications: Blood diseases like aplastic anaemia or pancytopenia; severe liver failure with jaundice. Combination with other potentially haematotoxic preparations (e. g. cytotoxic drugs, sulphonamides, phenothiazine, phenylbutazone, hydantoin etc.). The dose should be restricted in premature and full-term neonates.

Administration: Usually oral, as a syrup for children. I. v. for unconscious and seriously ill patients, as 10–20% chloramphenicol succinate solution. Topical administration of free chloramphenicol for infections of the skin, eyes and ears. Intramuscular and rectal administration is not recommended (absorption unreliable).

Dosage: *Adults:* 1.5–3 g a day in 3–4 divided doses. Do not give less than the minimum dose of 1.5 g. The same dose is used orally and parenterally, because chloramphenicol is almost completely absorbed. *Children and infants:* 50(−80) mg/kg a day, usually as a syrup or parenterally. *Neonates:* in 1st–2nd week: 25 mg/kg/day, in 3rd–4th week: 50 mg/kg/day, in two or three divided doses. Some authors (DAVIES) recommend 25 mg/kg/day for premature neonates in the first month of life, and 37.5–50 mg/kg/day for term neonates older than 7 days. MULHALL, de LOUVOIS, and HURLEY also recommend this dosage, supported by regular serum chloramphenicol assay every 48–72 hours to ensure that peak concentrations are in the range 20–30 mg/l, and trough concentrations remain less than 15 mg/l.

The total dose should generally be limited to 25–30 g for adults and 700 mg/kg for children, and should only be exceeded in life-threatening disease. Treatment with chloramphenicol should not, therefore, normally last longer than 14 days, except in neonatal septicaemia and meningitis where up to 3 weeks may be necessary. If the total dose is exceeded, the blood count, platelet and reticulocyte counts should be checked frequently. Regular tests are also advisable to detect any fall in haematocrit or increase in serum iron, so that treatment can be stopped immediately at the first sign of incipient blood disease. Bone-marrow depression, which usually develops only after a latent period, cannot be identified in time with this method. Dosage and length of treatment are not restricted in topical therapy with eye drops, ear drops or skin ointments.

Preparations: For *oral administration:* capsules of 250 mg, 330 mg and 500 mg, and coated tablets of 50 mg and 250 mg of chloramphenicol (non-esterified), as a paediatric syrup of 25 mg/ml chloramphenicol, either as the palmitate or the stearoyl glycollate.
Parenteral administration: as chloramphenicol succinate in 10–20% solution for slow i. v. injection but not i. v. infusion. *Topical chloramphenicol* as a skin (2%) and ophthalmic (1%) ointment and as ear drops (5%) may be used without reservation.

Summary: No longer considered for routine clinical use because of its rare but irreversible bone marrow toxicity. It is malpractice to give chloramphenicol systemically without clear indications of a potentially life-threatening condition, but this antibiotic is still very valuable in such circumstances. The total dose of 25–30 g in adults should not be exceeded.

References

CAVANAGH, P., C. A. MORRIS, N. J. MITCHELL: Chloramphenicol resistance in Haemophilus species. Lancet 1: 696 (1975).
DAVIES, P. A.: Neonatal bacterial meningitis. Brit. J. Hosp. Med. 18: 425 (1977).
HUGHES, D. W.: Studies on chloramphenicol. II. Possible determinants and progress of haemopoietic toxicity during chloramphenicol therapy. Med. J. Aust. 2: 1142 (1973).
KINMONTH, A. L., C. N. STORRS, R. G. MITCHELL: Meningitis due to chloramphenicol-resistant Haemophilus influenzae type b. Brit. med. J. 1: 694 (1978).
MULHALL, A., J. DE LOUVOIS, R. HURLEY: Efficacy of chloramphenicol in the treatment of neonatal and infantile meningitis: a study of 70 cases. Lancet I: 284 (1983).
OLES, A., B. STANIO-PYRKOSZ: Chloromycetin resistance of Salmonella typhi strains isolated from carriers and cases of typhoid fever. J. Hyg. Epid. Microb. Immunol. 8: 169 (1964).
SHAW, W. V., D. H. BOUANCHAUD, F. W. GOLDSTEIN: Mechanism of transferable resistance to chloramphenicol in Haemophilus parainfluenzae. Antimicrob. Ag. Chemother. 13: 326 (1978).

b) Thiamphenicol

Proprietary names: Fluimucil Antibiotic and Urfamycine. Thiamphenicol (methylsulphonylamphenicol) is an analogue of chloramphenicol and its *antimicrobial spectrum* is similar. It is less active, differs in *pharmacokinetic properties* (slower absorption, delayed excretion in the non-conjugated form, higher concentrations in urine and bile).

Side effects, indications: Careful haematological investigations show thiamphenicol to have more acute haematotoxicity than chloramphenicol, expressed as impaired erythropoiesis and inhibition of haemoglobin synthesis. With sensitive methods, this reversible depression of red-cell formation can be demonstrated in almost all patients treated with thiamphenicol, which has a valuable role, therefore, in the treatment of polycythaemia rubra vera. Despite its frequent use in Italy and France, irreversible bone marrow aplasia has not so far described. A short course of thiamphenicol may be justified in severe infections (e. g. acute pyelonephritis due to agents resistant to other antibiotics) and with regular blood counts. Treatment longer than 2 weeks is *strictly contra-indicated.* Thiamphenicol can be inhaled in combination with the mucolytic agent acetyl cysteine without the risk of blood dyscrasias.

Preparations: Capsules and tablets of 250 mg and 500 mg; a syrup containing 25 mg/ml and ampoules of 250, 500 and 750 mg.

References

AZZOLINI, F., A. GAZZANIGA, E. LODOLA: Thiamphenicol excretion in subjects with renal insufficiency. Int. Z. klin. Pharmakol. Ther. Toxikol. *3:* 303 (1970).

CORCOS, A., J. LEBEAU: Sur un cas d'agranulocytose transitoire par thiamphenicol. Sem. Hôp. Paris *47:* 1579 (1971).

DETTLI, L., P. SPRING: The dosage regimen of thiamphenicol in patients with kidney disease. Postgrad. med. J. *(Suppl. 5) 50:* 32 (1974).

HANSMAN, D.: Chloramphenicol-resistant pneumococci in West Africa. Lancet *1:* 1102 (1978).

KALTWASSER, B. SIMON, E. WERNER, U. LEUSCHNER, M. KHAN, H.-J. BECKER, W. STILLE: Hämatologische Nebenwirkungen von Thiamphenicol. Klin. Wschr. *51:* 347 (1973).

6. Aminoglycosides

Streptamine, desoxystreptamine, and certain other aminocyclitols are the common components of the aminoglycoside antibiotics which include kanamycin, neomycin, paromomycin, streptomycin, spectinomycin, gentamicin, tobramycin, sisomicin, dibekacin, netilmicin etc.

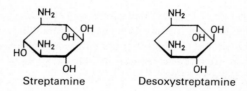

Streptamine   Desoxystreptamine

Mode of action: Glycosides are formed by the linkage of various naturally occurring sugars through hydroxyl groups. They show a certain degree of variation in their antibacterial activity and spectrum of action. Aminoglycosides formed by Streptomyces species are named with *"mycin"* as the last syllable, whereas those produced by Micromonospora species are designated *"micin"*. They are all broadspectrum, bactericidal antibiotics which inhibit the protein synthesis of grampositive and gram-negative bacteria.

Spectrum of action: Aminoglycosides generally have little activity against streptococci, Haemophilus influenzae or the non-sporing anaerobes (e. g. Bacteroides species). The antibacterial activity of the older aminoglycosides such as streptomycin, neomycin, and kanamycin is much poorer than that of newer aminoglycosides such as gentamicin, tobramycin, and amikacin. Amikacin has the advantage of retaining activity against the majority of gentamicin- and tobramycin-resistant strains. All the aminoglycosides are more active against proliferating bacteria than during the resting phase. Aminoglycosides are inactivated by certain bacterial enzymes through adenylation, phosphorylation and/or acetylation. This accounts for the incomplete cross-resistance in this group.

Aminoglycosides all have similar **pharmacokinetic properties** inasmuch as they are virtually not absorbed after oral administration and can be oto- and nephrotoxic when given parenterally.

a) Kanamycin

Properties: A very stable aminoglycoside, the sulphate of which is soluble in water. Bactericidal predominantly against actively proliferating bacteria.

Spectrum of activity: Active against staphylococci, Escherichia coli, Enterobacter aerogenes, Klebsiella pneumoniae and some strains of Proteus and Serratia. Streptococci (including enterococci), Bacteroides, clostridia, fungi, and most strains of Pseudomonas aeruginosa are resistant. Primary *resistance* with Escherichia coli and other gram-negative rods occurs frequently. Resistance can also arise during therapy. Cross-resistance is complete with neomycin and paromomycin and partial with streptomycin and gentamicin.

Preparations: Kanamycin has been largely superceded by other, more active and less toxic aminoglycosides for systemic use. In Britain, though no longer in Germany, however, a solution of kanamycin sulphate for injection is still available in two strengths of 250 mg/l (Kannasyn) and 333 mg/l (Kantrex). Capsules of 250 mg are also available for oral use, although there is no absorption by this route. In Germany, kanamycin is available commercially only as a skin ointment (Kanamyson), an ophthalmic ointment (Kanamytrex) and eye drops. These topical preparations are not available in the United Kingdom.

b) Neomycin

Properties: Neomycin B is identical with framycetin and is a topical, bactericidal antibiotic which is soluble in water and largely stable.

Principal activity is against gram-negative bacteria including salmonellae, shigellae, some strains of Proteus and Escherichia coli, but very rarely against Pseudomonas aeruginosa. Some staphylococci are sensitive but streptococci and enterococci are resistant. *Resistance* develops slowly in stages. Cross-resistance is complete with kanamycin and paromomycin and partial with streptomycin and gentamicin.

Little or no *absorption* after oral intake.

Side effects: Parenteral use is *contraindicated* because of the considerable *oto- and nephrotoxicity*. Sufficient absorption can also take place from extensive wounds and gastric or duodenal ulcers to create a risk of side effects. If high doses of neomycin are given for long periods during hepatic coma, small amounts can be absorbed from the bowel and, if there is simultaneous renal failure, accumulate and lead to deafness. Allergic skin rashes (contact dermatitis) are not uncommon with topical administration. Neomycin releases histamine from most cells *in vitro* and *in vivo*. An overgrowth of candida in the bowel sometimes follows oral administration and results in diarrhoea; prophylactic nystatin is therefore recommended. Severe enterocolitis caused by neomycin-resistant staphylococci has been observed after pre-operative preparation (sometimes mis-named "sterilisation") of the large intestine. A malabsorption syndrome with diarrhoea and steatorrhoea can result from mucosal damage after giving high doses by mouth for a long period. It is generally reversible after treatment has stopped.

Topical administration:
1. As an *ointment, spray, solution, eye and ear drops* and *ophthalmic ointment* for superficial infections of the skin and mucous membranes. Because of the risk of absorption, a maximum total topical dose of 15 mg/kg/day should not be exceeded; length of treatment: 1–3 days; reduce dose over longer periods.
2. *Instillation:* No longer necessary since effective antibiotics are now available which penetrate body cavities well. There is a risk of neuromuscular blockade (apnoea) with intraperitoneal and intrapleural instillation, particularly when muscle relaxants are given at the same time. *Antidote:* prostigmine and calcium gluconate i. v.
3. *Oral administration* for "bacterial diarrhoea" is no longer justifiable because of the lack of clinical effect and risk of side effects. Do not give to patients with ileus or renal failure because small quantities of neomycin absorbed from the bowel can accumulate. Neomycin is still used occasionally as part of the surgical bowel preparation (sometimes misnamed "sterilisation") prior to intestinal operations, in leukaemia and hepatic coma. Dosage: 2–4 g orally for adults, 30–60 mg/kg for children, in 4–6 divided doses, possibly in combination with nystatin (against candida).

Proprietary preparations: Framycin spray, Framygen, Graneodin, Myciguent, Myacine comp. (with formophthalylsulphacarbamide), Cysto-Myacine (with sulphaurea for bladder irrigation), Neomycin solution, Soframycin (framycetin with gramicidin), Batrax, Cicatrin and Nebacetin (in combination with bacitracin), Dispray Antibiotic, Polybactrin, Polyspectran and Tribiotic (in combination with polymyxin B and bacitracin) etc. A frequent additive in ointments containing corticosteroids.

References

BREEN, L. J., R. E. BRYANT, J. D. LEVINSON, S. SCHENKER: Neomycin absorption in man. Ann. intern. Med. 76: 211 (1972).
CLARK, L. W.: Neomycin in the prevention of postcatheterization bacteriuria. Med. J. Aust. 1: 1034 (1973).
WEINSTEIN, A. J., M. McHENRY, T. L. GAVAN: Systemic absorption of neomycin irrigating solution. JAMA 238: 152 (1977).

c) Paromomycin

Brand names: Humatin, Paromomycin. Not marketed in Great Britain.

A bactericidal aminoglycoside antibiotic, identical with *aminosidin* and *catenulin,* which is soluble in water as paromomycin base and should be used topically only.

Activity against Escherichia coli, Enterobacter aerogenes, Klebsiella pneumoniae, salmonellae, shigellae, Proteus and staphylococci. Paromomycin has little activity against Pseudomonas. Clostridia, streptococci, fungi and viruses are resistant. Hospital strains of resistant intestinal bacteria have been found. Cross-resistance is found with kanamycin, neomycin and partially with streptomycin also.

Unlike other aminoglycosides, paromomycin is active against Entamoeba histolytica and some helminths, particularly Taenia solium and T. saginata. Good results have been reported in the treatment of amoebic dysentery.

Absorption: Very little after oral administration.

Side effects: Parenteral use is contraindicated because of oto- and nephrotoxicity. Minor gastro-intestinal disorders can occur after oral administration.

Administration: For bacterial enterocolitis (no longer recommended as is neomycin): as capsules, syrup, powder. *Adults:* 1–2 g daily, *children:* 50 mg/kg daily, in 3–4 divided doses for 7 days. Also for preoperative intestinal preparation.

Reference

TANOWITZ, H. B., M. WITTNER: Paromomycin in the treatment of Diphyllobothrium latum infections. J. Trop. Med. 76: 151 (1973).

d) Gentamicin

Proprietary names: Bristagen, Cidomycin, Garamycin, Genticin, Gentigan, Retobacin, Sulmycin.

Description: Gentamicin (sometimes mis-spelled gentamycin) is an alkaline aminoglycoside complex of various fractions, the principal ones of which are C_1 and C_2. They are all water-soluble and stable.

Mode of action: Bactericidal activity in both the log and the lag phases of bacterial growth. Gentamicin potentiates *in vitro* the bactericidal activity of penicillins and cephalosporins even at low concentrations.

Spectrum of activity: Good activity against most strains of Pseudomonas aeruginosa, staphylococci, Enterobacter aerogenes, Klebsiella pneumoniae, Escherichia coli, Proteus vulgaris, uncommon species of Enterobacteriaceae, Serratia, Yersinia, pasteurellae, brucellae and campylobacters; moderate activity on gonococci, Listeria, Haemophilus influenzae, Proteus mirabilis and salmonellae. Group A streptococci, pneumococci, enterococci, meningococci, clostridia, Bacteroides species, Nocardia asteroides, Pseudomonas maltophilia and Pseudomonas pseudomallei are all relatively resistant. Marked synergistic activity is found with azlo- and piperacillin against Pseudomonas, with ampicillin against enterococci and with cephalosporins against Klebsiella.

Resistance: Primary resistance in gram-negative bacilli is rare but has become more frequent recently, especially in hospitals, where outbreaks of infection with gentamicin-resistant staphylococci, Serratia marcescens and Pseudomonas aeruginosa have been observed. Development of resistance during therapy is extremely rare. Partial cross-resistance is found with tobramycin, sisomicin, netilmicin, neomycin, kanamycin, amikacin, streptomycin and paromomycin. Gentamicin-resistant strains of Pseudomonas are now found with a frequency of 0.1–5% but are often still sensitive to tobramycin and amikacin.

Pharmacokinetics: Little *absorption* after oral and topical administration (up to 2% in gastro-enteritis); rapid absorption after i. m. administration. Maximal blood concentrations after 1 hour.
  Serum concentrations (Fig. 23): Maxima of 2.8 mg/l after 40 mg i. m. (0.5 mg/l after 6 h); and of 5.1 mg/l after 80 mg i. m. (0.6 mg/l after 6 h).
  Continuous i. v. infusion of 6.6 mg/h (i. e. 160 mg/24 h) gives a *blood concentration* of 1 mg/l. *Half-life:* 1½ h. No *plasma protein binding.* Cerebrospinal fluid penetration is very poor. Gentamicin diffuses into bronchial secretions and some passes into the fetal circulation. 30–50% of serum concentrations are found in pleural, peritoneal and synovial fluids.

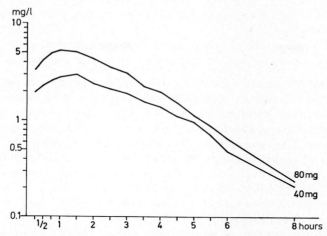

Fig. 23. Mean serum concentration-time curve in adults after 40 and 80 mg of gentamicin i. m.

Excretion: 85–95% in active form through the kidneys within 24 hours, predominantly by glomerular filtration. Urine concentrations in the first 3 hours are 60–115 mg/l after 40 mg i. m. and 90–500 mg/l after 80 mg i. m. As with other aminoglycosides, gentamicin is excreted in low concentrations in the urine for up to 1 month after the end of treatment (renal storage). A small amount passes out with the bile.

Side effects:
1. *Vestibular damage* (dizziness, tinnitus, spontaneous or provocation nystagmus, Menière's disease) and *lesions of the acoustic nerves* can occur when renal function is impaired or dosage is excessive (see below). Caloric tests show little or no excitability and audiometry shows loss of hearing at high frequencies, although speech is heard normally until very late.
2. *Nephrotoxicity* is detected by oliguria and the presence of casts, protein and enzymes in the urine, and increased concentrations of creatinine and uric acid in the blood. It is commoner at persistent high dosage and where there is pre-existent renal disease. Deposits in the renal cortex can lead at very high dosage to acute tubular necrosis. Combination with large doses of cephalothin and cephaloridine can be acutely nephrotoxic under certain circumstances such as shock, and the simultaneous administration of powerful diuretics such as frusemide and ethacrynic acid. The newer cephalosporins such as cefuroxime,

cefamandole and cefotaxime are much less likely to potentiate the nephrotoxicity of aminoglycosides.

3. *Allergic reactions,* such as rashes, urticaria and laryngeal oedema, are uncommon. Cross-resistance with other aminoglycosides (e. g. neomycin) is found.

Indications: Treatment of severe bacterial infections (pneumonia, septicaemia, peritonitis etc.) caused by susceptible gram-negative aerobic bacilli such as Enterobacteriaceae, Pseudomonas, Serratia. Gentamicin should be combined with azlocillin or piperacillin for severe infections with Pseudomonas aeruginosa, and with these or with one or more of the following antibiotics where the causative organism is not known, or likely to be mixed (e. g. faecal peritonitis, cholecystitis, other gut-related sepsis): metronidazole or clindamycin (for non-sporing anaerobes), or a cephalosporin of the cefotaxime group (see p. 87).

Gentamicin alone may be used in urinary infections with otherwise resistant bacteria (e. g. Pseudomonas) in hospital patients, but is not advised for such infections in the presence of an indwelling urinary catheter unless secondary septicaemia supervenes.

Preparations for topical use are available but are not recommended for the treatment of infected wounds, burns, chronic varicose ulcers, pressure sores, or chronic otitis media by this route since much use in hospitals encourages the development of resistance to aminoglycosides in Pseudomonas and other gram-negative organisms. Severe infections at such sites should be treated systemically; otherwise a local antiseptic (e. g. silver nitrate) or non-systemic antibiotic (e. g. neomycin, framycetin) should be used.

Incorrect use: Parenteral use in infections which should respond readily to less toxic antibiotics. Gentamicin should not be used alone in life-threatening infections, but should be combined as above.

Contra-indications: *Pregnancy* is a relative contra-indication because of the risk of ototoxicity in the fetus, although gentamicin crosses the placenta poorly and this risk is theoretical only when short or standard courses of treatment are given. Gentamicin should not, therefore, be withheld from a pregnant mother with a life-threatening infection, e. g. septicaemia. Do not combine with other potentially nephrotoxic antibiotics such as other aminoglycosides or, where avoidable, with rapidly acting diuretics such as frusemide (Lasix) or ethacrynic acid, since these potentiate the neurotoxicity.

Administration and dosage: Rapid i. v. injection results in brief but high peak concentrations which may enhance toxicity, though this is not proven. Slow intravenous injection, short i. v. infusion or i. m. injection are therefore preferred. Where the infection is caused by a very sensitive organism, doses of 80 mg

Table 18. Gentamicin dosage in renal failure.

Creatinine clearance (ml/min)	Serum creatinine (μmol/l)	Serum urea (mmol/l)	Dose interval (h)	Single dose
>70	<125	<3	8	
35–70	125–170	3–5	12	
24–34	171–250	5–6.5	18	
16–23	251–330	6.5–8	24	1 mg/kg
10–15	331–470	8–12.5	36	
5–9	471–640	12.5–17.0	48	

(approximately 1 mg/kg) every 12 hours may suffice, but should be given every 8 hours for less sensitive infections (normally 2–3 mg/kg/day for 7–10 days). In severe or life-threatening infections, give up to 5 mg/kg/day in 3 divided doses. The use of higher doses has been reported but carries an increased risk of ototoxicity, and lower doses may suffice when synergistic combinations with β-lactam antibiotics are used. Renal, auditory and vestibular function should be regularly checked when high doses are used for long periods. In renal failure, the single dose of 1 mg/kg (generally 80 mg in adults) should be given at longer intervals in relation to the severity of the renal impairment (Table 18). A useful guide to dosage based on body weight, age, sex, and plasma creatinine has been published by G. H. MAWER in the form of a nomogram which predicts the initial or loading dose, the maintenance dose and the appropriate dose interval.

Whenever gentamicin or another aminoglycoside is used, even where dosage has been based on a nomogram, serum concentrations should be assayed regularly to ensure that the maximal concentrations (peaks) lie within the therapeutic range (5–12 mg/l) and the troughs immediately prior to a dose are less than 2 mg/l, and preferably less than 1 mg/l. Peaks higher than 12 mg/l are in themselves less important associations with oto- or nephrotoxicity than high or progressively increasing troughs, which indicate accumulation. Aminoglycoside assays are now performed by most clinical microbiology departments either by conventional microbiological methods or by radio- or enzyme immunoassay. The frequency of assay depends on the patient's renal function and should be controlled where possible by a physician or microbiologist with the necessary experience.

Gentamicin is dialysable and can be given in a dose of 1 mg/kg at the end of each dialysis when two haemodialyses are performed each week. Intraperitoneal administration carries the risk of neuromuscular blockade with respiratory arrest while under anaesthetic, by functioning as a membrane stabiliser in the same way as curare.

Intrathecal instillation (more effective by the intraventricular than the intralumbar route): 5 mg for adults and 0.5–1 mg for the newborn and infants, of a preparation specifically for intrathecal administration which is free of the usual solvents. A solution of 5 mg/ml of gentamicin can be instilled intratracheally after each tracheal aspiration in patients on long-term ventilation. Subconjunctival injection for Pseudomonas infections of the eye is also possible. Gentamicin should not be mixed in vitro with other preparations, e.g. azlocillin, heparin, vitamins, because of the danger of mutual inactivation.

Gentamicin-PMMA-beads with a diameter of 7 mm can be used for the topical treatment of bone and soft-tissue infections. They consist of the tissue-compatible PMMA (polymethylmethacrylate) and the x-ray contrast medium zirconium dioxide (Septopal). The beads, which are implanted into the bone or soft-tissue defect, each contain 7.5 mg of gentamicin sulphate which is slowly released in bactericidal concentrations by diffusion. The beads are wired together as a chain which is inserted into the bone cavity. The last bead protrudes from the wound which has been closed by a suture. A tube drain without suction allows any exudate to escape. The beads can be removed without an anaesthetic during the first 2 weeks. In some cases, the beads can be implanted permanently within the bone as treatment of chronic and post-traumatic osteomyelitis and of infected osteosynthesis. The beads, which are available either loose or as a chain, can also be inserted in abscess cavities and infected soft-tissue lesions. Toxic side effects do not arise since only very low gentamicin concentrations are detected in the serum. The beads are assembled on a wire containing chromium and nickel, and topical hypersensitivity reactions have been reported. A bone cement containing gentamicin for prosthetic implants is also available combined with Palacos R, a radio-opaque synthetic cement which is used to fix internal prostheses into the bone at the hip, knees and other arthroplasties. Gentamicin has antimicrobial activity at the site of implantation and is used for the prophylaxis of infections.

Preparations: Ampoules of 10, 40, 80 and 120 mg for injection, ampoules for intrathecal instillation of 1 mg and 5 mg, skin ointment and powder, ophthalmic solution and ointment, gentamicin-PMMA beads and chains (Septopal), and gentamicin-Palacos bone cement.

Summary: The advantages of gentamicin are its broad spectrum of activity (including Pseudomonas aeruginosa and staphylococci) and its bactericidal action. It is not active against streptococci or anaerobes and has weak activity against Haemophilus. Its main uses are in combination with other antibiotics in septicaemia (particularly where gut-related) and endocarditis, gram-negative pneumonia and alone in severe urinary infections with susceptible organisms. Gentamicin is the standard aminoglycoside in use at present.

References

APPEL, G. B., H. C. NEU: The nephrotoxicity of antimicrobial agents (second of three parts). New Engl. J. Med. *296:* 722 (1977).

BYGBJERG, I. C., R. MØLLER: Gentamicin-induced nephropathy. Scand. J. infect. Dis. *8:* 203 (1976).

ECHEVERRIA, P., G. R. SIBER, J. PAISLEY, A. L. SMITH, N. JAFFE: Age-dependent dose response to gentamicin. J. Pediat. *87:* 805 (1975).

EDWARDS, C. O., C. R. SMITH, K. L. BAUGHMAN, J. F. ROGERS, P. S. LIETMAN: Concentrations of gentamicin and amikacin in human kidneys. Antimicrob. Ag. Chemother *9:* 925 (1976).

GARY, N. E., L. BUZZEO, J. SALAKI, R. P. EISINGER: Gentamicin-associated acute renal failure. Arch. intern. Med. *136:* 1101 (1976).

HALPREN, B. A., S. G. AXLINE, N. S. COPLON, D. M. BROWN: Clearance of gentamicin during hemodialysis: Comparison of four artificial kidneys. J. infect. Dis. *133:* 627 (1976).

HYAMS, P. J., T. SMITHIVAS, R. MATALON, L. KATZ, M. S. SIMBERKOFF, J. J. RAHAL Jr.: The use of gentamicin in peritoneal dialysis. II. Microbiologic and clinical results. J. infect. Dis. (Suppl.) *124:* 84 (1971).

JONES, R. A. K.: Ototoxicity of gentamicin ear-drops. Lancet *1:* 1161 (1978).

LAWSON, D. H., R. F. MACADAM, H. SINGH, H. GAVRAS, S. HARTZ, D. TURNBULL, A. L. LINTON: Effect of furosemide on antibiotic-induced renal damage in rats. J. infect. Dis. *126:* 593 (1972).

MAWER, G. E., R. AHMAD, S. M. DOBBS, J. G. MCGOUGH, S. B. LUCAS, J. A. TOOTH: Prescribing aids for gentamicin. Brit. J. Pharmacol. *1:* 45 (1974).

PATEL, V., F. C. LUFT, M. N. YUM, B. PATEL, W. ZEMAN, S. A. KLEIT: Enzymuria in gentamicin-induced kidney damage. Antimicrob. Ag. Chemother. *7:* 364 (1975).

PICKERING, L. K., C. D. ERICSSON, G. RUIZ-PALACIOS, J. BLEVINS, M. E. MINER: Intraventricular and parenteral gentamicin therapy for ventriculitis in children. Amer. J. Dis. Child. *132:* 480 (1978).

SCHENTAG, J. J., W. J. JUSKO, M. E. PLAUT, T. J. CUMBO, J. W. VANCE, E. ABRUTYN: Tissue persistence of gentamicin in man. JAMA *238:* 327 (1977).

WAHLIG, H., E. DINGELDEIN: Gentamicin bei alloarthroplastischen Operationen. Chemotherapy *1:* 189 (1976).

YOSHIOKA, H., T. MONMA, S. MATSUDA: Placental transfer of gentamicin. J. Pediat. *80:* 121 (1972).

e) Tobramycin

Proprietary names: Gernebcin, Nebcin, Tobrasix.

Description: An aminoglycoside antibiotic (nebramycin factor 6), the sulphate of which is water-soluble and heat-stable.

Spectrum of activity: Comparable to gentamicin, but considerably more active against Pseudomonas aeruginosa including some gentamicin-resistant strains. Tobramycin is less active against Serratia marcescens, but similar to gentamicin

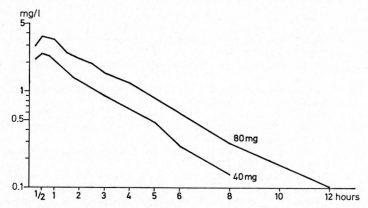

Fig. 24. Mean serum concentration-time curve after 40 and 80 mg of tobramycin i. m.

against other susceptible strains. Combination with penicillins (e. g. piperacillin) or cephalosporins is synergistic and potentiates the activity of both components.

Resistance: Some cross-resistance with gentamicin, sisomicin, netilmicin and amikacin. Gentamicin-resistant strains of Pseudomonas are often sensitive to tobramycin and mostly to amikacin as well.

Pharmacokinetics: *Maximal blood concentrations:* 3.7 mg/l after 80 mg i. m. (0.56 mg/l after 6 h) and 2.4 mg/l after 40 mg i. m. (0.26 mg/l after 6 h) (Fig. 24). Continuous i. v. infusion of 6.6 mg/h (160 mg/24 h) produces blood concentrations of 1 mg/l.

Half-life: 1½ h. *Not bound to protein. Excretion* of 93% of the dose in active form through the kidneys within 24 h.

Side effects: Less nephro- and ototoxic than gentamicin.

Indications: Proven and suspected infections with Pseudomonas aeruginosa. May be used as an alternative to gentamicin in the combined therapy of severe mixed infections.

Contra-indications: As gentamicin. Do not combine with gentamicin, another aminoglycoside, or a potent loop diuretic such as frusemide, ethacrynic acid or bumetanide.

Dose and administration: By injection i. m. every 8–12 h or by slow i. v. injection (15 min) or short i. v. infusion of 2–5 mg/kg/day according to the severity and site of the infection, generally for not longer than 10 days. The dose should be reduced, and the dose-interval prolonged in renal failure, as with gentamicin (see p. 137). In renal insufficiency, treatment should be monitored by assay.

Preparations: Ampoules of 20, 40 and 80 mg.

Summary: A similar aminoglycoside to gentamicin with improved activity against Pseudomonas. Should be combined with an antipseudomonal penicillin in severe infections with this organism.

References

BRUMMETT, R. D., K. E. FOX, T. W. BENDRICK, D. L. HIMES: Ototoxicity of tobramycin, gentamicin, amikacin and sisomicin in the guinea pig. J. Antimicrob. Chemother. (Suppl. A). *4:* 73 (1978).

DEE, T. H., F. KOZIN: Gentamicin and tobramycin penetration into synovial fluid. Antimicrob. Ag. Chemother. *12:* 548 (1977).

FEE, W. E., Jr., J. VIERRA, G. R. LATHROP: Clinical evaluation of aminoglycoside toxicity: Tobramycin versus gentamicin, a preliminary report. J. Antimicrob. Chemother. (Suppl. A) *4:* 31 (1978).

GILBERT, D. N., C. PLAMP, P. STARR, W. M. BENNETT, D. C. HOUGHTON, G. PORTER: Comparative nephrotoxicity of gentamicin and tobramycin in rats. Antimicrob. Ag. Chemother. *13:* 34 (1978).

HOECKER, J. L., L. K. PICKERING, J. SWANEY, W. G. KRAMER, J. VAN EYS, S. FELDMAN, S. KOHL: Clinical pharmacology of tobramycin in children. J. infect. Dis. *137:* 592 (1978).

KAPLAN, J. M., G. H. JR. MCCRACKEN, M. L. THOMAS, L. J. HORTON, N. DAVIS: Clinical pharmacology of tobramycin in newborns. Amer. J. Dis. Child. *125:* 656 (1973).

MARSH, F. P.: Do cephalosporins potentiate or antagonise aminoglycoside nephrotoxicity? J. Antimicrob. Chemother. *4:* 103 (1978).

SCHENTAG, J. J., G. LASEZKAY, T. J. CUMBO, H. E. PLAUT, W. J. JUSKO: Accumulation pharmacokinetics of tobramycin. Antimicrob. Ag. Chemother. *13:* 649 (1978).

SIMON, C., E. U. MÖSINGER, V. MALERCZYK: Pharmakokinetic studies of tobramycin and gentamicin. Antimicrob. Ag. Chemother. *3:* 445 (1973).

WILSON, P., R. T. RAMSDEN: Immediate effects of tobramycin on human cochlea and correlation with serum tobramycin levels. Brit. med. J. *1:* 259 (1977).

WHELTON, A., G. G. CARTER, T. J. CRAIG, H. H. BRYANT, D. V. HERBST, W. G. WALKER: Comparison of the intrarenal disposition of tobramycin and gentamicin. J. Antimicrob. Chemother. (Suppl.) *4:* 13 (1978).

f) Sisomicin

Proprietary names: Extramycin, Pathomycin, Siseptin. Sisomicin is not commercially available at present in Great Britain.

Description: A similar aminoglycoside to gentamicin C_{1a}, from which it differs only by the presence of a double bond in one of the glycoside rings. Colourless or slightly yellow, water-soluble as the sulphate and stable. Sometimes spelt sissomicin.

Structural formula:

Mode of action: Bactericidal in the log phase of bacterial growth but not in the resting phase. Acts by inhibition of protein synthesis.

Spectrum of action: Almost identical with that of gentamicin. Sisomicin is, however, more active against Proteus species (especially Proteus vulgaris), and Pseudomonas aeruginosa and some strains of Citrobacter, Klebsiella and Serratia. Less effective than tobramycin against Pseudomonas. Synergistic with ampicillin against Escherichia coli, with carbenicillin against Pseudomonas and Proteus and with cephalosporins against Klebsiella.

Resistance: Incomplete cross-resistance with gentamicin and tobramycin because of differences in activity against certain species. Like gentamicin, sisomicin is inactivated by 5 of the 9 most important bacterial enzymes. Bacterial strains which elaborate the aminoglycoside acetyltransferase-6' (AAC-6') enzyme, are resistant to both sisomicin and amikacin, and amikacin-resistant bacteria are almost all sisomicin-resistant as well. Resistance does not develop rapidly during therapy.

Pharmacokinetics:

Absorption after oral administration is minimal, but is rapid after i.m. injection.

Serum concentrations: Maximum serum concentrations of 3–4 mg/l are found about 45 min after 80 mg i.m. and decline to 0.5 mg/l after 6 h. Continuous infusion of 6.6 mg/h (160 mg/day) gives a serum concentration of 0.64 mg/l in the steady state.

Half-life: 1½ h. Not bound to *plasma protein.* Poor cerebrospinal fluid penetration. Tissue penetration comparable to that of gentamicin.

Excretion: About 80% through the kidneys in 24 h; storage in the renal parenchyma results in measurable urine concentrations for up to 2 weeks after cessation of therapy. Urine concentrations in the first 2 h after 80 mg i.m.: 100–500 mg/l (at 6–9 h: 20–50 mg/l).

Side effects: As for gentamicin. Potentially nephro- and ototoxic; dosage should therefore be carefully controlled. Reduce dosage in renal failure (see p. 137).

Indications and contra-indications: As for gentamicin (p. 136).

Administration: I.m. injection, very slow i.v. injection or short i.v. infusion over 30 min. Do not mix with other drugs in the solution, particularly with carbenicillin (inactivation). The infusion solution (preferably 5% glucose) should not contain magnesium or calcium. A solution for inhalation containing 4 mg/ml may be given to a total dose of 40–60 mg without significant absorption.

Dosage: As for gentamicin (2–5 mg/kg/day) in 2–3 divided doses. For details see p. 136.

Preparations: Ampoules of 10, 20, 50, 75 and 100 mg.

Summary: A variant of gentamicin with somewhat better activity against Proteus vulgaris, Klebsiella pneumoniae, Serratia marcescens and Pseudomonas aeruginosa.

References

CROWE, C. C., E. SANDERS: Sisomicin: Evaluation in vitro and comparison of gentamicin and tobramycin. Antimicrob. Ag. Chemother. *3:* 24 (1973).
DOERCK, M., G. FRICKE, G. GRUENWALDT, H. M. VON HATTINGBERG, M. SCHEER: Pharmakokinetische und klinische Untersuchungen mit Sisomicin in der Paediatrie. Infection *8:* 107 (1980).
LODE, H., B. KEMMERICH, R. KOEPPE, H. LANGMAACK: Vergleichende Pharmakokinetik und klinische Erfahrungen mit einem neuen Aminoglycosid-Derivat: Sisomicin. Dtsch. med. Wschr. *100:* 2144 (1975).
NAUMANN, P., H. ROSIN, E. REINTJENS, M. KÖHLER: Sisomicin versus Gentamicin. Dtsch. med. Wschr. *101:* 1277 (1976).

NICOT, G., L. MERLE, J.-P. VALETTE, J.-P. CHARMES, J. TOURNOIS, G. LACHATRE: Toxicité tubulaire renale induite par la sisomicine chez l'homme. J. Pharmacol. (Paris) *12:* 76 (1981).
RICHMOND, J. M., R. G. WALKER, P. KINCAID-SMITH: Sisomicin in the treatment of urinary tract infections Med. J. Aust. *2:* 375 (1979).
SCHEER, M.: Antibakterielle Wirkung von Sisomicin im Vergleich zu Gentamicin. Arzneimittel-Forsch. *26:* 12 (1976).
SIMON, C., V. MALERCZYK, W. AHLENDORF: Sisomicin: in vitro activity and pharmacokinetics. Int. J. clin. Pharmacol. *16:* 143 (1978).
WEINGAERTNER, L., U. SITKA, R. PATSCH, U. BURCHARDT, I. RICHTER: Erfahrungen mit Sisomicin in der Paediatrie. Infection *7:* 119 (1979).

g) Netilmicin

Proprietary names: Certomycin, Netillin, Netromycin.

Properties: Developed in the USA by the Schering Corporation. Netilmicin is the N-ethyl derivative of sisomicin and, as the sulphate, is water-soluble and stable.

Spectrum of action: Largely the same as gentamicin, though some gentamicin-resistant strains of Escherichia coli, Proteus mirabilis, Enterobacter species, Klebsiella pneumoniae, Citrobacter freundii and Serratia marcescens are sensitive to netilmicin. On the other hand, most gentamicin-resistant strains of Pseudomonas are resistant to netilmicin, which is only inactivated by four of the nine known bacterial inactivating enzymes, while gentamicin is inactivated by six enzymes. Netilmicin is less active against Pseudomonas aeruginosa but more active against Serratia marcescens than gentamicin.

Resistance: There is incomplete cross-resistance with gentamicin and partial (one-sided) cross-resistance with amikacin (amikacin-resistant strains are always netilmicin-resistant, but not vice versa).

Pharmacokinetics and side effects: Similar to gentamicin. Oto- and nephrotoxicity in animal tests are less than with gentamicin, but disturbances of hearing, balance and renal function (reversible) have also been observed in man.

Dosage in adults is 2–5 mg/kg/day in 2 or 3 divided doses. The manufacturers recommend that renal function, hearing and balance be monitored in patients treated for longer than 14 days, and that peak serum concentrations of more than 16 mg/l be avoided.

Conclusion: Netilmicin has few advantages in bacterial sensitivity and general tolerance over gentamicin and is less likely to be effective against gentamicin-resistant bacteria than amikacin.

References

BOWMAN, R. L., F. J. SILVERBLATT, G. J. KALOYANIDES: Comparison of the nephrotoxicity of netilmicin and gentamicin in rats. Antimicrob. Ag. Chemother. *12:* 474 (1977).

BRAVENY, I., J. VOECKL, K. MACHKA: Antimicrobial activity of Netilmicin in comparison with Gentamicin, Sisomicin, Tobramycin and Amikacin and their resistance patterns. Arzneimittel-Forsch. *3, 30:* 491 (1980).

CHIU, P. J. S., G. H. MILLER, A. D. BROWN, J. F. LONG, J. A. WAITZ: Renal pharmacology of netilmicin. Antimicrob. Ag. Chemother. *11:* 821 (1977).

KANTOR, R. J., C. W. NORDEN: In vitro activity of netilmicin, gentamicin, and amikacin. Antimicrob. Ag. Chemother. *11:* 126 (1977).

KLASTERSKY, J., F. MEUNIER-CARPENTIER, L. COPPENS-KAHAN, D. DANEAU, J. M. PREVOST: Clinical and bacteriological evaluation of netilmicin in Gram-negative infections. Antimicrob. Ag. Chemother. *12:* 503 (1977).

MEYERS, B. R., S. Z. HIRSCHMAN, G. WORMSER, D. SIEGEL: Pharmacokinetic study of netilmicin. Antimicrob. Ag. Chemother. *12:* 122 (1977).

PANWALKER, A. P., J. B. MALOW, V. M. ZIMELIS, G. G. JACKSON: Netilmicin: Clinical efficacy, tolerance, and toxicity. Antimicrob. Ag. Chemother. *13:* 170 (1978).

PHILLIPS, I., A. SMITH, K. SHANNON: Antibacterial activity of netilmicin, a new aminoglycoside antibiotic, compared with that of gentamicin. Antimicrob. Ag. Chemother. *11:* 402 (1977).

TRESTMAN, I., J. PARSONS, J. SANTORO, G. GOODHART, D. KAYE: Pharmacology and efficacy of netilmicin. Antimicrob. Ag. Chemother. *13:* 832 (1978).

WELLING, P. G., A. BAUMUELLER, C. C. LAU, P. O. MADSEN: Netilmicin pharmacokinetics after single intravenous doses to elderly male patients. Antimicrob. Ag. Chemother. *12:* 328 (1977).

YAN, B.-S., D. STEWART, G. P. BODEY: Clinical pharmacology of netilmicin: Antimicrob. Ag. Chemother. *12:* 717 (1977).

h) Amikacin

Proprietary names: Amikin, Biklin, Fabianol.

Properties: A semi-synthetic derivative of kanamycin which, as the sulphate, is a colourless or slightly yellow solution which is stable at room temperature for at least 2 years.

Mode of action: Bactericidal against actively proliferating, and possibly also non-proliferating, bacteria by inhibition of protein synthesis.

Range of action: Since amikacin is not affected by most of the bacterial aminoglycoside-inactivating enzymes, it has a broader spectrum than gentamicin, sisomicin, tobramycin and netilmicin and inhibits most gentamicin-resistant strains of Escherichia coli, Klebsiella, Enterobacter, Serratia, Proteus species (including Proteus rettgeri), Providencia, Acinetobacter, Citobacter freundii and Staphylococcus aureus. Nocardia asteroides is always sensitive. Amikacin-resistance is extremely rare in gentamicin-sensitive bacteria (gram-negative bacilli and staphylococci). Amikacin is synergistic with azlocillin and ticarcillin against Pseudomonas aeruginosa and other Enterobacteriaceae, but is less active, weight for weight, than gentamicin and so has to be given at the same high dosage as kanamycin. Streptococci (including pneumococci) and Haemophilus influenzae are not sensitive. Amikacin is not active against most anaerobes, Pseudomonas cepacia and Pseudomonas maltophilia.

Resistance: Resistance during treatment is not quite as rare as was thought earlier. Partial cross-resistance in one or both directions with the other aminoglycosides.

Pharmacokinetics:
Absorption after oral administration is minimal, and is somewhat slower than gentamicin after i. m. injection (maximum serum concentration after 1½ h).
Serum concentrations: 21 mg/l (1 h) and 2.1 mg/l (10 h) after 500 mg (0.75 mg/kg) i. m. A short infusion of 500 mg over ½ h gives a mean serum concentration of 38 mg/l at the end of infusion, 18 mg/l 1 h later, and 0.75 mg/l after 10 h. There is no accumulation during a course of treatment when renal function is intact. *Half-life:* 2.3 h (7 h for the newborn in the first week of life). *Plasma protein binding:* 4–10%. Limited *CSF penetration* of 10–20% of the serum concentrations, and up to 50% in meningitis. Amikacin crosses the placenta and is concentrated in amniotic fluid.
Excretion: More than 90% excreted through the kidneys in the first 8 h in active form, primarily by glomerular filtration, and 95–100% in 24 h. Mean urinary concentrations during the first 6 h after 500 mg i. m.: 800 mg/l.

Side effects: Like other aminoglycosides, amikacin is potentially nephro-, oto- and neurotoxic.
1. *Nephrotoxicity* (urinary loss of protein, cells and casts, azotaemia and oliguria) at normal dosage in the presence of normal renal function and an adequate fluid intake is uncommon and usually reversible.
2. *Ototoxicity* (labyrinthine deafness, dizziness) usually only occurs when the recommended dose is exceeded (see below), with prolonged treatment (longer than 10 days) or with renal failure without a compensatory reduction of dosage.

A peak serum concentration of 35 mg/l should not be exceeded. Permanent auditory damage is rare. When related to the normal therapeutic dosage, the ototoxicity of amikacin (1 g a day) is comparable with that of gentamicin (240–320 mg a day).

3. *Neurotoxicity* (neuromuscular blockade and respiratory paralysis) occurs in combination with anaesthetics and muscle relaxants.

4. *Rare side effects* are skin rashes, drug fever, tremor, nausea, vomiting, eosinophilia etc.

Main indications: Severe infections where other aminoglycosides have failed and hospital isolates of gentamicin-resistant gram-negative bacilli are common. Specific treatment of severe infections with gentamicin-resistant organisms, particularly Proteus rettgeri or Providencia stuartii, Serratia marcescens and Pseudomonas aeruginosa. Initial treatment of septicaemia and severe organ infections before the causative organism is known in immunologically compromised patients, particularly with malignancies. Also useful in peritonitis, neonatal sepsis and neonatal meningitis, always given in combination with other agents.

Inappropriate use: Mild infections, and severe infections where gentamicin or tobramycin would be equally effective. Infections with streptococci, pneumococci or enterococci.

Care must be taken in renal failure, when a different aminoglycoside has been given immediately before, when the patient has inner ear damage, and in pregnancy. Amikacin should not be combined with other potentially nephro- or ototoxic antibiotics, with other aminoglycosides or with potent loop diuretics such as ethacrynic acid, frusemide or mannitol, because of the increased risk of ototoxicity.

Administration: Generally by intramuscular injection, i. v. infusion over 1 h, or very slow i. v. injection. Do not mix other drugs with amikacin in the infusion solution (preferably 5% glucose).

Dosage: Daily dose of 15 mg/kg up to a maximum of 1.5 g, given as 2 or 3 i. m. injections or i. v. infusions (7.5 mg/kg every 12 h or 5 mg/kg every 8 h). Length of treatment: up to 7–10 days. If longer courses cannot be avoided, auditory and vestibular function should be checked regularly, performing audiography if possible. If renal function is impaired, extend the dose interval between single doses of 7.5 mg/kg according to the following rule: Divide the patient's serum creatinine value in µmoles/l by 10. You will then have the correct dose interval in hours (e. g. creatinine value of 180 µmol/l divided by 10 = 18, i. e. give 7.5 mg/kg every 18 h). In chronic renal failure, where the maintenance dose to be given every 12 hours is to be determined and the creatinine clearance is known, apply the following formula:

$$\frac{\text{patient's creatinine clearance (ml/min)}}{\text{normal creatinine clearance (ml/min)}} \times 7.5 \text{ mg/kg,}$$

e. g. creatinine clearance of patient (30), divided by normal creatinine clearance (140), × 7.5 mg/kg = maintenance dose of 1.6 mg/kg/12 h. The initial dose should always be 7.5 mg/kg. New, rapid assay methods such as enzyme and radioimmunoassays are now available as kits and greatly facilitate the control of serum concentrations during therapy, particularly in severe renal failure. The peak serum concentration should not exceed 35 mg/l and the trough 3 mg/l. Give 7.5 mg/kg every 12 h in the newborn during the first week of life to avoid accumulation. In the very premature, the dose interval may have to be prolonged to 24 h.

Topical use: Intrapleural or intra-articular instillation at a concentration of 2.5 mg/ml and an aerosol containing 250 mg/ml are available.

Preparations: Ampoules of 100, 250, 350, and 500 mg.

Summary: A broad-spectrum, bactericidal antibiotic which is generally reserved for severe systemic infections such as suspected gram-negative septicaemia, when it can be life-saving, particularly when combined with an anti-pseudomonal penicillin (e. g. azlocillin) in patients with impaired immunity. Often active against organisms resistant to gentamicin. A valuable agent in severe hospital-acquired infection with gentamicin-resistant bacteria, but the dosage must be carefully controlled because of the risk of toxic side effects.

References

AMIRAK, I. D., R. J. WILLIAMS, P. NOONE, M. R. WILLS: Amikacin resistance developing in a patient with Pseudomonas aeruginosa bronchopneumonia. Lancet *1:* 537 (1977).

BLOCK, C. S., R. CASSEL, H. J. KOORNHOF, R. G. ROBINSON: Klebsiella meningitis treated with intrathecal amikacin. Lancet *1:* 137 (1977).

CRAVEN, P. C., J. H. JORGENSEN, R. L. KASPAR, D. J. DRUTZ: Amikacin therapy of patients with multiple antibiotic-resistant Serratia marcescens infections. Development of increasing resistance during therapy. US Amikacin Symposium, Amer. J. Med. *62 (Suppl.):* 66 (1977).

HAMORY, B., P. IGNATIADIS, M. A. SANDE: Intrathecal amikacin administration. Use in the treatment of gentamicin-resistant Klebsiella pneumoniae meningitis. JAMA *236:* 1973 (1976).

KANTOR, R. J., C. W. NORDEN: In vitro activity of netilmicin, gentamicin, and amikacin. Antimicrob. Ag. Chemother. *11:* 126 (1977).

MYERS, M. G., R. J. ROBERTS, N. J. MIRHIJ: Effects of gestational age, birth weight and hypoxemia on pharmacokinetics of amikacin in serum of infants. Antimicrob. Ag. Chemother. *11:* 1027 (1977).

PARSLEY, T. L., R. B. PROVONCHEE, C. GLICKSMAN, S. H. ZINNER: Synergistic activity of trimethoprim and amikacin against Gram-negative bacilli. Antimicrob. Ag. Chemother. *12:* 349 (1977).

SELIGMAN, S. J.: Frequency of resistance to kanamycin, tobramycin, netilmicin and amikacin in gentamicin-resistant Gram-negative bacteria. Antimicrob. Ag. Chemother. *13:* 70 (1978).

SHAH, P. M., G. HEETDERKS, W. STILLE: Activity of amikacin at subinhibitory levels. J. Antimicrob. Chemotherapy. *2:* 97 (1976).

SMITH, C. R., K. L. BAUGHMAN, C. Q. EDWARDS, J. F. ROGERS, P. S. LIETMAN: Controlled comparison of amikacin and gentamicin. New Engl. J. Med. *296:* 349 (1977).

VOGELSTEIN, B., A. A. KOWARSKI, P. S. LIETMAN: The pharmacokinetics of amikacin in children. J. Pediat. *91:* 333 (1977).

i) Dibekacin

Proprietary name: Orbicin (not commercially available in Great Britain).

Properties: A kanamycin derivative (3'4'-dideoxykanamycin B) and hence an aminoglycoside. The sulphate is stable, soluble in water but virtually insoluble in organic solvents.

Mode of action: Bactericidal, by inhibition of bacterial protein synthesis.

Spectrum of activity: Similar to gentamicin. Inactive against streptococci (including pneumococci and enterococci), Clostridia and Bacteroides species. Somewhat more active than gentamicin against some strains of Pseudomonas aeruginosa, but less active than tobramycin in this respect. Similar activity to gentamicin against Klebsiella, Enterobacter and Proteus species, but somewhat less active than amikacin.

Resistance: Partial cross-resistance with gentamicin, sisomicin, tobramycin, netilmicin and amikacin.

Pharmacokinetics:
Serum concentrations: Maxima of 4–6 mg/l are found 1½ h, after 80 mg i. m. or immediately after 1 hour of i. v. infusion. *Half-life:* 1½–2 h.

Excretion: 60–80% excreted in active form in the urine in 12 h. An unknown amount is stored in the kidneys and excreted after a delay.

Side effects: Oto- und nephrotoxicity, as with to gentamicin.

Indications and contra-indications: Similar to gentamicin (see p. 136).

Administration and dosage: As i. m. or slow i. v. injection or short i. v. infusion over 30–60 min. Daily dose 2–5 mg/kg, according to the severity of the disease. In renal impairment, reduce dosage as with gentamicin (see p. 137).

Preparations: Ampoules of 50, 75 and 100 mg.

Summary: A broad-spectrum, bactericidal antibiotic similar to gentamicin. Useful in severe infections where β-lactam antibiotics would have less or no activity.

References

BOPP, S., R. MARRE, E. SCHULZ, K. SACK: Tierexperimentelle Studien zur Nierenverträglichkeit, Pharmakokinetik und therapeutischen Effektivität von Dibekacin-Arzneimittel-Forsch. 31, *3:* 473 (1981).

FUJITA, M.: Absorption, excretion, distribution and metabolism of 3',4'-dideoxykanamycin B. Jap. J. Antibiotics 26: 55 (1973).

IWASAWA, T.: Fundamental and clinical studies on 3',4'-dideoxykanamycin B in otorhinolaryngologic field. Chemotherapy 22: 967 (1973).

KOZAKEI, N., T. OGURI: On the antibacterial activity of 3,4-dideoxykanamycin B against various pathogenic bacteria. Chemotherapy (Tokyo) 22: 771 (1974).

MITSUHASHI, S.: Bacteriological study on 3',4'-dideoxykanamycin B. Jap. J. Antibiotics 26: 89 (1973).

UMEZAWA, H.: 3',4'-dideoxykanamycin B active against kanamycin-resistant Escherichia coli and Pseudomonas aeruginosa. J. Antibiotics 24: 485 (1971).

YAMASAKU, F., H. TAKEDA, M. NOWAYAMA, S. KAWASHIMA, J. WADA, F. GEIO, Y. KINOSHITA: Fundamental land clinical study on 3',4'-dideoxykanamycin B (Dibekacin). Chemotherapy 22: 804 (1974).

7. Polymyxins (Colistin and Polymyxin B)

Proprietary names: Aerosporin, Colimycine, Colistin, Colomycin, Coly-Mycin, Polybactrin (with neomycin and bacitracin), Polymyxin B.

Description: Basic cyclic polypeptides which are unrelated to other antibiotics. Colistin is polymyxin E and so is chemically related to polymyxin B. The two are therefore presented together. Colistin is available as colistin sulphate for oral use and as colistin sulphomethate for parenteral administration. Polymyxin B is produced as the sulphate for both oral and parenteral use. Colistin is dosed by units (1 unit = 0.033 μg of colistin base; 1 mg of colistin base = approx. 30,000 units). Polymyxin B is dosed according to weight (1 mg polymyxin B base = 10,000 U). The sulphates of colistin and polymyxin B are water-soluble and relatively stable.

Mode of action: Bactericidal in both the lag and log phases of bacterial growth, acting on the cytoplasmic membrane as cationic detergents. The polymyxins mainly affect extracellular bacteria and have little or no action on organisms within cells.

Spectrum of activity: Active only against gram-negative bacteria such as Pseudomonas aeruginosa, Escherichia coli, Enterobacter, Klebsiella and Brucella, though some resistant strains are found within these species. Salmonellae, shigellae, pasteurellae and Haemophilus influenzae are always sensitive, while Proteus, gonococci, meningococci and gram-positive bacteria are resistant. In-vitro tests of sensitivity, particularly disc tests, are unreliable because of antagonists in the culture medium.

Resistance develops slowly in vitro and is rare during therapy. Complete cross-resistance between colistin and polymyxin B.

Pharmacokinetics:

Absorption is minimal after oral administration and high concentrations are found in the intestines. Colistin sulphomethate is absorbed more slowly after i. m. injection than polymyxin B sulphate. *Maximum blood concentration* after 1–2 hours. The *half-life* of colistin is 2 h and of polymyxin B 4 h. *Plasma protein binding* is slight. Polymyxins accumulate with repeated doses. A considerable fraction is metabolised.

Tissue diffusion is poor, and low concentrations are found in the bile, pleural and synovial fluids. *CSF penetration* is very poor. Colistin crosses the placenta and enters the fetal circulation.

Excretion up to 60% in the urine where the concentrations are 20–40 times those in the blood. Polymyxins are not dialysable.

Side effects *(after parenteral administration):*
1. *Neurotoxicity* may follow excessive dosage or accumulation in renal impairment, and is expressed as paraesthesiae, headaches, lethargy, irritability, ataxia and impairment of vision and speech. These symptoms are reversible and are generally only found at higher dosage.
2. *Nephrotoxicity,* particularly with pre-existing renal damage or where the daily dose exceeds 120,000 units/kg of colistin or 2.5 mg/kg of polymyxin-B-sulphate or where treatment is given for longer than one week. This toxicity is shown by proteinuria, casts, haematuria and a raised blood urea and is reversible after stopping treatment.
3. *Allergic reactions* with urticaria, rashes, and fever (rare). Cross-sensitivity between colistin and polymyxin B. Polymyxin B releases histamine in the skin.

4. *Neuromuscular* blockade and apnoea after intraperitoneal or i. m. administration in patients with impaired renal function or given muscle relaxants at the same time. Neostigmine does not antagonise this effect. Cramps and paralysis may follow the intrathecal administration of doses of polymyxin B greater than 5 mg.

5. *Local irritation* (pain) after i. m. injection of polymyxin B sulphate is more frequent and more severe than after i. m. injections of colistin sulphomethate.

Indications: Given by mouth for intestinal decontamination in leukaemic patients, and topically for superficial infections. Systemic administration is no longer justifiable now that more active and less toxic preparations are available.

Contra-indications: Renal failure. Do not inject i. v. because of the danger of neuromuscular blockade and respiratory arrest. Do not combine with other potentially nephrotoxic or neurotoxic drugs.

Administration: By mouth for intestinal decontamination. As an ointment of powder for burns, superficial wound infections etc. and also as eye and ear drops. Instillation into the pleural cavity or joints is not recommended because of the possibility of absorption. Intrathecal administration is contraindicated because of the risk of the cauda equina syndrome.

Dosage: Average daily dose by mouth of *colistin sulphate:* 8 million units for adults, 4 million units for children between 1 and 12 y. and 0.25 million units/kg in the newborn; *polymyxin B sulphate:* Adults and children from 6–12 y.: 300–400 mg; children between 2 and 5 y.: 150–225 mg; neonates: 20 mg/kg.

Solutions of 1–10 mg of polymyxin B in 2 ml are used for *inhalation therapy,* since polymyxin irritates the mucosa.

Preparations: Colistin is available as ampoules of 1 million units ($= 33.3$ mg) for parenteral use and of 3 million units ($= 100$ mg) for infusion, and as tablets of 0.5 million units ($= 16.7$ mg). Polymyxin B is available in ampoules of 50 mg for parenteral use and as tablets of 25 mg by mouth. Polymyxin B is contained in many topical preparations used in dermatology, ENT and ophthalmological practice.

Summary: Polymyxins should only be used now as topical antibiotics. They should no longer be given systemically, since more effective and better tolerated antibiotics are now available.

8. Erythromycin

Proprietary names: Arpimycin, E.E.S., E-Mycin, Ermysin, Erycen, Erycinum, Erythrocin and Erythroped, Erythromid, Ethril, Ilosone, Ilotycin, Paediathrocin, Retcin.

Properties: A narrow-spectrum macrolide antibiotic with much greater activity than either *oleandomycin* or *spiramycin*, both of which are now obsolete. The base, estolate, ethylsuccinate and stearate are poorly soluble in water, but erythromycin glucoheptonate and lactobionate are readily soluble and suitable for parenteral use. Stable at alkaline pH, but rapidly inactivated in acid pH.

Mode of action: Inhibition of bacterial protein synthesis. Bacteriostatic at therapeutic concentrations; bactericidal only in higher concentrations and against proliferating organisms.

Spectrum of activity:
Sensitive (minimal inhibitory concentration = MIC 0.1–1 mg/l): streptococci, pneumococci, gonococci, Listeria, Erysipelothrix rhusiopathiae, Actinomyces israeli, Bacillus anthracis, Clostridium tetani and perfringens, non-sporing anaerobes (except Bacteroides fragilis and fusobacteria), Bordetella pertussis, Chlamydia trachomatis, Mycoplasma pneumoniae and Ureaplasma urealyticum (T-mycoplasma).
Moderately sensitive (MIC 2–5 mg/l): Campylobacter, Legionella pneumophila, spirochaetes, enterococci, meningococci and Corynebacterium.
Resistant (MIC greater than 5 mg/l): Enterobacteriaceae, Chlamydia psittaci, Mycoplasma hominis and Nocardia asteroides. Some strains of Staphylococcus aureus and Haemophilus influenzae are sensitive, others are resistant.

Resistance: Primary resistance in streptococci and pneumococci is rare; about 10% of enterococci are resistant. About 5% of hospital staphylococci are resistant though the proportion may be as high as 30% in some hospitals. Almost all strains isolated outside hospital are sensitive. Penicillin-resistant gonococci are usually resistant to erythromycin as well. There is partial cross-resistance between erythromycin and lincomycin. Resistance in staphylococci can develop *in vitro* after relatively few subcultures.

Pharmacokinetics:
Absorption after oral administration is better with erythromycin estolate and ethylsuccinate than with the stearate ester, which is less well absorbed when taken with food. Erythromycin base is inactivated by hydrochloric acid and is therefore given as enteric coated tablets with an acid-proof coating which does not dissolve

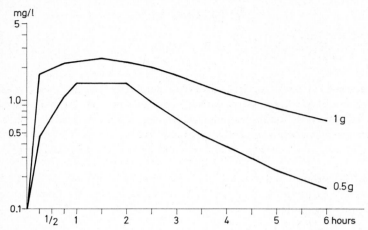

Fig. 25. Mean serum concentrations in 10 healthy adults after 500 mg and 1 g of erythromycin ethylsuccinate by mouth 1 hour after a standard breakfast.

until it reaches the duodenum. *Maximal serum concentrations* are found after 2–3 h, and after 1½ h with the ethylsuccinate.

Serum concentrations are 0.7–3 mg/l at 1–2 h and 0.8–2 mg/l at 3–4 h after 500 mg of erythromycin estolate by mouth, of which 20% is present in the serum as active base and 80% as the inactive ester. The two forms are distinguishable only by chromatography and not by microbiological methods, because when the latter are used, the ester is hydrolysed in vitro into the base. The *ethylsuccinate* is absorbed with no particular individual variation and gives rise to a maximum serum concentration of 1.8 mg/l after 500 mg and 2.4 mg/l after 1 g, which decline to 0.15 mg/l and 0.64 mg/l respectively after 6 h (Fig. 25). After the i. v. infusion of 500 mg of *lactobionate* over 60 min, serum concentrations of 10 mg/l are found at the end of infusion, 3 mg/l at 2 h and 1 mg/l at 5 h after the end of infusion. *Half-life:* 2 hours, but 4 times as long in anuric patients.

Plasma protein binding: 60%.

CSF penetration: Small (2–5%), but 10–20% of serum concentrations with inflamed meninges.

Tissue concentrations: Good. Rapid passage into the saliva (constant relationship to the serum of 1:2). 30% of serum levels in bronchial secretions 3 and 6 h after taking the stearate by mouth.

15–30% of serum concentrations are found in pleural, peritoneal and synovial fluids. Only 10% of the mother's blood concentration is detected in the cord blood. The erythromycin concentrations in breast milk are about 50% of the serum values.

Excretion varies according to the preparation: 20–30% passes out through the bile where concentrations of 6–50 mg/l are found after oral administration and of 50–300 mg/l after an i. v. dose, where hepatic function is normal. Only 2–8% passes into the urine after oral administration, and 12–15% after i. v. administration, giving concentrations of 5–60 mg/l. Concentrations of 300–600 mg/kg are found in the faeces. Erythromycin is rapidly metabolised by demethylation into the antibacterially inactive N-methyl erythromycin.

Side effects are remarkably few. About 5% of patients experience mild gastrointestinal disorders after oral administration (abdominal pain, nausea, loose stools), mainly with high doses. Allergic skin rashes are rare. When given over 2–3 weeks, erythromycin estolate and lauryl sulphate give rise relatively frequently to intrahepatic cholestasis with or without jaundice and colicky abdominal pain, particularly with preexisting liver damage, repeated courses and in already sensitised patients. This is a hypersensitivity reaction. The abdominal pain can be severe enough to mimic cholelithiasis, pancreatitis or ulcer perforation. For this reason, erythromycin estolate is now little used; the course should be limited to 7–10 days and the estolate not given to patients with liver disease or general allergies. Jaundice does not apparently occur with the other erythromycin derivatives.

Indications: Acute respiratory infections, particularly with staphylococci, streptococci, pneumococci and mycoplasma; otitis media; skin infections with sensitive organisms; erythrasma. The drug of choice in legionellosis (due to Legionella pneumophila) for which it should be given at high dosage, preferably in combination with rifampicin. Useful in severe cases of campylobacter enteritis, where it shortens the period of excretion of the organisms, though not necessarily the duration of symptoms. Erythromycin is an alternative to penicillin in penicillin-allergic patients with scarlet fever, erysipelas, gonorrhoea, syphilis or diphtheria. Effective in trachoma, lymphogranuloma inguinale, non-gonococcal urethritis due to chlamydia, and as a prophylaxis for whooping cough.

Inappropriate use: Generalised sepsis and osteomyelitis, against which penicillins, cephalosporins or aminoglycosides act more rapidly and effectively.

Contra-indications: Erythromycin estolate in patients with liver damage, other allergies and repeated courses (risk of cholestatic jaundice).

Administration: Erythromycin ethylsuccinate is preferable for oral use. In severe infections and where the oral route is not possible, erythromycin glucoheptonate or lactobionate may be given parenterally, preferably by short intravenous infusion or slow i. v. injection. Reconstitute the powder in sterile double distilled water or 5% dextrose solution strictly as instructed, as solutions which are too concentrated can cause thrombophlebitis. Nausea and vomiting may follow slow i. v. injection of the diluted solution. Intramuscular injection is often painful and therefore not recommended.

Dosage:

Oral erythromycin ethylsuccinate or stearate: 1 (–2) g a day for adults, 30 (–50) mg/kg for children, in 4 divided doses. The dose should not be reduced in renal failure.

Intravenous administration of erythromycin glucoheptonate or lactobionate as a short infusion (250–500 mg in 30 min) or continuous infusion (1–2 g in 500–1000 ml fluid): 1–2 g a day for adults, 20–30 mg/kg a day for children.

Instillation (intrapleural, intraperitoneal or intra-articular) of erythromycin glucoheptonate or erythromycin lactobionate, dissolved as instructed and then further dissolved to a final concentration of 10 mg/ml (intrapleural), 2.5 mg/ml (intraperitoneal), and 1.25–2.5 mg/ml (intra-articular).

Preparations:

Tablets of 125, 250 and 500 mg as erythromycin ethylsuccinate.

Granules for reconstitution as syrup or drops containing 40 mg/ml, suspension and drops ready for use containing 40 mg/ml. Tablets of 250 and 500 mg and an oral suspension (20 mg/dl) as erythromycin stearate.

Coated tablets of 250 mg as erythromycin base.   ʼ

Capsules of 250 and 500 mg as estolate.

Suppositories of 250 mg as ethylsuccinate.

Ampoules of 250 mg as glucoheptonate.

Ampoules of 300 mg as lactobionate.

Ampoules of 100 mg erythromycin ethylsuccinate for i. m. injection.

Summary:

Advantages: Selective activity against gram-positive bacteria and Haemophilus influenzae; well tolerated (except the estolate).

Disadvantages: Some resistance amongst staphylococci and Haemophilus influenzae; secondary resistance can arise during prolonged treatment. Erythromycin stearate and base are less well absorbed than the ethylsuccinate. Many confusing forms available. There are other macrolides closely resembling erythromycin. e. g. midacamycin, josamycin and rosamicin, which are not superior to erythromycin in clinical activity.

References

ALTEMEIER, W. A. III, E. M. AYOUB: Erythromycin prophylaxis for pertussis. Pediatrics *59:* 623 (1977).

BASS, J. W., R. W. STEELE, R. A. WIEBE, E. P. DIERDORF: Erythromycin concentrations in middle ear exudates. Pediatrics *48:* 417 (1971).

BELL, S. M.: A comparison of absorption after oral administration of erythromycin estolate and erythromycin stearate. Med. J. Aust. *2:* 1280 (1971).

BOGGIANO, B. G., M. GLEESON: Gastric acid inactivation of erythromycin stearate in solid dosage forms. J. pharm. Sci. *65:* 497 (1976).

DIXON, J. M. S., A. E. LIPINSKI: Resistance of group A beta-hemolytic streptococci to lincomycin und erythromycin. Antimicrob. Ag. Chemother. *1:* 333 (1972).

JELLARD, C. H., A. E. LIPINSKI: Corynebacterium diphtheriae resistant to erythromycin and lincomycin. Lancet *1:* 156 (1973).

GINSBURG, C. M., G. H. MCCRACKEN Jr., M. C. CULBERTSON Jr.: Concentrations of erythromycin in serum and tonsil: Comparison of the estolate and ethylsuccinate suspensions. J. Pediatrics *89:* 1011 (1976).

MANNISTO, P., J. TOUMISTO, R. RASANEN: Absorption of erythromycin. Arzneimittel-Forsch. *25:* 1828 (1975).

MCCORMACK, W. M., H. GEORGE, A. DONNER, L. F. KODGIS, S. ALPERT, E. W. LOWE, E. H. KASS: Hepatotoxicity of erythromycin estolate during pregnancy. Antimicrob. Ag. Chemother. *12:* 630 (1977).

OLIVER, L. E., J. H. ISER, G. F. STENING, R. A. SMALLWOOD: Biliary colic and Ilosone. Med. J. Aust. *1:* 1148 (1973).

PHILIPSON, A., L. D. SABATH, D. CHARLES: Transplacental passage of erythromycin and clindamycin. New Engl. J. Med. *288:* 1219 (1973).

SIMON, C., J. CLASEN: Sputum concentrations of erythromycin after single and repeated oral administration in adult patients with bronchitis, p. 652. International Society of Chemotherapy. Published by American Society for Microbiology. Reprinted from Current Chemotherapy 1978.

TOLMAN, K. G., J. J. SANELLA, J. W. FRESTON: Chemical structure of erythromycin and hepatotoxicity. Ann. intern. Med. *81:* 58 (1974).

WEISBLUM, B., C. SIDDHIKOL, C. J. LAI, V. DEMOHN: Erythromycin-inducible resistance in staphylococcus aureus: Requirements for induction. J. Bacteriol. *106:* 835 (1971).

9. Josamycin

Proprietary name: Wilprafen.

Properties: Josamycin is a macrolide and consists of a macrocyclic lactone ring to which sugars are attached. It was developed in 1964 in Japan where it is widely used. It was introduced in Germany in 1984. Josamycin is available as the propionate (antibacterially inactive) which is hydrolyzed in the body to the active base. Poorly soluble in water but readily soluble in ethanol and other organic solvents.

Spectrum of activity: Similar to that of erythromycin (also active against Bordetella pertussis and Mycoplasma pneumoniae) but campylobacter and some strains of clostridia and fusobacteria are resistant. Josamycin is 2–4 times less active than erythromycin against staphylococci, pneumococci, other streptococci and Haemophilus influenzae. About 3–6% of staphylococcal strains and most haemophilus strains are resistant. There is a partial cross-resistance with other macrolides.

Pharmakokinetics resemble that of erythromycin: incomplete absorption after oral administration, half-life 90 min, low urinary recovery (<10%), highly metabolised in the liver.

Gastrointestinal **side effects** (4–5%) are usually mild.

Indication: Acute bacterial infections of the upper respiratory tract.

Contra-indication: Impaired liver function.

Daily dose: 1–2 g for adults, 30–50 mg/kg for children, divided in 3–4 doses.

Preparation: Suspension (30 mg/ml).

Summary: No advantages in comparison to erythromycin. Not effective in haemophilus infections.

References

BOCK, D., W. RITZERFELD: Studien zur Resistenzentwicklung von Staphylokokken gegenüber Erythromycin und Josamycin. Arzneimittel-Forsch. (Drug Res.) 24 2: 140 (1974).
LONG, S. S., S. MUELLER, R. M. SWENSON: In vitro susceptibilities of anaerobic bacteria to josamycin. Antimicrob. Ag. Chemother. 9: 859 (1976).
MITSUHASHI, S. (ed.): Drug Action and Drug Resistance in Bacteria. University Park Press, Tokyo 1971.
NITTA, K. et al.: A new antibiotic, josamycin II. Biological studies. J. Antibiot. (Tokyo) 20: 181 (1976).
OSONO, T. et al.: A new antibiotic, josamycin I. Isolation and physico-chemical characteristics. J. Antibiot. (Tokyo) 20: 174 (1967).
REESE, E. R.: In vitro suspectibility of common clinical anaerobic and aerobic isolates against josamycin. Antimicrob. Ag. Chemother. 10: 253 (1976).
SANTORO, J., D. KAYE, M. E. LEVISON: In vitro activity of josamycin and rosamycin against Bacteroides fragilis compared with clindamycin, erythromycin and metronidazole. Antimicrob. Ag. Chemother. 10: 188 (1976).
SHADOMY, S., M. TIPPLE, L. PAXTON: Josamycin and rosamicin: In vitro comparisons with erythromycin and clindamycin. Antimicrob. Ag. Chemother. 10: 773 (1976).

SIMON, C.: Wirksamkeit von Josamycin auf bakterielle Erreger von Atemwegsinfektionen. Pädiat. Praxis *30:* 57 (1984).

STRAUSBAUGH, L. J., J. A. DILWORTH, J. M. GWALTNEY, Jr., M. A. SANDE: In vitro susceptibility studies with josamycin and erythromycin. Antimicrob. Ag. Chemother. *9:* 546 (1976).

STRAUSBAUGH, L. J., W. K. BOLTON, J. A. DILWORTH, R. L. GUERRANT, M. A. SANDE: Comparative pharmacology of josamycin and erythromycin stearate. Antimicrob. Ag. Chemother. *10:* 450 (1976).

WENZEL, R. P., J O. HENDLEY, W. K. DODD, J. M. GWALTNEY, Jr.: Comparison of josamycin and erythromycin in the therapy of Mycoplasma pneumoniae pheumonia, Antimicrob. Ag. Chemother. *10:* 899 (1976).

WETSERMAN, E. L., T. W. WILLIAMS, jr., N. MORELAND: In vitro activity of josamycin against aerobic Gram-positive cocci and anaerobes. Antimicrob. Ag. Chemother. *9:* 988 (1976).

10. Lincomycins

a) Lincomycin

Proprietary names: Albiotic, Cillimycin, Lincocin.

Properties: A pyranoside, which is chemically unrelated to other antibiotics, except clindamycin. The hydrochloride is water-soluble.

Mode of action: Lincomycin inhibits bacterial protein synthesis and is bacteriostatic at therapeutically achievable concentrations but can be bactericidal at higher concentrations.

Spectrum of activity: Active against staphylococci, including penicillinase-producing strains, streptococci, pneumococci, Corynebacterium diphtheriae, clostridia, Bacteroides species and Mycoplasma hominis; not active against enterococci, Neisseria or gram-negative bacilli (except Bacteroides and Veillonela).

Resistance: Stepwise increase in resistance occurs *in vitro* but is rare during therapy. Primarily resistant strains of staphylococci and Bacteroides occur at varying frequencies. Pneumococci and group A streptococci are very rarely resistant. Partial cross-resistance is found with erythromycin and clindamycin. Lincomycin-resistant strains of Bacteroides fragilis can be clindamycin-sensitive.

Pharmacokinetics:
Absorption after oral administration depends very much on food intake (Fig. 26). The fasting absorption rate is 73% but with food it is less than 25%. *Peak blood levels* occur after 4 hours and are higher with repeated administration. *Serum concentrations* after 600 mg i.m. are 9–12 mg/l (1 h) and 3–4 mg/l (12 h).

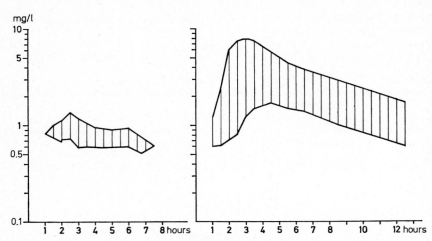

Fig. 26. Serum concentrations of lincomycin in adults after 500 mg of lincomycin by mouth 30 min after a standard breakfast (left) and fasting, i.e. 2 hours before breakfast (right).

The mean serum concentration after a short i.v. infusion over 1 h of 600 mg are 21.5 mg/l at the end of the infusion and 1.7 mg/l at 12 h. *Plasma protein binding:* 20–30%. *Half-life* 5 h (doubled in renal failure). Good *penetration* of tissues, including bone. Poor CSF penetration with up to 40% of the plasma concentrations in the CSF in meningitis. 10–60% in cord blood and amniotic fluid and 50–100% of the mother's serum values in breast milk.

Excretion: 38% urine recovery after i.v. administration (9–10% after oral administration on an empty stomach). A small part is excreted in the bile. Rapidly metabolised (more than 50%). Not dialysable.

Side effects: Gastrointestinal upset in 5–20% (glossitis, stomatitis, nausea, vomiting, diarrhoea) which can continue after treatment has finished, partly due to the suppression of the anaerobic flora and their replacement by enterococci. Pseudomembranous enterocolitis with persistent mucosanguinous diarrhoea and abdominal pain can be severe and sometimes fatal. It is related to the proliferation of toxin-producing strains of Clostridium difficile in the large bowel and is resistant to penicillins, cephalosporins, aminoglycosides, tetracyclines, erythromycin, lincomycin and often to clindamycin also. Toxin, which is formed in larger quantities and p-cresol, which is formed from tyrosine, cause mild or severe diarrhoea after 2–25 days which usually stops within 3 weeks but which can recur. Oral vancomycin or metronidazole, to which Clostridium difficile is sensitive, is effective therapy. The frequency of these side effects varies regionally, being less frequent in Europe and varying between less than 1% and 10% in the USA. Pseudomembranous enterocolitis is more frequent in the elderly and after intestinal operations. It may also occur during treatment with amino penicillins and other antibiotics. Allergic reactions also occur. Cardiovascular disturbances (collapse and cardiac arrest) are reported after rapid i. v. injection because of potassium imbalance. Care should be taken in renal and hepatic impairment because of the risk of accumulation.

Indications: Staphylococcal infections in patients with penicillin allergy, with methicillin resistance, and other infections with gram-positive bacteria (e. g. osteomyelitis), if other well tolerated antibiotics are ineffective.

Inappropriate use: Infections due to gram-positive bacteria against which penicillins or erythromycin are equally active.

Administration: Oral doses should be given at least 2 hours before or 2 hours after meals. I. m. injection and i. v. infusion are also available.

Dosage: 2 g a day by mouth for adults, and 30–40 mg/kg for children, preferably fasting, in 4 divided doses. I. m. administration (2–4 times a day) or i. v. infusion: 1.2–1.8 g a day for adults, 10–20 mg/kg for children; as a short infusion: 600 mg in 250 ml of 5% dextrose solution (for ½ hour) 2–3 times a day. Reduce dosage in renal and liver impairment.

Preparations: Capsules of 500 mg, ampoules of 600 mg and 3 g, and a syrup (50 mg/ml).

Summary: An effective antibiotic against staphylococci though oral absorption is unreliable. Because of the risk of enterocolitis, lincomycin should only be given where clearly indicated.

References

Burdon, D. W., R. H. George: Pseudomembranous colitis. Lancet *1:* 444 (1978).
Clark, C. E., H. Thompson, A. R. McLeisch, S. J. A. Powis, N. J. Dorricott, J. Alexander-Williams: Pseudomembranous colitis following prophylactic antibiotics in bowel surgery. J. Antimicrob. Chemother. *2:* 167 (1970).
Dornbusch, K., A. Carlström, H. Hugo, A. Lidström: Antibacterial activity of clindamycin and lincomycin in human bone. J. Antimicrob. Chemother. *3:* 153 (1977).
Dyck, W. P., A. L. Viteri, P. H. Howard: Lincomycin, clindamycin, and colitis. Lancet *1:* 272 (1974).
George, R. H., J. M. Symonds, F. Dimock, H. D. Brown, Y. Arabi, N. Shinagawa, M. R. B. Keighley, J. Alexander-Williams, D. W. Burdon: Identification of Clostridium difficile as a cause of pseudomembranous colitis. Brit. med. J. *1:* 695 (1978).

GEORGE, W. L., V. L. SUTTER, E. J. C. GOLDSTEIN, S. L. LUDWIG, S. M. FINEGOLD: Aetiology of antimicrobial-agent-associated colitis. Lancet *1:* 802 (1978).
GORBACH, S. L., J. G. BARTLETT: Pseudomembranous enterocolitis: A review of its diverse forms. J. infect. Dis. (Suppl.), *135:* 89 (1977).
LINZENMEIER, G., P. SCHÄFER, H. VOLK, M. GATOS: Bestimmung der Konzentration von Lincomycin in chronisch entzündetem Knochen- und Weichteilgewebe. Arzneimittel-Forsch. *18:* 204 (1968).
PICHLER, H., H. MITSCHKE: Klinischer Anwendungsbereich der Lincomycine. Infection *5:* 42 (1977).
PITTMAN, F. E., J. C. PITTMAN, C. D. HUMPHEY: Lincomycin and pseudomembranous colitis. Lancet *1:* 451 (1974).
SCOTT, A. J., G. I. NICHOLSON, A. R. KERR: Lincomycin as a cause of pseudomembranous colitis. Lancet *2:* 1232 (1973).

b) Clindamycin

Proprietary names: Cleocin, Dalacin C, Sobelin.

Properties: Clindamycin (chlordesoxy lincomycin) is a derivative of lincomycin with a similar spectrum of action but a tenfold improvement in *in vitro* activity against staphylococci, pneumococci and Bacteroides fragilis. Among the anaerobes, there are sensitive strains of Bacteroides, fusobacteria, Actinomyces species, anaerobic streptococci, most strains of Clostridium perfringens and Campylobacter. Almost all strains of Bacteroides fragilis are inhibited at concentrations of 3 mg/l or less. Other clostridia, enterococci (Streptococcus faecalis and faecium), Neisseria, all aerobic gram-negative bacilli and Mycoplasma are resistant. Clindamycin is available as the hydrochloride for oral administration (coated tablets) or the palmitate (granules) and the phosphate for parenteral administration.

Resistance: About 3% of all staphylococci, including a number of the methicillin-resistant strains, are resistant to clindamycin. Resistance is rare amongst streptococci of groups A, B and C, and pneumococci. There is partial cross-resistance with lincomycin and erythromycin. Resistance develops *in vitro* only slowly, except with erythromycin-resistant strains of staphylococci which become resistant to clindamycin after a few subcultures.

Pharmacokinetics:
Clindamycin is 75% absorbed by the *oral route,* independent of food intake. More rapidly absorbed than lincomycin (*maximal blood concentration* after 45–60 min, though later after meals). Peaks after 150 mg and 300 mg by mouth (Fig. 27) are 2.8 mg/l, and 4.5 mg/l respectively, falling to 0.2 mg/l and 0.7 mg/l respectively after 8 hours. No accumulation with repeated administration.

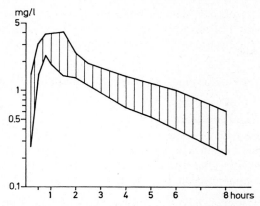

Fig. 27. Serum concentrations of clindamycin in adults after a single oral dose of 150 mg of clindamycin.

Maximum serum levels of 6 mg/l, 3 h after 300 mg i.m., 3.3 mg/l 1 h after 150 mg i.v. and 0.5 mg/l after 8 hours. *Half-life:* 2¾ hours. *Plasma protein binding* 84%. Good *tissue penetration* and relatively good penetration into bone. Passes into the fetal circulation but not into the CSF. Extensively metabolised. Active metabolites are found in the urine in addition to clindamycin (particularly N-dimethyl-clindamycin and clindamycin sulphoxide). *Urinary recovery:* 20–40% compared to 15–35% with oral administration. Not dialysable.

Side effects: Loose stools in 5–20%. A severe ulcerating pseudomembranous enterocolitis with persistent diarrhoea with blood and mucus and abdominal cramps can be fatal (see p. 160). Skin rashes and anaphylactic reactions are rare. Jaundice and abnormal liver function tests also occur during clindamycin therapy. Pain or induration at the site may follow i.m. injection and thrombophlebitis i.v. administration; circulatory collapse or cardiac arrest can result from the rapid i.v. injection of a large dose.

Indications: Bacteriologically proven or clinically suspected anaerobic infections (empyema, lung abscess, peritonitis, intraabdominal abscess, pelvic, tubular, ovarian abscess or endometritis). Staphylococcal infections with methicillin-resistant strains or in patients with penicillin allergy, and osteomyelitis when better tolerated antibiotics are ineffective.

Clindamycin is also very effective in the treatment of streptococcal infections (pharyngitis, otitis media, cellulitis) and for the prophylaxis of anaerobic infections, particularly in association with intraabdominal sepsis or the female genital tract. Concern about pseudomembranous enterocolitis has greatly reduced this use, particularly in less severe infections, but effective control of the latter complication with oral vancomycin (p. 169) has increased confidence in clindamycin once again.

Inappropriate use: Infections against which penicillins or erythromycin are equally effective.

Administration and dosage: 600 mg–1.2 g a day by mouth in 3–4 divided doses, and 10–20 mg/kg/day for children. Same dose for parenteral use (i. m. injection, short or continuous i. v. infusion, but not rapid i. v. injection). If liver function is seriously impaired (acute hepatitis), the half-life is sometimes prolonged. Reduce dose to ¼–⅓ of normal in severe renal failure.

Preparations: Capsules of 75 and 150 mg, syrup (15 mg/ml) and ampoules of 300, 600 and 900 mg.

Summary: An important antibiotic for the treatment of severe infections with anaerobes and with staphylococci resistant to other agents. Only use when clearly indicated because of the risk of pseudomembranous enterocolitis.

References

BAILEY, R. R., E. DANN, B. PEDDIE: The effect of impairment of renal function and dialysis on the serum and urine levels of clindamycin. Aust. N. Z. J. Med. *4:* 434 (1974).

BRANDL, R., C. ARKENAU, C. SIMON, V. MALERCZYK, G. EIDELLOTH: Zur Pharmakokinetik von Clindamycin bei gestörter Leber- und Nierenfunktion. Dtsch. med. Wschr. *97:* 1057 (1972).

DOUGLAS, R. L., J. W. KISLAK: Treatment of Bacteroides fragilis bacteremia with clindamycin. J. infect. Dis. *128:* 569 (1973).

HUGO, H., K. DORNBUSCH, G. STERNER: Studies on the clinical efficacy, serum levels and side effects of clindamycin phosphate administered intravenously. Scand. J. infect. Dis. *9:* 221 (1977).

KAPPAS, A., N. SHINAGAWA, Y. ARABI, H. THOMPSON, D. W. BURDON, F. DIMOCK, R. H. GEORGE, J. ALEXANDER-WILLIAMS, M. R. B. KEIGHLEY: Diagnosis of pseudomembranous colitis. Brit. med. J. *1:* 675 (1978).

LARSON, H. E., A. B. PRICE, P. HONOUR, S. P. BORRIELLO: Clostridium difficile and the aetiology of pseudomembranous colitis. Lancet *1:* 1063 (1978).

LEDGER, W. J., C. L. GEE, W. P. LEWIS, J. R. BOBITT: Comparison of clindamycin and chloramphenicol in treatment of serious infections of the female genital tract. J. infect. Dis. (Suppl.) *135:* 30 (1977).

LEIGH, D. A., K. SIMMONS, S. WILLIAMS: The treatment of abdominal and gynaecological infections with parenteral clindamycin phosphate. J. Antimicrob. Chemother. *3:* 493 (1977).

LEVISON, M. E., J. L. BRAN, K. RIES: Treatment of anaerobic bacterial infections with clindamycin-2-phosphate. Antimicrob. Ag. Chemother. *5:* 276 (1974).

NEU, H. C., A. PRINCE, C. O. NEU, G. J. GARVEY: Incidence of diarrhea and colitis associated with clindamycin therapy. J. infect. Dis. *(Suppl.) 35:* 120 (1977).

NICHOLAS, P., B. R. MEYERS, R. N. LEVY, S. Z. HIRSCHMAN: Concentration of clindamycin in human bone. Antimicrob. Ag. Chemother. *8:* 220 (1975).

PRICE, A. B., D. R. DAVIES: Pseudomembranous colitis. J. clin. Path. *30:* 1 (1977).

RODRIGUEZ, W., S. ROSS, W. KHAN, D. McKAY, P. MOSKOWITZ: Clindamycin in the traetment of osteomyelitis in children. A report of 29 cases. Amer. J. Dis. Child. *131:* 1088 (1977).

ROSE, H. D., M. W. RYTEL: Actinomycosis treated with clindamycin. JAMA *221:* 1052 (1972).

SALAKI, J. S., R. BLACK, F. P. TALLY, J. W. KISLAK: Bacteroides fragilis resistant to the administration of clindamycin. Amer. J. Med. *60:* 426 (1976).

SIMON, C., V. MALERCZYK, E. EIDELLOTH: Zur Pharmakokinetik von Lincomycin und Clindamycin. Med. Welt (N. F.) *27:* 1096 (1976).

TEDESKO, F. J., J. STANLEY, D. H. ALPERS: Diagnostic features of clindamycin-associated pseudomembranous colitis. New Engl. J. Med. *290:* 841 (1974).

WELLS, R. F., L. E. COHEN, C. J. McNEILL: Clindamycin and pseudomembranous colitis. Lancet *1:* 66 (1974).

11. Fusidic Acid

Proprietary names: Fucidin, Fucidine.

Properties: Fusidic acid is a surface-active, lipophilic steroid which bears no relationship to other common antibiotics. The sodium and diethenanolamine salts are stable and readily soluble in water and lipoids.

Mode of action: Predominantly bacteriostatic in therapeutically achievable concentrations by inhibition of protein synthesis.

Spectrum of activity: Active against staphylococci, including penicillinase-producing and methicillin-resistant strains (in very low concentrations), as well as against Corynebacterium diphtheriae, gonococci, meningococci, clostridia and Bacteroides fragilis. Most streptococci and pneumococci are only slightly sensitive, and gram-negative bacteria are resistant.

Resistance: Develops rapidly *in vitro* but rarely during therapy. Primary resistance in staphylococci is occasionally found. No cross-resistance with other antibiotics.

Pharmacokinetics: Absorption after oral administration is somewhat delayed, with *maximal concentrations* after 2–4 hours. *Serum concentrations* of 20 mg/l are found with 500 mg given twice a day over a period of time. *Plasma protein binding:* 90–97%. *Half-life:* 4–6 hours (Fig. 28). Good *tissue diffusion.* Relatively good *penetration* into inflamed and non-inflamed bone tissue. Synovial fluid

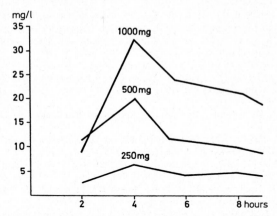

Fig. 28. Serum concentrations after 250, 500 and 1000 mg of fusidic acid by mouth.

concentrations: 70–80% of serum levels, and almost 100% when purulent. Virtually no penetration of non-inflamed meninges. Very low concentrations in aqueous humor. Repeated doses lead to accumulation through the enterohepatic circulation. Excretion is predominantly biliary at high concentrations. Very little (about 10%) is excreted in the urine. The major part is metabolised.

Side effects: Oral intake can give rise to epigastric pain, sometimes with nausea and even vomiting. These effects can be largely avoided by giving the drug with meals.

Indications: Staphylococcal infections (osteomyelitis, septicaemia, staphylococcal pneumonia, skin and wound infections), including follow-up treatment and as an alternative in penicillin allergy or where other anti-staphylococcal agents have failed. In severe cases, clindamycin may be usefully combined with a penicillin or cephalosporin.

Administration: By mouth, i.m. injection or as a slow i.v. infusion (up to 50 mg/kg/h) every 4 hours. Rapid i.v. injection may lead to circulatory collapse, hypotension and arrhythmias. Local treatment with fusidic acid ointment, gel, gauze, powder or solution is available in Germany but not in Britain, where the local use of systemic antibiotics is generally discouraged.

Dosage: *Adults:* 1.5 g a day, *children* 20–30 mg/kg/day in 3 divided doses for up to 2–3 weeks. The dose may be doubled in severe infection and need not be reduced for renal impairment.

Preparations: Capsules of 75 and 150 mg (250 mg in Germany), and ampoules for injection of 150 mg (as phosphate) per ml. Preparations for topical use are not available in Britain.

Summary: An antibiotic with good pharmacokinetic features for use as an alternative in severe staphylococcal infection (e. g. osteomyelitis), in patients with penicillin allergy, and against methicillin-resistant strains.

References

DEODHAR, S. D., F. RUSSEL, W. C. DICK, G. NUKI, W. W. BUCHANAN: Penetration of sodium fusidate (Fucidin) in the synovial cavity. Scand. J. Rheumatol. *1:* 33 (1972).

HIERHOLZER, G., H. KNOTHE, J. REHN: Penetration der Fusidinsäure in aseptisches Knochengewebe. Arzneimittel-Forsch. *20:* 1473 (1970).

RAO, R., A. B. D. WEBSTER, D. R. SUNDERLAND, W. F. SMITH, S. AMPLALAM, H. E. LEE: Cloxacillin and sodium fusidate in management of shunt infections. Brit. med. J. *3:* 618 (1972).

STIRLING, J., S. GOODWIN: Susceptibility of Bacteroides fragilis to fusidic acid. J. Antimicrob. Chemother. *3:* 522 (1977).

WRIGHT, G. L. T., J. HARPER: Fusidic acid and lincomycin therapy in staphylococcal infections in cystic fibrosis. Lancet *1:* 9 (1970).

12. Vancomycin

Proprietary names: Vancocin, Vancomycin.

Properties: A glycopeptide of large molecular size which is unrelated to other antibiotics. The hydrochloride is readily soluble in water, and stable.

Mode of action: Vancomycin inhibits bacterial cell wall formation and is bactericidal on growing bacteria.

Spectrum of action: Staphylococci, streptococci (including enterococci and pneumococci), Clostridium difficile, Corynebacterium diphtheriae and a few other gram-positive organisms are sensitive, but gram-negative bacilli are completely resistant.

Resistance: Does not develop during therapy; resistant staphylococcal strains are rare and cross-resistance with other antibiotics is not found.

Pharmacokinetics: Not absorbed by mouth. *Serum concentrations* after 1 g i.v. are therapeutically adequate for 12 h. *Half-life:* 6 hours. Accumulation can occur with repeated dosing. *Plasma protein binding:* 10%.

When excretion is impaired, repeated doses lead rapidly to toxic concentrations in the blood.

Poor *CSF penetration*, increasing to 10–20% in meningitis. 50–100% of serum concentrations in pleural, pericardial and synovial fluids.

Excretion after i.v. administration is 80–90% through the kidneys, giving urine concentrations of 100–300 mg/l. A small amount is excreted with the bile, giving concentrations up to 50% of serum values. Not dialysable.

Side effects: Occasional thrombophlebitis. Allergic reactions with fever, urticaria, rashes and even anaphylactic shock can occur more frequently. Ototoxicity, particularly when accumulation occurs in renal insufficiency, is a serious risk and renal function should be assessed carefully before treatment. Early reports of nephrotoxicity were apparently due to contamination of the first batches of the drug. Transient flushing may occur, when given too rapidly.

Indications: Severe staphylococcal infections such as septicaemia, endocarditis or osteomyelitis, where penicillinase-stable penicillins or cephalosporins are contra-indicated because of allergy or methicillin resistance. Vancomycin is also a useful bactericidal agent in endocarditis with staphylococci, streptococci or enterococci resistant to β-lactam antibiotics, especially when prosthetic heart valves become colonised with multiresistant strains of Staphylococcus epidermidis. It may be given by mouth in pseudomembranous enterocolitis due to Clostridium difficile and has been used in combination with other agents for intestinal decontamination. Not recommended for other infections.

Contra-indications: Acute renal failure, pre-existing deafness, pregnancy.

Administration: Because vancomycin is not absorbed by mouth, it must be given by continuous i.v. infusion or in 2–4 short infusions a day, either of which may cause phlebitis. Vancomycin should not be injected i.v. since it gives rise to flushes, nausea and paraesthesiae. Intramuscular administration is very painful and can cause necrosis. The hydrochloride is available as a powder for oral use in enterocolitis but has an unpleasant taste.

Dosage: 1–2 g a day *in adults* as a continuous i.v. infusion or 2–4 short i.v. infusions (500 mg in at least 200 ml of 5% glucose solution), 20–40 mg/kg daily in *children*, and reduced dosage in patients over 60 years of age. Because of the possibility of accumulation even where renal function is normal, the daily dose should be halved after the first week of treatment. Treatment should be no longer than 14 days, except in exceptional circumstances (e.g. endocarditis). Reduce dosage from the outset if renal function is impaired, and perform regular audiometric examination and monitor blood concentrations, keeping levels between 5 and 25 mg/l if possible, with maximum acceptable peaks of 40 mg/l. A single dose of 1 g of vancomycin gives adequate blood concentrations for at least 2 weeks in anuric patients on regular haemodialysis. Most cases of pseudomembranous enterocolitis respond to 500 mg a day in four divided doses of 125 mg.

Preparations: Ampoules for injection of 500 mg; powder for oral administration.

Summary: A bactericidal antibiotic for serious infections with gram-positive cocci when other, less toxic alternatives are ineffective. An important oral agent for pseudomembranous enterocolitis.

References

COOK, F. V., W. E. FARRAR, Jr: Vancomycin revisited. Ann. intern. Med. *88:* 813 (1978).

EYKYN, S., I. PHILLIPS, J. EVANS: Vancomycin for staphylococcal shunt site infections in patients on regular haemodialysis. Brit. med. J. *3:* 80 (1970).

HAWLEY, H. B., D. W. GUMP: Vancomycin therapy of bacterial meningitis. Amer. J. Dis. Child. *126:* 261 (1973).

LARSON, H. E., A. J. LEVI, S. P. BORRIELLO: Vancomycin for pseudomembranous colitis. Lancet *2:* 48 (1978).

MODIGLIANI, R., J. C. DELCHIER: Vancomycin for antibiotic-induced colitis. Lancet *1:* 97 (1978).

TEDESCO, F., R. MARKHAM, M. GURWITH, D. CHRISTIE, J. G. BARTLETT: Oral vancomycin for antibiotic-associated pseudomembranous colitis. Lancet *2:* 226 (1978).

WESTENFELDER, G. O., P. Y. PATERSON, B. E. REISBERG, G. M. CARLSON: Vancomycin-streptomycin synergism in Enterococcal endocarditis. JAMA *223:* 37 (1973).

13. Spectinomycin

Proprietary names: Stanilo, Trobicin.

Properties: An aminocyclitol. More effective and better tolerated locally as the hydrochloride than as the sulphate, which was formerly used.

Mode of action: A broad-spectrum antibiotic with relatively low activity except against gonococci (minimal inhibitory concentration 7.5–20 mg/l) which is of clinical use. Ureaplasma urealyticum is also sensitive, but not Chlamydia trachomatis (both can cause nongonococcal urethritis).

Resistance amongst gonococci has been reported, but is rare and there is no cross-resistance with penicillins and cephalosporins.

Pharmacokinetics: Not absorbed by mouth. *Serum concentrations* of 100 mg/l and 15 mg/l occur 1 and 8 h respectively after 2 g i. m., and 160 and 31 mg/l are found 2 and 8 h respectively after 4 g i. m. *Half-life:* 2½ h. High urine concentrations. *Urinary recovery:* 80%.

Side effects occur in less than 1% of patients after a single dose, but headache, dizziness, nausea, vomiting and pain at the site of injection have been reported.

Indications: Single-dose therapy of gonorrhoea especially in patients with allergy to penicillin or where penicillin has failed. Such treatment is ineffective against gonococcal pharyngitis.

Inappropriate use: Other infections. Avoid in pregnancy and the newborn.

Dosage: A single deep i. m. injection of 2 g in 35 ml of water for injection is recommended for gonorrhoea of the urethra in the male, and 4 g i. m. in 6.5 ml of water for injection, possibly divided between 2 sites in gonorrhoea of the female, proctitis, epididymitis and where other therapy has failed. 90% cure rates are achieved. Syphilis is not affected by spectinomycin and so is not masked either.

Preparations: Ampoules of 2 g.

Summary: An alternative to benzyl penicillin as a single treatment of gonorrhoea, but with a failure rate of about 10%.

References

ASHFORD, W. A.: Spectinomycin-resistant penicillinase-producing Neisseria gonorrhoeae. Lancet *8254:* 1035 (1981 II).
FIUMARA, N. J.: The treatment of gonococcal proctitis. An evaluation of 173 patients treated with 4 g of spectinomycin. JAMA *239:* 735 (1978).
MCCORMACK, W. M., M. FINLAND: Drugs five years later. Spectinomycin. Ann. intern. Med. *84:* 712 (1976).
PORTER, I. A., H. W. RUTHERFORD: Treatment of uncomplicated gonorrhoea with spectinomycin hydrochloride (Trobicin). Brit. J. vener. Dis. *53:* 115 (1977).
Report of a WHO Scientific Group: Neisseria gonorrhoeae and gonococcal infections. Wld. Hlth. Org. techn. Rep. Ser., No. 616 (1978).
THORNSBERRY, C., H. JAFFEE, S. T. BROWN, T. EDWARDS, J. W. BIDDLE, S. E. THOMPSON: Spectinomycin-resistant Neisseria gonorrhoeae. JAMA *273:* 2405 (1977).

14. Fosfomycin

Proprietary name: Fosfocin (not yet available in Britain).

Properties: This broad-spectrum antibiotic has been developed in the USA and has the following structural formula:

$$H_3C - C - C - PO_3H_2$$

Fosfomycin is an epoxide and bears no chemical relationship to other antibiotics. It is readily soluble in water but insoluble in ethanol. 1 g fosfomycin contains 14.5 milliequivalents of sodium.

Mode of action: Bactericidal in the phase of bactericidal growth. Cell wall synthesis is inhibited by a different mechanism from that of β-lactam antibiotics.

Spectrum of activity: Active *in vitro* against staphylococci, gonococci, Haemophilus influenzae, Escherichia coli, Proteus mirabilis, salmonellae, shigellae, particularly in the presence of glucose-6-phosphate in the medium. Glucose and phosphate inhibits its activity in vitro. Moderately active against streptococci, Pseudomonas aeruginosa and Serratia marcescens. Many strains of Proteus morganii, Klebsiella pneumoniae and Enterobacter species are resistant. Fosfomycin is inactive against all species of Bacteroides. Activity in vitro is very dependent on the culture, inoculum medium and method of testing.

Resistance: Secondary resistance is found *in vitro* and *in vivo* and is due to inhibition of active transport of fosfomycin in the bacterial cell wall. Cross-resistance with other antibiotics is not found.

Pharmacokinetics: Poorly absorbed after oral administration. *Serum concentrations* are 40 mg/l after the i.v. infusion of 3 g and 70 mg/l after 5 g (2 h after the end of the infusion in each case). *Half-life:* 2 h. Not bound to plasma proteins. Good *tissue penetration*. Passes into the CSF and fetal circulation. *Urine recovery:* 90%. High urine concentrations. Little or no metabolism. Dialysable.

Side effects: Local pain after i.m. and phlebitis after i.v. injection; nausea and gastric discomfort are reported in 8% of cases, but vomiting, diarrhoea, headache and allergic reactions are less frequent. *Beware* of sodium load.

Indications: Bacterial infections with sensitive organisms in patients allergic to penicillins and cephalosporins. Do not give as a single agent in severe or life-threatening infection.

Contra-indications: Pregnancy.

Recommended dosage: 3–5 g 2–3 times a day *in adults* (according to the sensitivity of the organisms treated). Reduced dosage in renal failure. Give as a short i. v. infusion over 30 min. Monitor serum electrolytes at higher dosage because of the risk of hypernatraemia.

Preparations: Ampoules of 3 and 5 g.

Summary: A broad-spectrum antibiotic which is well tolerated but has been little used to date. Many questions are still unanswered. Watch for development of resistance during therapy and for hypernatraemia.

References

FOLTZ, E. L., H. WALLICK: Pharmacodynamics of phosphonomycin. Antimicrob. Ag. Chemother. *316:* 968 (1969).

GRIMM, H.: In vitro-Investigations with Fosfomycin on Mueller-Hinton-Agar with and without Glucose-6-Phosphate. Infection 7, No. *5:* 256 (1979).

HIRSCHL, A., M. ROTTER: Einfluß von Glukose-6-Phosphat und anorganischem Phosphat auf die Resistenz von Klebsiellen und E. coli gegen Fosfomyzin. Zbl. Bakt. Hyg., I. Abt. Orig. A. *973:* 222 (1979).

KAHAN, F. M., J. S. KAHAN, P. J. CASSIDY, H. KROPP: The mechanism of action of Fosfomycin. Ann. N. Y. Acad. Sci. *235:* 364 (1974).

KIRBY, W. M. M.: Pharmacokinetics of fosfomycin. Chemotherapy 23 *(Suppl. 1):* 141 (1977).

PETERS, G., F. SCHUHMACHER-PEDREAU, G. PULVERER: Vergleich der Staphylokokken- und Mikrokokken-Wirksamkeit von Fosfomycin, Oxacillin und Penicillin G. Dtsch. med. Wschr. *105:* 1541 (1980).

ULLMANN, U., B. LINDEMANN: In vitro investigations on the action of fosfomycin alone and in combination with other antibiotics on Pseudomonas aeruginosa and Serratia marcescens. Arzneim.-Forsch./Drug Res. *30:* 1247 (1980).

WOODRUFF, H. B., J. M. MATA, S. HERNANDEZ, S. MOCHALES, A. RODRIGUEZ, E. O. STABLEY, H. WALLICK, A. K. MILLER, D. HENDLIN: Fosfomycin: laboratory studies. Chemotherapy 23 *(Suppl. 1):* 1 (1977).

15. Local Antibiotics

a) Bacitracin

Properties: For topical use only; a toxic polypeptide antibiotic which is bactericidal to gram-positive bacteria including staphylococci and enterococci, to

Neisseria and Haemophilus influenzae but not other gram-negative bacteria or fungi. Resistance develops only slowly, and there is no cross-resistance with other antibiotics. Not absorbed by mouth. No longer used parenterally because of nephrotoxicity.

Topical administration: Alone or in combination with neomycin as a skin ointment, powder, spray or eye ointment. Instillation of bacitracin in combination with neomycin is not recommended because of side effects. Systemic antibiotic therapy with other agents is preferable.

Preparations: Nebacetin, Cicatrin (in combination with neomycin); Polybactrin (in combination with neomycin and polymyxin B).

b) Tyrothricin

Properties: A topical bactericidal antibiotic containing gramicidin and tyrocidin. It is a very stable polypeptide, is only partly soluble in water but dissolves in alcohol and propylene glycol. Predominant activity against gram-positive cocci and bacilli and some fungi. No cross-resistance with other antibiotics. Because of its high toxicity, it is not used parenterally or instilled into body cavities.

Administration: External only, on superficial infections as an ointment, powder, spray, solution and lozenges. Several commercial preparations. It should never be used alone in streptococcal sore throat since it is inadequate therapy and does not prevent secondary complications.

16. Antifungal Agents

a) Amphotericin B

Proprietary names: Ampho-Moronal, Fungilin, Fungizone.

Properties: An amphoteric heptaene which, like nystatin and pimaricin, is a member of the polyene group. The amphotericin-B-sodium-desoxycholate complex with phosphate buffer is more water-soluble and so is preferred for intravenous use.

Mode of action: Alteration of cytoplasmic membrane permeability (antagonism of sterol synthesis).

Spectrum of action: Active in candidiasis (Candida albicans and other candida species), histoplasmosis, sporotrichosis, cryptococcosis (torulosis), blastomycosis, mucormycosis, aspergillosis and coccidioidomycosis. No effect against dermatophytes (Microsporum, Trichophyton and Epidermophyton species) or bacteria, viruses or most protozoa. Synergistic in combination with flucytosine but antagonistic with miconazole.

Resistance has not developed during therapy. Primary resistance in strains of candida is very rare. Cross-resistance occurs with other polyenes such as nystatin but not always with pimaricin.

Pharmacokinetics: There is virtually no *absorption* after oral administration. *Serum concentrations* of about 2–3 mg/l follow an i. v. infusion of 0.7–1 mg/kg, and these levels fall slowly. *Half-life:* 20 hours. *Plasma protein binding:* 10%. Poor *CSF penetration,* somewhat improved in meningitis (0.1–0.5 mg/l). Slow renal *excretion* (5% in 24 h, 20–40% in 1 week), urine concentrations between 1 and 5 mg/l. Serum levels are not increased even in severe renal failure. Not dialysable.

Side effects:
1. *Nephrotoxicity:* The increased blood urea is reversible at first, but permanent renal damage can follow higher dosage. Symptoms: haematuria, proteinuria, hyposthenuria, azotaemia, hyperkaliuria and hypokalaemia.
2. *Systemic manifestations:* Fever, rigors, vomiting, circulatory collapse.
3. *Thrombophlebitis* at site of injection.
4. *Rare side effects:* Convulsions, hypomagnesaemia, liver damage, reversible paresis.

Indications: Generalised fungal infections such as histoplasmosis, candida septicaemia and meningitis, cryptococcal meningitis, granulomatous candidiasis, coccidioidomycosis. Sometimes effective in aspergillosis with A. fumigatus. Test sensitivity beforehand and combine with flucytosine if necessary.

Inappropriate use: Parenteral administration for superficial fungal skin infections or without good evidence of generalised fungal infection.

Contra-indication: Impending renal failure (nephrotoxicity).

Administration:
Intravenous infusion in accordance with strict instructions: prepare primary solution by adding 10 ml of distilled water, then dilute with 5% glucose to a concentration of 0.1 mg/ml. Other solutions must not be used as diluents, and the infusion should last at least 6 h.

Topical administration: As ointment, cream, pessaries, vaginal cream, or tablets.

Dosage in parenteral administration:
Give a *test dose* of 1 mg on day 1, 5 mg on day 2 *(adults)*, 10 mg on day 3, followed by a daily increase of 5–10 mg (1–2 mg in *children*) until the full dose of 1 mg/kg/day is reached. A more rapid regime for acute clinical situations is 0.25 mg/kg body weight initially, increased daily by 0.25 mg/kg up to the daily dose of 1 mg/kg. A smaller dose may be adequate when combined with flucytosine (0.3–0.6 mg/kg/day), if sensitivity to flucytosine in vitro has already been established. A total adult dose of 2–4 g should not be exceeded, and treatment will normally be required for 4–8 weeks. Dosage interval: 24 hours, extended to 48 hours when improvement begins. Toxicity should be monitored 2–3 times weekly by blood urea, creatinine, potassium, magnesium, a full blood count, liver function tests and urinalysis. Where febrile reactions occur, hydrocortisone (50 mg initially) or prednisone may be added to the infusion. Small quantities of heparin (1000 U) in the infusion may reduce the risk of thrombophlebitis. If signs of nephrotoxicity emerge, stop amphotericin B until they improve.

Lumbar intrathecal administration in meningitis: Give 10 mg prednisone initially, followed by a slow injection of 0.5 mg amphotericin B diluted with CSF in the syringe. Repeat after 2 or 3 days. If possible increase the dose progressively (0.1 mg on 1st day, increasing by 0.1 mg every second day to 0.5 mg). Side effects: paraesthesiae, transient paralysis, arachnoiditis, and spinal nerve root inflammation.

Intrapleural and intrapericardial instillation is possible (3 mg) as is intra-articular (5–20 mg every 48 h); in the latter case 25 mg of hydrocortisone at the same time improves tolerance.

Bladder instillation (in candida cystitis): Dissolve 50 mg in 1 litre of sterile water and infuse for a day through a 3-way catheter.

Peritoneal lavage with amphotericin B (1 µg/ml) may be performed in candida peritonitis.

Aerosol (5 mg/ml every 6 h) in fungal respiratory infections including pneumonia; absorption through the mucosa does not occur.

Topical administration for gastrointestinal fungal infection: one 100 mg tablet 4 times a day (1 ml suspension 4 times a day in the newborn); for oral thrush: 1 mg lozenge 4 times a day; for vaginal thrush: 10 mg pessary 1–2 times a day, or the introduction of a proprietary applicator filling of vaginal cream.

Preparations: Ampoules for injection containing 50 mg, tablets of 100 mg, lozenges of 10 mg, suspension of 100 mg/ml as well as a lotion, cream, ointment, dry substance (with diluting solution), pessary and vaginal cream. An ointment and cream in combination with triamcinolone, neomycin and gramicidin, and a combination with tetracycline as mystecline (capsules of 250 mg with the addition of 50 mg of amphotericin B).

Summary: A highly effective parenteral anti-fungal antibiotic which carries a risk of serious side effects. Systemic administration is only justifiable in systemic mycoses and severe organ infections where the diagnosis can be made with reasonable certainty.

References

ATKINSON, A. J., jr. J. E. BENNETT: Amphotericin B pharmacocinetics in humans. Antimicrob. Ag. Chemother. *13:* 271 (1978).

BENNETT, J. E.: Chemotherapy of systemic mycoses. New Engl. J. Med. *290:* 30 (1974).

BLOCK, F. E., J. E. BENNETT, L. G. LIVOTI, W. J. KLEIN Jr., R. R. McGREGOR, L. HENDERSON: Flucytosine and amphotericin B: Hemodialysis effects on the plasma concentration and clearance. Studies in man. Ann. intern. Med. *80:* 613 (1974).

EDMONSON, R. P., S. S. EYKYN, D. R. DAVIES, I. W. FAWCETT, I. PHILLIPS: Disseminated histoplasmosis successfully treated with amphotericin B. J. clin. Path. *27:* 308 (1974).

FELDMAN, H. A., J. D. HAMILTON, R. A. GUTMAN: Amphotericin B therapy in an anephric patient. Antimicrob. Ag. Chemother. *4:* 302 (1973).

HAYDEN, G., C. LAPP, F. LODA: Arthritis caused by Monosporium apiospermum treated with intra-articular amphotericin B. Amer. J. Dis. Child. *131:* 927 (1977).

KELLER, M. A., B. B. Jr. SELLERS, M. E. MELISH, G. W. KAPLAN, K. E. MILLER, S. A. MENDOZA: Systemic candidiasis in infants. A case presentation and literature review: Amer. J. Dis. Child *131:* 1260 (1977).

SMITH, J. W.: Synergism of amphotericin B with other antimicrobial agents. Ann. intern. Med. *78:* 450 (1973).

SUTLIFF, W. D.: Histoplasmosis cooperative study. V. Amphotericin B dosage for chronic pulmonary histoplasmosis. Amer. Rev. resp. Dis. *105:* 60 (1972).

TOBIAS, J. S., P. F. M. WRIGLEY, E. SHAW: Combination antifungal therapy for cryptococcal meningitis. Postgrad. med. J. *52:* 305 (1976).

WISE, G. J., S. WAINSTEIN, P. GOLDBERG, P. J. KOZINN: Candidal cystitis. Management by continuous bladder irrigation with amphotericin B. JAMA. *224:* 1636 (1973).

b) Nystatin

Proprietary names: Candex, Fungicidin, Korostatin, Moronal, Mycostatin, Mykogynal, Nilstat, Nyspes, Nystadermal, Nystaform, Nystavescent, Timodine etc.

Properties: An amphoteric tetraene of the polyene group. Insoluble in water but soluble in propylene glycol.

Mode of action: Nystatin increases the permeability of the cytoplasmic membrane of fungi.

Spectrum of action: Active against Candida albicans and other candida species, Blastomyces dermatitidis and brasiliensis, Coccidioides immitis, Cryptococcus neoformans, Histoplasma capsulatum, Geotrichum, Aspergillus. No effect on bacteria, viruses or actinomycetes.

Resistance: Development of resistance during therapy has not been observed. Primary resistant strains are very rare. Cross-resistance with amphotericin B occurs.

Pharmacokinetics: No significant *absorption* after oral or topical administration. A parenteral form is not available.

Side effects: Uncommon (nausea, vomiting and loose stools may all follow a large oral dose).

Indications: Candidiasis of the skin, mouth, genital or intestinal mucosa, candida balanitis, other topical fungal diseases (see spectrum of action), topical treatment in generalised fungal infection. Long-term therapy for susceptible patients such as the newborn, infants treated with antibiotics, diabetics and patients with malignancies, particularly leukaemia.

Administration: As an oral suspension containing 100000 units/ml, or sugar-coated tablets, as a powder or ointment for topical use and as a pessary in vaginitis. A suspension for irrigation and aerosol treatment can be made from an ampoule of sterile pure substance by shaking with 5 ml of physiological saline. The patient inhales 1 ml (= 100,000 u) twice a day as an aerosol. Since nystatin is inactivated by heat, a pressurised inhaler should be used.

Dosage: Adults and children with intestinal candidiasis should be given 1.5–3 million units a day, in three divided doses (0.5–1 million units in the newborn). 1–2 pessaries a day for at least 2 weeks are recommended for candida vaginitis, and in pregnancy this should be started 3–6 weeks before the estimated date of delivery. Used in this way, prophylaxis of neonatal candidiasis can be achieved.

Preparations: Coated tablets, oral suspension, ointment, paste, powder, pessaries, vaginal cream, pure substance, vaginal tablets, eye drops, ear drops, compound gel and ointment (with neomycin, gramicidin and triamcinolone acetonide), paste with zinc oxide etc. Combined with demethyl chlortetracycline as capsules of 300 mg with 500,000 units of nystatin added.

Summary: An antifungal agent for local use only in candidiasis of the skin and mucous membranes, with a low risk of side effects.

c) Natamycin (Pimaricin)

Properties: Natamycin is a tetraene of the polyene group and is mainly fungistatic; it is sensitive to light and insoluble in water. It may be used in skin infections with Candida, Trichophyton and Microsporum species, and is active against trichomonads also.

Administration: As a cream, powder, lozenge, coated tablet, suspension, vaginal tablets; as an eye ointment in combination with neomycin + hydrocortisone; as a cream in combination with benzalkonium chloride and hydrocortisone for anal mycosis and anal fissures.

Reference

RAAB, W.: Natamycin (Pimaricin). Thieme, Stuttgart 1972.

d) Pecilocin

A *topical* antifungal which is inactive against Candida but effective against Trichophyton, Microsporum and Epidermophyton. An unstable oily substance, which, although a tetraene, is not a macrolide.

Proprietary names: Leofungine, Supral, Variotin.

e) Griseofulvin

Proprietary names: Fulcin-125, Fulcin S, Fulvicin, Gricin, Grifulvin, Grisactin, Griseostatin, Grisovin, Lamoryl, Likuden M.

Properties: A benzofuran derivative which is soluble in water but stable at acid pH.

Mode of action: Fungistatic (affects fungal guanine metabolism). No antibacterial activity.

Spectrum of action: Active against all Trichophyton species, Microsporum audouinii, M. canis, M. gypseum, M. distortum, Epidermophyton floccosum and

Tinea species except Tinea (Pityriasis) versicolor. Ineffective against Blastomyces, Candida, Aspergillus, Coccidioides, Cryptococcus, Histoplasma and Mucor. No activity in actinomycosis or erythrasma.

Resistance: Rarely arises during therapy. Cross-resistance with other antibiotics has not been observed.

Pharmacokinetics:

Absorption after oral administration depends on particle size (optimal diameter 0.8–2.7 µ) and is better after a high-fat meal than fasting. *Maximum blood level* occurs 4–5 hours after oral administration.

Serum concentrations: 1–1.5 mg/l with 0.25 g 4 times daily (after 4 h). *Half-life:* about 20 hours.

There is selective deposition in the newly formed keratin of the hair root, nail matrix and epidermis, but only gradual progression from these deep layers to the skin surface. Prolonged therapy is therefore required to eradicate the fungal infection. *Excretion* is largely faecal, with about 1% in the urine.

Side effects (relatively rare despite prolonged administration):
1. Central nervous disorders such as headaches, dizziness, fatigue, psychological disturbances, impaired vision, alcohol intolerance.
2. Gastrointestinal upset.
3. Allergic exanthema or photosensitivity.
4. Reversible leucocytopenia, monocytosis.
5. Transient albuminuria.

Indications: Infections with filamentous fungi, i. e. trichophytosis, microsporosis, onychomycosis, favus and epidermophytosis, where the fungi concerned are sensitive.

Incorrect usage: Candida infections, Tinea versicolor and mild dermatophytoses which should respond to tolnaftate or miconazole.

Contra-indications: Pregnancy, severe liver disease, porphyria.

Dosage: 0.5 g daily for *adults,* 10(−15)mg/kg for *children,* in (1–)2 and preferably 4 single doses. Higher initial dose for extensive lesions (0.75–1 g daily). Half dose upon first signs of improvement, or continue full dose on alternate days. Length of therapy: 1–6 months according to localisation and severity of fungal infection; about 4–6 weeks for tinea capitis, 2–4 weeks for tinea corporis, 4–8 weeks for tinea pedis, 4 months for finger nails, and 6 months for toe nails. Monitor therapy by regular fungal culture. Simultaneous topical therapy with other antifungal agents and keratolytic agents is always recommended, and the removal of the infected hair may be necessary. Barbiturates given at the same time may inhibit the activity of griseofulvin by the induction of hepatic enzymes; the simultaneous administration of coumarin derivatives can impair anticoagulant activity. Avoid extensive exposure to light during therapy because of possible skin photosensitivity.

Preparations: Tablets of 125, 250 or 500 mg.

Summary: A suitable agent for the systemic treatment of severe fungal infections such as trichophytosis, epidermophytosis, microsporosis and onychomycosis, but not for yeast or mould infections. Good results can only be achieved with prolonged treatment. The presence of infection with one of the filamentous fungi should always be confirmed by prior mycological examination.

References

ANDERSON, D. W.: Griseofulvin. Biology and clinical usefulness: a review. Ann. Allergy 23: 103 (1965).
CULLEN, S. I., P. M. CATALANO: Griseofulvin-warfarin antagonism. JAMA. 199: 582 (1967).
FIEDLER, H.: Zur Beeinflussung des Porphyrinstoffwechsels durch Griseofulvin. Biochemische Grundlagen. Derm. Mschr. 157: 79 (1971).
GOLDMANN, L.: Griseofulvin. Med. Clin. North Amer. 54: 1339 (1970).
SHAH, V. P., S. RIEGELMAN, W. L. EPSTEIN: Determination of griseofulvin in skin, plasma and sweat. J. Pharm. Sci 61: 634 (1972).

f) Flucytosine

Proprietary names: Alcobon, Ancobon, Ancotil.

Properties: Flucytosine (5-Fluorocytosine) is a fluorinated pyrimidine (see below for structural formula) and acts as an antimetabolite of cytosine by being transformed into the cytotoxic agent 5-fluorouracil within the cells of sensitive fungi. Flucytosine metabolism is not increased in man. Very little metabolite is excreted in the urine.

Structural formula:

Spectrum of action: Good or excellent activity against Candida albicans, most other species of candida, Cryptococcus neoformans, Geotrichum candidum, some of the aspergilli (particularly Aspergillus fumigatus) and the pathogens of chromoblastomycosis (Phialophora, Cladosporium). There is synergy with amphotericin B against Candida, Cryptococcus and Aspergillus. There is no activity against Histoplasma capsulatum, Blastomyces dermatitidis, Coccidioides immitis, Sporotrichon, Epidermophyton, Mucor and other filamentous fungi, nor against any bacteria.

Resistance: Primary resistance is found in candida (from 20–50%), Cryptococcus, and Aspergillus strains. Disc-sensitivity testing is therefore advisable prior to therapy using antagonist-free culture media in order to avoid false negative results. Secondary resistance often arises during treatment (risk of relapse), especially with infections due to Candida species and Cryptococcus neoformans. No cross-resistance with other antifungal agents.

Pharmacokinetics:

Serum levels of 10–30 mg/l (for 6–10 h) follow the oral administration of 100 mg/kg daily (single dose of 2 g), and CSF levels of 8–20 mg/l. Flucytosine is well distributed and penetrates the aqueous humor, peritoneal exudate and synovial fluid. Maximum serum concentrations of 30–50 mg/l follow the i. v. administration of 1.5–2 g. *Half-life:* 3–4 hours. Little *plasma protein binding.* *Urinary recovery:* 90% (as the unchanged substance). 1–10% eliminated with the faeces. Considerable accumulation in renal failure.

Side effects: Fairly well tolerated even at high dosage. Reversible blood dyscrasias (leukocytopenia, thrombocytopenia and/or anaemia) in about 10% and temporary rise in blood liver enzymes. Gastrointestinal upset, hallucinations, dizziness, headache and fatigue are rare, and fatal cases of agranulocytosis and hepatic necrosis have been described.

Indications: Disseminated infection and severe organ involvement with Cryptococcus neoformans, Candida albicans, Aspergillus fumigatus, Candida glabrata etc., and chromoblastomycosis. Fungal infections in bone-marrow insufficiency (leukaemia etc.) sometimes require urgent treatment without prior testing, although there is then a risk that treatment will fail if the pathogen is resistant. Combined treatment with amphotericin B prevents the emergence of secondary resistance in cryptococcosis, aspergillosis and candidiasis, allows a lower dosage of amphotericin B and gives the best clinical results.

Contra-indication: Pregnancy. Use with caution in renal failure (increased risk of blood toxicity), in liver damage and in pre-existing bone-marrow suppression (due to malignancy).

Administration and dosage: Oral administration of 100–150 (and exceptionally 200) mg/kg body weight daily (6–10 g in adults) in 4 divided doses. Taking the tablets over 15 min reduces nausea and vomiting. Length of treatment: 4–6 weeks, up to 12 weeks for cryptococcosis (risk of relapse). Blood count and liver function need regular monitoring. The tablets dissolve readily in water and can then be taken as a tasteless suspension. Dosage for short i. v. infusion (30 min) as for oral administration. The low concentration (1%) necessitates a high volume of infusion. No other drugs should be mixed with the infusion solution. Reduce dosage in impaired renal function to a single dose of 50 mg/kg 12-hourly (creatinine clearance 20–40 ml/min) and 24-hourly (creatinine clearance 10–20 ml/min). Where there is severe renal impairment, the dose interval must be established by measuring serum concentrations which should lie between 25–40 mg/l and not exceed 80 mg/l. Flucytosine is readily dialysable. A peritoneal lavage with flucytosine (50 mg/l) is useful in candida peritonitis, which sometimes complicates peritoneal dialysis.

For combined therapy with amphotericin B, give 150 mg/kg/day of flucytosine on day 1 with 0.05 mg/kg/day of amphotericin B, 0.10 mg/kg/day on day 2 and 0.25 mg/kg/day on day 3. The 10% ointment is only recommended to supplement the oral or i. v. treatment of chromoblastomycosis, preferably with an occlusive dresssing.

Preparations: Tablets of 0.5 g, infusions of 2.5 g in 250 ml, ointment (10%).

Summary: A reliable antimycotic agent against susceptible strains which is quite well tolerated when used systemically in fungal infections. Should not be used prophylactically because of the risk of secondary resistance. Crosses well into the cerebrospinal fluid. Best effect in combination with amphotericin B.

References

BENNETT, J. E.: Flucytosine. Ann. intern. Med. *86:* 319 (1977).
BLOCK, E. R., J. E. BENNETT: Pharmacological studies with 5-fluorocytosine. Antimicrob. Ag. Chemother. *1:* 476 (1972).
BRYAN, C. S., J. A. McFARLAND: Cryptococcal meningitis. Fatal marrow aplasia from combined therapy. JAMA *239:* 1068 (1978).
DIASIO, R. B., D. E. LAKINGS, J. E. BENNETT: Evidence for conversion of 5-fluorocytosine to 5-fluorouracil in humans: Possible factor in 5-fluorocytosine clinical toxicity. Antimicrob. Ag. Chemother. *14:* 903 (1978).
HOLDSWORTH, S. R., R. C. ATKINS, D. F. SCOTT, R. JACKSON: Management of Candida peritonitis by prolonged peritoneal lavage containing 5-fluorocytosine. Clin. Nephrol. *4:* 147 (1975).
IMBEAU, S. A., L. HANSON, G. LANGEJANS, D. D'ALESSIO: Flucytosine treatment of Candida arthritis. JAMA *238:* 1395 (1977).

KAUFFMANN, C. A., P. T. FRAME: Bone marrow toxicity associated with 5-fluorocytosine therapy. Antimicrob. Ag. Chemother. *11:* 244 (1977).

MEDOFF, G., M. COMFORT, G. S. KOBAYASHI: Synergistic action of amphotericin B and 5-fluorocytosine against yeast-like organisms. Proc. Soc. exp. Biol. *138:* 571 (1971).

MEYER, R., J. L. AXELROD: Fatal aplastic anaemia resulting from flucytosine. JAMA *228:* 1573 (1974).

NORDSTRÖM, L., S. ÖISTÄMO, F. ÖLMEBRING: Candida meningoencephalitis treated with 5-fluorocytosine. Scand. J. infect. Dis. *9:* 63 (1977).

NORMARK, S., J. SCHÖNBECK: In vitro studies of 5-fluorocytosine resistance in Candida albicans and Torulopsis glabrata. Antimicrob. Ag. Chemother. *2:* 114 (1972).

SHADOMY, S., C. B. KIRCHHOFF, A. E. INGROFF: In vitro activity of 5-fluorocytosine against candida and torulopsis species. Antimicrob. Ag. Chemother. *3:* 9 (1973).

SPELLER, D. C. E., M. G. DAVIES: Sensitivity of yeasts to 5-fluorocytosine. J. Med. Microbiol. *6:* 315 (1973).

STANTON, K. G., C. R. SANDERSON: The treatment of systemic cryptococcosis with 5-fluorocytosine. Aust. N. Z. J. Med. *4:* 262 (1974).

g) Clotrimazole

Proprietary names: Canesten, Empecid, Eparol, Lotrimin, Mycelex, Panmicol.

Properties: A tritylimidazole derivative, slightly alkaline, insoluble in water but soluble in lipoid solvents.

Spectrum of action: Fungistatic against dermatomycetes (Trichophyton and Microsporum species, Epidermophyton floccosum), Blastomycetes (Candida), Chromomycetes (Hormodendrum and Phialophora species) and some causes of systemic mycoses. Inactive against most bacteria.

Resistance: Apparently no primary resistance of Candida albicans and Trichophyton. Secondary resistance has not been observed so far.

Indications: Suitable for topical treatment (with a 1% solution, ointment or spray) of dermatomycoses due to Candida, Trichophyton, Microsporum, Epidermophyton floccosum and Malassezia furfur, as well as erythrasma and pityriasis versicolor. Pessaries and vaginal cream are available for the local treatment of candida vaginitis.

Duration of treatment: 4–6 weeks for skin infections with Candida and Trichophyton. About 3 weeks for erythrasma and pityriasis; at least 4 months for onychomycosis.

Preparations: As a solution, ointment, powder, vaginal tablet, vaginal cream and spray. In some countries, also combined with antibiotics (e. g. thiamphenicol) and steroids (e. g. dexamethasone).

Summary: A highly effective topical antimycotic with a broad spectrum and good local tolerance.

References

FREDERIKSSON, T.: Topical treatment of superficial mycoses with clotrimazole. Postgrad. med. J. (Suppl.) *50:* 62 (1974).

HOLT, R. J., R. L. NEWMAN: Laboratory assessment of the antimycotic drug clotrimazole. J. clin. Pathol. *24:* 1089 (1977).

MASTERTON, G., I. R. NAPIER, J. N. HENDERSON, J. E. ROBERTS: Three-day clotrimazole treatment in candidal vulvovaginitis. Brit. J. vener. Dis. *53:* 126 (1977).

PLEMPEL, M., K. BARTMANN: Experimentelle Untersuchungen zur antimykotischen Wirkung von Clotrimazol in vitro und bei lokaler Applikation in vivo. Arzneimittel-Forsch. *22:* 1280 (1972).

UTZ, J. P.: New drugs for the systemic mycoses: Flucytosine and clotrimazole. Bull. N. Y. Acad. Med. *51:* 1103 (1975).

h) Miconazole

Proprietary names: Daktar, Daktarin, Dermonistat, Gyno-Daktar, Gyno-Daktarin, Gyno-Monistat, Monistat.

Properties: Miconazole is a poorly water-soluble imidazole derivative with less *in-vitro* activity than clotrimazole. It also has a wide range of action including Epidermophyton, Trichophyton, Candida and Aspergillus species as well as Malassezia furfur (the cause of tinea versicolor). Histoplasma capsulatum, Coccidioides immitis and some gram-positive bacteria (e. g. nocardia, streptococci) are also sensitive. No activity against gram-negative bacteria. Structural formula:

Pharmacokinetics:
Miconazole is not absorbed when applied to skin or mucous membranes and only slightly absorbed when given orally. Intravenous dosage achieves *maximal*

serum concentrations which are tenfold greater than after oral administration (5–7 mg/l after 0.8 g i.v.). *Half-life:* 20 hours. *Plasma protein binding:* 98%. *Urinary recovery:* 10% (only 1% unchanged). Highly metabolised in the body. Low concentrations in CSF and aqueous humor. Half-life is not prolonged in renal failure. Only dialysable to a small extent.

Side effects: Thrombophlebitis not uncommonly complicates administration. Vomiting, diarrhoea, allergic reactions, fever and flushes are also reported. Tachycardia and arrhythmias can follow rapid injection. The proprietary solvent Cremophor in the intravenous preparation can cause hyperlipaemia and changes in the blood picture (erythrocyte rouleaux, anaemia and thrombocytosis). Generally well tolerated.

Indications: Topical treatment of infections with dermatomycetes and candida. Systemic treatment of localised organ involvement, disseminated fungal infection and severe cutaneous mycoses, especially candidiasis, aspergillosis, cryptococcosis, as well as blastomycosis and coccidioidomycosis. Should not be combined with amphotericin B in systemic use because of the possibility of antagonism.

Administration and dosage: Powders and ointment may be used for the *topical treatment of skin infections.* Prolonged treatment with occlusive dressings is necessary for nail infections. *Candidal vaginitis* should be treated for at least 2 weeks, despite rapid improvement, to prevent recurrence. Miconazole gel may be given for *oral thrush* for 1–2 weeks (1.25 ml four times a day in the newborn, and 2.5 ml four times daily for older children). Adults with oral thrush should dissolve a tablet in the mouth several times a day.

Systemic and organic mycoses in adults are treated with a daily dose of 0.6 g by i.v. infusion in 60 min; children should receive 15–20 mg/kg. The dosage can be increased without risk up to 1.8 g a day in 2 or 3 doses. Phlebitis may be avoided by adequate dilution or by infusion through a central venous line. Treatment should last at least 12 days. Miconazole should not be given orally in systemic mycoses.

Bladder instillations: 200 mg in 20 ml of undiluted solution 2–4 times a day.
Sinus instillations: 20 ml of solution twice a day.
Aerosol inhalations: 50 mg in 5 ml of undiluted solution 2–4 times a day.
Intrathecal instillations: 20 mg in 2 ml of undiluted solution once a day.

Preparations: Powder, ointment (2%), gel, lotion, solution, vaginal cream, pessaries, tampons, solution for i.v. infusion in 0.2 g ampoules, tablets of 125 mg and 250 mg.

Summary: An effective broad-spectrum antimycotic for topical and systemic use. Treatment should last long enough to prevent recurrence. Some failures of treatment of systemic fungal infections are reported. A valuable alternative to amphotericin B because of its better tolerance. Will probably be superceded by ketoconazole for systemic treatment.

References

BANNATYNE, R. M., R. CHEUNG: Susceptibility of Candida albicans to miconazole. Antimicrob. Ag. Chemother. *13:* 1040 (1978).

DERESINSKI, S. C.: Treatment of fungal meningitis with miconazole. Amer. Rev. resp. Dis. *113:* 71 (1976).

FISCHER, T. J.: Miconazole in the treatment of chronic mucocutaneous candidiasis: a preliminary report. J. Pediat. *91:* 815 (1977).

HATALIA, M.: Miconazole in systemic candidosis. Proc. roy. Soc. Med. (Suppl. 1) *70:* 20 (1977).

HOLT, R. J., A. AZMI: Miconazole-resistant Candida. Lancet *1:* 50 (1978).

IWAND, A., D. DEPPERMANN: Miconazole in systemic mycosis. Proc. roy. Soc. Med. *(Suppl. 1) 70:* 43 (1977).

KATZ, M. E., P. A. CASSILETH: Disseminated candidiasis in a patient with acute leukaemia. Successful treatment with miconazole. JAMA *237:* 1124 (1977).

LEWI, P. J., J. BOELAERT, R. DANEELS, R. DE MEYERE, H. VAN LANDUYT, J. J. HEYKANTS, P. SYMOENS, J. WYNANTS: Pharmacokinetic profile of intravenous miconazole in man. Comparison of normal subjects and patients with renal insufficiency. Europ. J. clin. Pharmacol. *10:* 49 (1976).

MARMION, L. C., K. B. DESSER, R. B. LILLY, D. A. STEVENS: Reversible thrombocytosis and anemia due to miconazole therapy. Antimicrob. Ag. Chemother. *10:* 447 (1976).

SCHACTER, L. P., R. J. OWELLEN, H. K. RATHBUN, B. BUCHANAN: Antagonism between miconazole and amphotericin B. Lancet *2:* 318 (1976).

STEVENS, D. A., H. B. LEVINE, S. C. DERESINSKI: Miconazole in coccidioidomycosis II. Therapeutic and pharmacologic studies in man. Amer. J. Med. *60:* 191 (1976).

STILLE, W., E. HELM, W. KILP: Treatment of fungal infections with miconazole. Proc. roy. Soc. Med. *70:* 40 (1977).

SYMOENS, J.: Clinical and experimental evidence on miconazole for the treatment of systemic mycosis: A review. Proc. roy. Soc. Med. (Suppl. 1) *70:* 4 (1977).

VERHAEGEN, H.: Miconazole treatment in candidal oesophagitis. Proc. roy. Soc. Med. (Suppl. 1) *70:* 47 (1977).

i) Econazole

Proprietary names: Ecostatin, Epi-Pevaryl, Gyno-Pevaryl, Mycopevaryl, Skilar.

Properties: Imidazole derivative, closely related chemically to miconazole (1 chlorine atom less). Structural formula:

Econazole is somewhat more active *in vitro* against fungi than miconazole. Effective in topical treatment of cutaneous mycoses and vaginal thrush.

Administration: Topical as a powder, ointment, lotion, pessaries and spray.

Reference

THIENPONT, D., J. VAN CUTSEM, J. M. VAN NUETEN, C. J. E. NIEMEGEERS, R. MARSBOOM: Biological and toxicological properties of econazole, a broad spectrum antimycotic. Arzneimittel-Forsch. *25:* 224 (1975).

j) Ketoconazole

Proprietary name: Nizoral.

Properties: An imidazole dioxolane derivative with a similar range of activity to miconazole, namely dermatophytes, candida and other fungal pathogens. Poorly water-soluble except at a pH of 3.0 or less, highly lipophilic and with the following structural formula:

Pharmacokinetics:
Absorption with and after meals is considerably better than fasting. *Serum levels* after 0.2 g oral administration: 3 mg/l (1–2 h), 0.08 mg/l (12 h) and 0.03 mg/l (24 h). *Half-life:* 8 hours. *Plasma protein binding:* 99%. *Urine recovery:* 2–4% (unchanged). 20–65% is excreted with the faeces. Highly metabolised.

Side effects: Itching, nausea, vomiting, or diarrhoea in about 10%; dizziness, headaches, liver damage and rashes are less frequent.

Indications: Deep cutaneous mycoses, also pityriasis versicolor and chronic mucocutaneous candidiasis, as well as systemic and organic mycoses (candidiasis, coccidioidomycosis, histoplasmosis), and chronic and recurrent vaginal mycoses. Prophylaxis in leukaemia.

Contra-indications: Pregnancy. Should not be used for uncomplicated infections which will respond to topical treatment.

Dosage: 200 mg by mouth once a day, always with meals, and 3 mg/kg for children. Dosage can be increased to 600 mg (9 mg/kg) once a day. Duration of therapy: 10 days for thrush, 1–2 months for deep cutaneous mycoses and systemic candidiasis, and 2–6 months for coccidioidomycosis and histoplasmosis.

Preparation: Tablets of 200 mg.

Summary: The first antifungal imidazole to be relatively well absorbed with few side effects. The effectiveness of this agent in therapy still needs further evaluation.

References

BORELLI, D., J. FUENTES, E. LEIDERMAN, M. A. RESTREPO, J. L. BRAN, R. LEGENDRE, H. B. LEVINE, D. A. STEVENS: Ketoconazole, an oral antifungal: laboratory and clinical assessment of imidazole drugs. Postgrad. med. J. *55:* 657 (1979).

BOTTER, A. A.: Skin and nail mycoses, treatment with ketoconazole. Mykosen *22:* 274 (1979).

FIBBE, W. E., J. W. M. VAN DER MEER, J. THOMPSON, R. P. MOUTON: CSF concentrations of ketoconazole. J. Antimicrob. Chemother. *6(5):* 681 (1980).

GRAYBILL, J. R., J. H. HERNDON, W. T. KNIKER, H. B. LEVINE: Ketoconazole treatment of chronic mucocutaneous candidiasis. Arch. Derm. *116:* 1137 (1980).

JONES, H. E., J. G. SIMPSON, W. M. ARTIS: Oral ketoconazole: an effective and safe treatment for dermatophytosis. Arch. Derm. *117:* 129 (1981).

ROSENBLATT, H. M., W. BYRNE, M. E. AMENT, J. GRAYBILL, E. R. STIEHM: Successful treatment of chronic mucocutaneous candidiasis with ketoconazole. J. Pediat. *97:* 657 (1980).

ZELLWEGER, J. P.: Traitement oral au ketoconazole d'un cas d'histoplasmose pulmonaire. Schweiz. med. Wschr. *111:* 190 (1980).

k) Isoconazole

Proprietary names: Bi-Vaspit, Fazol, Gyno-Travogen, Travocort, Travogen, Travogyn.

Properties: An imidazole derivative with activity against candida, dermatophytes and moulds. A 1% cream or solution in polyethylene glycol may be used for superficial fungal infections of the skin, erythrasma and pityriasis versicolor. A combined ointment containing corticosteroids is available but should not be used for longer than 2 weeks. Hypersensitivity to cetyl and stearyl alcohols in the ointment or polyethylene glycol in the solution sometimes occurs. Avoid eye contact. Vaginal pessaries containing 300 mg and a vaginal cream are available for the topical treatment of vulvovaginal mycoses.

Side effects: Skin and mucosal inflammation.

l) Ciclopiroxolamine

Proprietary name: Batrafen.

Properties: A topical antifungal agent. It is not an imidazole but a pyridone derivative, and so is unrelated to other antimycotics. When given as the aminoethyl salt, it is active against dermatophytes and pathogenic yeasts and moulds. Penetrates the deeper layers of the skin and nails well. Percutaneous absorption: about 1%. Absorbed better from the vaginal mucosa, so should be avoided in pregnancy. Generally well tolerated; itching and skin burning are rare. Avoid contact with eyes. The ointment and vaginal cream contain cetyl and stearyl alcohols which may cause hypersensitivity. Effective against superficial cutaneous fungal infections, mycosis of the nail, and vaginal thrush. Available as a lotion, ointment, and vaginal cream (apply sparingly 2–3 times a day). Treat dermatomycoses for 2 weeks and vaginal thrush for 6 days. Prolonged therapy is only justified for infections of the nails.

Summary: A non-imidazole broad-spectrum antimycotic for the treatment of dermatomycoses.

References

ADAM, W.: Klinische Ergebnisse mit dem Antimykotikum Ciclopiroxolamin. Arzneimittel-Forsch. *31:* 1360 (1981).
ALPERMANN, H. G., E. SCHÜTZ: Zur Pharmakologie und Toxikologie von Ciclopiroxolamin. Arzneimittel-Forsch. *31:* 1328 (1981).

DITTMAR, W.: Offene, außereuropäische Studien zur Wirksamkeit und Verträglichkeit von Ciclopiroxolamin bei Dermatomykosen. Arzneimittel-Forsch. *31:* 1381 (1981).
DITTMAR, W.: Mikrobiologische Laboruntersuchungen mit Ciclopiroxolamin. Arzneimittel-Forsch. *31:* 1317 (1981).
KOCH, H.: Ciclopiroxolamin: antifungal agent. Pharmacy international *3:* 46 (1982).
QUADRIPUR, S.-A.: Zur Lokalwirksamkeit von Ciclopiroxolamin bei Nagelmykosen. Arzneimittel-Forsch. *31:* 1369 (1981).

m) Tolnaftate

Proprietary names: Tinactin, Tinaderm, Tonoftal.

Properties: A colourless, flavourless, synthetic antifungal agent. Fungicidal against Trichophyton, Microsporum, Epidermophyton, Aspergillus niger, but not Candida species.

Indications: Skin infections with filamentous fungi, pityriasis versicolor, erythrasma and onychomycosis. Alternate treatment with 10% salicylic acid ointment in hyperkeratosis. Available as an ointment, solution and powder. Combined preparations containing nystatin, against candida, are also available.

17. Chemotherapeutic Agents

a) Sulphonamides

Classifications and common proprietary names:
Short-acting sulphonamides: Sulphasomidine (Aristamid, Elcosine, Elkosin, Isosulf), sulphaurea (Euvernil, Uromide), sulphafurazole (Gantrisin), sulphamethizole (Urolucosil), sulphadimidine (Sulphamezathine).
Medium-acting sulphonamides: Sulphadiazine, sulphamoxole (Justamil, Sulphmidil, Sulfuno), sulphamethoxazole (Gantanol).
Long-acting sulphonamides: Sulphamethoxypyridazine (Lederkyn), sulphadimethoxine (Deposul, Madribon), sulfaperin (Pallidin), sulfamethoxydiazine (Bayrena, Durenate, Kiron, Ultrax), sulfaclomide, sulfamerazine (Mebacid).
Ultra-long-acting sulphonamides: Sulfametopyrazine (Kelfizine, Longum), sulfadoxine (Fanasil).
Polysulphonamides: Sulphaethidole + sulphamethizole (Harnosal).
Poorly absorbed sulphonamides: Formosulphathiazole (Formo-Cibazol), formophthalylsulphacarbamide (Intestin-Euvernil), sulphaguanidine (Resulfon), sul-

phaguanole (Enterocura), phthalylsulphathiazole (Neo-Sulfazon, Talisulfazol, Thalazole).

Properties: All sulphonamides are derivatives of para-aminobenzene-sulphonamide with a benzene nucleus consisting of an amino (NH_2) and an amido (SO_2NH_2) group. The structural formula of sulphanilamide is:

$$H_2N-\langle\ \rangle-SO_2NH_2$$

Mode of action: Bacteriostatic for proliferating bacteria by inhibition of folic acid synthesis (blocking the enzyme which forms folic acid from para-aminobenzoic acid), and partly also by inactivation of other enzymes, e. g. dehydrogenase or carboxylase (inhibition of bacterial respiration).

Spectrum of action: Good activity against streptococci (except enterococci), pneumococci, meningococci, actinomycetes and chlamydia.

Moderate, slight or variable activity against Escherichia coli, Proteus, Klebsiella pneumoniae, Enterobacter aerogenes, Haemophilus influenzae, Pseudomonas aeruginosa, Brucella, enterococci, gonococci, staphylococci, shigellae etc. Rickettsiae, spirochaetes, mycobacteria and fungi are *completely resistant*.

Resistance: Streptococci, pneumococci and gonococci can become resistant during prolonged therapy (more than 3 weeks). Meningococci are nowadays often resistant to sulphonamides (up to 75%) as are Shigella, Proteus, Escherichia coli etc. There is almost total cross-resistance between individual sulphonamides but no cross-resistance with antibiotics. *In vitro* tests, particularly disc-sensitivity determinations, are unreliable with sulphonamides; the marked inoculum effect and influence of antagonists in the culture medium can give a false picture of resistance.

Pharmacokinetics:
Sulphonamides are *well absorbed* in the stomach and small intestine (80–100%) after oral administration, with a maximal blood concentration after 4–6 hours.

Blood concentrations of individual sulphonamides after oral administration vary between 50 and 150 mg/l; the decisive factor is the content of free, non-acetylated and non-protein-bound sulphonamide. Very low blood levels (10–30 mg/l or less) are found with the poorly absorbable sulphonamides.

The *half-life* in the blood is less than 8 hours for short-acting sulphonamides, 24 to 48 hours for the long-acting sulphonamides and about 65 hours for sulphametopyrazine. Half-lives of the polysulphonamides vary but are mostly between 10 and 20 hours.

Plasma protein binding: Some sulphonamides are reversibly bound to protein in the blood and have no antibacterial activity; the irreversibly acetylated sulphonamides behave similarly. The level of protein binding depends on the blood level and is generally lower in short-acting sulphonamides than in most of the medium-acting and long-acting sulphonamides (70–90% and above). However, sulphametopyrazine, which is an ultra-long-acting sulphonamide, has a protein binding of only 34%. The *degree of acetylation* of sulphonamides in the blood varies between 5 and 20%.

Cerebrospinal fluid penetration is quite good with sulfasomidine, sulphamethoxydiazine and sulfamoxole, but is best with sulphadiazine (CSF serum distribution coefficient: 0.3–0.8). The sulphonamides pass more readily into the CSF when the meninges are inflamed and the protein content of the CSF is increased.

Tissue concentrations: Sulphonamides are concentrated well in the stomach, kidneys, and skin, moderately in the liver, lungs, uterus and muscle and poorly in the brain, bones, adrenal and intestines. They diffuse well into the aqueous humor of the eye, readily into the fetal circulation, but pass poorly into the breast milk. 50–70% of the serum values are found in pleural and pericardial effusions and ascites. Varying concentrations are found in the liver and gall-bladder according to the preparation given and the state of liver function.

Excretion: Predominantly urinary (60–90% with most preparations) and the remainder in the faeces. Present in urine as free sulphonamide and also as an antibacterially inert acetyl derivative and glucuronide. Excretion is mostly by glomerular filtration but partly by tubular secretion, and free sulphonamide is reabsorbed through the tubules. There is rapid excretion of the short-acting sulphonamides and almost no reabsorption through the kidneys, while the excretion of long-acting sulphonamides is retarded and reabsorption is greater (e. g. 60–85% with sulphamethoxydiazine). Urine concentrations of short-acting sulphonamides (daily dose of 3 g): about 1–2 g/l; long-acting sulphonamides (daily dose of 0.5 g): about 0.1–0.5 g/l. About 90% of the poorly absorbable sulphonamides pass in the faeces (only 30% of sulfaguanidine).

Side effects:
1. *Allergic reactions:* Occur in 1–3% of cases as fever, conjunctivitis and rashes (macular, nodular or urticarial), mostly between the 5th and 9th day of treatment. They may be more severe with medium and long-acting sulphonamides than with the rapidly excreted short-acting compounds and were more frequent when sulphonamides were used for the topical treatment of the

skin. Sulphonamide allergy can be demonstrated by patch tests with sulphonamide ointment performed after scarification of the skin. Sulphonamide medication can also cause photosensitivity of the skin, the Stevens-Johnson syndrome, erythema multiforme, erythema nodosum, exfoliative dermatitis and toxic epidermolysis (Lyell's syndrome).

2. *Renal damage:* Deposition of crystals of poorly soluble sulphonamides and particularly of acetyl derivatives in the kidneys can cause renal colic, haematuria, the passage of casts, albuminuria, oliguria and anuria. The occurrence of these side effects depends on the solubility of the related sulphonamide in the urine, which is normally acid (pH 5.5–6.5), the rate of acetylation in the urine (preferably not more than 50%), the dosage and the fluid intake. Modern sulphonamides carry almost no risk of renal damage by crystallisation because of the low degree of acetylation and improved solubility, even in slightly acid urine. Crystalluria can still occur with the poorly soluble sulphadiazine, however. Great care must be taken in patients with dehydration and renal insufficiency. Premature and newborn babies should not be treated with sulphonamides because of their immature renal and hepatic function.

3. *Gastrointestinal upset* with nausea and vomiting are less frequent with the new sulphonamides because of their reduced dosage.

4. There is a risk of *hyperbilirubinaemia* in premature and full-term neonates because the bilirubin is insufficiently bound to glucuronic acid, and so is excreted in this form. Bilirubin is also displaced by sulphonamides from its albumin-binding site and can therefore diffuse more easily through the vascular walls.

5. *Abnormal blood counts* resulting from toxic or allergic bone marrow lesions (agranulocytosis, aplastic anaemia) are rare; they generally develop after longer courses of treatment, from the third week onwards, and are also occasionally associated with long-acting sulphonamides.

6. *Cyanosis* due to sulph- or methaemoglobinaemia is very uncommon nowadays except in cases of congenital erythrocyte glucose-6-phosphate dehydrogenase deficiency and haemoglobinopathies, e. g. Hb Köln and Hb Zürich.

7. Cholestatic *jaundice* is rare.

Indications: Toxoplasmosis (in combination with pyrimethamine), trachoma, nocardiosis (in combination with another agent such as ampicillin) and chloroquine-resistant malaria (in combination with pyrimethamine etc.). Long-term treatment with sulphamethoxypyridazine or diaminodiphenylsulphone (Dapsone) has been effective against dermatitis herpetiformis. Other indications mentioned earlier are generally no longer valid because of the frequency of bacterial resistance and the superiority of co-trimoxazole and antibiotics. Urinary infections used to be treated with sulphadimidine, sulphafurazole, sulphasomidine and sulphaurea because of their rapid absorption and excretion, mainly as free sulphonamide. Because of their cheapness, there is still a place for these agents in the initial treatment of acute, uncomplicated cystitis in women presenting outside hospital. Drugs used earlier in gastroenteritis, such as formosulphathiazole and formophthalylsulphacarbamide, which are hardly absorbed and produce no tissue levels, are no longer indicated and are replaced by co-trimoxazole. Sulfaguanidine is about 40% absorbed, but the achievable serum concentrations are only 20–50 mg/l, of which 25–40% is acetylated and hence ineffective. Entero-pathogenic bacteria are now generally resistant to sulphonamides, although these drugs are still used, largely empirically and often in combination (e. g. triple sulphonamide) for the treatment of travellers' diarrhoea.

The *long-acting sulphonamides* sulphamethoxypyridazine, sulphadimethoxine and sulfaperin are rapidly absorbed and very slowly excreted. A single daily dose produces adequate blood levels, but approximately 90% is bound to plasma protein. Since a low dosage is sufficient because of the slow excretion, the risk of gastrointestinal upset and renal damage is reduced, but allergic reactions and blood dyscrasias are more frequent than with the short-acting sulphonamides. The same is true for sulphamethoxydiazine which is only 75% bound to plasma protein. Sulphametopyrazine has a low plasma protein binding of 34% and the longest half-life (65 h). After a 5-fold initial dose, a daily dose of 100 mg (every 24 h) is adequate, and in uncomplicated urinary infections with sensitive organisms, the initial dose will suffice.

The position of the cheap and stable sulphonamides is more important in developing countries with a restricted supply of other agents. Here they belong to the WHO list of essential drugs.

Sulphasalazine (Salazopyrine), a compound of sulphapyridine and salicylic acid, is useful in ulcerative colitis both in the acute attack and to prevent relapse. After absorption from the upper gastrointestinal tract, sulphasalazine is mainly excreted through the bile into the intestines, from where it is split by intestinal bacteria into 5-aminosalicylic acid (the active substance) and sulphapyridine. After oral administration, the sulphonamide is only partially absorbed from the intestinal tract and leads, in patients who are rapid acetylators, to relatively low blood levels (10–20 mg/l) after 3–4 g daily. Slow acetylators produce levels of more than 50 mg/l and suffer more frequent side effects. Slow acetylators should therefore only receive 2.5–3 g daily. Allergic rashes and fever are not uncommon.

Sulphasalazine is also used for the treatment of Crohn's disease. It can be given as an enema.

Mafenide was an early discovery and, although too weak for general use, is active against Pseudomonas and therefore used as a 10% cream for the topical treatment of burns. Side effects include intense pain (due to hypertonic concentration), the inhibition of carbonic anhydrase (with subsequent acidosis and hyperventilation), and a 5% allergy rate. Silver sulphadiazine 1% cream (Flamazine) and silver nitrate chlorhexidine cream are also used to treat bums locally, but have been associated with the emergence of resistant strains of Enterobacteriaceae.

Inappropriate use of sulphonamides: Infections against which antibiotics are more effective, e. g. streptococcal sore throat, scarlet fever, gonorrhoea, pneumonia, septicaemia, endocarditis, staphylococcal infection, ENT infections etc.

Contra-indications: Hypersensitivity to sulphonamides, renal failure, liver damage, late pregnancy, the premature and full-term newborn, hereditary erythrocytic glucose-6-phosphate-dehydrogenase deficiency, haemoglobinopathies such as Hb Köln and Hb Zürich.

Table 19. Dosage of sulphonamides.

	Age	Average daily dose	Maximum daily dose
Short-acting sulphonamides (e. g. sulphadimidine, sulphamethizole, sulphasomidine, sulphaurea)	Adults Children of 6 – 12 y. 1 – 6 y. 0 – 1 y.	4.0 – 6.0 g 3.0 – 4.0 g 2.0 – 3.0 g 1.0 – 2.0 g	6.0 – 8.0 g 4.0 – 5.0 g 3.0 – 4.0 g 2.0 g
Medium-acting sulphonamides (e. g. sulphadiazine, sulphamoxole)	Adults Children of 6 – 12 y. 1 – 6 y. 0 – 1 y.	1.0 g^1 1.0 g^1 0.5 g^1 0.25 g^1	2.0 g 1.5 g 1.0 g 0.5 g
Long-acting sulphonamides (e. g. sulphamethoxypyridazine, sulfaperin)	Adults Children of 6 – 12 y. 1 – 6 y. 0 – 1 y.	0.5 g^1 0.37 g^1 0.25 g^1 $0.06 – 0.12 \text{ g}^1$	1.0 g 0.5 g 0.25 g 0.12 g
Poorly absorbable sulphonamides (e. g. formosulphathiazole, formophthalylsulphacarbamide)	Adults Children Newborn	4.0 – 5.0 g 1.5 – 2.0 g 0.75 g	
Ultra-long-acting sulphonamides (sulfadoxine, sulfametopyrazine)	Adults	2.0 g 1 dose per week	

[1] Double dose initially.

Administration:
Intravenous administration often gave rise to thrombophlebitis because of the alkaline reaction of the solutions and used in exceptional cases to be given at the start of therapy and also in somnolence and vomiting.

Intramuscular administration is not recommended because of local irritation. Rectal administration is unreliable and intralumbar administration dangerous. Intrapleural and intraperitoneal instillation are poorly tolerated and have been superceded by bactericidal antibiotics. They are not used topically on the skin or mucous membranes because of the risk of sensitisation (exception: ophthalmic infections).

Oral administration is the route of choice, provided there is adequate fluid intake.

Dosage *for oral administration* varies for short-, medium- and long-acting sulphonamides (Table 19). The upper dosage limit should not be exceeded because of the risk of accumulation, particularly with the long-acting sulphonamides. The intervals depend on the rates of excretion: 4–6 hours with short-acting sulphonamides, 12 hours with medium-acting sulphonamides, 24 hours with long-acting sulphonamides and 6–8 hours with poorly absorbable sulphonamides. A single dose of 2 g of sulphametopyrazine generates an adequate level for one week.

Preparations: Tablets of 500 mg and 750 mg, of 2 g (sulphametopyrazine only). Coated tablets of 400 mg. Solution for injection in ampoules of 500 mg, 1 g and 2 g. 5% and 10% syrups. 10% suspension. 12.5% and 20% drops. 5% solution for bladder instillation. Eye drops. Eye ointment.

Summary:
Advantages: Broad spectrum of action, well absorbed by mouth, good diffusion into CSF (with some sulphonamides), rare side effects when administered correctly (except for some allergic reactions).

Disadvantages: Not bactericidal, and generally less active than antibiotics; slow onset of action (latent period); inactivation by serum, pus and tissue autolysate; increasing resistance of pathogens; difficult evaluation of *in vitro* sensitivity tests.

Because of their much poorer activity and the development of antibiotics and the trimethroprim-sulphonamide combination, sulphonamides have become less important and now have few indications in Europe and the USA.

References

Azad Khan, A. K., J. Piris, S. C. Truelove: An experiment to determine the active therapeutic moiety of sulphasalazine. Lancet 2: 892 (1977).
Bridges, K., E. J. L. Lowbury: Drug resistance in relation to use of silver sulphadiazine cream in a burns unit. J. clin. Path. 30: 160 (1977).
Buchanan, N.: Sulphamethoxazole, hypoalbuminaemia, crystalluria, and renal failure. Brit. med. J. 2: 172 (1978).
Cowan, G. O., K. M. Das, M. A. Eastwood: Further studies of sulphasalazine metabolism in the treatment of ulcerative colitis. Brit. med. J. 2: 1057 (1977).
Craft, A. W., J. T. Brocklebank, R. H. Jackson: Acute renal failure and hypoglycaemia due to sulphadiazine poisoning. Postgrad. med. J. 53: (1977).
Goldman, P. M. A. Peppercorn: Drug therapy: Sulfasalazine. New Engl. J. Med. 293: 20 (1975).
Griffiths, I. D., S. P. Kane: Sulphasalazine-induced lupus syndrome in ulcerative colitis. Brit. med. J. 2: 1188 (1977).
Kane, S. P., M. A. Boots: Megaloblastic anaemia associated with sulphasalazine treatment. Brit. med. J. 2: 1287 (1977).
Lowbury, E. J. L., J. R. Baab, K. Bridges, D. M. Jackson: Topical chemoprophylaxis with silver sulphadiazine and silver nitrate chlorhexidine creams: Emergence of sulphonamide-resistant Gram-negative bacilli. Brit. med. J. 1: 493 (1976).
Mihas, A. A., D. J. Goldenberg, R. L. Slaughter: Sulfasalazine toxic reactions, hepatitis, fever, and skin rash with hypocomplementemia and immune complexes. JAMA 239: 2590 (1978).
Tydd, T. F., N. H. Dyer: Sulphasalazine lung. Med. J. Aust. 1: 570 (1976).
van Hees, P. A. M., J. H. M. van Tongeren, J. H. Barke, H. J. J. van Lier: Active therapeutic moiety of sulphasalazine. Lancet 1: 277 (1978).

b) Co-trimoxazole

Proprietary names: Bactrim, Cotrimox, Eusaprim, Fectrim, Nodilon, Oecotrim, Septra, Septrin, Sulfatrim, Sulptrim.

Description: A combination of the chemotherapeutic agent trimethoprim with the sulphonamide sulphamethoxazole. Trimethoprim is a weak base, is poorly water-soluble, and is, like the antimalarial drug pyrimethamine, a diaminopyrimidine. It has the following structural formula:

Sulphamethoxazole is closely related to sulphisoxazole but is excreted more slowly and so is regarded as a medium-acting sulphonamide. Other sulphonamides, such as sulphadiazine, sulphametrole and sulphamoxole (see page 202) are used in place of sulphamethoxazole.

Mode of action: Inhibition of bacterial folic acid synthesis. Sulphamethoxazole inhibits the use of the p-aminobenzoic acid and trimethoprim blocks the reduction of dihydrofolic acid to tetrahydrofolic acid. Sulphamethoxazole and trimethoprim alone act bacteriostatically and the combination of both has been claimed by some to produce a bactericidal effect although this claim has been disputed. Certainly, the antibacterial activity of the combination is greater than that of the individual components. The activity against most pathogens is increased with a concentration of 1 part trimethoprim and 20 parts of sulphamethoxazole which, after oral administration, the body absorbs in a ratio of 1:5. The synergistic (potentiated) activity is explained by the sequential sites of action of each component in the bacterial metabolic pathway. This synergy is greatest when the pathogen is sensitive to both drugs. The potentiation of trimethoprim activity by the sulphonamide (and vice versa) varies in intensity with the bacterial species and also within the same species, i.e. it can differ from strain to strain. Synergy is sometimes absent, even when the bacteria are sensitive to both agents. Folic acid deficiency does not generally arise in man because the body's folic acid requirement is supplied in the food and human folic acid reductase is not inhibited until trimethoprim concentrations are 50,000 times in excess.

Spectrum of action: Trimethoprim is active against a broad range of pathogenic bacteria except clostridia, Treponema pallidum, leptospiras, rickettsiae, Chlamydia psittaci, tubercle bacilli and Pseudomonas aeruginosa; it has no effect against mycoplasmas and fungi. The combination extends the range of activity of the sulphonamide component.

An increasing percentage of local and urinary infections may be resistant to co-trimoxazole, however, and sensitivities should be tested before beginning treatment. Species in which resistance is found include Staphylococcus aureus, enterococci, pneumococci, Klebsiella and Enterobacter. Resistant strains of Haemophilus influenzae are rare. Co-trimoxazole is also active against malarial parasites, but not as effective as chloroquine. It is active, in combination, against chloroquine-resistant falciparum malaria, and also against Pneumocystis carinii.

Resistance: Secondary resistance *in vitro* can be selected for by serial passage through trimethoprim-containing media. Resistance has developed during treatment of infections caused by Escherichia coli and Haemophilus. Culture media free of antagonists (e.g. Oxoid DST medium) must be used when testing bacterial sensitivity in vitro. They should have as low a thymidine content as possible.

Pharmacokinetics: *Trimethoprim* is almost completely absorbed after oral administration. *Maximal blood levels* occur after 1½–3½ hours (0.9–1.2 mg/l after

100 mg orally, and about 2 mg/l after 160 mg). During therapy with i. v. infusion of 0.16 g trimethoprim +0.8 g sulphamethoxazole (over 1 h) repeated devery 8 hours serum concentrations are 2 mg/l (trimethoprim) and 30 mg/l (free sulphamethoxazole). *Protein binding* 45%, *half-life* 12 hours. High tissue levels, especially in the lungs and kidneys. Diffuses relatively well in the saliva, bronchial secretions, aqueous humor, bile and prostatic secretions. Relatively high concentrations are found in the lungs, kidneys, prostate and bones. Low *CSF concentrations*, but antibacterial activity present. Up to 60% glomerular and tubular *excretion* by the kidneys (in 24 h), 8% as conjugated, inactive forms. Urine concentrations are about 100 times higher than serum levels. A small quantity is excreted through the bile, and part is metabolised in the body.

The pharmacokinetic characteristics of *sulphamethoxazole* resemble those of trimethoprim, and this maintains the good activity of both components in the body. *Half-life:* 10 hours, *plasma protein binding:* 70%, without displacement by trimethoprim or vice versa. 80–90% excreted in the urine in 24 h, ⅓ as the unconjugated form. Dialyses well.

Side effects: Trimethoprim has very little toxicity in man. There is no haemotoxicity in the short term, though reversible bone-marrow depression (granulo- or thrombocytopenia) can occur with prolonged administration. Fatal agranulocytosis and anaemia (aplastic, haemolytic or megaloblastic) are extremely rare. Thrombocytopenia with purpura has been observed in older patients who received diuretics simultaneously, especially thiazides. As with other sulphonamides, allergic reactions may occur with sulphamethoxazole, including the very serious Stevens-Johnson syndrome. Where renal function is already impaired, co-trimoxazole can worsen renal function reversibly, and some recovery occurs after discontinuation. There have been individual cases of gastrointestinal upset (nausea, vomiting). Infusions may cause local pain or phlebitis.

Indications: Acute and chronic urinary infections, including pyelonephritis, acute and chronic bronchitis, sinusitis, wound and biliary infections, prostatitis and prostatic abscess. Co-trimoxazole is as active as chloramphenicol in typhoid and paratyphoid fever and may be preferable because of the reduced risk of side effects. The combination is also effective in enteric infections (dysentery, cholera and salmonellosis), as well as in brucellosis, nocardiosis and skin granulomas due to Mycobacterium marinum. The simultaneous administration of an antibiotic such as amikacin, may help in infections with gram-negative bacilli of low sensitivity (e. g. Serratia marcescens). Treatment and prophylaxis of proven or clinically typical pneumocystis pneumonia, for which 3 times the dose is required.

Incorrect use: Viral pneumonia, Pseudomonas infections, ornithosis, syphilis, tuberculosis, streptococcal sore throat (penicillin is more effective).

Contra-indications: Allergy against sulphonamides, acute hepatitis and severe hepatic diseases, blood dyscrasias, megaloblastic anaemia, pregnancy, 1st month of life (in USA also 2nd month), lactation (during child's first four weeks). Caution should be exercised in cases of granulocytopenia and severe renal failure as well as in long-term treatment, which should be monitored with regular blood and platelet counts. Sulphamethoxazole may enhance the anticoagulant activity of coumarins in patients with a low content of albumin in the blood; clotting tests should be frequently carried out in such cases.

Administration and dosage: Tablets, syrup and suspension for oral use. 2 tablets of 480 mg twice a day for adults (maximum of 3 tablets twice a day, and 1 tablet twice a day for long-term treatment). A syrup is available for adults (5 ml = 1 adult tablet) as well as forte tablets (= 2 normal adult tablets). 4 paediatric tablets twice a day for children aged 6–12 months, and 2.5 ml of paediatric syrup twice a day for children aged 2–5 months (5 ml = 2 paediatric tablets).

May also be administered as a one-hour *i. v. infusion* (2 ampoules twice a day in adequate dilution for up to 3 days). Regular full blood counts should be checked when administered for more than 10 days.

Use half the daily dose (2 tablets once a day) in *renal failure* (creatinine clearance 15–30 ml/min). Co-trimoxazole should not be given in severe renal failure. In practice, adjusting dosage by weight is complicated in renal failure and it would be better if the tablets contained 500 mg of co-trimoxazole instead of 480 mg (because of possible errors due to non-metric dosage).

For *Pneumocystis carinii pneumonia,* give 3–4 times the usual dose, i. e. 20 mg/kg of trimethoprim and 100 mg/kg sulphamethoxazole daily by mouth in 4 divided doses; for prophylaxis, give a daily dose of 8 mg/kg of trimethoprim and 40 mg/kg sulphamethoxazole in 2 divided doses.

Preparations: Tablets and ampoules containing 80 mg trimethoprim and 400 mg sulphamethoxazole;

syrup or suspension for adults (5 ml contain 80 mg trimethoprim and 400 mg sulphamethoxazole;

tablets of 160 mg trimethoprim and 800 mg sulphamethoxazole;

paediatric syrup and suspension (5 ml contain 40 mg trimethoprim and 200 mg sulphamethoxazole).

Summary: A rational combination of chemotherapeutic agents with a broad spectrum of activity and good clinical results. A valuable agent in urinary tract infections, although trimethoprim alone is now preferred by many (see below). Preferred by some in the treatment of typhoid fever, although chloramphenicol is still regarded by many as the treatment of choice for chloramphenicol-sensitive strains. A therapeutic alternative in acute and chronic bronchitis, sinusitis, bacillary dysentery and infections of the biliary tract. Co-trimoxazole is a well tolerated oral chemotherapeutic agent which has to some extent filled the gap created when chloramphenicol ceased to be frequently used.

References

ADAM, W. R., M. HENNING, J. K. DAWBORN: Excretion of trimethoprim and sulphamethoxazole in patients with renal failure. Aust. N. Z. J. Med. *3:* 383 (1973).

ANDERSON, J. D., R. W. LACEY, E. L. LEWIS, M. A. SELLIN: Failure to demonstrate an advantage in combining sulphamethoxazole with trimethoprim in an experimental model of urinary tract infection. J. clin. Path. *27:* 619 (1974).

ANDERSON, J. D.: Application of non-animal models to studies of the chemotherapy of bacterial urinary tract infections. J. Antimicrob. Chemother. *12:* 297 (1983).

BARKER, J., D. HEALING, J. G. P. HUTCHISON: Characteristics of some cotrimoxazole-resistant Enterobacteriaceae from infected patients. J. clin. Path. *25:* 1086 (1972).

BERGAN, T., E. K. BRODWALL: Human pharmacokinetics of a sulfamethoxazole trimethoprim combination. Acta med. scand. *192:* 483 (1972).

BERNSTEIN, L. S., J. COOPER: Co-trimoxazole and Stevens-Johnson syndrome. Lancet *1:* 988 (1978).

BRUMFITT, W., J. M. T. HAMILTON-MILLER, D. GREY: Trimethoprim-resistant coliforms. Lancet *2:* 926 (1977).

CAMERON, A., M. THOMAS: Pseudomembranous colitis and cotrimoxazole. Brit. med. J. *1:* 1321 (1977).

CHATTOPADHYAY, B.: Co-trimoxazole resistant Staphylococcus aureus in hospital practice J. Antimicrob. Chemother. *3:* 371 (1977).

CHIEN, L. T.: Intracranial hypertension and sulfamethoxazole. New Engl. J. Med. *283:* 47 (1970).

FRISCH, J. M.: Clinical experience with adverse reactions to trimethoprim-sulfamethoxazole. J. infect. Dis. *(Suppl.) 128:* 607 (1973).

HAMILTON-MILLER, J. M. T., D. GREY: Resistance to trimethoprim in Klebsiellae before its introduction. J. Antimicrob. Chemother. *1:* 213 (1975).

HART, C. A., M. F. GIBSON, E. MULVIHILL, H. T. GREEN: Co-trimoxazole resistant coliforms. Lancet *2:* 1081 (1977).

HOWARD, A. J., C. J. HINCE, J. D. WILLIAMS: Antibiotic resistance in Streptococcus pneumoniae and Haemophilus influenzae: Report of a study group on bacterial resistance. Brit. med. J. *1:* 1657 (1978).

HOWE, J. G., T. S. WILSON: Co-trimoxazole-resistant pneumococci. Lancet *2:* 184 (1972).

HUGHES, W. T., S. KUHNS, S. CHAUDHARY, S. FELDMAN, M. VERZOSA, R. J. A. AUR, C. PRATT, S. L. GEORGE: Successful chemoprophylaxis for Pneumocystis carinii pneumonitis. New Engl. J. Med. *297:* 1419 (1977).

HUGHES, W. T., S. FELDMAN, S. C. CHAUDHARY, M. J. OSSI, F. COX, S. K. SANYAL: Comparison of pentamidine isothionate and trimethoprim-sulfamethoxazole in the treatment of Pneumocystis carinii pneumonia. J. Pediat. *92:* 285 (1978).

KALOWSKI, S., R. S. NANRA, T. H. MATHEW, P. KINCAID-SMITH: Deterioration in renal function in association with co-trimoxazole therapy. Lancet *1:* 394 (1973).

LAWSON, D. H., D. A. HENRY: Fatal agranulocytosis attributed to cotrimoxazole therapy. Brit. med. J. *2:* 316 (1977).

LEWIS, E. L., R. W. LACEY: Present significance of resistance to trimethoprim and sulphonamides in coliforms, Staphylococcus aureus, and Streptococcus faecalis. J. clin. Path. *26:* 175 (1973).

MAY, J. R., J. DAVIES: Resistance of Haemophilus influenzae to trimethoprim. Brit. med. J. *3:* 376 (1972).

NOLTE, H., H. BÜTTNER: Pharmacokinetics of trimethoprim and its combination with sulfamethoxazole in man after single and chronic oral administration. Chemotherapy *18:* 274 (1973).

PALVA, I. P., O. KOIVISTO: Agranulocytosis associated with trimethoprim-sulphamethoxazole. Brit. med. J. *4:* 301 (1971).

SHOUVAL, D., M. LIGUMSKY, D. BEN-ISHAY: Effect of co-trimoxazole on normal creatinine clearance. Lancet *1:* 244 (1978).

SIGEL, C. W., M. E. GRACE, C. A. NICHOL: Metabolism of trimethoprim in man and measurement of a new metabolite: A new fluorescence assay. J. infect. Dis. (Suppl.) *128:* 580 (1973).

YUILI, G. M.: Megaloblastic anaemia due to trimethoprim-sulphamethoxazole therapy in uraemia. Postgrad. med. J. *49:* 100 (1973).

c) Other Diaminopyrimidine-Sulphonamide Combinations

Trimethoprim has also been **combined with sulphonamides other than sulphamethoxazole** (Table 20). Their characteristics are similar to sulphamethoxa-

Table 20. Diaminopyrimidine-sulphonamide combination. Initial dose of 2 tablets for trimethoprim plus sulphamoxole, trimethoprim plus sulphadiazine, and tetroxoprim plus sulphadiazine.

Generic name	Combination	Recommended daily dose (g)			
		Diamino-pyrimidine	Sulphon-amide	Total	No. of tablets per day of common proprietary preparation
Co-trimoxazole	Trimethoprim + sulphamethoxazole	0.32	1.6	1.92	2 × 2
Co-trimetrole	Trimethoprim + sulphametrole	0.32	1.6	1.92	2 × 2
Co-trimoxole	Trimethoprim + sulphamoxole	0.16	0.8	0.96	2 × 1
Co-trimazine	Trimethoprim + sulphadiazine	0.18	0.82	1.0	1 × 1
Co-tetroxazine	Tetroxoprim + sulphadiazine	0.2	0.5	0.7	2 × 1

zole: *Sulphametrole* has a half-life of 8 h, is 80% bound to serum protein and 90% is excreted in the urine (18% in an unchanged form). *Sulphamoxole* has a half-life of 10 h and a serum protein binding of 90%; 50% appears as free sulphonamide in the urine. *Sulphadiazine* has the same half-life but is less protein-bound (50%) and 65% are excreted unchanged in the urine. The water-solubility *in vitro* of sulphamethoxazole, sulphametrole and sulphamoxole is better than that of sulphadiazine; it is of course dependent on pH and temperature. The primary metabolite of sulphadiazine is more water-soluble at acid pH than that of sulphamethoxazole. Smaller daily doses may be sufficient in urinary infections.

Tetroxoprim has a shorter half-life (6 h) than trimethoprim, is less bound to serum protein (15%) and has a higher rate of excretion (50% in an active form); 30% of the dose passes out with the faeces. Tetroxoprim is less active *in vitro* on gram-negative rods than trimethoprim and in combination with sulphadiazine is 2–3 times less effective than co-trimoxazole. Tetroxoprim is only licensed in Germany and Switzerland for urinary and respiratory tract infections and is not licensed in Great Britain at present. More active diaminopyrimidine derivatives (e. g. brodimoprim) are expected to be developed.

d) Trimethoprim

Trimethoprim alone is *less active in vitro* than in a combination with a sulphonamide and its main use is for the treatment of urinary infections. It is said to have fewer *side effects*; but there is the theoretical risk that resistance may develop during therapy. It should be considered as an alternative to co-trimoxazole where there is allergy to sulphonamides. Licensed in the USA for treatment of initial episodes of uncomplicated urinary tract infections by enterobacteria.

Dosage: 100 mg twice a day for at least 1 week for *adults,* and 50 mg twice a day for *children* of 6–12 years. Adults are given 50 mg each evening for *long-term treatment,* and children of 6–12 years 25 mg.

References

DONICKE, M., P. W. LÜCKER, B. SIMON: Klinisch-pharmakologische Untersuchungen zur Pharmakokinetik einer Trimethoprim-Sulfamethoxazol-Zubereitung. Arzneimittel-Forsch. *27:* 2373 (1977).
ECKSTEIN, E., M. ETZEL, W. WESENBERG: Klinische Prüfung der antibakteriellen Kombination Sulfamoxol/Trimethoprim. Arzneimittel-Forsch. *26:* 665 (1976).
ETZEL, M., F. NEUHOF, W. WESENBERG: Klinische Prüfung der antibakteriellen Kombination Sulfamoxol/Trimethoprim. Arzneimittel-Forsch. *26:* 661, 671, 674, 678 (1976).

GLADTKE, E.: Trimethoprim und Sulfonamid: Eine chemotherapeutisch wirksame Kombination mit zwei Ansatzpunkten. Münch. med. Wschr. *120:* 1059 (1978).
HAHN, H., A. KIROV: Antibakterielle Aktivität von Trimethoprim/Sulfamethoxazol (Cotrimoxazol) und Tetroxoprim/Sulfadiazin in vitro. Arzneimittel-Forsch. 30 *(II):* 1047 (1980).
HELWIG, H., M. BULLA, W. SITZEMANN, K. SCHREIER, K. LOH, A. WODETZKY: Wirksamkeit und Verträglichkeit einer Trimethoprim-Sulfamoxol-Kombination im Kindesalter. Klin. Pädiat. *188:* 518 (1976).
KNOTHE, H.: The antibacterial efficacy of two trimethoprim-sulfonamide combinations. Chemotherapy *22:* 62 (1975).
KUHNE, J., F. W. KOHLMANN, J. K. SEYDEL, E. WEMPE: Pharmakokinetik der Kombination Sulfamoxol/Trimethoprim (CN 3123) bei Tier und Mensch. Arzneimittel-Forsch. *26:* 651 (1976).
NABERT-BOCK, G., H. GRIMS: Bakteriologie des Chemotherapeutikums Sulfametrol-Trimethoprim. Arzneimittel-Forsch. *27:* 1109 (1977).
NIJSSEN, J., J. SCHIEMANN, W. WESENBERG: Klinische Prüfung der antibakteriellen Kombination Sulfamoxol/Trimethoprim. Arzneimittel-Forsch. *26:* 676 (1976).
SEYDEL, J. K., E. WEMPE: Untersuchungen zum synergistischen Verhalten und zur Pharmakokinetik von Sulfonamid-Trimethoprim-Kombinationen. Arzneimittel-Forsch. *27:* 1521 (1977).
SIETZEN, W., E. W. RUGENDORFF: Co-trimazine once daily in urinary tract infections in comparison with co-trimoxazole given twice daily. – A double-blind randomized study. Infection *9:* 91 (1981).

e) Nitrofurans

α) Nitrofurantoin

Proprietary names: Berkfurin, Ceduran, Furadantin and Furadantin retard, Furan, Ituran, Macrodantin, Nifurantin, Nifuretten, Urantoin, Uvamin retard.

Properties: A synthetic nitrofuran derivative, N-(5-nitro-2-furfuryliden)-1-aminohydantoin, which is only slightly water-soluble, is stable and has a bitter taste. It is unrelated to other antibacterially active drugs except for its close chemical relative hydroxymethyl-nitrofurantoin, with which it is almost identical.

Mode of action: Bacteriostatic at low concentrations but bactericidal on actively proliferating and resting bacteria at the higher concentrations achieved therapeutically in the urine. Less active at alkaline pH.

Spectrum of action: Active against most causes of urinary infection (Escherichia coli, Klebsiella, Enterobacter, enterococci, staphylococci) but ineffective against Pseudomonas aeruginosa and candida. Nitrofurantoin cannot be relied upon in infections with Proteus because the urea-splitting effect of the urease of Proteus spp. makes the urine alkaline.

Resistance: No or little development of resistance during therapy. Primarily resistant strains of Escherichia coli, enterococci, Enterobacter and Proteus occur.

Pharmacokinetics: Well absorbed after oral administration; *absorption* may be retarded with macrocrystalline preparations of nitrofurantoin (e.g. Macrodantin, Furadantin retard) in order to improve the tolerance. *Blood and tissue levels* are too low for systemic therapy. Rapid, almost complete *excretion* in the urine, up to 40% during the first 6 h in an unchanged, bacterially active form and partly also as inactive metabolites (causing the yellowish colour of the urine). Maximal excretion after 3–4 hours. Urine concentrations between 300 and 400 mg/l. About 17% of the excreted nitrofurantoin is filtered by the glomeruli and the remaining 83% is secreted by the tubules.

Nitrofurantoin may diffuse back by "non-ionic diffusion" from the distal tubules into the renal parenchyma when the urine is acid and there is sufficient proximal secretion of nitrofurantoin.

Side effects:

1. *Nausea* and *vomiting* are predominantly central nervous effects, especially at high dosage (in 15% of cases given more than 7 mg/kg). These symptoms are less frequent when the dose is small, divided into several single doses, or given as macrocrystalline nitrofurantoin (slow-release), which is better tolerated because of its slower absorption.
2. *Central nervous symptoms* such as ataxia, headaches etc.
3. *Allergies* (rashes, fever, eosinophilia) are relatively frequent and anaphylactic shock can occur. Cholestatic jaundice, chronic active hepatitis and allergic lung infiltration ("nitrofurantoin-pneumonia"), exudative pleurisy and asthmatic attacks are all rare. Pulmonary fibrosis can develop.
4. *Peripheral polyneuritis* with some irreversible paralysis occurs particularly in renal failure (in up to 18% of cases where the blood urea is greater than 15 mmol/l and at large dosage.
5. Very occasional *blood dyscrasias* have been observed (anaemia, leucocytopenia), as has *haemolytic anaemia* with congenital glucose-6-phosphate-dehydrogenase deficiency (favism).

While the central nervous disorders mostly disappear after reducing the dose, the other side effects are indications to stop treatment immediately. The occurrence in recent years of dangerous and sometimes fatal side effects has led to a reluctance to use nitrofurantoin nowadays when other agents are equally suitable.

Indications: Treatment of urinary infections which cannot be treated with alternative drugs because of resistance. Other agents are preferable in the prophylaxis of recurrent or ascending urinary infections.

Incorrect uses: As a single agent in acute pyelonephritis requiring effective blood and tissue levels. Infections other than of the urinary tract.

Care should be taken in moderate renal failure (urea between 6 and 15 mmol/l) when the daily dosage should be reduced to 50–100 mg. Do not use in the newborn, in babies during the first year of life or in pregnant women (until delivery) because of the risk of haemolytic anaemia (due to enzymatic immaturity). Teratogenic damage has not been observed but in animal experiments nitrofurantoin was teratogenic and mutagenic and should therefore not be given during pregnancy.

Contra-indications: Anuria, severe renal failure a with urea above 15 mmol/l and creatinine clearance below 40 ml/min, favism (glucose-6-phosphate-dehydrogenase deficiency), and neuritis. Contra-indicated during the first month of life because of the risk of haemolytic anaemia (enzymatic immaturity), and in pregnant women (shortly before delivery). Avoid alcohol during therapy (because of possible alcohol intolerance due to disorders of acetaldehyde metabolism).

Administration: Oral administration as tablets, syrup, drops or suspension for children, preferably after meals (better tolerance). Possible instillation in the bladder.

Dosage: Standard dosage for *adults:* daily 150–300 mg; for *children:* 5 mg/kg in 3–6 divided doses for 7–10 days. A reduced dosage of 100(–200) mg daily (2.5 mg/kg) is generally sufficient for prolonged treatment, but not in case of prior infection caused by relatively insensitive species such as Proteus or Enterobacter. Long-term oral therapy for months or years is possible if medically controlled. 50 mg a day are sufficient for the prophylaxis of ascending infection.

The *combination* of nitrofurantoin with sulphadiazine is no better than treatment with nitrofurantoin alone.

Preparations: Tablets and capsules of 50 mg, 100 mg and 150 mg; coated tablets of 50 mg and 75 mg, 1% syrup, drops, capsules of 75 mg and 100 mg (macrocrystalline form), and instillations in ampoules of 100 mg for dilution with 100 ml physiological saline.

Summary:
Advantages: Broad spectrum of action, resistance infrequent, and long term treatment possible.
Disadvantages: Relatively frequent, sometimes severe side effects, no effective blood and tissue levels, not active against Pseudomonas aeruginosa.

A drug dating back to the early days of chemotherapy with considerable side effects (pulmonary fibrosis etc.). Better tolerated agents are available today.

References

Bäck, O., R. Lundgren, L.-G. Wiman: Nitrofurantoin induced pulmonary fibrosis and lupus syndrome. Lancet *1:* 930 (1974).

McCalla, D. R.: Biological effects of nitrofurans. J. Antimicrob. Chemother. *3:* 517 (1977).

Enzensberger, R., W. Stille: Die Stellung des Nitrofurantoins heute. Dtsch. med. Wschr. *108:* 1330 (1983).

Israel, K. S., R. E. Brashear, H. M. Sharma, M. N. Yum, J. L. Glover: Pulmonary fibrosis and nitrofurantoin. Amer. Rev. resp. Dis. *108:* 353 (1973).

Kalowski, S., N. Radford, P. Kincaid-Smith: Crystaline and macrocrystaline nitrofurantoin in the treatment of urinary tract infection. New Engl. J. Med. *290:* 385 (1974).

Koch-Weser, J., V. W. Sidel, M. Dexter, C. Parish, D. C. Finer, P. Kanarek: Adverse reactions to sulfisoxazole, sulfamethoxazole, and nitrofurantoin. Arch. intern. Med. *128:* 399 (1972).

Stefanini, M.: Chronic hemolytic anemia association with erythrocyte enolase deficiency exacerbated by ingestion of nitrofurantoin. Amer. J. clin. Path. *58:* 408 (1972).

Toole, J. F., M. L. Parrish: Nitrofurantoin polyneuropathy. Neurology *23:* 554 (1973).

β) Nitrofurazone

Proprietary name: Furacin.

Properties: A good topical drug, poorly soluble and not absorbed. When used topically, higher concentrations and bactericidal activity against staphylococci, streptococci, Escherichia coli, Enterobacter, Klebsiella and Proteus may be expected, but not against Pseudomonas aeruginosa or Candida albicans. Sensitisation (allergic contact dermatitis) sometimes occurs.

Administration and indications: Used as ointment or powder for skin and wound infections and as ear drops in otitis.

γ) Nifuratel

Proprietary name: Inimur (Germany). No longer marketed in Great Britain. Nifuratel has the same *range of action* as nitrofurantoin, but is also active against Candida albicans and Trichomonas vaginalis. Vaginal application is used daily for Candida and Trichomonas vaginitis, and a coated tablet is used for yeast infections of the urinary tract.

Dosage: 200–400 mg 3 times a day for 1 week.

f) Gyrase Inhibitors (Quinolones)

All agents of this group are similar in that they have a carboxylic acid and neighbouring oxygen atoms needed for antibacterial activity (Fig. 29). They inhibit bacterial DNA topoisomerases (or gyrases) and are called DNA gyrase inhibitors (other names are quinolones or quinolocarboxylic acids). Higher concentrations act on bacterial RNA as well. There are a number of compounds with different spectra of activity and different potencies; they may be divided into four groups on the basis of their chemical structure:

1. naphthyridines (e. g. nalidixic acid),
2. oxacines (e. g. cinoxacin),
3. 4-quinolones with a piperazinyl group (e. g. pipemidic acid),
4. fluorinated compounds with a piperazinyl group (e. g. norfloxacin).

The addition of a piperazinyl radical to the molecule confers activity against Pseudomonas and the addition of a fluorine atom at the 6-position improves the activity of the newer compounds and extends the spectrum to include gram-positive bacteria. In contrast to the older gyrase inhibitors (nalidixic acid group), the newer agents (norfloxacin group) are bactericidal and lower doses are sufficient for therapy; all members of the group are absorbed more or less incompletely from the mouth, however, leading to relatively low serum levels. They are also metabolised to varying extents in the liver. Norfloxacin was the first of the fluorinated compounds to be introduced and had fewer side effects than nalidixic acid. Further members of this group are currently undergoing in clinical trials and will be used for a wider range of infections. They can all be given by mouth and some newer compounds (e. g. ciprofloxacin) may be given parenterally as well.

α) Nalidixic Acid

Proprietary names: Mictral, Negram, Neg-Gram, Nevigramon, Nogram.

Properties: A synthetical naphthyridine derivative, unrelated to any antibiotic, poorly water-soluble, and stable. Structural formula in shown in Fig. 29.

Spectrum of action: Most gram-negative bacteria are sensitive (Escherichia, coli, Enterobacter, Klebsiella, Proteus etc.), although a few resistant strains are found. Pseudomonas aeruginosa and gram-positive bacteria (staphylococci, streptococci, enterococci etc.) are completely resistant.

Resistance: Secondary resistance develops rapidly. Cross-resistance is found with oxolinic acid and other older gyrase inhibitors.

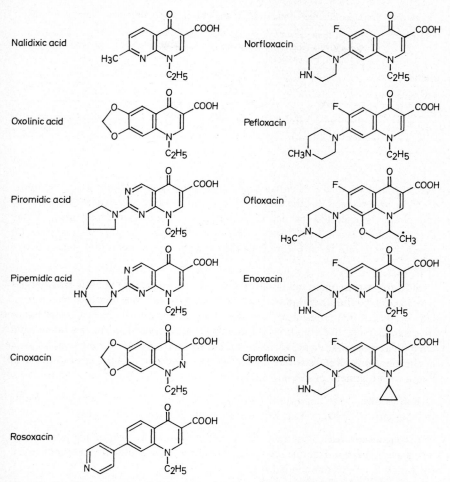

Fig. 29. Chemical structure of the older quinolones (left) and the new quinolones (right).

Pharmacokinetics (Table 21):

Almost completely *absorbed* after oral administration. Maximal *blood levels* (after 1–2 h): 20–40 mg/l in adults after 1 g, 50 mg/l in small children after 20 mg/kg. *Half-life:* 1½ hours; 2½ hours during first 3 months of life (due to renal immaturity). *Plasma protein binding:* 93% (63% as the active metabolite

Table 21. Pharmacokinetics of the older quinolones (gyrase inhibitors) after oral intake.

Drug	Mean serum levels (mg/l) after 1 h (dose)	Half-life (min)	Plasma protein binding (%)	Urinary recovery (%)
Nalidixic acid	20–40 (1 g)	90	93	10
Oxolinic acid	0.8 (0.75 g)	360	85	1–5
Pipemidic acid	3 (0.4 g)	90	20	60
Cinoxacin	6 (0.25 g)	90	80	50–60

hydroxynalidixic acid). Nalidixic acid is extensively metabolised in the body. 85–90% is excreted in the urine in a conjugated ineffective form, and the remainder is excreted as active nalidixic and hydroxynalidixic acid. Urine concentrations (with 1 g 4 times a day) vary between 50 and 500 mg/l and are lower in moderate renal failure, but they are still in the microbiologically active range.

Side effects: Frequent mild gastrointestinal upsets (nausea, vomiting). Allergies (rashes, eosinophilia) and phototoxic reactions are less frequent, as are cramps, depression of the respiratory centre, fatigue, psychosis, visual disturbance (nystagmus, defective colour vision, diplopia), metabolic acidosis, leucopenia and haemolytic anaemia. Acute increases of intracranial pressure have been observed in the newborn. Relapses due to secondarily resistant bacteria are reported in long-term treatment of chronic infections.

Indications: Uncomplicated urinary infections due to sensitive agents (Escherichia coli, Klebsiella, Enterobacter and particularly Proteus).

Inappropriate use: Treatment of acute pyelonephritis, where adequate tissue levels are required. Treatment of other infections, especially intestinal infections, for which it was recommended formerly.

Caution in severe liver damage (nalidixic acid is metabolised by the liver), renal failure (critical level: a blood urea of 12 mmol/l) and during the first three months of pregnancy. Avoid direct sunlight. Nalidixic acid can displace coumarin anticoagulants from their protein binding sites, and hence potentiate their activity.

Contra-indications: Oliguria, anuria, epilepsy and cerebral arteriosclerosis. Generally contra-indicated in children and young people because of the possibility of joint changes, which have so far been shown to occur with all naphthyridine derivatives in animal experiments only. Do not give to lactating mothers.

Administration: Oral only.

Dosage: Standard dose for adults: 4 g daily in 4 divided doses. Length of therapy: generally 7–10 days. Long-term treatment possible, at full or half dosage.

Summary: Advantages are activity against Escherichia coli, Enterobacter and Proteus and good general tolerance. Disadvantages are the unreliability of activity in tissues, the extensive transformation into inactive metabolites and the rapid development of resistance during therapy. Nalidixic acid is therefore mainly recommended for the treatment of uncomplicated urinary infections caused by Proteus, Escherichia coli, or Enterobacter. Ineffective against Pseudomonas aeruginosa. It has now been largely replaced by norfloxacin.

References

BOURGUIGNON, G. J., M. LEVITI, R. STERNGLANZ: Studies on the mechanism of action of nalidixic acid. Antimicrob. Ag. Chemother. *4:* 479 (1973).
GILBERTSON, C., D. R. JONES: Haemolytic anaemia with nalidixic acid. Brit. med. J. *4:* 493 (1972).
GREENWOOD, D., F. O'GRADY: Factors governing the emergence of resistance to nalidixic acid in treatment of urinary tract infections. Antimicrob. Ag. Chemother. *12:* 678 (1977).
HOFFBRAND, B. I.: Interaction of nalidixic acid and warfarin. Brit. med. J. *2:* 666 (1974).
NAUMANN, P.: The value of antibiotic levels in tissue and in urine in the treatment of urinary tract infections. J. Antimicrob. Chemother. *4:* 9 (1978).

β) Piromidic Acid

Proprietary name: Septural. Not available in Great Britain.

Description: Naphthyridine derivative with good activity against gram-negative rods but none against gram-positive cocci. Only indicated in lower urinary tract infections.

Side effects: Impairment of hepatic and renal function, gastro-intestinal upset, allergic reactions and dizziness. Acute renal failure has been reported.

Contra-indications: Children, adolescents, elderly patients, disorders of hepatic and renal functions.

Dosage: 100 mg twice daily for 1–2 weeks.

γ) Pipemidic Acid

Proprietary name: Deblaston. Not available in Great Britain.

Description: A derivative of piromidic acid, chemically closely related to nalidixic acid. Very poorly soluble in water and ethyl alcohol, soluble in acid and alkaline solvents. For structural formula, see Fig. 29, p. 209.

Antibacterial activity: Inhibition of DNA synthesis. The spectrum includes all the gram-negative rods which are commonly found in urinary infections, but not enterococci and only some staphylococci.

Resistance: There are few resistant strains amongst the enterobacteria and Pseudomonas aeruginosa. Pipemidic acid has a generally greater antibacterial activity than nalidixic acid (Table 22). Resistance can develop *in vitro* but is rare *in vivo*. There is extensive cross-resistance with nalidixic acid (except for Pseudomonas).

Table 22. Minimal inhibitory concentrations of older and newer quinolones required to inhibit 90% of the strains (MIC$_{90\%}$) isolated at the University Children's Hospital, Kiel (650 strains).

Species	MIC$_{90\%}$ (mg/l) of				
	Nalidixic acid	Pipemidic acid	Norflox-acin	Cipro-floxacin	Oflox-acin
Escherichia coli	8	4	0.06	0.016	0.06
Klebsiella pneumoniae	64	32	0.5	0.06	0.5
Enterobacter aerogenes	16	8	0.25	0.03	0.12
Proteus mirabilis	16	4	0.12	0.03	0.12
Proteus vulgaris	4	2	0.12	0.03	0.12
Pseudomonas aeruginosa	>128	64	2.0	0.5	2.0
Serratia marcescens	4	4	0.5	0.12	0.5
Streptococcus faecalis	>128	>128	8.0	2.0	2.0
Staphylococcus aureus	>128	128	2.0	0.5	0.5
Mycoplasma pneumoniae	>100	>100	12.5	–	1.5
Ureaplasma urealyticum	>100	>100	12.5	3.0	3.0
Chlamydia trachomatis	1600	100	16	1.0	–
Bacteroides fragilis	512	–	32	8.0	8.0
Other Bacteroides species	512	–	8.0	8.0	4.0
Anaerobic gram-positive cocci	512	–	8.0	2.0	2.0

Pharmacokinetics: *Serum levels* of 3 mg/l (1 h) after 400 mg by mouth and 1 mg/l (6 h). *Half-life:* 1½ h. 20–30% bound to *serum protein*. 50–70% excreted unchanged in the urine, about 25% with the faeces (Table 22). Urinary concentrations of 200–800 mg/l (during the first 6 h) follow a 400 mg oral dose. Acetyl, formyl, and oxopipemidic acid are found as metabolites. Therapeutically active concentrations have been found in prostatic secretion and prostatic tissue. Haemodialyses well.

Side effects: Quite well tolerated. Occasional nausea, vomiting, allergic skin reactions and phototoxic reactions. Since degenerative joint changes (proliferation and erosion of the cartilage) have been detected in beagle dogs aged 4–6 months after a daily dose of 100 mg/kg, pipemidic acid is contra-indicated in children and adolescents.

Indications: Urinary tract infections.

Contra-indications: Oliguria, anuria, epilepsy, pregnancy, children and adolescents. *Caution* with long-term treatment.

Dosage: 400 mg orally twice a day for 5–10 days.

Preparation: 200 mg capsules.

Summary: Pipemidic acid is superior to nalidixic acid because of its low rate of metabolism and the high urine concentrations. It is an alternative chemotherapeutic agent for the treatment of urinary infections with Pseudomonas.

References

GRIMM, H.: Vergleichende bakteriologische In-vitro-Untersuchungen mit Pipemidsäure und Nalidixinsäure. Med. Welt *31:* 1189 (1980).
INOUE, S., T. OHUE, J. YAMAGISHI, S. NAKAMURA, M. SHIMIZU: Mode of incomplete cross-resistance among pipemidic, piromidic and nalidixic acids. Antimicrob. Ag. Chemother. *14/2:* 240 (1978).
LAJUDIE DE, P.: L'acide pipémidique nouvel antibactérien de synthése. J. pharmacol. Clin. *1:* 155 (1974).
NASU, M., M. NAKATOMI, A. SAITO, K. HARA: Fundamental and clinical evaluation of Pipemidic acid in respiratory tract infections. Chemotherapy *23:* 2861 (1975).
PETERS, G., H. FREIESLEBEN, R. MARRE, H. METZ, H. TANNENBERG, G. PULVERER: Antibakterielle In-vitro-Wirksamkeit von Pipemidsäure und Nalidixinsäure. Dtsch. med. Wschr. *104:* 946 (1979).
SHIMIZU, N., Y. TAKASE, S. NAKAMURA: Pipemidic acid, a new antibacterial agent active against Pseudomonas aeruginosa. In vitro properties. Antimicrob. Ag. Chemother. *8:* 132 (1975).
SHIMIZU, M., S. NAKAMURA, Y. TAKASE, N. KUROBE: Pipemidic acid: absorption, distribution and excretion. Antimicrob. Ag. Chemother. *7:* 441 (1975).

δ) Oxolinic Acid

Proprietary names: Nidantin, Oxotrid, Utibid. No longer available in Great Britain.

Properties: A quinolone derivative and a weak organic acid. Range of action similar to nalidixic acid, but the development of secondary resistance is slower. Poorly absorbed after oral administration. Low serum levels but good urinary concentrations which last for more than 12 hours. For structural formula, see Fig. 29, p. 209.

Administration in urinary infections in the relatively low dosage of 750 mg twice a day, but central nervous side effects are more frequent than with nalidixic acid.

Contra-indications: Similar to nalidixic acid. Do not give to children and adolescents.

Preparations: Tablets of 750 mg.

References

KERSHAW, N. J., D. A. LEIGH: The antibacterial and pharmacological activity of oxolinic acid (Prodoxol). J. Antimicrob. Chemother *1:* 311 (1975).

KLEIN, D., J. M. MATSEN: In vitro susceptibility comparison and recommendations for oxolinic acid. Antimicrob. Ag. Chemother *9:* 649 (1976).

MADSEN, P. O., P. R. RHODES: Oxolinic acid, a new chemotherapeutic agent in the treatment of urinary tract infection. J. Urol. *105:* 870 (1971).

MEERS, P. D.: Oxolinic acid in urinary infections. Lancet *2:* 721 (1974).

NEUSSEL, H., G. LINZENMEIER: In vitro investigations with oxolinic acid, a new chemotherapeutic agent. Chemotherapy *18:* 253 (1973).

SCHEIDT, J., H. SCHACH: Therapie chronischer Harnwegsinfekte mit Oxolinsäure. Dtsch. med. Wschr. *96:* 1242 (1971).

SHAPERA, R., M. MATSEN, M. JOHN: Oxolinic acid for urinary tract infections in children. Amer. J. Dis. Child. *131:* 34 (1977).

ε) Cinoxacin

Proprietary names: Cinobac, Cinobactin.

Description: A quinoline derivative, water-soluble as sodium salt, stable. Structural formula see Fig. 29, p. 209.

Mode of action: A bacteriostatic agent, which may be bactericidal when the concentration is doubled or quadrupled.

Spectrum of activity similar to nalidixic and oxolinic acids; active against almost all aerobic gram-negative rods (except Pseudomonas aeruginosa), but not against gram-positive bacteria.

Resistance: Primary resistance is rare among those gram-negative rods which commonly cause urinary infections. Secondary resistance may develop during therapy in less than 1% of cases, but apparently less often than with nalidixic acid. Complete cross-resistance between nalidixic and oxolinic acids.

Pharmacokinetics: Rapid and complete *absorption* after oral administration. *Serum levels* after 250 mg by mouth 4 times a day: 6–8 mg/l (1 h) and 1–2 mg/l (6 h); after 500 mg twice a day: 16 mg/l (1 h) and 3 mg/l (6 h). *Half-life:* 1½ h (Table 21). *Urinary recovery:* 50% in an active form, the remainder as inactive metabolites (a catechol metabolite and a glucuronide). Urinary concentrations are 3–4 times higher than those found with nalidixic acid, allowing an interval of 12 h after 500 mg by mouth. Lower doses are necessary in *renal failure*.

Side effects: Nausea, dizziness, gastric discomfort and rashes in about 8% of cases. Diarrhoea, vomiting, fatigue, tinnitus and photophobia occur less frequently. Treatment need not be stopped in most cases; symptoms disappear rapidly when treatment is interrupted.

Indication: Uncomplicated urinary infections due to sensitive gram-negative bacilli.

Administration and dosage: By mouth, either 500 mg twice a day or 250 mg 4 times a day for 7–10 days.

Preparation: Capsules of 500 mg.

Summary: Cinoxacin is much less extensively metabolised in the body than nalidixic acid, and is less protein-bound. A low daily dose (1 g) is therefore sufficient in urinary infection.

References

BLACK, H. R., K. S. ISRAEL, R. WOLEN, G. BRIER, B. OBERMEYER, E. ZIEGE: Pharmacology of cinoxacin in humans. Antimicrob. Ag. Chemother. *15:* 165 (1979).

BRIEDIGKEIT, H., R. SCHIMMELPFENNIG, R. BRUDER, K. PRECHT, H. DRÖSELER: Vergleich von Cinoxacin und Nalidixinsäure bei der Behandlung von chronischen Harnwegsinfektionen. Infection *10:* 219 (1982).

COX, C. E., J. R. SIMMONS: Cinoxacin in therapy of urinary tract infections. Urology *17:* 539 (1981).

LANDES, R. R.: Long-term low-dose cinoxacin therapy for the prevention of recurrent urinary tract infections. J. Urology *123:* 47 (1980).

MADSEN, P. O., N. FRIMODT-MÖLLER, S. MAIGAARD: Cinoxacin in urinary tract infections. Urology *17:* 496 (1981).
PAULSON, D. F.: Comparison of cinoxacin and nalidixic acid in patients with cystitis. Urology *20:* 138 (1982).
SCHAEFFER, A. J., S. FLYNN, J. JONES: Comparison of cinoxacin and trimethoprim-sulfamethoxazole in the treatment of urinary tract infections. J. Urol. *125:* 825 (1981).
SZWED, J. J., D. E. BRANNON et al.: Pharmacokinetics of cinoxacin in patients with renal failure. J. Antimicrob. Chemother. *4:* 451 (1978).
VUYE, A.: In vitro comparison of norfloxacin with nalidixic acid, cinoxacin and oxolinic acid. Arzneimittel-Forsch./Drug Res. *33:* 1623 (1983).

ζ) Norfloxacin

Proprietary names: Barazan, Utinor.

Properties: A fluorinated newer gyrase inhibitor with a piperazinyl group (Fig. 29, p. 209). Inhibits synthesis of DNA and RNA in the bacterial cell. Bactericidal action.

Spectrum of activity: Active against all aerobic gram-negative and gram-positive bacteria including Pseudomonas aeruginosa, Proteus vulgaris, Serratia marcescens and Enterobacter species (Table 22, p. 212). Ureaplasma urealyticum, Gardnerella vaginalis and Chlamydia trachomatis are also inhibited. There is less activity against anaerobes, Acinetobacter, Providencia and pneumococci. The in vitro activity of norfloxacin in comparison to other compounds is shown in Table 22. The antibacterial activity of norfloxacin is 10–20 times as great as that of nalidixic and pipemidic acids. Gonococci (β-lactamase-producing strains) are sensitive. Resistant strains of other bacteria are rare.

Resistance: There is no tendency for secondary resistance to develop, unlike nalidixic acid. Partial cross-resistance is found between the older and newer gyrase inhibitors. Enterobacteria resistant to nalidixic acid are generally moderately sensitive to norfloxacin.

Pharmacokinetics:
Incomplete absorption after oral intake. *Serum levels* differ in the fasting and non-fasting states. After 0.2 g orally, the mean serum concentration is 1.1 mg/l (1 h). *Half-life:* 150 min. *Protein binding:* 20%. Good *tissue penetration.*
Urinary recovery: 30% (as unmetabolised drug); six active metabolites and small amounts of an inactive glucuronide conjugate have been found in the urine. *Urine concentrations:* 150–200 mg/l in the first 2 h (after 0.2 g by mouth). An unkown amount of the drug is excreted in the faeces.

Side effects: Gastrointestinal disorders (2–11%), central nervous symptoms such as ataxia, headaches, drowsiness, visual disturbances, photophobia, paraesthesiae, depression (2–10%) and allergic skin reactions (4–5%). These side effects are always reversible.

As with other gyrase inhibitors, norfloxacin may cause degenerative joint changes in beagle dogs aged 4–6 months at higher dosages; it is therefore not licensed for use in children and adolescents in Germany.

Indications: Urinary tract infection.

Contra-indications: Oliguria, anuria, pregnancy, children and adolescents. Caution in patient with impaired liver function. Do not give during lactation because of transfer into the breast milk.

Administration and dosage: 400 mg orally twice a day for 3–10 days.

Preparation: Tablets of 400 mg.

Summary: A highly active compound with a broad spectrum (including Pseudomonas) for the oral therapy of urinary infections. Not for use in children and adolescents.

References

BODY, B. A., R. A. FROMTLING, S. SHADOMY, H. J. SHADOMY: In vitro antibacterial activity of norfloxacin compared with eight other antimicrobial agents. Eur. J. clin. Microbiol. *2:* 230 (1983).

CAESAR, M., W. STILLE: Substanzen der Nalidixinsäure-Gruppe ("Gyrase-Hemmer"). Zuckschwerdt, München 1983.

CHARTRAND, ST. A., R. K. SCRIBNER, A. H. WEBER, D. F. WELCH, M. I. MARKS: In vitro activity of CI-919 (AT-2266), an oral antipseudomonal compound. Antimicrob. Ag. Chemother. *23:* 658 (1983).

EANDI, M., I. VIANO, F. DI NOLA, L. LEONE, E. GENAZZANI: Pharmacokinetics of norfloxacin in healthy volunteers and patients with renal and hepatic damage. Eur. J. clin. Microbiol. *2:* 253 (1983).

HAASE, D., B. URIAS, G. HARDING, A. RONALD: Comparative in vitro activity of norfloxacin against urinary tract pathogens. Eur. J. clin. Microbiol. *2:* 235 (1983).

HIRAI, K.: Comparative activities of AM-715 and pipemidic and nalidixic acids against experimentally induced systemic and urinary tract infections. Antimicrob. Ag. Chemother. *1:* 188 (1981).

ITO, A.: In vitro antibacterial activity of AM-715, a new nalidixic acid analog. Antimicrob. Ag. Chemother. *2:* 103 (1980).

KHAN, M. Y.: Comparative in vitro activity of Mk-0366 and other selected oral antimicrobial agents against Neisseria gonorrhoeae. Antimicrob. Ag. Chemother. *2:* 265 (1981).

MEIER-EWERT, H., G. WEIL, G. MILLOTT: In vitro activity of norfloxacin against Chlamydia trachomatis. Eur. J. clin. Microbiol. *2:* 271 (1983).

NAKAMURA, S., A. MINAMI, H. KATAE, S. INOUE, J. YAMAGISHI, J. TAKASE, M. SHIMIZU: In vitro antibacterial properties of AZ-2266, a new pyridonecarboxylic acid. Antimicrob. Ag. Chemother. *23:* 641 (1983).
NAKAMURA, SH., KATSUHISA NAKATA, H. KATAE, A. MNAMI, S. KASHIMOTO: Activity of AT-2266 compared with those of norfloxacin, pipemidic acid, nalidixic acid, and gentamicin against various experimental infections in mice. Antimicrob. Ag. Chemother. *23:* 742 (1983).
NISHIMURA, Y.: Clinical evaluation of AM-715 on urological infections. Europ. J. Chemother. Antibiot. *1:* 25 (1981).
SIMON, C.: Im Tierexperiment beobachtete Knorpelschädigung durch Chinolone. Fortschr. antimikr. Chemother. "Gyrase-Hemmer". Futuramed, Munich 1984.
SIMON, C., U. LINDNER: In vitro activity of norfloxacin against Mycoplasma hominis and Ureaplasma urealyticum. Eur. J. clin. Microbiol. *2:* 479 (1983).

g) Nitroimidazoles

Proprietary names:
For *metronidazole:* Arilin, Clont, Flagyl, Tricho Cordes, Tricho-Gynaedron, Vagimid, Vaginyl;
   for *tinidazole:*   Fasigyn, Simplotan;
   for *ornidazole:* Tiberal;
   for *nimorazole:* Esclama, Nagoxin 500, Nulogyl.

Properties: Nitroimidazoles are a group of heterocyclic compounds based on a 5-membered nucleus (Fig. 30) with certain similarities to the nitrofurans. Metronidazole and its related compounds tinidazole, ornidazole and nimorazole act by oxygen deprivation, which explains their activity against protozoa and anaerobic bacteria and also as radiosensitisers. All agents of this group may be carcinogenic in laboratory animals and are mutagenic in the Ames test, but have not so far been found to have similar effects in humans.

Mode of action: Inhibition of nucleic acid synthesis of anaerobic bacteria. Strongly bactericidal.

Spectrum of action: Protozoa (Entamoeba histolytica, Trichomonas vaginalis, Giardia lamblia) are inhibited *in vitro* by metronidazole at concentrations of 2 mg/l or less. Tinidazole, ornidazole and nimorazole have about the same activity against trichomonads, Entamoeba and Giardia as metronidazole. All anaerobic bacteria except Propionibacterium and the actinomycetes are killed by the nitroimidazoles at concentrations of 6.2 mg/l or less, and many at lower concentrations (0.4–0.8 mg/l). The spectrum of activity includes Bacteroides species (including B. fragilis), Fusobacterium, anaerobic cocci (Peptococcus, Peptostreptococcus, Veillonella) and clostridia (including Clostridium difficile), campylobacters and eubacteria. Metronidazole, tinidazole and ornidazole are similar in their antibacterial activity, while nimorazole is less active. All aerobic and facultatively anaerobic bacteria are resistant.

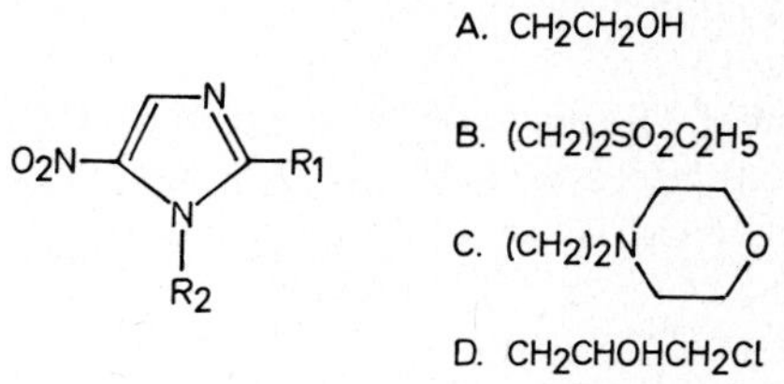

A. CH_2CH_2OH

B. $(CH_2)_2SO_2C_2H_5$

C. $(CH_2)_2N$⟨ ⟩O

D. $CH_2CHOHCH_2Cl$

Fig. 30. Structures of metronidazole ($R_1 = CH_3$; $R_2 = A$); tinidazole ($R_1 = CH_3$; $R_2 = B$); nimorazole ($R_1 = H$; $R_2 = C$) and ornidazole ($R_1 = H$; $R_2 = D$).

Resistance: Primary resistance is very rare in sensitive species of anaerobes. Resistance or failure of therapy sometimes occurs with Trichomonas vaginalis and Entamoeba histolytica. There is complete cross-resistance between the four nitroimidazoles, but no cross-resistance with antibiotics. Resistance does not develop during treatment.

Pharmacokinetics:
Well *absorbed* after oral administration. *Maximal serum concentrations* of 15 mg/l after 500 mg of metronidazole and 40 mg/l after 2.4 g; 40 mg/l with tinidazole and 37 mg/l with ornidazole (after 2 g). Serum concentrations of 13–15 mg/l can be achieved after 500 mg of metronidazole i.v. by short infusion over 20 min. Repeated doses do not lead to accumulation. *Half-life:* 7 hours (metronidazole), 13 h (tinidazole, ornidazole), 10 h (nimorazole). *Plasma protein binding:* 15% (metronidazole), 12% (tinidazole, ornidazole), 15% (nimorazole). Very good *tissue penetration* (particularly in the brain, liver, uterus, adipose tissue, skin, and abscess cavities). High concentrations in CSF, saliva, peritoneal fluid, vaginal secretions, amniotic fluid and breast milk. Metronidazole is extensively oxidised and conjugated in the liver to products with less antimicrobial activity. Tinidazole is less metabolised in the liver than metronidazole; the effective concentrations are therefore higher in the tissue and body fluids.

Excretion is mainly renal, both unchanged and as metabolites. Total urinary recovery: 30% (metronidazole), 15% (tinidazole), 63% (ornidazole), 55% (nimorazole). Metronidazole causes a reddish-brown discolouration of the urine.

Side effects: Dose-dependent, and apparently not as frequent after tinidazole or ornidazole as after metronidazole. Gastrointestinal upset in 3% (nausea, vomiting, diarrhoea). Some patients complain of an unpleasant metallic taste. The following symptoms sometimes occur during prolonged therapy and after high dosage: Central nervous disorders (dizziness, ataxia, clouding of consciousness, seizures etc.), paraesthesiae, glossitis, stomatitis, urticaria, rashes, itching, dysuria, cystitis, a sensation of pressure in the pelvis and reversible neutropenia. There is marked intolerance to alcohol (antabuse-like effect). Potentiation of oral anticoagulants can occur. No increase in congenital abnormalities, premature deliveries or postnatal disorders has been observed after administration at different stages of pregnancy. However, because they are carcinogenic in animals, nitroimidazoles should be avoided in pregnancy and for long-term treatment unless their use is essential.

Indications:
1. Drug of choice in trichomoniasis and vaginitis due to Gardnerella vaginalis (treat infected partner as well).
2. Amoebic dysentery (all types, and amoebic liver abscess).
3. Intestinal infections with Giardia lamblia and Balantidium coli.
4. Anaerobic bacterial infections including mixed infections with aerobic bacteria, e. g. septicaemia associated with thrombophlebitis, aspiration pneumonia, liver abscess, cerebral, pulmonary or pelvic abscesses, other intraabdominal abscesses, peritonitis, pelvic infections, endometritis, puerperal sepsis, febrile abortion, gangrene. For mixed infections, always combine with a broad-spectrum antibiotic active against aerobes (e. g. an aminoglycoside or cephalosporin). In ulcerative stomatitis or gingivitis, peridontitis and gas gangrene, combine with benzyl penicillin.
5. Prophylaxis for major gynaecological and colon surgery and appendicectomy.
6. Sometimes effective in antibiotic-induced pseudomembranous enterocolitis (due to Clostridium difficile), if vancomycin cannot be given.
7. In Crohn's disease with a draining fistula, long-term treatment with metronidazole may be useful but peripheral neuropathy (usually reversible) occur in 10–20% of cases.

Contra-indications: Active central nervous diseases, blood dyscrasias, 1st trimester of pregnancy. *Caution* in serious liver disease (reduce dosage). Avoid alcohol during treatment. Replace breast milk temporarily with cow's milk when mother is treated during lactation.

Administration and dosage:
For *amoebic dysentery* (all types): 800 mg 3 times a day (about 10 mg/kg 3 times a day in children) for 5–10 days after meals. For ornidazole, 0.5–1 g every

12 hours is sufficient. A sequential course of diloxanide furoate, 500 mg three times a day is recommended for ten days to eliminate luminal forms of the parasite.

For *trichomoniasis* and *giardiasis:* 250 mg 3 times a day (about 3 mg/kg 3 times a day for children) for 6 days, or a single dose for trichomoniasis with metronidazole, tinidazole or nimorazole: 2.0 g (4 tablets) in a single dose, preferably after meals. 1.5 g (3 tablets) of ornidazole as a single dose is sufficient for this indication. An alternative short oral course of metronidazole is 2 doses of 1 g, 6 hours apart, on the 1st day, followed by 1 g the next morning (total dose 3 g). Repeat after 4–6 weeks. Simultaneous topical treatment with vaginal tablets, pessaries or vaginal gel is sometimes recommended but not essential. Stop treatment if ataxia or other signs of intolerance develop.

For *anaerobic infections* (not nimorazole): 400 mg of metronidazole 3 times a day for adults, 7 mg/kg 3 times a day for children. For prophylaxis in gynaecological and colonic surgery, give a short course of 400 mg 3 times a day beginning on the day of operation. The same dose is used for i. v. administration (infuse 500 mg in 100 ml of solvent over 20 min). Accumulation may occur in severe renal failure but these agents are largely cleared by haemodialysis. In gynaecological and abdominal surgical prophylaxis, give 500 mg metronidazole i. v. or by suppository, or 400 mg by mouth, shortly before the operation, and continue the same dose 3 times a day for 24 hours. Longer courses should be regarded as treatment rather than prophylaxis.

Tinidazole is given orally for anaerobic infections in doses of 1 g once a day and ornidazole 500 mg twice a day. The i. v. dose of tinidazole is 800 mg once a day and of ornidazole 500 mg twice a day.

Preparations: Tablets and capsules of 250 mg and 400 mg (metronidazole), of 500 mg (ornidazole, nimorazole), of 1 g (tinidazole), suppositories (metronidazole) of 500 mg and 1 g, also vaginal tablets, suppositories or capsules (metronidazole, ornidazole), ampoules of 500 mg (metronidazole, ornidazole), of 800 mg (tinidazole).

Summary: A group of reliable chemotherapeutic agents in trichomoniasis, amoebic and anaerobic infections with an unknown carcinogenic risk and occasional serious side effects.

References

Bäck, E., L. Hermanson, M. Wickman: Metronidazole treatment of liver abscess due to Bacteroides fragilis. Scand. J. infect. Dis. *10:* 152 (1978).
Bradley, W. G., I. J. Karlsson, C. G. Rassol: Metronidazole neuropathy. Brit. med. J. *2:* 610 (1977).

CADOZ, M.: The treatment of bacteroides fragilis meningitis using injectable ornidazole. Nouv. Presse méd. *6:* 2438 (1977).

CHRISTENSSON, B., S. A. HEDSTROEM, B. URSING: Treatment of anaerobic infections with metronidazole. Scand. J. infect. Dis. *11:* 68 (1979).

DINH, H. T., S. KERNBAUM, J. FROTTIER: Treatment of antibiotic-induced colitis by metronidazole. Lancet *1:* 338 (1978).

FRYTAK, S., C. G. MOERTEL, D. S. CHILDS, J. W. ALBERS: Neurologic toxicity associated with high-dose metronidazole therapy. Ann. intern. Med. *88:* 361 (1978).

GIAMARELLOU, H., K. KANELLAKOPOULOU, D. PRAGASTIS, N. TAGARIS, G. K. DAIKOS: Treatment with metronidazole of 48 patients with serious anaerobic infections. J. Antimicrob. Chemother. *3:* 347 (1977).

HILLSTRÖM, L., L. PETTERSSON, E. PALSSON: Comparison of ornidazole and tinidazole in single-dose treatment of trichomoniasis in women. Brit. J. vener. Dis. *53:* 193 (1977).

JOKIPII, L., A. M. M. JOKIPII: Bactericidal activity of metronidazole, tinidazole and ornidazole against Bacteroides fragilis in vitro. J. Antimicrob. Chemother. *3:* 571 (1977).

JOKIPII, A. M. M., E. MYLLYLÄ HOKKANEN, L. JOKIPII: Penetration of the blood brain barrier by metronidazole and tinidazole. J. Antimicrob. Chemother. *3:* 239 (1977).

LEVI, G. C., C. A. DE AVILA, V. A. NETO: Efficacy of various drugs for treatment of giardiasis. A comparative study. Amer. J. trop. Med. Hyg. *26:* 564 (1977).

MATUCHANSKY, C., J. ARIES, P. MAIRE: Metronidazole for antibiotic-associated pseudomembranous colitis. Lancet. *2:* 580 (1978).

PRAKASH, C., B. C. BANSAL, M. R. BANSAL: Tinidazole in symptomatic intestinal amoebiasis. J. trop. Med. Hyg. *77:* 165 (1974).

REYNOLDS, A. V., J. M. T. HAMILTON-MILLER, W. BRUMFITT: A comparison of the in vitro activity of metronidazole, tinidazole and nimorazole against gram-negative anaerobic bacilli. J. clin. Path. *28:* 775 (1975).

RIPA, T., L. WESTRÖM, P.-A. MÅRDH, K.-E. ANDERSSON: Concentrations of tinidazole in body fluids and tissues in gynaecological patients. Chemotherapy *23:* 227 (1977).

ROE, F. J. C.: Metronidazole: Review of uses and toxicity. J. Antimicrob. Chemother. *3:* 205 (1977).

ROSS, S. M.: Single and triple dose treatment of Trichomonas infection of the vagina. Brit. J. vener. Dis. *49:* 475 (1973).

SCHWARTZ, D. E., F. JEUNET: Comparative pharmacokinetic studies of ornidazole and metronidazole in man. Chemotherapy *22:* 19 (1976).

SEGGIE, J.: Fusobacterium endocarditis treated with metronidazole. Brit. med. J. *1:* 960 (1978).

SKOLD, M.: Ornidazole: a new antiprotozoa: compounds for treatment of trichomonas vaginalis infection. Brit. J. vener. Dis. *53:* 44 (1977).

SMITH, B. J. D., J. WELLINGHAM: Metronidazole in treatment of empyema. Brit. med. J. *1:* 1074 (1976).

THURNER, J., J. G. MEINGASSNER: Isolation of Trichomonas vaginalis resistant to metronidazole. Lancet *2:* 738 (1978).

ULLMANN, U.: Die Aktivität von Metronidazol, seiner Hauptmetaboliten und ausgewählter Betalactamantibiotika gegenüber klinisch bedeutsamen anaeroben Bakterien. Z. antimikrob. Chemother. *1:* 73 (1983).

WALLIN, J., J. FORSGREN: Tinidazole – a new preparation for Trichomonas vaginalis infections. II. Clinical evaluation of treatment with a single oral dose. Brit. J. vener. Dis. *50:* 148 (1974).

WELLING, P. G., A. M. MONRO: The pharmacokinetics of metronidazole and tinidazole in man. Arzneimittel-Forsch. *22:* 2128 (1972).

WHEELER, L. A., M. DE MEO, M. HALULA, L. GEORGE, P. HESELTINE: Use of high-pressure liquid chromatography to determine plasma levels of metronidazole and metabolites after intravenous administration. Antimicrob. Ag. Chemother. *13:* 205 (1978).

WILLIS, A. T., I. R. FERGUSON, P. M. JONES: Metronidazole in the prevention and treatment of bacteroides infections following appendectomy. Brit. med. J. *1:* 318 (1976).

WOOD, B. A., A. M. MONRO: Pharmacokinetics of tinidazole and metronidazole in women after single large oral doses. Brit. J. vener. Dis. *51:* 51 (1975).

WÜST, J.: Susceptibility of anaerobic bacteria to metronidazole, ornidazole, and tinidazole and routine susceptibility testing by standardized methods. Antimicrob. Ag. Chemother. *11:* 631 (1977).

h) Povidone Iodine

Proprietary names: Batticon, Betadine, Betaisodona, Braunol, Braunosan, Braunovidone, Disadine, Povidine, Videne.

Properties: An organic polyvinyl-pyrrolidone complex of the iodophore group. Polyvinyl-pyrrolidone (PVP) is a water-soluble synthetic polymer which binds elemental iodine reversibly by an electrostatic mechanism. It is more stable than tincture of iodine. Application of the 10% solution, which contains 1% free iodine, releases iodine directly on the skin or mucous membrane in a manner which is less painful or irritant than with the 1% iodine tincture. Povidone iodine is a brown, washable solution which is free of smell.

Activity: Kills bacteria rapidly and bacterial spores much more slowly. Viruses, fungi, and trichomonads are also killed at low concentrations (0.1%). The minimal inhibitory concentrations are high in comparison with antibiotics (about 1000 mg/l). Povidone iodine reduces the bacterial count on infected skin and mucosa but cannot be relied upon to sterilise since pathogens may be sequestered in collections of pus or under crusts. Failure of therapy is more frequent in severe skin infections, for which systemic antibiotic therapy is preferable. Some inactivation by organic substances (peptone, pus etc.). Interactions with iodine-sensitive antibiotics (e. g. penicillin) may occur. Resistance has yet not been observed.

Side effects: Generally well tolerated on the skin. The high risk of allergy by the tincture of iodine, which is the main objection to its use, does not, apparently, exist with povidone iodine. Iodine applied to the skin is rapidly absorbed, and the serum levels of iodine can increase after excessive administration. Disorders of thyroid function have only rarely been observed. Transient dermatitis has been very occasionally reported.

Administration: In various forms (see below) for surgical hand disinfection and pre-operative skin cleansing, for topical treatment of wounds and burns, decubitus ulcers, pressure sores and vaginitis. There are serious reservations about its instillation in body cavities (e.g. for peritonitis) and about long-term application to large wounds because of the possibility of absorption of larger quantities of iodine and possibly of povidone as well. Povidone iodine should not be given to patients with allergy to iodine or with thyroid disease.

Preparations: Solution, liquid soaps, ointment, vaginal suppositories, vaginal jelly.

References

ALDEN, E. R., P. V. CAPOROSSI, G. C. LATHAM, R. G. SCHERZ: Effect of prenatal povidone iodine perineal antisepsis on serum protein bound iodine. Obstet. and Gynec. *35:* 253 (1970).

HAUSER, G. A.: Neues, die Döderleinflora schonendes Vaginaldesinfiziens zur Therapie unspezifischer Vaginitiden. Schweiz. Rundsch. Med. (Praxis) *64:* 1289 (1975).

KING, I. R., A. W. DIDDLE: Protein-bound iodine and T4 tests after vaginal application of povidone-iodine. Amer. J. Obstet. Gynec. *108:* 1175 (1970).

LINKNER, L. M., D. T. CLOUD, D. S. TRUMP, G. W. DORMAN: Prevention of bacterial growth and local infection in burn wounds. J. Pediat. Surg. *7:* 310 (1972).

MÜNTENER, M., H. SCHWARZ, H. REBER: Zur chirurgischen Händedesinfektion mit einem Jodophor (Betadine). Schweiz. med. Wschr. *102:* 699 (1972).

ZELLNER, P. R., E. METZGER: Asepsis und Antisepsis bei der Behandlung des Brandverletzten. Infection *5:* 36 (1977).

i) Bicozamycin

Properties: An antibiotic developed in Japan (also called bicyclomycin) with activity against salmonellae, shigellae, Yersinia enterocolitica, campylobacters, enterotoxigenic Escherichia coli, vibrios and aeromonads.

Activity: Oral bicozamycin is virtually not absorbed from the gastrointestinal tract and shortens considerably the duration of diarrhoea in cases of bacterial gastro-enteritis. Not effective against gram-positive bacteria or Bacteroides species (except Bacteroides fragilis), or protozoa (amoebae, giardia). No cross-resistance with other antibiotics. Secondary resistance does not develop. Primarily resistant strains of salmonella are rare. Well tolerated.

Recommended dosage: 500 mg 4 times a day for 3 days for gastro-enteritis and travellers' diarrhoea. Planned brand name: N.N. (Ciba).

Preparation: Tablets of 500 mg.

References

ERICSSON, CH. D., H. L. DUPONT, P. SULLIVAN: Bicozamycin, a poorly absorbable antibiotic, effectively treats travelers' diarrhea. Ann. intern. Med. *98:* 20 (1983).
HARFORD, P. S., B. E. MURRAY, H. L. DUPONT, CH. D. ERICSSON: Bacteriological studies of the enteric flora of patients treated with bicozamycin (CGP 3543/E) for acute nonparasitic diarrhea. Antimicrob. Ag. Chemother. *23:* 630 (1983).
MIYOSHI, T., N. MIYAIRI, H. AOKI, M. KOSHAKA, H. SAKAI, H. IMANAKA: Bicyclomycin, a new antibiotic. J. Antibiotics *25:* 569 (1972).
NISHIDA, M., Y. MINE, T. MATSUBARA: Bicyclomycin, a new antibiotic. III. In vitro and in vivo antimicrobial activity. J. Antibiotics *25:* 582 (1972).
VANHOOF, R., H. COIGNAU, G. STAS, H. GOOSSENS, J. P. BUTZLER: Activity of bicozamycin (CGP 3543/E) on different enteropathogenic micro-organisms: comparison with other antimicrobial agents. J. Antimicrob. Chemoth. *10:* 343 (1982).
WATT, B., F. V. BROWN: The in-vitro-activity of bicozamycin against anaerobic bacteria of clinical interest. J. Antimicrob. Chemother. *12:* 549 (1983).

18. Antituberculous Agents

a) Isoniazid (INH)

Proprietary names: Isozid, Neoteben, Nitrazid, Rimifon, Tebilon.

Properties: Isonicotinic acid hydrazide, a water-soluble, synthetic chemotherapeutic agent, which is bactericidal to extra- and intracellular bacteria.

Mode of action: Inhibition of bacterial nucleic acid and mycolic acid synthesis. Bacteriostatic to tubercle bacilli at concentrations of 0.05–0.2 mg/l, and bactericidal at 4 to 5 times that concentration, during the phase of active bacterial growth.

Spectrum of activity: Effective against Mycobacterium tuberculosis only, and not atypical mycobacteria (except M. kansasii to a small extent), nor any other bacterial species.

Resistance: Primary resistance in M. tuberculosis is rare (1–4%), but resistance develops rapidly with single drug therapy. No cross-resistance with other antituberculous agents.

Pharmacokinetics:

Absorption occurs within 1–2 hours of an oral dose.

Metabolism: Human populations show genetically determined differences in the rate at which isoniazid is inactivated by acetylation. Rapid inactivators have the dominant genotype in homozygous or heterozygous form, whereas slow inactivators are homozygous recessives. Certain ethnic groups, particularly the Japanese and many Eskimos, are predominantly rapid inactivators. In others, e. g. Caucasians and Negroes, about half are slow inactivators. Rapid inactivators have lower blood concentrations, a shorter half-life and less frequent side effects such as neuritis. Isoniazid is partly metabolised in the body to acetyl-isoniazid to an extent which is determined genetically as above, but other metabolites such as isonicotinic acid, isonictinuric acid, hydrazine and hydrazone derivatives are independent of genetic factors. All of these metabolites except the hydrazones are inactive.

Plasma concentrations after 200 mg by mouth are 2–3 mg/l after 1–2 h and 1.1 mg/l after 6 h in slow inactivators; after 300 mg orally they are 3–9 mg/l after 1–2 h and 1.4 mg/l after 6 h. These serum concentrations are 30–40% lower after 1 and 2 h in rapid inactivators, and this factor must be taken into account in the intermittent chemotherapy of tuberculosis. PAS is also acetylated and so the acetylation of isoniazid is reduced when PAS is given at the same time; correspondingly higher serum concentrations are then found.

Plasma protein binding 20–30%.

Half-life: 3 hours in slow inactivators and 1 hour in rapid inactivators. The half-life is prolonged in liver dysfunction. Only about 30–60% of the total dose of isoniazid remains active in the body.

Good *CSF penetration* with 50–80% of the serum concentration in meningitis. 50–100% of the serum concentration in pleural, peritoneal and synovial fluid. About 50% enters the fetal circulation. Good tissue diffusion. Also penetrates areas of caseous necrosis and macrophages.

Excretion is predominantly through the kidneys by glomerular filtration, almost entirely as metabolites, and in smaller amounts with the faeces. Urinary concentrations of active isoniazid are 20–80 mg/l.

Side effects (relatively rare with daily doses of up to 300 mg):
1. *Central nervous disorders and peripheral neuropathy* (dizziness, headaches, restlessness, psychological disorders, muscular fibrillation, cramps, paraesthesiae, retrobulbar neuritis). These occur more frequently with alcoholics, diabetics and slow inactivators and at higher dosage. Pyridoxine (vitamin B_6), 100–200 mg daily, can be given for the prophylaxis and treatment of isoniazid neuropathy. Somnolence or incoordination often occur when barbiturates or

diphenylhydantoin are given at the same time, because of delayed catabolism. Intolerance to alcohol is not uncommon.

2. *Gastrointestinal disorders and transient elevations of transaminases,* with hepatitis with or without jaundice in 1% of cases which can occasionally be fatal, particularly in people over 50. These are more frequent in combination with rifampicin than with ethambutol. The drug should be discontinued immediately at the first sign of hepatitis.

3. *Allergic rashes, fever* and *arthropathy.*

4. *Blood dyscrasias* (leucocytopenia, occasionally agranulocytosis, anaemia and thrombocytopenia).

5. *Bleeding tendency* due to damage to vessel walls, *cardiovascular disturbances, pellagra* and *acne.*

Indications: The most important drug in the combined treatment of tuberculosis, in prophylaxis in contacts whose tuberculin test is positive or has converted (particularly in immunosuppressive therapy, prolonged corticosteroid treatment, leukaemia, and Hodgkin's disease) and in the chemoprophylaxis of contacts, particularly infants.

Isoniazid should never be used alone to treat clinical tuberculosis.

Contra-indications: Acute hepatitis. Use with caution in alcoholics, epileptics, diabetics and patients with chronic liver disease or renal insufficiency.

Administration: Usually by mouth. The i.v. route is rarely necessary.

Dosage: *Oral:* 4–5 (–10) mg/kg a day, i.e. 200–300 (–600) mg for adults, 6(–10) mg/kg for children, 5–10 mg/kg for infants, but only 5 mg/kg in 1 or more divided doses during the first month of life, on account of metabolic immaturity. With higher dosage, give supplementary pyridoxine (10–20 mg per 100 mg isoniazid). Liver function, blood count and neurological status should be monitored regularly.

Intravenous route: Slow injection of 2–5% solution. The single dose should not exceed 200 mg, and continuous intravenous infusion is preferable.

Intrathecal route (rarely necessary): 20–40 mg a day for adults, and 5–30 mg (about 1 mg/kg) for children.

Local instillation: About 300 mg every 2–4 days into the pleura, 50–100 mg into joints and 50–100 mg into the bladder. Take the quantity of locally instilled isoniazid into account when calculating the total dose.

Treatment by inhalation is possible: 2 ml of 5% solution (= 100 mg) several times a day.

Preparations: 50, 100 and 200 mg tablets; an elixir containing 50 mg/5 ml, and 250 mg ampoules for injection.

Summary: A very effective antituberculous agent which is quite well tolerated. Use only in combination with other antituberculous agents to avoid the rapid development of resistance.

References

BAILEY, W. C., S. L. TAYLOR, H. E. DASCOMB, H. B. GREENBERG, M. M. ZISKIND: Disturbed hepatic function during isoniazid chemoprophylaxis. Amer. Rev. resp. Dis. *107:* 523 (1973).

BLACK, M.: Editorial. Isoniazid and the liver. Amer. Rev. resp. Dis. *110:* 1 (1974).

EIDUS, L., M. M. HODGKIN: Screening of isoniazid inactivators. Antimicrob. Ag. Chemother. *3:* 130 (1973).

BRASFIELD, D. M., T. B. GOODLOE, R. E. TILLER: Isoniazid hepatotoxicity in childhood. Pediatrics *58:* 291 (1976).

HSU, K. H. K.: Isoniazid in the prevention and treatment of tuberculosis. A 20-year study of the effectiveness in children. JAMA. *229:* 528 (1974).

HURWITZ, A., D. L. SCHLOZMAN: Effects of antacids on gastrointestinal absorption of isoniazid in rat and man. Amer. Rev. resp. Dis. *109:* 41 (1974).

JENNE, J. W., W. H. BEGGS: Correlation of in vitro and in vivo kinetics with clinical use of isoniazid, ethambutol and rifampin. Amer. Rev. resp. Dis. *107:* 1013 (1973).

JUNGBLUTH, H.: Isoniazid-Dosierung bei Niereninsuffizienz. Pneumologie *145:* 382 (1971).

KOPANOFF, D. E., D. E. SNIDER Jr., G. J. CARAS: Isoniazid-related hepatitis A. U.S. Public Health Service Cooperative Surveillance Study. Amer. Rev. resp. Dis. *117:* 991 (1978).

MADDREY, W. C., J. K. BOITNOTT: Isoniazid hepatitis. Ann. intern. Med. *79:* 1 (1973).

RAVIKRISHNAN, K. P., B. F. MULLER, A. NEUHAUS: Toxicity to isoniazid and rifampin in active tuberculosis patients. Amer. Rev. resp. Dis. (Suppl.) *115:* 405 (1977).

SCHRÖDER, J. M.: Zur Pathogenese der Isoniazid-Neuropathie. Acta neuropath. *16:* 301 (1970).

STEAD, W. W., E. C. Jr. TEXTER: Isoniazid hepatitis. Ann. intern. Med. *79:* 125 (1973).

VANDERHOFF, J. A., M. E. AMENT: Fatal hepatic necrosis due to isoniazid chemoprophylaxis in a 15-year-old girl. J. Paediatrics *88:* 867 (1976).

b) Streptomycin

Properties: Aminoglycoside aminocyclitol, which is stable, readily soluble in water and marketed as the sulphate.

Mode of action: More actively bactericidal in the proliferative than in the resting phase of bacterial growth (in the presence of metabolic activity).

Range of action: Mycobacterium tuberculosis, Brucella, Haemophilus ducreyi, Francisella tularensis and Yersinia pestis are usually sensitive. There is variable sensitivity (some strains being resistant) amongst streptococci, enterococci, staphylococci, Escherichia coli, Klebsiella, Proteus species, Pseudomonas aeruginosa, Actinomyces israeli and certain other species.

Atypical mycobacteria, clostridia, Bacteroides and rickettsiae are completely resistant.

Resistance: Primary resistance in strains of Mycobacterium tuberculosis is found with varying frequency (2–30%), but is rare in advanced countries. It is commoner, however, in patients from developing countries where tuberculosis is common and often inadequately treated. Resistance can develop rapidly within a few days by mutation (one-step resistance). There is cross-resistance in tubercle bacilli between streptomycin on the one hand and kanamycin, viomycin, and capreomycin on the other, but it is usually one-way, so that strains which have become resistant to streptomycin are generally still sensitive to these other drugs, but not the other way round.

Pharmacokinetics:

Virtually *not absorbed* by mouth.

Serum concentrations after i.m. injection of 500 mg are 14–30 mg/l after 1–2 h and 2–3 mg/l after 11–12 h; after 1 g, they are 20–45 mg/l after 1–2 h and 4–6 mg/l after 11–12 h (Fig. 31).

Half-life: 2½ hours which is prolonged in renal failure and in the newborn. *Plasma protein binding:* 30%.

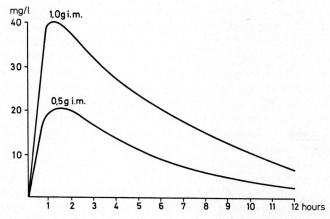

Fig. 31. Blood concentrations after a single i.m. injection of streptomycin.

CSF penetration: Very poor (2–4%) of serum concentrations, increased to 10–20% in acute meningitis.

Tissue diffusion: Adequate concentrations are attained in lung, muscle, uterus, intestinal mucosa, adrenals and lymph nodes. Diffusion into bone, brain and aqueous humor is poor. Increasing concentrations of 30–100% of peak plasma levels can be achieved on repeated dosing in pleural, peritoneal, and synovial fluids. The breast milk has the same concentration as serum. 50% of the mother's serum concentrations are found in cord blood and amniotic fluid.

Excretion: 50–60% excreted in the urine, predominantly by glomerular filtration. Urinary concentrations after 500 mg i. m. are 200–1500 mg/l in the first 6 hours. About 2% of the dose is excreted in the bile and faeces. Slowly haemodialysable.

Side effects:

1. *Neurotoxicity:* Vestibular damage can be caused by streptomycin in about 30% of cases, and cochlear damage by dihydrostreptomycin in about 26%. These toxic effects depend on the dose and length of treatment and are commoner when the daily dose of 1 g or the total dose of 60 g are exceeded. *Dihydrostreptomycin* should no longer be used because of its greater ototoxicity, although it continues to be marketed in Germany. In rare cases (about 6%) streptomycin may cause deafness. Renal, vestibular and auditory function should be monitored regularly throughout streptomycin therapy, preferably every 2 weeks. If audiometry is not possible, for example in small children, assay blood concentrations of streptomycin to detect accumulation due to impaired excretion, as shown by rising "trough" (pre-dose) concentrations. Do not exceed a maximum ("peak") concentration of 25 mg/l. These precautions also apply to combinations of streptomycin with pantothenic acid, which has the same neurotoxicity, and to combinations with benzyl penicillin, which were once commonly used but are now obsolete. The patient can only be protected from permanent damage by careful dosage, the regular monitoring of oto- and neurological function, and the prompt cessation of streptomycin at the first signs of any disorder of balance or hearing. Streptomycin given during pregnancy may damage the hearing of the baby, and so should only be used then if there is no alternative.

2. *Nephrotoxicity* can be acute in overdose and is shown by an increased blood urea, proteinuria, microhaematuria and casts.

3. *Allergic reactions* are relatively common, as shown by eosinophilia and rashes but rarely as anaphylactic shock or exfoliative dermatitis. Nursing staff sometimes suffer from contact dermatitis.

4. *Immediate reactions* (perioral paraesthesia, blurred vision, dizziness, behavioural disturbances) are harmless and are probably caused by the release of histamine from tissue mast cells.
5. *Others:* Hepatotoxic effects, eye muscle damage, scotoma, aplastic or haemolytic anaemia, agranulocytosis, leukocytopenia and thrombocytopenia are extremely rare.
6. The *intraperitoneal injection* of streptomycin may lead to a dangerous neuromuscular blockade with respiratory arrest, which can also occur after i. m. injection prior to anaesthesia or in conjunction with a muscle relaxant. Patients with myasthenia gravis are at particular risk. Treat with artificial respiration and inject prostigmine (0.1 mg i. v. every 2 min up to a total dose of 1 mg) and calcium gluconate.

Indications: Combination with other antibiotics to treat tuberculosis, subacute bacterial endocarditis (particularly when caused by enterococci), tularaemia and brucellosis. Less toxic aminoglycosides such as gentamicin, tobramycin or netilmicin are now preferable to streptomycin for the treatment of the last three (i. e. non-tuberculous) infections, however.

Incorrect use: As a single agent in tuberculosis. Treatment with a fixed penicillin-streptomycin combination.

Contra-indications: Anuria, severe renal failure and pregnancy. Use with care in the elderly (reduce daily dose). Avoid dihydrostreptomycin. Do not combine streptomycin with capreomycin, gentamicin, other aminoglycosides, colistin, or rapidly acting diuretics such as ethacrynic acid or frusemide (Lasix), which are also ototoxic.

Administration:
Parenteral route: Generally by i. m. injection of streptomycin sulphate at concentrations which do not exceed 500 mg/ml, i. e. 1 g in 2 ml, but occasionally as a continuous i. v. infusion (concentration 1 mg/ml) delivering 1 (–2) g over 7–8 hours in order to achieve a constant high blood level. There is a theoretical risk of toxic peaks of concentration with i. v. injection, although infusion carries the risk of thrombophlebitis. Do not instil streptomycin into the peritoneum because of the risk of respiratory arrest.

The *oral route* has been used for intestinal "sterilisation" and the treatment of gastroenteritis. Streptomycin is ineffective in both these roles and carries the risks of sensitisation and of possible overgrowth of resistant bacteria. It should not, therefore, be given by mouth.

Topical administration: Only in exceptional cases (e.g. in the eye) because of the risk of sensitisation. Include the amount given as part of the total dosage, because of the possibility of absorption.

Dosage: *I.m. route* (adults) 700 mg–1.5 g (14–20 mg/kg) a day, with a maximum daily dose of 2 g; for children (3 months – 12 y.): 20–30 mg/kg/day with a maximum of 1 g; for infants aged up to 3 months: 10 mg/kg/day up to a maximum of 50 mg in 3 divided doses. 1 injection per day is sufficient for tuberculosis. The daily dose for patients over 50 should not exceed 500 mg. Duration of treatment: 1–2 months in tuberculosis, with a maximum total dosage of 30–60 g for adults, 15–20 g for children and 10 g for infants. Longer courses of treatment are permissible, provided regular audiometry and vestibular tests are performed and treatment is stopped at the onset of any signs of inner ear damage, which is generally reversible at that stage. If renal insufficiency is not severe, prolong the dosage interval to
48 h (creatinine clearance of 60 ml/min),
72 h (creatinine clearance of 40 ml/min),
96 h (creatinine clearance of 30 ml/min).

The following concentrations may be used for *intrapleural* and *intraarticular* instillation: 0.5–1 g in 20–25 ml (25-50 mg/ml), and less in children according to their age.

Intrathecal administration is irritant and can give rise to other side effects. The advent of newer antituberculous agents which penetrate the CSF well means that intrathecal streptomycin is now almost never necessary.

Preparations: Ampoules of 500 mg, 1 g.

Summary:
Advantages: Bactericidal on tubercle bacilli when used in combination with other agents.
Disadvantages: Rapid development of resistance when used alone, neurotoxicity and risk of hypersensitivity.

Streptomycin should now be regarded as an agent for use in combination with others in tuberculosis only. It is rarely necessary for infections with other resistant bacteria (e.g. with benzyl penicillin in bacterial endocarditis) since newer, less toxic aminoglycosides are now preferred. Dihydrostreptomycin is still available in some countries (not Britain) but should no longer be used because of its toxicity.

Reference

MARTIN, W. J.: The present status of streptomycin in antimicrobial therapy. Med. Clin. North Amer. *54:* 1161 (1970).

c) Ethambutol

Proprietary names: EMB, Etibi, Myambutol. Combined with isoniazid in various dose ratios as Mynah.

Description: A stable, synthetic, water-soluble, dextrorotatory ethylene-diamine derivative.

Spectrum of activity: Bacteriostatic on proliferating, but not resting bacteria.

Active against Mycobacterium tuberculosis, Mycobacterium kansasii but not Mycobacterium fortuitum. Resistance develops slowly during therapy. No cross-resistance with other antituberculous agents. Primary resistance is found in about 4% of strains of M. tuberculosis.

Pharmacokinetics:
Absorption after oral intake: 70–80%, with maximum blood concentrations after 2 hours.
Serum concentrations (after 25 mg/kg by mouth) 4.4 mg/l (2 h) and 2.3 mg/l (8 h).
Half-life: 4–6 h. Concentrated in the erythrocytes which contain 2–3 times as much ethambutol as the plasma. Little *serum protein binding. Cerebro-spinal fluid* concentrations of 1–2 mg/l are found in tuberculous meningitis (after 25 mg/kg daily by mouth).
Slow *renal excretion* of 70–80% of the dose, including 8–15% as inactive metabolites. About 20% passes out with the faeces.

Side effects: Retrobulbar neuritis of the optic nerve, shown initially as disturbance of green vision followed by general weakness of vision, hemianopia and finally optic nerve atrophy. This effect is commoner at doses above 25 mg/kg/day and over a long course of treatment. It rarely occurs with normal dosage (see below). These changes are initially reversible but regress slowly and are seldom irreversible. Their frequency at normal dosage is 0–6%. Peripheral neuropathy, central nervous disorders, allergic rashes, attacks of gout (due to increased uric acid) and transient disturbances of liver function are rare.

Indications: Combined treatment of pulmonary tuberculosis, and in infections caused by atypical mycobacteria or where the organisms are resistant to other antituberculous agents.

Contra-indications: Optic atrophy or a history of retrobulbar neuritis. Reduce dose in renal failure.

Administration and dosage: The initial dose of 25 mg/kg once a day by mouth for 2 months can then be reduced to 15 mg/kg a day, but should always be combined with 1 or 2 other effective antituberculous agents. The dose by the i. m. or i. v. route is the same as by mouth. An ophthalmic examination should be performed before the start and then every 4 weeks during treatment, and should test colour vision, visual fields, visual acuity and the appearance of the fundus. A fundus check alone is not sufficient. Give the maintenance dose every 36 hours when the creatinine clearance is 10–50 ml/min, and every 48 hours with creatinine clearances of less than 10 ml/min.

Preparations: Tablets of 100 and 400 mg and ampoules of 200 and 400 mg and 1 g. A combined oral preparation with isoniazid is available in four dose ratios of ethambutol to isoniazid, namely 200 mg: 100 mg (Mynah 200), 250 mg: 100 mg (Mynah 250), 300 mg: 100 mg (Mynah 300) and 365 mg: 100 mg (Mynah 365).

Summary: An effective first-line antituberculous agent.

References

BOBROWITZ, I. D.: Ethambutol in tuberculous meningitis. Chest *61:* 629 (1972).
BOBROWITZ, I. D.: Ethambutol-isoniazid versus streptomycin-ethambutol-isoniazid in original treatment of cavitary tuberculosis. Amer. Rev. resp. Dis. *109:* 548 (1974).
CLARKE, G. B. M., J. CUTHBERT, R. J. CUTHBERT, A. W. LEES: Isoniazid plus ethambutol in the initial treatment of pulmonary tuberculosis. Brit. J. Dis. Chest *66:* 272 (1972).
COLLIER, J., A. M. JOEKES, P. E. PHILALITHIS, F. D. THOMPSON: Two cases of ethambutol nephrotoxicity. Brit. med. J. *2:* 1105 (1976).
DOSTER, B., F. J. MURRAY, R. NEWMAN, S. F. WOOLPERT: Ethambutol in the initial treatment of pulmonary tuberculosis. Amer. Rev. resp. Dis. *107:* 177 (1973).
GIRGIS, N. I., M. W. YASSIN, J. E. SIPPEL, K. SORENSEN, A. HASSAN, W. F. MINER, Z. FARID, A. ABU EL ELLA: The value of ethambutol in the treatment of tuberculous meningitis. J. trop. Med. Hyg. *79:* 14 (1976).
PILHEU, J. A., F. MAGLIO, R. CETRANGOLO, A. D. PLEUS: Concentrations of ethambutol in cerebrospinal fluid after oral administration. Tubercle *52:* 117 (1971).
POSTLETHWAITE, A. E., A. G. BARTEL, W. N. KELLEY: Hyperuricemia due to ethambutol. New Engl. J. Med. *286:* 761 (1972).
REIMERS, D.: Irreversible Augenschäden durch Ethambutol. Prax. Pneumol. *26:* 445 (1972).
SHARBARO, J. A., L. D. HUDSON: High dose ethambutol; an oral alternate for intermittent chemotherapy. Amer. Rev. resp. Dis. *110:* 91 (1974).
SOMNER, A. R., J. B. SELKON, M. WALTON, A. B. WHITE: Drug resistant pulmonary tuberculosis treated with ethambutol and rifampicin in North East England. Tubercle *54:* 141 (1973).
TUGWELL, P., S. L. JAMES: Peripheral neuropathy with ethambutol. Postgrad. med. J. *48:* 667 (1972).

d) Rifampicin

Proprietary names: Rifa, Rifadin, Rifamate, Rifoldin, Rimactane.

Description: Rifampicin (rifampin in the USA) is a semi-synthetic ansamycin antibiotic of the rifamycin group. It is soluble in organic solvents, and in water at acid pH, having a yellow-red colour. The ansamycins bear no relationship to other antibiotics.

Mode of action: Inhibition of bacterial RNA polymerase. Intensely bactericidal on proliferating bacteria including tubercle bacilli.

Spectrum of activity: Tubercle bacilli are very sensitive (minimal inhibitory concentration only 0.5 mg/l), as are gram-positive bacteria (staphylococci, streptococci, enterococci etc.), gonococci and meningococci, Legionella pneumophila and Chlamydia trachomatis. Some atypical mycobacteria (M. kansasii, M. marinum) are moderately sensitive and gram-negative strains are relatively insensitive (except for Haemophilus influenzae which is very sensitive). Rifampicin is effective in leprosy. Penicillin-resistant pneumococci are generally sensitive to rifampicin.

Resistance: Primary resistance against tubercle bacilli is rare (less than 1%). Resistance of the streptomycin type (one-step resistance) develops rapidly in staphylococci, gonococci, meningococci and other bacteria, but only after several weeks of single drug therapy in tubercle bacilli. No cross-resistance with other antituberculous agents.

Pharmacokinetics:
Absorption is good after oral intake. *Peak blood concentrations* occur after 2–4 hours. *Serum concentrations* after 600 mg by mouth are 7–14 mg/l at 2 h and 2 mg/l at 12 h. *Half-life* 3 hours, which is shortened on continuous treatment, probably due to increased biliary excretion, and prolonged to 4–7 hours in liver disorders but unaffected by *renal failure*. Rifampicin does not accumulate. *Plasma protein binding* 75 to 80%. This highly lipophilic antibiotic diffuses rapidly into the lungs, kidneys, adrenal glands and liver, where the concentration can even be higher than in the blood, depending on the time of administration. Rifampicin penetrates cells (e. g. leucocytes) as well as bronchial secretion, pleural and peritoneal fluid. Poor *CSF penetration* (0–11%), but better in meningitis (10–90%). Rifampicin gives a red colour to saliva, sputum, lacrimal fluid, sweat, faeces and urine.
Excretion (after 900 mg orally) of about 40% in the bile and up to 30% in the urine, 30–50% of which is unchanged. The principal metabolite is desacetyl rifampicin, which also has antibacterial activity. The urinary recovery decreases

with smaller doses, and a larger proportion is excreted in the bile, much of which is then reabsorbed in the intestines; this enterohepatic recirculation is partly responsible for the maintenance of therapeutic blood concentrations for 12 hours or more after each dose. Not eliminated during haemodialysis.

Side effects: Increases in liver transaminases (aminotransferases) are found in about 5–20% of cases, although values often return to normal in spite of continued treatment. Rifampicin therapy must be stopped immediately if the transaminases rise higher than 100 international units/litre or the serum bilirubin increases, since fatal acute hepatitis has been reported. Most patients will tolerate the resumption of rifampicin after an interval. This hepatotoxicity necessitates the regular monitoring of serum transaminases.

Other side effects include gastrointestinal upset, cutaneous symptoms (pruritus and flushes with or without a rash) and transient leucocytopenia or thrombocytopenia. Central nervous disorders are shown as drowsiness, ataxia, visual disturbances, muscle weakness, pain in the extremities and a sensation of deafness. Rifampicin very occasionally causes renal failure, apparently as a result of hypersensitivity and shown as interstitial nephritis, acute tubular necrosis or severe cortical necrosis. This can result from the interruption and subsequent resumption of rifampicin therapy.

Rifampicin interferes with oral contraception with ovulation inhibitors and anticoagulant therapy; the latter must therefore be controlled more frequently in long-term treatment with coumarin anticoagulants. The breakdown of tolbutamide can be shortened by enzyme induction during a course of rifampicin; withdrawal symptoms also appear in persons taking methadone because of increased breakdown of this drug in the liver.

Indications: All stages of tuberculosis, including initial treatment in combination with isoniazid and ethambutol or streptomycin; infections with atypical mycobacteria; leprosy. Although activity on gram-positive cocci and neisseria is very good, the risk of rapid development of resistance is high in nontuberculous infections so treatment with rifampicin alone should generally be avoided. The drug is valuable, however, in combination with other agents (e.g. trimethoprim) to treat chronic or inaccessible infections with organisms resistant to other antibiotics, e.g. chronic infections of implanted heart valves or ventriculoperitoneal shunts with multi-resistant strains of Staphylococcus epidermidis. Rifampicin is licensed in the USA for the prophylaxis of meaningococcal infections.

Contra-indications: Acute hepatitis, obstructive jaundice, other severe liver diseases, pregnancy.

Caution when combined with hepatotoxic antituberculous drugs (prothionamide, pyrazinamide), in alcoholism, pre-existing liver disease and previous intolerance of rifampicin.

Administration and dosage: 10 mg/kg (600–750 mg) a day by mouth for adults; 10–20 mg/kg for children (300–460 mg) a day between the ages of 6 and 12, and 150–300 mg a day up to age 6 in one or two divided doses 1 hour before meals.

Preparations: 150 and 300 mg capsules; a mixture containing 100 mg/5 ml; ampoules of 300 and 600 mg for injection (not in Britain). Combinations of rifampicin 150 mg plus isoniazid 100 mg (Rimactazid 150) and rifampicin 300 mg plus isoniazid 150 mg (Rimactazid 300) are also available.

Summary: Rifampicin is a very active oral first-line antituberculous agent which should always be used in combination with 1 or 2 other antituberculous agents (e. g. isoniazid and ethambutol) in order to prevent the development of secondary resistance. Rifampicin is not recommended for infections other than tuberculosis except in severe or inaccessible infections where no alternative is available.

References

ACOCELLA, B. G., L. BONOLLO, M. MAINARDI, P. MARGAROLI, L. T. TENCONI: Serum and urine concentrations of rifampicin administered by intravenous infusion in man. Arzneimittel-Forsch./Drug Res. *27:* 1221 (1977).

BOLT, H. M., H. KAPPUS, M. BOLT: Rifampicin and oral contraception. Lancet *1:* 1280 (1974).

CASTEELS-VAN DAELE, M., L. IGODT-AMEYE, L. CORBEEL, R. FECKELS: Hepatotoxicity of rifampicin and isoniazid in children. J. Pediat. *86:* 739 (1975).

CHAN, W. C., M. G. O'MAHONEY, D. Y. G. YU, R. Y. H. YU: Renal failure during intermittent rifampicin therapy. Tubercle *56:* 191 (1975).

COCHRAN, M., P. J. MOORHEAD, M. PLATTS: Permanent renal damage with rifampicin. Lancet *1:* 1428 (1975).

EDWARDS, O. M., R. J. COURTENAY-EVANS, J. M. GALLEY, J. HUNTER, A. D. TAIT: Changes in cortisol metabolism following rifampicin therapy. Lancet *2:* 549 (1974).

GABOW, P. A., J. W. LACHER, T. A. NEFF: Tubulointerstitial and glomerular nephritis associated with rifampicin. JAMA *235:* 2517 (1970).

GIRLING, D. J.: Adverse reactions to rifampicin in antituberculosis regimens. J. Antimicrob. Chemother *3:* 115 (1977).

KISSLING, M., N. BERGAMINI, M. XILINAS: Parenteral rifampicin in tuberculous and severe non-mycobacterial infections. Chemotherapy *28:* 229 (1982).

MANDELL, F., P. E. WRIGHT: Treatment of atypical mycobacterial cervical adenitis with rifampin. Pediatrics *55:* 39 (1975).

NESSI, R., G. L. BONOLDI, B. REDAELLI, G. DI FILIPPO: Acute renal failure after rifampicin: A case report and survey of the literature. Nephron *16:* 148 (1976).

NILSSON, B. S., G. BOMAN: Intravenous use of rifampicin. Amer. J. resp. Dis. *62:* 212 (1981).

NITTI, V., R. VIRGILIO, M. R. PATRICOLO, A. IULIANO: Pharmacokinetic study of intravenous rifampicin. Chemotherapy 23: 1 (1977).
NYIRENDA, R., G. V. GILL: Stevens-Johnson syndrome due to rifampicin. Brit. med. J. 2: 1189 (1977).
O'REILLY, R. A.: Interaction of chronic daily warfarin therapy and rifampin. Ann. intern. Med. 83: 506 (1975).
SIPPEL, J. E., I. A. MIKHAIL, N. I. GIRGIS, H. H. YOUSSEF: Rifampin concentrations in cerebrospinal fluid of patients with tuberculous meningitis. Amer. Rev. resp. Dis. 109: 579 (1974).
SKOLNICK, J. L., B. S. STOLER, D. B. KATZ, W. H. ANDERSON: Rifampin, oral contraceptives, and pregnancy. JAMA 236: 1382 (1976).
STANFORD, J. L., I. PHILLIPS: Rifampicin in experimental Mycobacterium ulcerans infection. J. Med. Microbiol. 5: 39 (1972).
STERN, J. S. M., D. M. STAINTON-ELLIS: Rifampicin in pregnancy. Lancet 2: 604 (1977).
SYVÄLAHTI, E. K. G., K. K. PIHLAJAMÄKI, E. J. JISALO: Rifampicin and drug metabolism. Lancet 2: 232 (1974).
WILKINSON, F. F., J. GAGO, E. SNATABAYA: Therapy of leprosy with rifampicin. Int. J. Leprosy 40: 53 (1972).
WOODLEY, C. L., J. O. KILBURN, H. L. DAVID, V. A. SILCOX: Susceptibility of myocobacteria to rifampin. Antimicrob. Ag. Chemother. 2: 245 (1972).

e) Para-Aminosalicylic Acid (PAS)

Proprietary names: Inapasade, PAS, Nicopas (in combination with isoniazid).

Description: p-Amino salicylic acid is a synthetic chemotherapeutic agent, the sodium salt of which is soluble in water. A brown colour develops on inactivation.

Mode of action: The relatively weak bacteriostatic action is due to competitive antagonism of p-amino benzoic acid.

Spectrum of action: PAS acts only on tubercle bacilli and not on atypical mycobacteria or on other bacteria.

Resistance: Primary resistance is rare. Secondary resistance develops slowly and there is no cross-resistance with other antituberculous drugs.

Pharmacokinetics:
Absorption: The sodium or potassium salt is 75–80% absorbed after oral intake, giving maximal blood concentrations after 2 hours.
Serum concentrations of free PAS after 4 g by mouth are 50–100 mg/l during the first 2 hours. *Plasma protein binding:* 50–60%. Only the free PAS (about 55–80% in the serum) is active, and the metabolites acetyl-PAS and glycocol-PAS have no antituberculous activity. *Half-life:* 1 hour.

Tissue concentrations: Not very high, and low concentrations are found in the pleural, peritoneal and synovial fluids as well as in the cerebrospinal fluid, although 30–50% of the serum values occur in meningitis.

Excretion is predominantly through the kidneys (about 80%), 15–30% as free PAS and the rest as ineffective metabolites. Urinary concentration of free PAS are 3–7 mg/ml.

Side effects: Frequent gastro-intestinal upset and allergic reactions (eosinophilia, fever, rashes, and occasional leucocytopenia; renal abnormalities are quite common (haematuria, leucocyturia, casts, albuminuria), and hepatotoxicity and hypothyroidism. Malfunction of iodine metabolism, goitre and myxoedema are occasionally found.

Indications: In combination with other antituberculous agents against sensitive strains of Mycobacterium tuberculosis. PAS is bacteriostatic in vivo and its intrinsic antituberculous activity is not very great, so its main role is the prevention of development of resistance to other major compounds given at the same time.

Contra-indications: Severe liver damage or renal failure, gastritis and gastric or duodenal ulcer; use sodium-PAS with caution in hypertension and oedema and potassium-PAS with care in renal disease and adrenal insufficiency.

Administration and dosage: Adults should be given 12–16 g a day and children 200–300 mg/kg by mouth in 2–4 divided doses, preferably with meals.

Preparations: Coated tablets of 410 mg (sodium salt).

Summary: A weak antituberculous agent with considerable gastrointestinal side effects which is only bacteriostatic in the body at high dosage. It is regarded nowadays as a reserve agent. Tissue diffusion is poorer than with INH, but there is no risk of the rapid development of resistance. May be given as the third component of a potent triple combination, but is generally replaced today with ethambutol or rifampicin.

f) Thioamides (Ethionamide and Prothionamide)

Proprietary names: Prothionamide is marketed as Ektebin and Peteha in Germany, where ethionamide is no longer available, and was formerly marketed as Trevintix in Great Britain, where ethionamide was formerly sold as Trescatyl. Both agents are still available in Britain but not as proprietary drugs.

Description: Ethionamide is an α-ethylthioisonicotinamide (a derivative of isonicotinic acid), and prothionamide is a propyl-2-thionicotinic acid amide; both are unstable, poorly soluble in water but readily soluble in dimethyl sulphoxide.

Mode of action: Bacteriostatic at therapeutic concentrations, but bactericidal at higher concentrations.

Spectrum of action: Tubercle bacilli and some atypical mycobacteria (particularly M. kansasii).

Resistance: Develops rapidly. Complete cross-resistance between ethionamide and prothionamide. No cross-resistance with isoniazid.

Pharmacokinetics:
Absorption after oral intake is more rapid with prothionamide than with ethionamide; the *serum concentration* of prothionamide after 1 hour is therefore almost twice as high as that of ethionamide (5.7 mg/l after 500 mg by mouth), but after 6 hours it is only one third of the ethionamide concentration (0.9 mg/l). *Half-life:* 3 hours. *Tissue diffusion* and *CSF penetration* are both good (30–60%), as is penetration into cells. Metabolism is almost complete (more than 95%). One of the numerous metabolites is sulphoxide, which has antituberculous properties itself.
Excretion: Primarily renal, but less than 1% in active form; the mean urinary concentration of active ethionamide after 500 mg by mouth is 10–20 mg/l.

Side effects: Gastrointestinal disorders are less frequent with prothionamide than with ethionamide, and are less frequent after i. v. injection. Other side effects include neurotoxic and psychic disturbances (headache, dizziness, restlessness, sleep disturbances, peripheral neuropathy, depression, and convulsions in epileptics), acne and pellagra, photosensitisation of the skin, liver damage (particularly in diabetics), hypoglycaemia in diabetics, hypothyroidism, eosinophilia, leucocytopenia, gynaecomastia and menstrual disorders. Prophylaxis and treatment of these effects with pyridoxine (50–150 mg a day) is sometimes effective.

Indication: Used in combination with other antituberculous agents, particularly when there is resistance to isoniazid.

Contra-indications: Early pregnancy, severe liver damage, gastric complaints. Use with care in epilepsy and psychotic patients. Avoid alcohol. Avoid combination with isoniazid and cycloserine wherever possible, because of the potentiation of side effects.

Dosage:

By mouth, give ethionamide and prothionamide in small doses initially and slowly increase to:

Adults	750 mg (–1 g)	
Children up to 4 y.	25 mg/kg	in 3–4 divided
Children 4–8 y.	20 mg/kg	doses
Children of 8 y. and above	15 mg/kg	

For *intravenous infusion* of prothionamide do not exceed 500–750 mg in 500 ml for 5–6 h and use only freshly prepared solutions. Every patient treated with prothionamide should have serum transaminases monitored to detect incipient hepatotoxicity.

Preparations: Tablets and coated tablets of 250 mg, and ampoules of 500 mg for infusion.

Summary: A reliable antituberculous agent which diffuses well into tissues but which causes frequent side effects and carries the risk of rapid development of bacterial resistance; only use in small doses, combined with other agents, as a second-line drug when others have failed or not been tolerated.

References

LEES, A. W.: Ethionamide, 500 mg daily, plus isoniazid 500 mg or 300 mg daily in previously untreated patients with pulmonary tuberculosis. Amer. Rev. resp. Dis. *95:* 109 (1967).

NARANG, R. K.: Acute psychotic reaction probably caused by ethionamide. Tubercle *53:* 137 (1972).

SCHÜTZ, I., K. BARTMANN, K. L. RADENBACH, W. SIEGLER: Vergleich der Verträglichkeit von Prothionamid und Ethionamid im Doppelblindversuch. Beitr. klin. Tuberk. *140:* 296 (1969).

SIMON, E., E. VERES, G. BANKI: Changes in SGOT activity during treatment with ethionamide. Scand. J. resp. Dis. *50:* 314 (1969).

SWASH, M., A. J. ROBERTS, D. J. MURNAGHAN: Reversible pellagra-like encephalopathy with ethionamide and cycloserine. Tubercle *53:* 132 (1972).

g) Pyrazinamide

Proprietary names: Pyrafat, Zinamide.

Description: Pyrazine carbonic acid amide, a stable, moderately water-soluble chemotherapeutic agent.

Mode of action: Bactericidal on human but not bovine tubercle bacilli, nor usually on atypical mycobacteria. pH-dependent, being more active at acid pH, i. e. particularly good in caseous necrosis. Almost inactive at neutral pH. No cross-resistance with other antituberculous agents.

Pharmacokinetics:

Absorption: Maximum blood concentrations occur after 1–2 hours.

Serum concentrations (after a single oral dose of 1 g) are 40–45 mg/l after 2 hours and 10 mg/l after 15 hours. *Half-life:* 6 hours. Highly metabolised. Good *tissue diffusion* and *CSF penetration.*

Excretion: Through the kidneys, partly as the weakly antibacterial compound pyrazinoic acid.

Side effects: The risk of liver damage has been overestimated. Functional disorders of the liver were apparently mostly caused by the simultaneous administration of PAS. As well as jaundice, there may be gastrointestinal complaints, hyperuricaemia with attacks of gout, and hyperglycaemia.

Indications: Initial therapy of caseous tuberculosis. Treatment for longer than 2 months is not recommended.

Contra-indications: Severe liver damage and gout. Reduce dose in renal impairment.

Administration and dosage: 1.5–2.5 g daily by mouth for *adults*, and 20–35 mg/ kg a day for *children* in 2 or 3 divided doses. Check the serum transaminases every 2–3 weeks during treatment and stop therapy at the first sign of liver damage.

Preparations: Tablets of 500 mg.

Summary: A bactericidal antituberculous agent for initial chemotherapy which has become re-established in the 1970s.

References

BRANDER, E.: A simple way of detecting pyrazinamide resistance. Tubercle *53:* 128 (1972).

DICKINSON, J. M., D. A. MITCHISON: Observations in vitro on the suitability of pyrazinamide for intermittent chemotherapy of tuberculosis. Tubercle *51:* 389 (1970).

FORGAN-SMITH, R., G. A. ELLGARD, D. NEWTON, D. A. MITCHISON: Pyrazinamide and other drugs in tuberculous meningitis. Lancet *2:* 374 (1973).

HESS, W., H. JUNGBLUTH, R. KROPP: Prospektive kooperative Prüfung der Lebertoxizität des Pyrazinamids. Prax. Pneumol. *24:* 486 (1970).

HORSFALL, P. A. L.: Treatment of resistant pulmonary tuberculosis in Hong Kong with regimes of second-line drugs. Tubercle *53:* 166 (1972).

MacCurdy, R. K., E. R. Simon: Thrombocytopenia and sideroblastic anemia with pyrazinoic acid amide (pyrazinamide) therapy. Chest. *57:* 378 (1970).
Mitchison, D. A.: Symposium on drug resistant tuberculosis. Reserve drug combinations. J. Ir. med. Ass. *63:* 86 (1970).
Toida, J.: Pyrazinamide deamidase in tuberculous infection. Amer. Rev. resp. Dis. *107:* 639 (1973).
Yu, T. F., J. Perel, L. Berger, J. Roboz, Z. H. Israili, and P. G. Dayton: The effect of the interaction of pyrazinamide and probenecid on urinary uric acid excretion in man. Amer. J. Med. *63:* 723 (1977).

h) Capreomycin

Proprietary names: Capastat, Capstat, Ogostal.

Description: An aminoglycoside. The sulphate is stable and water-soluble. Bacteriostatic on tubercle bacilli, but little action on other bacteria; generally less active than streptomycin in vitro and in vivo.

Resistance: Primary resistance is rare. Resistance develops quite rapidly during treatment, and there is partial cross-resistance with kanamycin.

Pharmacokinetics:
Not *absorbed* by mouth.
Maximum blood *concentrations* occur 1–2 hours after i.m. injection. *Serum concentrations* after 1 g i.m. are 29 mg/l after 2 h and 4 mg/l after 10 h. *Half-life:* 5 hours.
Excretion is about 50—70% in active form with the urine.

Side effects: Ototoxicity is possibly somewhat less than with streptomycin and kanamycin, as is nephrotoxicity. Fever, skin rashes and eosinophilia can occur.

Indications: Treatment of tuberculosis with strains resistant to streptomycin. May also be used as initial therapy of recurrent tuberculosis.

Contra-indications: Severe renal insufficiency, pre-existing middle ear damage, pregnancy.

Dosage: 1 g a day for *adults*, 20 mg/kg a day for *children*, for 1–2 months, later twice or three times a week. Regular audiometric and renal functions tests are necessary. Use only in combination with two other antituberculous agents, but not with streptomycin, kanamycin or the highly toxic agent *viomycin* (additive toxicity). In renal impairment, prolong the dose interval to 48 hours when the creatinine clearance is 60 ml/min, to 72 hours with a creatinine clearance of 40 ml/min and to 96 hours when the creatinine clearance is 30 ml/min.

Preparations: Ampoules of 1 g.

Summary: A very effective second-line antituberculous agent which carries a risk of ototoxicity. Only of minor importance today.

References

ANDREWS, R. H., P. A. JENKINS, J. MARKS, A. PINES, J. B. SELKON, A. R. SOMNER: Treatment of isoniazid-resistant pulmonary tuberculosis with ethambutol, rifampicin and capreomycin: A co-operative study in England and Wales. Tubercle 55: 105 (1974).

Drug commentary: Evaluation of a new antituberculous agent. Capreomycin sulfate (capastat sulfate). JAMA 233: 179 (1973).

JUNGE, O.: Dünnschichtchromatographische Auftrennung der Antibiotika Carbenicillin, Polymyxin und Capreomycin. Intern. J. clin. Pharmacol. 6: 67 (1972).

KROPP, R., I. DÜCKER, H. JUNGBLUTH: Intravenose Infusion von Capreomycin. Pneumologie 144: 312 (1971).

McCLATCHY, J. K., W. KANES, P. T. DAVIDSON, T. S. MOULDING: Crossresistance in M. tuberculosis to kanamycin, capreomycin and viomycin. Tubercle 58: 29 (1977).

i) Cycloserine

Proprietary names: Cycloserine, D-Cycloserine, Seromycin.

Description: D-4-amino-3-isoxazolidinone (antibiotic), water-soluble, relatively stable. Inactivated by D-alanine.

Mode of action: Bacteriostatic on intra- and extracellular bacteria. Competitive inhibition of the incorporation of D-alanine in the mucopeptide of the bacterial cell wall.

Spectrum of activity: Active against tubercle bacilli and some atypical mycobacteria (M. avium and others) in concentrations of 10–20 mg/l; other gram-positive and gram-negative bacteria are inhibited at higher concentrations only.

Resistance develops slowly, if at all, during treatment.

Pharmacokinetics:
Complete and rapid *absorption* after oral intake. Maximum blood levels after 2 hours.

Serum concentrations after 250 mg 4 times a day by mouth reach a maximum of 15–25 mg/l. *Half-life:* about 10 hours.

Diffuses well in tissues and body fluids (50–80% in cerebrospinal fluid, 50–100% of serum concentrations in pleural and peritoneal fluid). 30–35%

converted into antibacterially inactive metabolites. *Terizidone* is a cycloserine derivative which acts as cycloserine in the body.

Excretion: 60–70% excreted in active form by the kidneys over 2–3 days, with urinary concentrations between 30 and 300 mg/l. Cycloserine is not found in the faeces.

Side effects are mostly reversible and particularly occur when a daily dose of 1 g is exceeded and when the dose is increased too rapidly at the beginning of the treatment. Neurotoxicity is shown as drowsiness, agitation, disorientation, headache, tremor, visual disturbances, depression, paresis, psychosis or convulsions. Intolerance to alcohol occurs. Gastrointestinal disorders and allergic symptoms are rare. At the beginning of the treatment, transient inflammatory reactions such as increased temperature, increase in sputum production, focal reactions, leucocytosis and an increased erythrocyte sedimentation rate are sometimes found.

Indications: Used in combination with other agents, particularly when there is bacterial resistance to isoniazid, PAS or streptomycin. Active on atypical mycobacteria.

Contra-indications: Renal insufficiency, epilepsy, previous psychosis, alcoholism.

Administration: Preferably by mouth (well absorbed).

Dosage: 750 mg–1 g a day for *adults*, and 20 mg/kg for *children*, in 3–4 divided doses with meals; dosage 250 mg initially, followed by a gradual increase by 250 mg every 2 days up to the full dose after 1 week. Side effects can be minimised by giving 200 mg of pyridoxine a day (pyridoxine loss is adjusted by the urine). Avoid alcohol completely.

Preparations: Tablets of 250 mg.

References

BAILEY, W. C., J. W. RALEIGH, A. P. TURNER: Treatment of mycobacterial disease. Amer. Rev. resp. Dis. *115:* 185 (1977).

EDER, J. L., F. G. B. EDWARDS, E. W. ABRAHAMS: Tuberculosis due to Mycobacterium kansasii. Aust. N. Z. J. Med. *7:* 8 (1977).

SWASH, M., A. H. ROBERTS, D. J. MURNAGHAN: Reversible pellagra-like encephalopathy with ethionamide and cycloserine. Tubercle *53:* 132 (1972).

C. General Rules of Antibiotic Therapy

1. Choice of Antibiotic

The right choice of antibiotic will determine the success or otherwise of antibiotic therapy. The drug chosen should combine the best chance of success with the least likelihood of side effects. This choice *should be based wherever possible on a reliable clinical and bacteriological diagnosis.* In severe infections, some risk of toxicity may be acceptable if a particular drug is clearly superior to others in its antibacterial activity.

In certain diseases, the bacterial cause and antibiotic sensitivity are always known; treatment of these can begin before results of culture and sensitivity are available. In pneumonia, pyelonephritis and many other infections, however, a number of pathogens with varying antibiotic sensitivity patterns must be considered, and the choice of antibiotic is based on the antibiotic sensitivity pattern.

The decision to use a particular antibiotic is influenced not only by the causative organism and its sensitivity, but also by its mode of action, pharmacokinetic properties, site and severity of the infection, and the patient's age, hepatic and renal function. Other important factors are the ease of administration and therapeutic range of the antibiotic, which must achieve adequate concentrations in the tissue or fluid where the infection is localized.

The antibiotic sensitivity patterns of the most important pathogens are shown in Tables 23 and 24. Table 25 lists possible ways of treating common infections by facultative pathogens with antibiotics. Apart from antibiotic prophylaxis, there are **three frequently recurring situations in clinical practice:**

1. **Culture results are not available,** or bacterial examination is not possible or not necessary. Treatment must be effective against the likeliest bacterial cause. This is relatively easy when the clinical picture is typical and the cause well known, as in scarlet fever or syphilis where the drug of choice is benzyl penicillin, or in typhoid fever, where the drug of choice is chloramphenicol or co-trimoxazole. If one or more of a range of pathogens may cause an organ infection, those most frequently encountered will receive priority. Cholecystitis is caused by Escherichia coli, other members of the Enterobacteriaceae, streptococci (including faecal streptococci), but rarely by Clostridium, Bacteroides or Pseudomonas species and never by staphylococci. Treatment with mezlocillin, is therefore suitable even though this agent is not effective against most strains of staphylococci. Lobar pneumonia is generally caused by pneumococci, but occasionally in the elderly by Klebsiella pneumoniae. *If initial antibiotic*

Table 23. Clinical use of the more important antibiotics.

Bacterial species	Benzyl penicillin	Ampicillin	Azlocillin	Mezlocillin	Piperacillin	Flucloxacillin	Cefazolin	Cefuroxime	Cefoxitin	Cefotaxime	Tetracycline	Chloramphenicol	Gentamicin, Tobramycin	Amikacin	Erythromycin	Clindamycin	Fusidic acid	Nitrofurantoin	Nalidixic acid	Co-trimoxazole
Corynebacterium diphtheriae	●	+	+	+	+	+	+	+	+	+	⊕	+	⊕	+	⊕	+	+	○	○	+
Streptococci	●	+	+	+	+	+	+	⊕	+	+	+	+	+	+	⊕	⊕	+	⊕	○	⊕
Pneumococci	●	+	+	+	+	+	+	⊕	+	+	+	+	○	○	⊕	⊕	+	+	○	⊕
Enterococci	+	●	⊕	●	⊕	○	○	○	○	○	⊕	+	○	○	⊕	○	○	⊕	○	+
Staphylococci	⊕	+	+	+	+	●	⊕	⊕	⊕	+	+	+	+	+	+	⊕	●	⊕	+	○	+
Gonococci	●	+	+	+	+	+	+	+	●	+	●	⊕	+	+	+	⊕	○	+	○	+
Meningococci	●	+	+	+	+	+	+	⊕	+	+	+	⊕	+	+	⊕	○	+	+	+	+
H. influenzae	○	●	●	+	●	○	+	⊕	+	●	●	●	+	+	⊕	○	○	○	+	⊕
Legionella pneumophila	○	○	○	○	○	○	○	○	○	○	+	+	○	○	○	●	○	○	○	○
Brucella	○	+	+	+	+	○	+	+	+	+	●	⊕	+	+	○	○	○	○	+	⊕
Bacteroides fragilis	○	○	⊕	+	⊕	○	○	○	●	○	⊕	⊕	○	○	+	●	○	○	○	+
Bacteroides melaninogenicus	●	+	+	+	+	○	○	+	●	+	⊕	+	○	○	+	●	○	○	○	+
M. tuberculosis	○	○	○	○	○	○	○	○	○	○	+	○	+	+	○	○	○	○	○	○
Treponema pallidum	●	+	+	+	+	+	⊕	⊕	+	+	⊕	+	○	○	+	○	○	○	○	○
Listeria	⊕	●	+	⊕	⊕	○	○	○	○	○	+	+	+	+	+	+	○	○	○	+
Clostridia	●	+	+	+	+	+	+	+	+	+	⊕	+	○	○	⊕	+	+	○	○	+
Ps. aeruginosa	○	○	●	⊕	●	○	○	○	○	+	+	+	●	●	○	○	○	○	○	○
Escherichia coli	○	⊕	⊕	●	●	○	⊕	●	●	●	⊕	⊕	⊕	⊕	○	○	○	⊕	⊕	●
Klebsiella pneumoniae	○	○	○	+	⊕	○	+	⊕	●	●	⊕	●	●	●	○	○	○	⊕	⊕	●
Enterobacter aerogenes	○	○	○	○	+	○	+	⊕	⊕	⊕	⊕	+	●	●	○	○	○	⊕	⊕	●
Proteus vulgaris	+	+	⊕	●	●	○	+	⊕	●	●	+	+	●	●	○	○	○	+	●	●
Proteus mirabilis	+	●	●	●	●	○	⊕	⊕	●	●	+	+	●	●	○	○	○	+	⊕	●
Salmonella typhi	+	⊕	+	+	+	○	+	+	+	+	+	●	+	+	○	○	○	○	○	●
Salmonella typhimurium	+	●	+	+	+	○	+	+	+	⊕	⊕	⊕	+	+	○	○	○	+	+	●
Shigella	+	●	+	+	+	○	+	+	+	+	⊕	⊕	+	+	○	○	○	+	+	●
Rickettsia	○	○	○	○	○	○	○	○	○	○	●	●	○	○	+	○	○	○	○	○
Mycoplasma pneumoniae	○	○	○	○	○	○	○	○	○	○	●	⊕	○	○	⊕	+	○	○	○	○
Chlamydia psittaci	○	○	○	○	○	○	○	○	○	○	●	⊕	○	○	+	○	○	○	○	○
Chlamydia trachomatis	○	○	○	○	○	○	○	○	○	○	●	⊕	○	○	●	○	○	○	○	⊕

● = very active, first choice for treatment, ⊕ = good activity, second line antibiotic, + = active but only recommended in special cases, or not at all, ○ = inactive.

Table 24. Clinical use of the more important antibiotics against less common pathogens.

Bacterial species	Benzyl penicillin	Ampicillin	Cefazolin	Cefoxitin	Cefotaxime	Streptomycin	Tetracycline	Chloramphenicol	Erythromycin	Kanamycin	Gentamicin	Polymyxin	Sulphonamide	Co-trimoxazole
Acinetobacter	∅	±	∅			±	⊞⊞	∅	±	+	+	+		+
Actinomyces israeli	⊞	++	++	++	+	±	±	±	±	∅		∅	+	
Aeromonas hydrophila	∅	±	∅	+	+	±	++	++	∅	±	±	+		+
Bacillus anthracis	⊞⊞	+	++	+	+	+	+	+	+	+	+	∅		+
Bordetella pertussis	∅	⊞⊞	∅		+	±	++	++	⊞⊞	±	±	±	∅	+
Borrelia recurrentis	+	+	+	+	+	+	⊞⊞	+						
Campylobacter jejuni	+				+	+	⊞⊞	⊞⊞	⊞⊞		⊞⊞			
Citrobacter	∅	+	+	∅	+	+	+	++	∅	++	⊞	++	+	⊞
Enterobacter cloacae	∅	+	+	±	±	+	++	++	∅	++	⊞⊞	++	+	+
Erwinia	∅	±	±	+	⊞⊞	+	+	++	∅	++	+	+		
Erysipelothrix rhusiopathiae	⊞	+	++	+	+	∅	+	+	+	∅	∅	∅	∅	
Francisella tularensis	∅					⊞⊞	++	++	∅	+	+	+	∅	∅
Fusobacterium species	⊞⊞	+	+	+	+	+	+	+	+	∅	∅			
Haemophilus ducreyi	+					+	+	+	+				⊞	
Hafnia	∅	+	+	+	⊞⊞	+	++	++	∅	++	⊞⊞	++	+	
Leptospira	⊞	+	+	+	+	±	⊞⊞	±	+				∅	∅
Moraxella lacunata	∅		+	+	+	+	⊞⊞	++	∅					
Nocardia asteroides	∅	∅	∅	∅	∅		⊞⊞	+					⊞⊞	
Pasteurella multocida	⊞	+	+	+	+	±	⊞⊞	+	++	∅	+	++	+	+
Providencia	∅	∅	∅	⊞	⊞⊞	∅	∅	±	∅	+	++	∅	∅	⊞
Ps. cepacia	∅	∅	∅	∅	+	∅	∅	+	∅	∅	∅	∅	+	+
Ps. mallei	∅					+	⊞⊞	+	∅				∅	
Ps. maltophilia	∅	∅	∅	∅	+	∅		+	∅	∅	∅	∅	∅	+
Ps. pseudo-mallei	∅				+	⊞	⊞	∅		+	+	∅	+	+

Table 24 (continued).

Bacterial species	Benzyl penicillin	Ampicillin	Cefazolin	Cefoxitin	Cefotaxime	Streptomycin	Tetracycline	Chloramphenicol	Erythromycin	Kanamycin	Gentamicin	Polymyxin	Sulphonamide	Co-trimoxazole
Serratia marcescens	∅	∅	∅	⊞	⊞⊞	∅	∅	∅	∅	⊞	⊞	∅	∅	⊞
Streptobacillus moniliformis	⊞⊞	+	+	+	+	+	⊞⊞	+	+				⊞	
Vibrio cholerae	∅	+	+	+	+	±	⊞⊞	+	+				⊞	⊞
Y. entero-colitica	∅	∅	∅	+	+	+	⊞⊞	⊞⊞	∅	+	+	+		
Y. pestis	∅					⊞⊞	++	++	∅	+	+	∅	+	+
Y. pseudo-tuberculosis	∅			+	+	+	⊞⊞	⊞⊞	∅	++	+	+		

⊞⊞ = Antibiotic of choice, + + = very active, + = moderately active, ± = doubtful activity, ∅ = inactive, Ps. = Pseudomonas, Y. = Yersinia, H. = Haemophilus.

treatment fails, rare causes such as tuberculosis should be considered. The bacterial causes of other forms of pneumonia vary; Bacteroides species and anaerobic streptococci can cause aspiration pneumonia, staphylococci post-operative pneumonia, and Pseudomonas and enterobacteria can cause inhalation pneumonia. If the first choice of antibiotic is unsuccessfuly, change to an antibiotic which is effective against the less common causes of the infection (see Table 24, p. 251).

This *calculated* ("best-guess") *chemotherapy* can be changed as soon as relevant bacteriological results are available.

2. **The disease is life-threatening.** Effective treatment is then urgent, and the drugs given initially have to be effective against *all* the likely causes of the infection. For example, septicaemia in a leukaemic patient may be due to any potentially pathogenic organism including opportunists, and (after blood culture) treatment must start with as broadly effective an antibiotic combination as possible, e. g. a combination of cefotaxime (or cefoxitin) with piperacillin (or azlocillin), possibly with gentamicin also, or metronidazole where anaerobic organisms may be involved. Such a combination not only extends the spectrum of activity; it can also be synergistic (when all the drugs are active) and bactericidal in the infected tissues and cells.

Table 25. Facultative pathogens, common infections and antibiotic therapy.

Name and synonyms	Usual site of occurrence	Typical infections	Effective antibiotics
Staphylococcus aureus Coagulase-positive staphylococci	Skin, upper respiratory tract	Boils, infected wounds, mastitis, purulent parotitis, suppurative pneumonia, antibiotic-induced enterocolitis, food poisoning, infections associated with foreign bodies, osteomyelitis	*Flucloxacillin, clindamycin,* (when sensitive, *benzyl penicillin),* erythromycin, fusidic acid, cefazolin, vancomycin
Staphylococcus epidermidis, coagulase-negative staphylococci, Staphylococcus albus	Always on the skin, nasal mucosa	Occasional cause of endocarditis, infections associated with foreign bodies (e. g. valve implants)	As Staphylococcus aureus (see above)
Streptococcus pyogenes, β-haemolytic streptococci, group A streptococci	Throat	Erysipelas, scarlet fever, angina, rheumatic fever, puerperal sepsis, cellulitis, septicaemia	*Benzyl, penicillin,* phenoxymethyl penicillin, in cases of allergy erythromycin, cefazolin, oral cephalosporins
Streptococcus pneumoniae, pneumococci	Upper respiratory tract	Lobar pneumonia, bronchitis, sinusitis, corneal ulcer, meningitis, empyema, septicaemia, otitis media	As Streptococcus pyogenes (see above)
Group B streptococci, Streptococcus agalactiae	Genital tract, intestines, cause of animal infections	Neonatal septicaemia and meningitis, gynaecological infections, pyelonephritis	*Benzyl penicillin,* cefuroxime, cefotaxime
Group D streptococci, enterococci, Strep. faecalis, Strep. faecium, faecal streptococci etc.	Intestines, urethra	Urinary infections, mixed infections of intestinal origin, septicaemia, endocarditis	*Ampicillin,* erythromycin, tetracycline, vancomycin, mezlocillin, cefazedone
Other aerobic streptococci, viridans and non-haemolytic streptococci	Upper respiratory tract, intestines	Subacute bacterial endocarditis	*Benzyl penicillin,* cefazolin, lincomycins, vancomycin

Table 25 (continued).

Name and synonyms	Usual site of occurrence	Typical infections	Effective antibiotics
Anaerobic streptococci, pepto-streptococci	Mouth, intestines, vagina	Mixed infections of intestinal or genital origin, dental infections, brain and lung abscess	*Benzyl penicillin,* also tetracycline, clindamycin, erythromycin in mixed infections
Escherichia coli	Intestines, possibly also the mouth and vagina	Urinary infections, pyelonephritis, neonatal meningitis, cholangitis	*Ampicillin, mezlocillin, piperacillin,* (where sensitive) *co-trimoxazole,* cephalosporins, gentamicin, sulphonamides, norfloxacin
Organisms of the Klebsiella enterobacter group	Respiratory tract, intestines	As with E. coli, also Klebsiella pneumoniae	*Cefoxitin, cefotaxime, gentamicin, amikacin,* co-trimoxazole, tetracycline, chloramphenicol, norfloxacin
Proteus species Pr. vulgaris, Pr. mirabilis, Pr. morganii, Pr. rettgeri	Intestines	Urinary infections, and occasionally in pyelonephritis, burns, wound infections, chronic otitis	*Ampicillin, mezlocillin, cefoxitin, amikacin,* gentamicin, co-trimoxazole, norfloxacin
Pseudomonas aeruginosa	Not normally on skin or mucous membranes, but common in sewage and dirt, sometimes found in the intestines	Wound infections, particularly burns, chronic otitis, urinary infections, septicaemia, chronic bronchitis, ecthyma gangrenosum, umbilical infections	*Tobramycin, gentamicin, amikacin, azlocillin,* piperacillin, ceftazidime, cefsulodin, norfloxacin
Haemophilus influenzae	Respiratory tract	Chronic bronchitis, bronchopneumonia, otitis media, sinusitis, conjunctivitis, meningitis, septicaemia, epiglottitis	*Ampicillin, cefuroxime, cefotaxime, chloramphenicol* in meningitis, also erythromycin, azidocillin, tetracycline

Table 25 (continued).

Name and synonyms	Usual site of occurrence	Typical infections	Effective antibiotics
Bacteroides melanino-genicus	Upper respiratory tract, rare in the intestines	Dental sepsis, lung abscess, empyema, brain abscess	*Benzyl penicillin, metronidazole*
Bacteroides fragilis	Mouth, intestines	Mixed infections of intestinal origin, appendicitis, pylephlebitis, septic thrombophlebitis, genital infections, abscesses with fetid pus	*Metronidazole, cefoxitin, clinda-mycin,* chloramphenicol, also mezlocillin or piperacillin (in large dosage)
Candida albicans	Skin, mouth, intestines	Candida stomatitis (thrush), vaginitis, balanitis, occasional pneumonia, oesophagitis, septica-emia. Common in skin infections, e. g. as intertrigo and nail infections	*Clotrimazole, nystatin, micona-zole, ketocona-zole, amphoteri-cin B,* flucytosine or miconazole i. v. in systemic infection

3. **The results of bacteriological culture and sensitivities are already available.** The best choice is then the *most effective antibiotic with the narrowest spectrum* (e. g. amoxycillin for urinary infections with Escherichia coli, or benzyl penicillin for pneumococcal pneumonia).

References

CONN, H. F. (ed.): Current Therapy 1984. Saunders, Philadelphia 1984.

GARROD, L. P., F. O'GRADY: Antibiotic and Chemotherapy. 5th Ed. Livingstone, Edinburgh 1981.

MONIF, G. R. G.: Infectious Diseases in Obstetrics and Gynecology. Harper and Row, Hagerstown, Maryland 1974.

SELWYN, S. (ed.): The Beta-Lactam Antibiotics: Penicillins and Cephalosporins in Perspective. Hodder and Stoughton, London 1982.

SIMON, C.: Anwendungsmöglichkeiten neuerer Antibiotika. Mschr. Kinderheilk. *127:* 171 (1979).

SPELLER, D. C. E.: Antifungal Chemotherapy. John Wiley, Chichester 1980.

WIEDEMANN, B.: Wirksamkeit von Chemotherapeutika. Z. antimikrob. Chemother. *1:* 113 (1983).

2. Administration

The decision of whether to give an antibiotic orally, parenterally or topically depends on the clinical picture, the condition of the patient and the general circumstances. Some antibiotics can only be given orally (e.g. phenoxymethyl penicillin, propicillin, and oral esters such as talampicillin), while others (e.g. amikacin) are only given parenterally, because they are not absorbed in the intestine. Because of their toxicity, some antibiotics, e.g. neomycin, paromomycin, nystatin, bacitracin etc., are unsuitable for systemic use and can only be applied topically. Many antibiotics may be given both orally and parenterally.

The **parenteral route** generally gives more complete absorption than the oral. This is why antibiotic treatment of serious infections should be *started intravenously* as a slow injection or short infusion, to achieve rapid, high and where possible bactericidal blood and tissue concentrations. Once the patient starts to improve, treatment is continued by mouth. *Continuous i.v. infusion* is only recommended with bacteriostatic drugs to obtain sustained high concentrations. High peaks of concentration, as after i.v. injection, give more favourable tissue concentrations of penicillins and cephalosporins than the longer and more sustained concentrations which result from constant i.v. infusion of the same daily dose. Tissue concentrations depend not only on the mode of action, however, but also on the rate of diffusion and other factors such as half-life, protein-binding, lipophilia, molecular size etc. Isotonic solutions are often better tolerated when given i.v. They are produced in volumes which vary with the individual preparation (see Table 26).

Intramuscular injection achieves a depot effect with poorly soluble antibiotics such as procaine penicillin. The absorption of the antibiotic can, however, be delayed in shock or dehydration. If the patient has poor veins, an antibiotic normally given i.v. may have to be injected i.m. (e.g. rolitetracycline). I.m. injection is not advisable in patients with a bleeding tendency; certain antibiotics (e.g. cephalothin and erythromycin) cause marked local inflammation when given i.m., and increase the serum LDH and CPK. Antibiotics should not be mixed with other drugs (vitamins, heparin etc.), with plasma concentrates or with amino acid infusions because of the possible risk of inactivation. When an antibiotic powder is dissolved in the fluid in the ampoule, the resultant volume will be larger than that of the original solvent. The solution thus contains a different concentration than could be assumed (see capreomycin sulphate, for example, Table 27). Table 28 lists the different concentrations of various penicillins after the substance has dissolved.

Absorption after **oral administration,** varies considerably with different antibiotics. While sulphonamides, chloramphenicol, minocycline etc. are almost

Table 26. Production of an isotonic solution of ampicillin, carbenicillin, flucloxacillin and methicillin (after LYNN 1973).

Antibiotic	Content of ampoule (g)	Concentration of isotonic solution (w/v)	Quantitiy of water (ml) for isotonic solution
Ampicillin	0.5	5 %	10.0
Carbenicillin	1.0	3.5%	28.5
Flucloxacillin	0.25	6.0%	4.0
Methicillin	1.0	5.5%	17.0

completely absorbed by mouth, the absorption of phenoxymethyl penicillin, ampicillin, cloxacillin and tetracycline is only partial. The *rate of absorption* also depends on the galenic preparation, which can vary between preparations of the same antibiotic (e. g. phenoxymethyl penicillin and tetracycline). Antibiotics should not be given by mouth to patients who are unconscious, vomiting, or who have dysphagia or gastric diseases. Unreliable patients, especially when treated as outpatients, are not suitable for oral therapy. The oral absorption of certain antibiotics also depends on whether the stomach is empty or full. Phenoxymethyl penicillin, cloxacillin and lincomycin, for example, should be given fasting, whereas griseofulvin is best absorbed after a fatty meal.

Because absorption is unreliable, antibiotics should not generally be given **rectally** by suppository. An exception is metronidazole which is well absorbed by this route.

The **dosage interval** required depends on the speed of absorption, metabolism and excretion. If the antibiotic is absorbed and eliminated rapidly, e. g. benzyl penicillin sodium injected i. v., the interval between doses must be shorter than for oral penicillins which are absorbed more slowly. The excretion of penicillins and cephalosporins can be delayed by giving probenecid, which inhibits tubular function, at the same time.

Table 27. Dissolving the contents of one ampoule of capreomycin (corresponding to 1 g base) in different amounts of solvent increases the volume of the solution and gives rise to varying concentrations per ml.

Initial volume of solvent	Final volume (ml) of capreomycin solution	Concentration (mg/ml)
2.15	2.85	350
2.63	3.33	300
3.3	4	250
4.3	5	200

Table 28. Content of ampoule, amount of water added and final volume of the resultant solution of various penicillins.

Antibiotic	Content of ampoule (g)	Volume of water (ml)	Final volume of solution
Ampicillin	0.5	1.5	1.9
Carbenicillin	1.0	2.0	2.75
Flucloxacillin	0.25	1.5	1.7
Methicillin	1.0	1.5	2.2
Ampicillin + Cloxacillin	0.5	1.5	1.9

The **tolerance** of an antibiotic can vary with different routes of administration. Rapid i. v. injection (e. g. of tetracycline) often causes venous inflammation and unwanted systemic effects, while gastrointestinal upset is more frequent after taking tetracycline by mouth. Local pain and inflammation are quite common after i. m. injection of almost all the cephalosporins, and should be avoided by mixing with a local anaesthetic or by giving i. v. Potentially toxic agents such as amphotericin are better given as a continuous infusion than as a rapid intravenous injection, which can give rise to high peaks of concentration and related side effects. Incompatibilities sometimes result from the addition of substances to the infusion fluid, or by its electrolyte content (Na).

Topical administration of an antibiotic is generally free of side effects except for allergy, and agents known to sensitise the patient, such as penicillins, should never be used topically for this reason. A certain degree of absorption and hence of systemic side effects is possible when antibiotics are applied locally to large wounds or instilled in large amounts into body cavities. Antibiotics which cannot be given systemically because of their toxicity are preferred for topical use because a systemic agent can still be given if resistant bacterial flora are selected. Local antibiotics are only likely to be effective in very superficial skin infections, and a spray or solution is generally better for this purpose than a cream or ointment; an oil-in-water emulsion is also preferable to an ointment. Eye, nose or ear drops containing antibiotics should be given at concentrations which are tolerated by the tissues. The same applies to aerosols and the intrathecal, intraarticular, intrapleural, intraperitoneal or intravesicular instillation of antibiotics. Topical antibiotics in the nasopharynx, still used in some countries, are of doubtful value because of their poor activity against streptococci, and inadequate penetration.

References

FEIGIN, R. D., K. S. MOSS, P. G. SHACKELFORD: Antibiotic stability in solutions used for intravenous nutrition and fluid therapy. Pediatrics *51:* 1016 (1973).
O'GRADY, F., W. R. L. BROWN, H. GAYA, I. P. MACKINTOSH: Antibiotic levels on continuous intravenous infusion. Lancet *2:* 209 (1971).
WYATT, R. G., G. A. OKAMOTO, R. D. FEIGIN: Stability of antibiotics in parenteral solutions. Pediatrics *49:* 22 (1972).

3. Dosage

The principal objective in giving an antibiotic is to achieve a concentration at the site of infection which is sufficient to kill or inhibit the growth of the bacteria present. The dosage required to achieve this aim cannot always be defined in fixed terms; it must often be adjusted to suit the special features of the individual case. Important factors which must be taken into account are the sensitivity of the causative organisms, the pharmacokinetics and tolerance of the antibiotic in relation to the patient's age and illness, and the site of the infection. The dose recommendations made by the manufacturers are sometimes also influenced by commercial considerations, with preference for underdosage (less expensive) or twice daily dosage (more convenient). Overdosage is less frequently recommended.

Tolerance of the antibiotic: If dose-related side effects are to be avoided, the *maximum* daily and total dosage should *not as a rule be exceeded*. The penicillins and, to a lesser extent, the cephalosporins, clindamycin, fusidic acid and rifampicin have such a broad therapeutic range that dose-related side effects are extremely uncommon. With most other antibiotics, however, side effects regularly occur when the maximum recommended dosage is exceeded.

A *moderate* dose is generally sufficient for less severe infections or when the causative organism is very sensitive, in which case the risk of dose-related side effects is less. If the infection does not respond, the dose can be increased up to the maximum recommended. With some antibiotics such as the tetracyclines, however, increasing the oral dose does not result in proportionately higher blood concentrations because gastrointestinal absorption is already taking place at the maximal rate.

The side effects of some antibiotics such as cycloserine in tuberculosis, chloramphenicol in typhoid fever and amphotericin B in systemic fungal infections can be minimised by starting with a low dose and progressively increasing it to the therapeutic dose or the limit of tolerance. Chloramphenicol should only be given at reduced dosage to premature neonates and full-term babies in the first two weeks of life because the immature liver fails to detoxify the drug adequately and progressive accumulation can lead to the "grey baby" syndrome. Aminoglycosides (gentamicin, tobramycin, netilmicin, amikacin) also have poor selective toxicity and accumulate at normal dosage in patients with renal impairment. Chloramphenicol or aminoglycosides should only be given to patients in these risk groups under regular assay control.

Sensitivity of the causative organism: The dosage of an antibiotic should be such that the minimal inhibitory concentration of that antibiotic against the organism concerned lies within the therapeutic range of that agent at the site of infection. Very sensitive bacteria such as Lancefield Group A streptococci are adequately treated with quite low daily doses of an antibiotic such as benzyl penicillin. Less sensitive organisms such as Pseudomonas may be better treated by a synergistic combination of antibiotics than by an excessive dosage of a single agent.

Difficult infections such as endocarditis, where the site of infection is relatively inaccessible to antibiotics, humoral antibodies and the body's cellular defences, may require the antibiotic dosage to be adjusted in relation to the sensitivity of the patient's isolate. Back-titration *in vitro* of the patient's serum during treatment is a useful means of ensuring that the dose given is adequately bactericidal against the organism originally isolated from the patient's blood culture.

Pharmacokinetics: Absorption, distribution, metabolism, conjugation and elimination differ according to the antibiotic, underlying disease and age of the patient. The dose and dose interval of a given antibiotic are generally determined from the *blood concentration-time curve* (absorption, half-life etc.) and the *urinary recovery*. Oral dosage must be higher than parenteral to achieve the same blood concentrations because oral absorption is generally poor, with the exception of the sulphonamides and chloramphenicol. To produce therapeutically effective blood and tissue concentrations rapidly at the beginning of treatment, the initial dose may be given intravenously or at double the usual dose. A lower dosage may be sufficient in cardiac failure or renal impairment (see p. 510). Regular assays may be necessary during therapy in difficult cases to avoid excessive concentrations, if possible, before they occur.

Site of infection: An important factor in successful treatment is the ability of the antibiotic to diffuse into the infected tissue. Infections in poorly accessible sites, such as bone, meninges, abscess cavities, may need to be treated by combining the maximum tolerated systemic dose with local instillation, intrathecal administration etc. The dose of penicillin or ampicillin necessary to treat bacterial meningitis may need to be 10–20 times higher than normal, particularly when meningeal inflammation subsides, since penicillins pass relatively poorly into the cerebrospinal fluid. High serum penicillin concentrations may also be achieved by using probenecid to delay renal tubular secretion.

Pediatric dosage may be based on the *average body surface area of* children, from which the following rules have been derived:

Age (years)	Fraction of adult dosage
1/4	1/6
1/2	1/5
1	1/4
3	1/3
7	1/2
12	2/3

In clinical practice, antibiotics are usually dosed according to *body weight*. The usual daily doses for children given in Table 29 apply to infants and small children. Applying the rules of body weight to older children could result in excessive doses, higher even than those recommended for adults. For this reason, *surface area* should be the determining factor for school children. Children between 6 and 9 years thus receive one half, and children between 10 and 12 years about two thirds of the dosage recommended for adults.

Dosage in premature and full term neonates and infants during the first month of life: At this age, the excretion of antibiotics whose main route of elimination is through the kidneys is *delayed* because of renal immaturity; the peak blood levels decline more slowly and the dose-intervals may need to be 2 to 3 times longer than with older children. Individual variations in the *degree of renal immaturity* between premature and full-term babies must, however, be taken into account. Special care is necessary in the first few days of life, whilst accumulation is less common after the first week. In particular, potentially toxic antibiotics should only be given in very low doses, or at extended dose-intervals. It may be helpful to assay the *serum concentration* immediately before the next dose (the trough or residual level). Commercial kits are now available for radio-immunoassay and enzyme immunoassay of aminoglycosides and require only very small samples of blood. Those antibiotics, such as penicillins, which are generally non-toxic, can be given without serious risk in the normal dosage for infants (Table 30).

Table 29. Daily dosage of important antimicrobial agents in adults and children.

Antibiotic	Adults	Children (except the newborns)	Route
Benzyl penicillin	1–5 (−40) megaunits	0.04–0.1 (−1) megaunits/kg	i. m., i. v.
Phenoxymethyl penicillin	1.5 (−8) megaunits	0.05 (−0.1) megaunits/kg	oral
Dicloxacillin	2–4 (−10) g	100 (−200) mg/kg	oral
Flucloxacillin	2–4 (−10) g	100 (−200) mg/kg	oral, i. v.
Ampicillin	3–4 g	100–150 (−200) mg/kg	oral
	1.5–2 (−20) g	100 (−400) mg/kg	i. m., i. v.
Amoxycillin	1–1.5 (−3) g	50 (−100) mg/kg	oral
Bacampicillin	2.4 g	60 mg/kg	oral
Azlo-, mezlocillin, piperacillin }	6–15 (−20) g	100–200 (−300) mg/kg	i. v.
Tetracycline, oxytetracycline }	1–1.5 (−2) g	20–30 mg/kg	oral
Rolitetracycline, oxytetracycline }	(0.25−) 0.5 (−0.75) g	10 mg/kg	i. v.
Doxycycline	0.1–0.2 g	2–4 mg/kg	oral, i. v.
Minocycline	0.2 g	4 mg/kg	oral, i. v.
Chloramphenicol	2–3 (−4) g	50 (−80) mg/kg	oral, i. v.
Cefoxitin, cefuroxime, cefotaxime, cefsulodin	3–6 g	60 (−150) mg/kg	i. v., i. m.
Oral cephalosporins	2–4 g	50–100 mg/kg	oral
Erythromycin	1–2 (−3) g	30–40 (−80) mg/kg	oral, i. v.
Clindamycin	0.6–1.2 g	10–20 mg/kg	oral, i. v., i. m.
Fusidic acid	1.5 (−3) g	20–30 mg/kg	oral
Genta-, tobramycin	160–240 (−320) mg	2–3 (−5) mg/kg	i. m.
Amikacin	1 g	15 mg/kg	i. m.
Vancomycin	1–2 g	20–40 mg/kg	i. v.
Nitrofurantoin	(0.1−) 0.2–0.3 g	(2−) 5 mg/kg	oral
Nalidixic acid	4 g	−	oral
Pipemidic acid	0.8 g	−	oral
Norfloxacin	0.8 g	−	oral
Co-trimoxazole	(0.9−) 1.9 (−2.8) g	20–30 mg/kg	oral
Metronidazole (anaerobic organisms)	1.5–2.25 g	30–40 mg/kg	oral

Duration of treatment: The duration of treatment depends on the course of the disease and the species of causative organism and should be long enough to eradicate the infection. *Longer courses of treatment* are needed for chronic infections such as tuberculosis, fungal infections etc., and also in septicaemic illnesses with a tendency to relapse or recur (e.g. staphylococcal septicaemia, brucellosis, endocarditis). *Prophylaxis* against recurrent infection is particularly recommended in rheumatic fever. Longer course of antibiotics are often necessary in patients with impaired immunity (leukaemia, immune deficiency diseases etc.) and who tend to relapse when treatment is discontinued.

Reference

v. HARNACK, G.-A.: Arzneimitteldosierung im Kindesalter. Thieme, Stuttgart 1982.

4. Side Effects

Side effects may be *toxic, allergic or biological.* Acute **toxicity,** as may occur after larger doses of colistin, should be distinguished from chronic toxicity (e.g. with chloramphenicol, which can cause anaemia and neutropenia after longer periods of treatment). Some antibiotics have little toxicity, such as penicillins,

Table 30. Dosage in premature and full-term neonates up to the end of the first month of life.

Antibiotic	Route	Daily dose per kg of body weight (in 2–3 divided doses)
Benzyl penicillin	i.v.	0.06–1 megaunits/kg
Phenoxymethyl penicillin	oral	30 mg/kg
Flucloxacillin	oral, i.v.	50–100 mg/kg
Ampicillin	i.v.	100–200 mg/kg
Azlo-, mezlo-, piperacillin	i.v.	100–200 mg/kg
Cefotaxime, cefsulodin, cefoxitin, cefuroxime	i.v.	60 mg/kg
Oral cephalosporins	oral	50–100 mg/kg
Gentamicin, tobramycin	i.m., i.v.	3 (–5) mg/kg
Amikacin	i.m., i.v.	10 mg/kg
Erythromycin	oral	30 mg/kg
Clindamycin	oral, i.v.	20 mg/kg
Chloramphenicol[1]	oral, i.v.	25 mg/kg

[1] 1st–2nd weeks of life (50 mg/kg from the 3rd week on)

cephalosporins, fusidic acid etc., while others are potentially very toxic, such as polymyxin, aminoglycosides, amphotericin B etc., all of which can cause both reversible and irreversible damage when given in excessive dosage. Side effects can also occur at normal dosage, however, particularly when the antibiotic accumulates as a result of inadequate detoxification by the liver or impaired excretion in cardiac and renal insufficiency. Potentially toxic antibiotics should therefore be used with care in patients with *metabolic, hepatic or renal disease, cardiac failure, pregnancy,* and in *premature and full term neonates.* Antibiotics which act at intracellular sites (e. g. rifampicin, co-trimoxazole, and isoniazid) are also often haemato- and hepatotoxic. Certain very toxic antibiotics are unsuitable for systemic use and can only be safely given topically, although even then some absorption can occur and give rise to toxic effects. The recommended dose should not, therefore, be exceeded, and highly concentrated solutions which could irritate or inflame tissues should be avoided. A curare-like respiratory paralysis by neuromuscular blockade can occur after the intraperitoneal or intrapleural instillation of neomycin, gentamicin, tobramycin, streptomycin or amikacin.

Table 31 lists the possible side effects of systemic antibiotic therapy. The **frequency** of their occurrence varies with different antibiotics and can only be estimated on the basis of the scientific evaluation of large series of patients. The danger of side effects, on the other hand, can be roughly assessed in the light of clinical experience, and this affects the indications for giving the drug. The only use nowadays for streptomycin, for example, is in the treatment of tuberculosis. Polymyxin B and colistin should only be used when other anti-pseudomonal agents have failed. Because of the albeit very small risk of severe marrow suppression, chloramphenicol should only be given in serious infections where other agents are less effective. Erythromycin estolate, but not the other forms of erythromycin, frequently causes allergic cholestatic hepatitis and so should not be given for more than 10 days, and should not be repeated. During *pregnancy*, ototoxic and potentially cytotoxic antibiotics and tetracyclines are only justifiable in life-threatening infections. Sulphonamides must not be given to pregnant women in the week before the estimated date of delivery, nor to newborn babies in the first few weeks of life, as this could cause hyperbilirubinaemia with the risk of kernicterus. Potentially toxic antibiotics (see Table 31) should be avoided in the *postnatal period* because of the immaturity of renal function and the risk of accumulation. Sometimes decades may pass before the risks of a drug are fully appreciated. For example, the complete range of serious side effects of nitrofurantoin has only recently been fully recognised.

Allergic side effects occur mainly with the *penicillins* and *cephalosporins* and are commoner when the drug has been given parenterally and topically than

Table 31. Important side effects of antimicrobial agents.

Antimicrobial	Side effects							Contra-indicated (except in life-threatening disease)		
Benzyl penicillin	++				+	±				
Methicillin	++	±	±							×
Flucloxacillin	++				±		1,2			
Ampicillin	⊞⊞				±	+	3			
Azlo-, mezlocillin, piperacillin	++	+			±	+	2			
Cephaloridine	+	±	⊞⊞			±				×
Cefazolin	+	±	±			±	1,2			
Cefoxitin	+	±				±	1			
Cefotaxime	+	±				±	1			
Latamoxef	+	±				±	1,7	?	?	
Cefoperazone	+	±				±	1,3,7	?	?	
Tetracyclines	±	±	±	+		+	2,3	×	×	×
Chloramphenicol	±	⊞			±	+	3	×	×	
Gentamicin	±		+		⊞⊞	±	4	×		×
Amikacin	+		+		⊞⊞	±	4	×	×	×
Polymyxins	+		+		⊞⊞		1			×
Erythromycin	±			+[1]		±	1,2,3			
Clindamycin	±			±		⊞	3			
Fusidic acid	±			+			1,3,5			
Vancomycin	++	±	±		+		1,2	×	×	×
Streptomycin	+	±	±		⊞⊞	±	4,5	×	×	×
Rifampicin	+	+	+	⊞⊞	+		3,5	×	×	
Capreomycin	+	±	±		⊞⊞		4,5	×	×	×
Isoniazid	±	±		+	⊞⊞		5			
Ethambutol	±			±	⊞⊞		5			
Amphotericin B	±	±	⊞⊞	±	±		1,2	×	×	×
Flucytosine		⊞⊞		++			3,5	×	×	×
Griseofulvin	+	±	±	±	±		3	×	×	×
Miconazole	+	±		+	+		3	×		
Sulphonamides	++	±	±	±			3		×	×
Co-trimoxazole	++	+	+	+		+	3	×	×	×
Nitrofurantoin	⊞⊞	±		+	⊞⊞		3,6	×	×	×
Nalidixic acid	±	±		±	+		3,5	×	×	×

[1]) as estolate

Key to side effects: ++ = relatively frequent, + = occasional, ± = rare, ⊞⊞ = principal complication and often the limiting factor in therapy, 1 = local intolerance with i. m. or s. c. injection, 2 = venous irritation with i.v. injection, 3 = gastrointestinal intolerance, 4 = histamine release, 5 = development of secondary resistance, 6 = pneumonia or pulmonary fibrosis, 7 = bleeding tendency, x = contra-indicated orally. The effects are variable and include different types of rash, urticaria, eosinophilia, oedema, fever, conjunctivitis, cutaneous photosensitivity reactions and immunological abnormalities in the blood. They can occur early in treatment when the patient is already allergic, or as a late reaction, usually after 9–11 days. The most serious allergic response is *anaphylactic shock*, which can be fatal. Sulphonamides also cause hypersensitivity reactions of various types such as rashes, Stevens-Johnson syndrome, exfoliative dermatitis and blood dyscrasias. Allergic reactions are not uncommon with *vancomycin, streptomycin* and the *nitrofurans*, but are rarely associated with the systemic use of antibiotics except for contact hypersensitivity after local application.

Biological side effects arise through the *influence of the antibiotic on the normal bacterial flora on the skin or mucous membranes.* They are commonly associated with broad-spectrum antibiotics such as the tetracyclines, but can occasionally complicate treatment with narrow-spectrum antibiotics as well. The overgrowth of fungi such as Candida albicans can produce stomatitis (oral thrush), and occasionally oesophagitis, pneumonia, balanitis, proctitis and vaginitis. The diagnosis of superficial candida infections should be confirmed microscopically.

Superinfection with multiresistant bacteria such as hospital staphylococci, Pseudomonas aeruginosa, Klebsiella pneumoniae or Serratia marcescens can cause stomatitis, pneumonia, wound infections, abscesses and occasionally septicaemia in immunosuppressed or severely debilitated patients.

Antibiotic-induced enterocolitis can follow treatment with ampicillin, tetracyclines, clindamycin and other broad-spectrum agents. It is a life-threatening condition with severe diarrhoea, dehydration, a pseudomembranous fibrinous exudate in the stool and shock, and is caused by the overgrowth of toxin-producing strains of Clostridium difficile. A clinically similar form of severe enterocolitis following antibiotic therapy is due to staphylococcal overgrowth and can be rapidly diagnosed by the demonstration of numerous clusters of gram-positive cocci in a gram-stained smear of the stool. The treatment of both conditions consists of rapid and intensive replacement of fluid and electrolyte losses, together with oral vancomycin. Other, less severe, forms of diarrhoea caused by disturbance of the intestinal flora regress rapidly when the antibiotic is discontinued and are also helped with dietary replacement, e. g. natural (live) yoghurt.

References

BAKER, C. E. (ed.): Physicians Desk Reference. 38th edition. Medical Economics Comp., Oradell, N. Y. 1984.

NEFTEL, K.: Verträglichkeit der hochdosierten Therapie mit Betalactam-Antibiotika – Pathogenese der Nebenwirkungen, insbesondere der Neutropenie. Fortschr. antimikrob. Chemother. *3–1:* 71 (1984).

TAUCHNITZ, CHR., W. HANDRICK: Schädigungen durch Antibiotika und Chemotherapeutika. Z. ges. inn. Med. *38 (24):* 653 (1983).

5. Antibiotic Combinations

An infection caused by a single, known pathogen should in principle be treated with a single antibiotic. Combinations of antibiotics are only occasionally justified. Some *bacteriological reasons* for the use of combinations are

1. to achieve synergy,
2. to extend the spectrum of activity,
3. to delay the development of resistance.

Synergy can develop in different ways, such as

1. blockade of sequential enzymes in the bacterial metabolic pathway (e.g. co-trimoxazole),
2. blockade of enzymes produced by bacteria (e.g. by penicillinase inhibitors such as clavulanic acid),
3. enhancement of the penetration of one antibiotic (e.g. gentamicin) by another (e.g. penicillin),
4. effect on different binding proteins (with β-lactam antibiotics).

Synergy may be expected on theoretical grounds with certain antibiotic combinations, but it must be demonstrated scientifically in vitro *and* in vivo before it can be relied on in treatment. *Antagonism* found in vitro is *not necessarily* present in vivo.

Combined antibiotic therapy is advised for the following **indications:**

A. Bacteriological

1. Benzyl penicillin alone has inadequate bactericidal activity for *enterococcal infections*; high doses of penicillin can even impair bactericidal activity (the Eagle phenomenon). Reliable bactericidal activity can only be obtained by combining the penicillin with an aminoglycoside, and such a combination should always be used when treating enterococcal endocarditis.
2. The combination of an aminoglycoside (e.g. tobramycin) with an acylamino or ureido penicillin (e.g. azlocillin) is superior to treatment with a single agent in severe *Pseudomonas infections*, as shown in vitro, in animals and in patients.

The combination of a cephalosporin with gentamicin is more effective than one or other as a single agent in the treatment of severe *Klebsiella infections* (septicaemia, pneumonia).

3. Combined treatment inhibits or delays the development of resistance in *tuberculosis* and increases the activity of antituberculous drugs on strains of tubercle bacilli with reduced sensitivity.

4. In *severe candida infections*, the combination of amphotericin B and flucytosine achieves better clinical results than one or other alone. Amphotericin B is very toxic and can be given in a lower dose.

5. In *toxoplasmosis*, pyrimethamine and sulphonamides inhibit sequential stages of the metabolic pathway of the parasites. Trimethoprim and sulphamethoxazole have an analogous synergistic activity on a number of potentially pathogenic bacteria.

B. Clinical

1. *Infections associated with foreign bodies or implants* can only be eliminated by a bactericidal antibiotic combination, if at all. Many such infections fail to resolve until the foreign material is removed.

2. *Endocarditis*. Infection is as difficult to eradicate from heart valves as it is from foreign bodies, and a bactericidal combination of antibiotics is almost always necessary.

3. *Severe impairment of host defences* (leukaemia, immunosuppression). Mixed infections often occur, which are difficult to treat. An antibiotic combination with a very broad spectrum (e.g. cefuroxime + azlocillin or gentamicin) is necessary because of the risk of rapid changes in infecting agent.

4. *Mixed infections,* e.g. in peritonitis or bronchiectasis, must be treated by antibiotic combinations if a single agent with activity against all the organisms involved is not available.

5. *Initial chemotherapy* given as a "best guess" in a life-threatening clinical situation before the results of culture are available. A combination of at least two antibiotics is usually required if all the likely infecting organisms are to be included.

Possible errors in combined therapy:

1. *Underdosage* of one or both components because of reliance on presumed synergistic activity.

2. Combination of two antibiotics which are *not fully effective* at the site of infection because of their different pharmacological properties.

3. *Cumulative toxicity* of two antibiotics in combination, each of which has related side effects, e.g. amikacin and gentamicin (both ototoxic).

Fixed combinations of antibiotics in commercial preparations are generally *undesirable* since individual dosage becomes more difficult and there is a risk of underdosage of individual components, as well as of stereotyping the antibiotic therapy. The following combinations are *not,* therefore, recommended: penicillin and streptomycin, penicillin and sulphonamide, penicillin and colistin, tetracycline and oleandomycin. The combinations of ampicillin or carbenicillin or mezlocillin with cloxacillin or oxacillin are seldom indicated as treatment of severe infections; many gram-negative bacilli (including Escherichia coli) are resistant to ampicillin and mezlocillin, and carbenicillin should be replaced by a more active anti-pseudomonal penicillin such as azlocillin or piperacillin. In Britain, the only fixed penicillin combination of this sort is of ampicillin and cloxacillin (Ampiclox, Magnapen).

References

BINT, A. J., D. S. REEVES: Interactions between antibiotics and other drugs. Antibiot. Chemother. *25:* 289 (1978).

KIOSZ, D., A. WATERMANN, C. SIMON: Untersuchungen zur Frage der Keimselektion während einer kombinierten Antibiotikatherapie bei Kindern. ZAC *1:* 85 (1983).

PEREA, E. J., M. C. NOGALES, J. AZNAR: Synergy between cefotaxime, cefsulodin, azlocillin, mezlocillin and aminoglycosides against carbenicillin resistant or sensitive Pseudomonas aeruginosa. J. Antimicrob. Chemother. *6:* 471 (1980).

STILLE, W., R. ELSSER: Kombination von Betalactam-Antibiotika. Zuckschwerdt, Munich 1981.

6. Cost of Treatment

The cost of antibiotic therapy can be considerable. Ideally, the choice of antibiotic should be based only on the best interests of the particular patient, with expense a secondary consideration. Inadequate treatment can in the long term cost more if an acute infection (e. g. sore throat) develops into a chronic process (e. g. endocarditis). On the other hand, once the decision to treat with antibiotics has been taken, there is no virtue in preferring a very expensive drug when a cheaper alternative is equally satisfactory, nor in giving excessive dosage or too long a course. Cost reductions are only acceptable when they are not made at the expense of quality of clinical judgement.

Antibiotics such as ampicillin, phenoxymethyl penicillin, tetracyclines and chloramphenicol have been shown to vary considerably in their bioavailability and incidence of side effects. Where preparations are otherwise similar, the drug with the maximum bioavailability should be chosen.

The price comparisons in Table 32 are made on the basic costs of the preparations as quoted in the British National Formulary (1983). The costs of the dispensed medicines are always greater, particularly when dispensing costs are included. Bulk orders by large hospitals, hospital districts or regional pharmacies can benefit from considerable discounts.

Table 32 a. Relative price bands of oral antibiotics based on the basic cost of each preparation in pounds sterling (British National Formulary, 1983, No. 6).

Antibiotic	Daily dose for adults	Price band*
Phenoxymethyl penicillin (oral)	1.0–2.0 g	A–C
Ampicillin (oral)	2.0 g	C–F
Amoxycillin	1.5 g	E–H
Cloxacillin (oral)	2.0 g	F–H
Flucloxacillin (oral)	1–2 g	E–H
Cephradine (oral)	2.0 g	E–G
Cephalexin	1.5 g	E–H
Cefaclor	1.5–3 g	F–G
Tetracycline (oral)	1–2 g	A–E
Doxycycline (oral)	0.1 g	D–H
Minocycline (oral)	0.2 g	F–H
Erythromycin (oral)	1–2 g	C–G
Clindamycin (oral)	0.6–1.2 g	E–G
Fusidic acid	1.5 g	E–I
Nitrofurantoin	0.2–0.4 g	A–F
Nalidixic acid	4.0 g	D–G
Cinoxacin	1.0 g	I
Short-acting sulphonamide	4.0 g	B–C
Long-acting sulphonamide	0.5 g	C
Poorly absorbable sulphonamide	3.0 g	B
Co-trimoxazole	1.92 g	C–F
Co-trifamole	0.96 g	E
Trimethoprim	0.4 g	C–G
Chloramphenicol	1.5–2 g	C–D
Metronidazole (oral)	1.2 g	D–F
(suppository)	2–3 g	G
Rifampicin	0.6 g	G–I
Isoniazid	0.3 g	A
Ethambutol	15 mg/kg	D–J
Pyrazinamide	20–30 mg/kg	D
Amphotericin B	0.8 g	D–E
Flucytosine	100–200 mg/kg	I
Griseofulvin	0.5–1 g	B–E
Ketoconazole	0.2 g	I
Nystatin	2×10^6 units	D–E

* Price bands in pounds sterling: A 0–0.20, B 0.21–0.50, C 0.51–1.00, D 1.01–1.80, E 1.81–3.00, F 3.01–4.50, G 4.51–6.50, H 6.51–9.00, I 9.01–12.00, J over 12.00.

Table 32 b. Relative price bands of parenteral preparations, based on the basic cost of each preparation in pounds sterling (British National Formulary, 1983, No. 6).

Antibiotic	Daily dose for adults	Price band*
Benzyl penicillin	4–10 megaunits	A–C
Procaine penicillin	0.6–4.8 g	B
Carbenicillin	6–30 g	H
Azlocillin	6–15 g	H–J
Mezlocillin	6–15 g	D–I
Piperacillin	6–16 g	E–I
Cephalothin	4–12 g	D–G
Cefazolin	1–6 g	D–E
Cephradine	2–8 g	C–E
Cefamandole	3–6 g	D–G
Cefuroxime	2.25–4.5 g	C–G
Cefoxitin	3–6 g	F–H
Cefotaxime	2–12 g	E–I
Latamoxef	2–12 g	F–J
Cefsulodin	3–6 g	G–J
Ceftazidime	1–6 g	I–J
Ampicillin + cloxacillin	2–6 g	B–E
Gentamicin	0.24–0.48 g	C–D
Tobramycin	0.24–0.48 g	C–E
Netilmicin	0.24–0.48 g	D–G
Amikacin	0.5–1.0 g	I
Injectable tetracycline	0.5 g	D–E
Vancomycin i. v.	2 g	J

* Price bands in pounds sterling: A 0–0.20, B 0.21–0.50, C 0.51–1.00, D 1.01–1.80, E 1.81–3.00, F 3.01–4.50, G 4.51–6.50, H 6.51–9.00, I 9.01–12.00, J over 12.00.

7. Laboratory Control

Antibiotic activity can be readily tested *in vitro*. The **minimal inhibitory concentration (MIC)** of an antibiotic is the most important index of its activity and is defined as that concentration which completely inhibits bacterial growth after 18–24 h; it is influenced by the size of the bacterial inoculum, the culture medium and the period of incubation. Partial inhibition is ignored, although in practice the end-point of titration may have to be taken as 99% inhibition of growth and the few surviving colonies disregarded. The MIC can be determined by serial doubling dilution in liquid media in tubes or on microtitre plates, or by incorporation of antibiotic solution at different concentrations into a series of agar plates. These different methods do not produce identical results and the MIC is a relatively imprecise measurement; an MIC of 5 mg/l lies in reality between 2.5 and 5 mg/l. To improve comparability between studies, the British Society for Antimicrobial

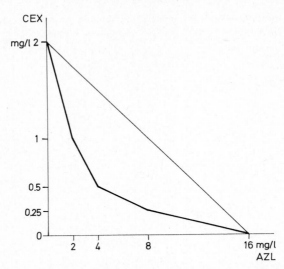

Fig. 32. Isobologram showing the minimal inhibitory concentrations of cefoxitin (CEX) and azlocillin (AZL) when combined in vitro at various concentrations against a strain of Klebsiella pneumoniae.

Chemotherapy now recommends that dilution series are based on 1 mg/l instead of 100 mg/l; dilutions greater than 1 are then always whole numbers (2, 4, 8, 16, 32, 64, 128 etc.). Since bacterial strains consist of a population with little variation in sensitivity, tests in liquid media determine the MIC of the most resistant cells.

Since MIC measurements are fairly laborious, antibiotic sensitivities are generally determined in clinical laboratories by **disc diffusion**, in which the antibiotic diffuses radially into a solid culture medium from a paper disc which contains a known quantity. Sensitive strains form a zone of inhibition of bacterial growth around the disc. These tests may be performed with discs containing a small or large antibiotic concentration and the development of a zone of inhibition is, with certain qualifications, the sign of sensitivity. *High-content discs* are used in the USA and in some European countries to perform the test under the standardised conditions described by ERICSSON and SHERRIS or by KIRBY and BAUER. Zones of inhibition smaller than a certain size indicate resistance. The *Kirby-Bauer test* is now the official method of the Food and Drug Administration in the USA. It requires the definition of a threshold concentration, the *»break point«*, and is performed under strictly defined conditions.

The disc diffusion test is very dependent on the bacterial inoculum, the medium, the thickness of the agar layer, the stability of the antibiotic and the rate at which it diffuses through the medium. A number of these variables can be eliminated by including a control organism of known sensitivity on the same test plate. Correlation between the MIC and the disc test is relatively poor; zones of 15–25 mm may be formed when the MIC is 2 mg/l. The character of the zone edge is also important; for organisms such as Staphylococcus aureus it is normally »soft«, that is, clearly defined but bounded by very small colonies, which enlarge to normal size a little further away from the centre of the disc. β-Lactamase-producing strains, however, can give apparently large zones of inhibition of growth with penicillins but have a »hard«, heaped-up edge which is characteristic of exogenous β-lactamase production and hence of penicillin resistance.

It is not wise, therefore, to draw too many conclusions from the results of disc diffusion, although the disc test remains the simplest, cheapest, most practicable and commonest method of assessing antibiotic sensitivity in clinical laboratories. The main purpose of this test is to detect resistant strains rapidly for clinical reasons, and not to compare different antibiotics scientifically.

Disc testing only shows the **effect of a combination of two antibiotics** on a bacterial strain when both components diffuse in a similar way, as do trimethoprim and sulphamethoxazole (co-trimoxazole). Discs containing more than one antibiotic are *not* generally useful. Fairly complex tests are needed to demonstrate antibiotic interactions in combination, such as *chessboard titration*, from which an isobologram (Fig. 32) can be derived (see above). If the activity of one component is potentiated by the other (synergy), the curve lies below a straight line joining the two upper concentrations used. It lies above this line if there is *antagonism*, and coincides with it when the effect is purely additive, or indifferent. Alternatively, the MIC of antibiotic A can be determined by *serial tube dilution* in the presence of one or more previously established subinhibitory concentrations of antibiotic B. Where the interactions of more than two combinations are to be tested on the same occasion, it is generally sufficient to use only a single concentration of each and to test each alone, and in every possible combination, arranged as a half chess-board. The disadvantages of this method are that only a single concentration of each drug is used and also that only a minute proportion of the original inoculum is subcultivated; both of these drawbacks can be overcome by a simple diffusion method, the *cellophane transfer technique* (tambour test, WATERWORTH, 1978). An alternative technique is the *β-lactamase method* of ANAND and PAULL (1976) in which two antibiotics are pre-diffused on an agar plate from blotting paper strips placed at right angles, following which the plate is flooded with a dilution of the test culture. After incubation for 6 hours, the plate is sprayed with β-lactamase and re-incubated. A zone of inhibition at the site of junction of the two strips indicates synergy and combined bactericidal activity, and this method is useful for assessing the clinical usefulness of penicillin-aminoglycoside combinations against streptococci.

Antibiotic assays: Antibiotic concentrations can be measured relatively easily in serum and other body fluids. Traditional methods have been microbiological and are based on the diffusion of various known and unknown concentrations of the antibiotic to be measured from discs or wells in a carefully poured, large, even agar plate. Plates with flat glass bases which are large enough to accomodate 30–60 standard and test wells in random order are best for this purpose. They are carefully poured on a level base with a known volume of agar which has either been pre-seeded with an indicator organism such as Bacillus subtilis, Sarcina lutea or Staphylococcus epidermidis, or is flooded when set and dry with a surface inoculum of a known concentration of a gram-negative indicator strain such as Klebsiella sp, Escherichia coli or Pseudomonas. Round wells of even diameter are then punched according to a standard pattern, carefully filled with a known volume of standard or unknown solution for assay, and the plate incubated overnight. The zones of inhibition are measured precisely with Vernier callipers or a magnifying zone reader, a standard curve on semi-logarithmic paper plotted of antibiotic concentration against zone diameter (linear) and the values of the unknown samples are read from this curve. Because the zone of inhibition is proportional to the logarithm of the concentration, this curve becomes a straight line over much of its range.

The *sensitivity, precision* and *reproducibility* of microbiological assays are generally good provided great care is taken to standardise all points of technical detail and to obtain strictly reproducible conditions. Some indicator organisms (e.g. Klebsiella) grow rapidly and, if incubated at 40° C provide a result within 4–5 hours. Prediffusion of the antibiotic for one hour before seeding also allows more rapid results, which are of clinical importance since they are most useful if known before the patient's next dose of antibiotic is due. Microbiological assays are the ultimate measurement of the antimicrobial activity of the serum or fluid in question, and their sensitivity is limited by the MIC of the test strain used.

Mixtures of antibiotics in the test fluid can cause difficulty, and are increasingly common in patients with severe illness receiving combined antibiotic therapy. β-Lactams can be removed by incorporating a broad-spectrum β-lactamase in the plate when poured; alternatively a multi-resistant indicator strain (e.g. Klebsiella) can be selected which is resistant to all components of the mixture except that to be assayed. Aminoglycosides can be absorbed from serum with chromatography paper. Some antibiotics, such as sulphonamides, co-trimoxazole and chloramphenicol, for which antagonists may be present in the medium, are not suitable for microbiological assay; moreover some antibiotic powders for clinical injection contain additives and some (e.g. chloramphenicol sodium succinate) are antibacterially inactive until hydrolysed in the body. The only suitable standard material therefore is pure powder of stated potency and provided by the manufacturer for assay purposes.

New methods: A number of new and rapid methods of varying degrees of technical sophistication and expense are now available and are already replacing microbiological assays for clinical purposes in many laboratories. These include the *urease method* for gentamicin, based on the measurement of the increase in pH produced by Proteus mirabilis in a medium containing urea, *enzymic methods*, measuring the uptake of radio-labelled substrates by aminoglycoside-inactivating enyzmes, *fluorescence quenching techniques, chromatography* (high pressure – high performance liquid chromatography), *chemical methods* and *immunoassays*. All have advantages and disadvantages. The urease method is very consumptive of technician time; enzymic methods often require liquid scintillation counters and hazardous radioactive materials, and HPLC, while assaying metabolites as well as active substance on microsamples with a high degree of precision, is expensive in equipment and requires specialist expertise.

Immunoassays are very specific and are now available as commercial kits. They are precise, simple and very rapid to perform, and require only minute samples, an important consideration in specialities such as neonatology. They are expensive, however, and radioimmunoassays have the disadvantage of requiring facilities for the handling and disposal of radio-isotopes. Enzyme immunoassays such as EMIT® (Syva) overcome the disadvantages of RIA and are now finding increasing application in clinical microbiological laboratories.

References

ANAND, C. M., A. PAULL: A modified technique for the detection of antibiotic synergism. J. clin. Path. *29:* 1130–1131 (1976).
ERICSSON, H. M., J. C. SHERRIS: Antibiotic sensitivity testing; report of an international collaborative study. Acta path. microbiol. scand., Section B, *Suppl. 217:1* (1971).
Federal Register 1972, *37:* 20525.
McCABE W. R., M. FINLAND: Contemporary Standards for Antimicrobial Usage. Futura, New York 1977.
REEVES, D. S., I. PHILLIPS, J. D. WILLIAMS, R. WISE: Laboratory Methods in Antimicrobial Chemotherapy. Churchill-Livingstone, Edinburgh 1978.
SMITH, J. A., J. H. NGUI-YEN, J. FOTHERGILL: Rapid method for determining antimicrobial susceptibility of Haemophilus influenzae. J. clin. Microbiol. *16:* 832 (1982).

STILLE, W.: The prognostic value of the antibiogram. Infection *11:* 66 (1983).

ULLMANN, U.: Correlation of minimum inhibitory concentration and β-lactamase activity. Infection *5:* 261 (1977).

STOKES, E. J., G. L. RIDGWAY: Clinical Bacteriology, 5th edition, p. 125. Arnold, London 1980.

WATERWORTH, P. M.: In: Laboratory Methods in Chemotherapy, p. 4. Churchill-Livingstone, Edinburgh, 1978.

WATT, P. J.: The Control of Chemotherapy. Churchill-Livingstone, Edinburgh, 1970.

D. Treatment of Infections and Infectious Diseases

1. Infections with Facultative Pathogenic Bacteria

Most antibiotics are used for the treatment of infections with facultative pathogens. These organisms occur naturally as part of the normal commensal flora at some sites in the body and as colonising flora at others. It is only when, under abnormal conditions, they obtain access to organs or tissues where they are not normally found that true infection arises. The rules for treatment of these infections differ from those applied to classical infectious diseases. For example, clinically similar infections of an organ such as the gall-bladder or urinary bladder can be caused by a number of different bacteria.

About one third of all infections of this type are caused by a mixture of species. Infections of some organs (e. g. pyelonephritis) are associated with a typical range of causative organisms. For example, Escherichia coli is the principle pathogen in acute pyelonephritis and is found more frequently than Proteus mirabilis or enterococci; pyelonephritis is very seldom caused by staphylococci.

Most infections are endogenous, that is, caused by invasion of organisms from the patient's own bacterial flora. They are much less commonly due to pathogens from the inanimate environment. Chains of infection are exceptional, although there is a considerable exchange of bacteria from the patient's body flora. The selection pressure exerted by certain antibiotics plays an important part in infections with facultative pathogens. Individual species can vary in their pathogenicity and certain strains within a single species can be particularly virulent. Staphylococci, members of the Enterobacteriaceae and Pseudomonas can have a variable antibiotic sensitivity pattern. Wherever possible, therefore, treatment should be based on laboratory reporting of appropriate antibiotic sensitivities.

a) Infections Caused by Enterobacteriaceae

Escherichia coli, Klebsiella, Enterobacter and *Proteus* are normally present in the human intestine. If they gain access to other organs, they can cause serious diseases such as pyelonephritis, cholecystitis or cholangitis, wound infections, septicaemia and meningitis. Such infections are therefore generally *endogenous*, that is, infection by the body's own flora of an organ which is functionally impaired by, for example, congenital abnormality, stones, or impaired defence mechanisms. Apparatus such as inhalers, humidifiers, and anaesthetic equipment can be a

Table 33. Differences in the *in vitro* activity of β-lactam antibiotics against various gram-negative bacilli (author's series of isolates from patients in the University Children's Hospital, Kiel, W. Germany). $MIC_{50\%}$ = minimal inhibitory concentration in 50% of strains. n = number of strains.

Anti-biotic	$MIC_{50\%}$ (mg/l) in						
	Esch. coli (n = 106)	Klebs. pneumoniae (n = 99)	Enterob. aerogenes (n = 108)	Prot. vulgaris (n = 86)	Citrob. freundii (n = 76)	Serr. marcescens (n = 92)	Pseudomonas aerug. (n = 119)
Ampicillin	3.1	100	>200	25	6.2	>200	>200
Mezlocillin	1.6	6.2	3.1	0.8	3.1	3.1	50
Azlocillin	6.2	100	25	3.1	6.2	>200	12.5
Piperacillin	1.6	6.2	1.6	0.4	1.6	1.6	6.2
Cephalothin	3.1	6.2	>200	>200	50	>200	>200
Cefuroxime	3.1	3.1	12.5	200	12.5	50	>200
Cefoxitin	3.1	3.1	50	6.2	50	12.5	>200
Cefotiam	0.1	0.2	0.4	25	50	100	200
Cefotaxime	0.05	0.05	0.2	<0.05	0.4	0.2	25
Ceftriaxone	0.02	<0.05	0.2	<0.05	0.4	0.2	25
Ceftizoxime	0.02	0.02	0.2	0.05	0.4	0.4	50
Latamoxef	0.1	0.1	0.1	<0.02	0.1	0.2	25
Cefoperazone	0.1	0.2	0.2	<0.8	0.8	0.4	6.2
Ceftazidime	0.1	0.1	0.2	<0.05	0.4	0.2	1.6

source of *exogenous* infection. A knowledge of likely pathogenic species and their antibiotic sensitivity is necessary for effective therapy, since bacteria acquired in this way from a hospital environment vary considerably in their sensitivity to antibiotics, and many are multiresistant.

In order to assess the differences in antibiotic sensitivity pattern of individual bacterial species better, Tables 33 and 34 summarise the minimal inhibitory concentrations found in 50% and 90% of a series of hospital isolates from patients in the University Children's Hospital, Kiel, W. Germany. The results are presented for three groups of antibiotics. The first group is composed of ampicillin and three acylamino (ureido) penicillins (mezlocillin, azlocillin and piperacillin). The second group comprises cephalothin, cefuroxime, cefoxitin and cefotiam, while the third group contains the newest cephalosporins (cefotaxime, ceftriaxone, ceftizoxime, latamoxef, cefoperazone and ceftazidime).

In the **ampicillin group**, mezlocillin and piperacillin are more effective on the basis of both MIC 50% and 90% against Escherichia coli than ampicillin and

Table 34. Differences of *in vitro* activity of various β-lactam antibiotics against gram-negative rods (author's series of isolates from patients in the University Children's Hospital, Kiel, W. Germany). $MIC_{90\%}$ = minimal inhibitory concentration in 90% of strains. n = number of strains.

Antibiotic	$MIC_{90\%}$ (mg/l) in						
	Esch. coli (n = 106)	Klebs. pneu- moniae (n = 99)	Enterob. aero- genes (n = 108)	Prot. vul- garis (n = 86)	Citrob. freundii (n = 76)	Serr. mar- cescens (n = 92)	Pseu- dom. aerug. (n = 119)
Ampicillin	200	>200	>200	50	>200	>200	>200
Mezlocillin	50	>200	12.5	3.1	100	12.5	200
Azlocillin	200	>200	>200	50	>200	>200	100
Piperacillin	50	200	6.2	0.8	50	12.5	12.5
Cephalothin	6.2	50	>200	>200	>200	>200	>200
Cefuroxime	3.1	6.2	50	>200	100	100	>200
Cefoxitin	3.1	6.2	200	12.5	200	25	>200
Cefotiam	0.4	0.4	1.6	50	>200	>200	>200
Cefotaxime	0.1	0.1	0.8	0.05	25	12.5	100
Ceftriaxone	0.1	0.1	0.8	0.05	25	25	100
Ceftizoxime	0.1	0.05	0.8	0.1	100	25	200
Latamoxef	0.1	0.5	0.2	0.2	3.1	12.5	50
Cefoperazone	1.6	6.2	0.8	1.6	12.5	12.5	12.5
Ceftazidime	0.2	0.4	0.4	0.1	25	12.5	6.2

azlocillin. The same is true with Klebsiella pneumoniae and Enterobacter aerogenes. Ampicillin is not generally active against Proteus vulgaris, and mezlocillin and piperacillin are more active than azlocillin. Citrobacter freundii is generally more sensitive to piperacillin than to the other acylamino penicillins. Some strains of Serratia marcescens are susceptible to piperacillin and mezlocillin but not azlocillin and ampicillin.

There are no major differences against Escherichia coli in the **cephalothin group**, apart from the greater effect of cefotiam. Cefuroxime and cefoxitin have similar activity against Klebsiella pneumoniae, while cephalothin is frequently ineffective. Cephalothin and cefoxitin are not usually effective against Enterobacter aerogenes; cefuroxime has some activity, and cefotiam is the best. Cefoxitin is superior to the other three agents against Proteus vulgaris. Citrobacter freundii is generally more sensitive to cefuroxime, while Serratia marcescens is more frequently inhibited by cefoxitin. Pseudomonas is always resistant to cephalothin, cefuroxime, cefoxitin and cefotiam.

In the **cefotaxime group**, ceftriaxone and ceftizoxime have the greatest activity against Escherichia coli. The minimal inhibitory concentrations of the other agents in this group are considerably lower than in the ampicillin and cephalothin group. All members of this group have similar activity against Klebsiella pneumoniae. At 6.2 mg/l, however, the $MIC_{90\%}$ of cefoperazone is much higher than that of the other drugs. Enterobacter aerogenes is inhibited by all drugs of the cefotaxime group in concentrations under 1 mg/l. Proteus vulgaris is most sensitive to cefotaxime, ceftriaxone and ceftazidime and less so to latamoxef and cefoperazone. The $MIC_{50\%}$ for all drugs of this group against Citrobacter freundii and Serratia marcescens is low, while the $MIC_{90\%}$ varies between 12.5 and 25 mg/l (but is 100 mg/l for ceftizoxime against Citrobacter). Only latamoxef has a lower $MIC_{90\%}$ against Citrobacter freundii. Pseudomonas aeruginosa is inhibited best by ceftazidime, followed by cefoperazone. Cefotaxime, ceftriaxone and latamoxef are less active against Pseudomonas, and ceftizoxime is inactive. These studies suggest that only a few species show therapeutically important differences in sensitivity, namely Pseudomonas, Serratia marcescens and Citrobacter freundii. Cefotaxime, ceftriaxone and cefoperazone are reported to be frequently ineffective against Enterobacter cloacae, while latamoxef is more active.

A **comparison of the activity** of these three groups shows members of the cefotaxime group to be the most active against most bacterial species. Since even these new agents have important gaps in their spectrum, however, life-threatening infections where the causative organisms are unknown should always be treated by a combination of antibiotics, to include an agent with reliable activity against Pseudomonas and/or anaerobes.

As seen in Table 33, penicillin treatment of **Escherichia coli infections** must be based on sensitivity testing because no penicillin is predictably effective. About 30–40% of hospital strains of Escherichia coli produce β-lactamase and so are resistant to ampicillin, and often to mezlocillin and piperacillin also. As with the staphylococci, a separation has developed between sensitive and multi-resistant strains. The newer aminoglycosides and β-lactamase-stable cephalosporins, on the other hand, are almost always active against Escherichia coli. The frequency of co-trimaxole-resistant strains has increased recently.

Klebsiella pneumoniae, Enterobacter aerogenes and **Enterobacter cloacae** are quite resistant to a number of antibiotics. Because they produce β-lactamase, they are usually resistant to all penicillins (except occasionally mezlocillin and piperacillin). Klebsiellae are mostly sensitive to the older parenteral cephalosporins. Enterobacter aerogenes is almost always inhibited by agents in the cefotaxime group. Enterobacter cloacae, however, is usually resistant to penicillins and cephalosporins. In recent years, Enterobacter cloacae has become an important organism in the hospital environment. These bacteria are often selected by treatment with newer cephalosporins such as cefoxitin or cefotaxime. Although frequently isolated, they rarely cause serious infections. Enterobacter cloacae is generally resistant to most β-lactams but sensitive to other antibiotics such as tetracycline, co-trimoxazole and aminoglycosides. The rate of resistance of members of the Klebsiella/Enterobacter group to aminoglycosides is low.

Proteus species are frequently found in urinary infections and also as secondary pathogens in the presence of chronic necrotic lesions such as decubitus ulcers and necrotising tumours. Proteus mirabilis (indole-negative) is commoner in pyelonephritis. Indole-positive species of Proteus (e.g. Proteus vulgaris) predominate in other infections. Most strains of Proteus mirabilis are sensitive to ampicillin and cephalothin. Ampicillin and the older parenteral cephalosporins are ineffective against indole-positive strains of Proteus, while cefotaxime, cefoxitin and amikacin are almost always active. Co-trimoxazole inhibits almost all strains of Proteus mirabilis, as well as most indole-positive strains, but not Providencia. Antibiotic sensitivity testing is important in Proteus infections because resistance can never be completely predicted. Of the urinary disinfectants nalidixic acid is frequently effective but nitrofurantoin rarely so, because it is inactive at the alkaline pH which results from the production of ammonia by the cleavage of urea by urease elaborated by Proteus spp.

Less common members of the Enterobacteriaceae: Multiresistant "coliforms" such as Hafnia, Erwinia, Citrobacter etc. are occasionally encountered; their sensitivity to antibiotics varies considerably. Citrobacters are often selected by cefoxitin treatment; their pathogenicity is low.

Reference

Paul-Ehrlich-Gesellschaft: Wirksamkeit von Chemotherapeutika. Z. antimikrob. Chemother. *1:* 113 (1983).

b) Serratia Infections

Occurrence and relevance: Serratia marcescens is an opportunistic bacterium which is normally non-pathogenic but can cause infection in patients with lowered resistance. Some strains of Serratia marcescens form a red pigment and are easily recognised; most significant clinical isolates are non-pigmented, however. Serratia marcescens is sometimes found in the intestinal flora of healthy patients, on the perineal skin and in the urethra. Urinary catheterisation, particularly when long-term, can allow Serratia to invade the bladder and cause severe infections which are difficult to treat. Such infections are particularly common in patients with a paraplegic bladder. Serratia marcescens bacteraemia is frequently caused by infection of a venous catheter (see Serratia septicaemia, p. 365). Necrotising pneumonia with Serratia marcescens is only found in patients with severe primary disease (chronic underlying lung or renal disease) and after treatment with corticosteroids or immunosuppressants. The bacteria can also enter the lungs during inhalation treatment and cause infection.

Resistance and antibiotic therapy: Serratia marcescens is resistant to most antibiotics and chemotherapeutic agents. Some strains are inhibited by co-trimoxazole, piperacillin and mezlocillin. Cefoxitin, cefotaxime, ceftazidime and amikacin are generally effective. In recent years, the percentage of gentamicin-resistant strains has increased. A single antibiotic is likely to be effective against fully sensitive strains, but combinations are usually necessary for more resistant isolates. Strains formerly called Enterobacter liquefaciens are now classified as Serratia and are also resistant to most antibiotics.

References

DASCHNER, F., Ch. SENSKA-EURINGER: Kontaminierte Infusionen als Ursache nosokomialer Serratia-marcescens-Sepsis bei Kindern. Dtsch. med. Wschr. *100:* 2324 (1975).

MEYER, R. D., R. P. LEWIS, J. HATTER, M. WHITE: Gentamicin-resistant Pseudomonas aeruginosa and Serratia marcescens in a general hospital. Lancet *1:* 580 (1976).

VERBIST, L., J. SPAEPEN, J. VANDEPITTE: In vitro sensitivity of hospital strains of Serratia marcescens to chemotherapeutic agents (with special reference to amikacin). Chemotherapy *22:* 43 (1975).

c) Pseudomonas Infections

Occurrence and relevance: Pseudomonas aeruginosa is found in wound and urinary infections and less commonly in pneumonia, septicaemia, skin diseases, ophthalmic and foreign body infections. These bacteria are important causes of infection because of their resistance to many antibiotics' ability to produce toxin and transmissibility. Control of the spread of Pseudomonas is a problem in many hospitals. Pseudomonas aeruginosa has been a major cause of secondary bacterial infection in patients with bone-marrow suppression for many years, possibly selected by the older cephalosporins. Pseudomonas is very common in the hospital environment, resistant to many disinfectants, and easily spread, particularly in surgical wards. Common reservoirs where the organism may be found are sinks, wash-basins, waste-bins, urinals and catheters. 10–30% of patients excrete Pseudomonas aeruginosa in the faeces, and small numbers have been found in hospital food, especially salads. Their spread in hospital should therefore be controlled by appropriate hygienic measures (asepsis, antisepsis, careful hand-washing, disinfection or sterilisation of apparatus, isolation etc.). Chemo-prophylaxis with antibiotics is of no value. Infections should be treated with an antibiotic appropriate to the site of infection and the sensitivity pattern.

Resistance and antibiotic therapy: The aminoglycosides are bactericidal and tobramycin is generally slightly more active than gentamicin. Both have a resistance rate of 0–8%. Amikacin, and to a lesser extent netilmicin, are active against gentamicin-resistant strains of Pseudomonas. Infections with Pseudomonas can be difficult to treat. Aminoglycosides are excreted by the kidneys and a single agent is often effective in urinary infection, but a combination of, for example, azlocillin and tobramycin should be used for systemic and tissue infections. Topical treatment (e. g. intrathecal gentamicin or tobramycin for Pseudomonas meningitis) can be useful for sites where systemic aminoglycosides penetrate poorly. Carbenicillin should be replaced by azlocillin or piperacillin, which are 4–8 times as effective and can be given in smaller doses. New cephalosporins with activity against Pseudomonas have extended the range of available treatment (Table 35), and cefsulodin is particularly useful for cases of

Table 35. Anti-pseudomonas activity of 11 β-lactam antibiotics against 119 clinical isolates from the University Children's Hospital Kiel. $MIC_{50\%}$ and $MIC_{90\%}$ = minimum inhibitory concentration (mg/l) of 50% and 90% of tested strains.

Antibiotic	Pseudomonas aeruginosa	
	$MIC_{50\%}$	$MIC_{90\%}$
Carbenicillin	100	>200
Mezlocillin	50	200
Ticarcillin	25	100
Ceftriaxone	25	100
Latamoxef	25	50
Cefotaxime	12.5	100
Azlocillin	12.5	100
Cefoperazone	6.2	12.5
Piperacillin	6.2	12.5
Cefsulodin	3,1	6.2
Ceftazidime	1.6	6.2

azlocillin resistance or allergy to penicillins. Ceftazidime is the only representative of the newer cephalosporins (except cefsulodin) so far to have strong activity against Pseudomonas; other members of that group are not sufficiently active for severe infections.

Polymyxins (colistin and polymyxin B) have poor tissue diffusion and unreliable activity, and should only be used locally. 5–10% of isolates are polymyxin resistant. The combination of polymyxins with gentamicin is antagonistic. Pseudomonas is generally resistant to chloramphenicol and tetracyclines. Topical treatment may be given with mafenide (see p. 194), povidone iodine (see p. 223), silver compounds (see p. 388), and occasionally neomycin or framycetin. Other pseudomonads (Ps. cepacia, Ps. maltophilia, Ps. putida, and Ps. fluorescens) have recently been reported as causing a number of wound infections, septicaemias and urinary infections. Some of these species are resistant to many antibiotics, particularly Ps. cepacia.

References

N. N.: Pseudomonas septicaemia (Pseudomonas-Septikaemie) Brit. med. J. *280:* 1240 (1980).

KAYSER, F. H.: Pseudomonaswirksame Betalactam-Antibiotika. Fortschr. antimikrob. Chemother. *3–1* 1–6 (1984).

SLACK, M. P. E.: Antipseudomonal β-lactams. J. Antimicrob. Chemother. *8:* 165–170 (1981).

YOUNG, V. M.: Pseudomonas aeruginosa: Ecological Aspects and Patient Colonization. Raven Press, New York 1977.

d) Staphylococcal Infections

Occurrence and importance: Severe infections with **Staphylococcus aureus** are commoner in hospital patients with impaired resistance than in outpatients. Infants and the elderly are at particular risk. Staphylococci are said to cause about 40% of cases of pneumonia, 20–40% of septicaemias and 30–90% of wound infections, although these rates vary with different hospitals and patient groups.

Resistance: While only 30–50% of staphylococci acquired in the community are resistant to benzyl penicillin and other non-penicillinase-stable penicillins, the frequency of resistance in hospital isolates is 60–80% (see Table 36a).

There are penicillin-tolerant staphylococci against which this antibiotic is bacteriostatic only, even at high concentration. Tolerant strains may appear sensitive *in vitro,* but the results of treatment are usually unsatisfactory. In such cases, rifampicin or gentamicin are usually effective. Penicillin-tolerant staphylococci are rare at present in Europe.

Table 36a. Resistance of Staphylococcus aureus to various antibiotics.

Antibiotic	Frequency of resistance of Staphylococcus aureus (in %)
Benzyl penicillin	(50–) 60–75 (–80)
Penicillinase-stable penicillins	0–2 (–15)
Cefazolin	0–2 (–15)
Erythromycin	5–15 (–30)
Lincomycin	1–5 (–12)
Chloramphenicol	(7–) 10–20 (–50)
Tetracycline	35–45 (–67)
Neomycin	10–20 (–30)
Gentamicin	0–10 (–30)
Vancomycin	0
Fusidic acid	0–2

The proportion of staphylococcal isolates resistant to penicillinase-stable penicillins (e.g. methicillin) and cephalosporins is small. Isolation with undue frequency from hospital patients suggests a special epidemiological situation such as the spread of a particular phage-type of staphylococcus. Differences in the antistaphylococcal activity of new cephalosporins are shown in Table 33b.

Even methicillin-resistant strains can be sensitive *in vitro* to other β-lactam antibiotics, although β-lactams are not generally advised in such cases. Methicillin-resistant staphylococci are generally sensitive to fusidic acid and vancomycin, and can often be treated with fosfomycin or rifampicin as well.

Table 36b. Activity of new cephalosporins against Staphylococcus aureus in comparison with cephalothin. GM = geometric mean minimal inhibitory concentrations (mg/l), $MIC_{50\%}$ and $MIC_{90\%}$ = minimal inhibitory concentrations (mg/l) against 50% and 90% of tested strains.

Antibiotic	GM	$MIC_{50\%}$	$MIC_{90\%}$
Cephalothin	0.2	0.1	0.4
Cefamandole	0.2	0.2	0.8
Cefotiam	1.4	0.4	0.8
Cefoxitin	1.6	1.6	3.1
Cefotaxime	2.0	1.6	3.1
Ceftizoxime	4.0	1.6	3.1
Ceftriaxone	4.1	3.1	6.3
Cefoperazone	3.8	3.1	6.2
Ceftazidime	6.8	4.0	8.0
Latamoxef	10.0	8.0	16.0

The rate of resistance varies between 5 and 30% with erythromycin and between 1 and 12% with lincomycin. Staphylococci resistant to vancomycin have not so far been found. Staphylococci resistant to fusidic acid are relatively rare. On the other hand, 7–50% are resistant to chloramphenicol, 35–67% to tetracycline, and 10–30% now to neomycin and gentamicin in some hospitals.

Staphylococcus epidermidis (albus) is normally found on the skin and mucous membranes, and is of low pathogenicity. Its isolation is often indicative of contamination rather than genuine infection. However, infections of intravenous vein catheters, implanted foreign bodies, Spitz-Holter valves, the urinary tract and abnormal heart valves do occur, and some strains are resistant to many antibiotics, including methicillin.

Unlike methicillin-resistant strains of Staphylococcus aureus, those of Staphylococcus epidermidis are mostly sensitive to cephalosporins. Staphylococcus saprophyticus, which occurs in acute urinary infections in young, sexually active women, is generally sensitive to penicillin.

Choice of antibiotic: Because of their good tolerance and low resistance rate, penicillinase-stable penicillins have been the drugs of choice. Oral flucloxacillin (1–2 g a day) can be given for mild staphylococcal infections, and parenteral flucloxacillin (5–10 g a day) or a cephalosporin for severe infections. Equally effective alternatives are oral cephalexin or clindamycin. Treatment should not be stopped too early because of the risk of abscess formation or relapse; 4–6 weeks of therapy may be necessary in severe infections. If the isolates are sensitive to benzyl penicillin, this agent is preferred because of its greater antibacterial activity. Patients allergic to penicillin should receive erythromycin or a cephalosporin. Certain second-line antibiotics such as fusidic acid, which is well tolerated, can be used in skin and bone infections but secondary resistance can develop rapidly when fusidic acid is used as a single agent. Vancomycin is recommended in cases of resistance or allergy to cephalosporins, but should not be given to patients with poor renal function because of the risk of ototoxicity. Broad-spectrum antibiotics such as tetracycline, ampicillin, azlocillin, mezlocillin and co-trimoxazole are not suitable for staphylococcal infections.

Reference

HAMMOND, G. W., H. G. STIVER: Combination antibiotic therapy in an outbreak of prosthetic endocarditis caused by Staphylococcus epidermidis. Canad. med. Ass. J. *118:* 524 (1978).

e) Streptococcal and Pneumococcal Infections

Group A streptococcal infections: Streptococcus pyogenes, that is, β-haemolytic streptococci of Lancefield Group A, are still of considerable importance as the cause of streptococcal sore throat, erysipelas and impetigo, although streptococci of groups B, C and G are found in this role also. Wound infections and puerperal sepsis with group A streptococci are rare nowadays, though they can be fulminant. Glomerulonephritis and rheumatic fever can both arise as complications of group A streptococcal infection.

Group A streptococcal infections should always be treated with antibiotics preferably with *penicillin*. Sore throat, erysipelas, impetigo and mild wound infections respond well to oral phenoxymethyl penicillin. Streptococcal septicaemia and severe wound infections should be treated with high doses of intravenous benzyl penicillin, which is still more active than any other penicillin or cephalosporin against group A streptococci; penicillin resistance has not yet been reported. Alternative antibiotics are only necessary in patients with penicillin allergy, when erythromycin or sometimes cephalosporins should be considered. Co-trimoxazole does not eradicate streptococci satisfactorily from tissue infection.

Viridans streptococci, which typically cause subacute bacterial endocarditis, and anaerobic streptococci (peptostreptococci), which cause infections of the uterine adnexae, diverticulitis, cerebral abscess and dental sepsis, are almost always sensitive to penicillin. Strains with reduced sensitivity (MIC 1 mg/l instead of 0.01 mg/l) are only very occasionally found in subacute bacterial endocarditis.

Pneumococci have until now been very sensitive to benzyl penicillin. Multiresistant strains occurred for the first time in epidemic fashion in South Africa in 1977 and were resistant to penicillin, cephalosporins, lincomycin, erythromycin, chloramphenicol and tetracycline. Penicillin-resistant pneumococci have recently also been reported from Mexico, Australia, the USA and Great Britain, and may well become important in the future. Between 2.5 and 50% of strains of streptococci (generally about 10%) and 4–20% of pneumococci are resistant to tetracycline. Erythromycin- and lincomycin-resistant strains occur only occasionally.

Group B streptococci (Streptococcus agalactiae) are an important cause of neonatal septicaemia and meningitis. The infection occurs before birth due to premature rupture of the membranes, or from the birth canal during birth, and leads to severe septicaemia of either early or late onset which should be treated urgently with benzyl penicillin. The early onset type appears within 24 hours of birth, and the late form often after 2–4 weeks. Group B streptococci are carried in the vagina of a proportion of healthy women and can occasionally cause urinary infection.

An increasing number of cases are being reported of group B streptococci causing septicaemia and other infections in immunocompromised and normal adults.

The **enterococci** (Streptococcus faecalis and other group D streptococci) are exceptional among streptococci in not being inhibited by moderate doses of benzyl penicillin. Enterococci are, however, always sensitive to ampicillin, mezlocillin and piperacillin but not, or only very slightly, to cephalosporins. The new cephalosporins such as cefoxitin, cefotaxime and ceftazidime are not active against enterococci which are frequently selected by their use. The most active β-lactam against enterococci is mezlocillin. The bactericidal activity of all penicillins is weak and killing is slow; increasing the concentration can further impair bacterial killing (the Eagle effect). Aminoglycosides alone are virtually inactive against enterococci but in combination with a penicillin show marked synergy and a rapid bactericidal effect. Severe enterococcal infections such as endocarditis must therefore be treated with a combination of agents such as ampicillin plus gentamicin, or high doses of penicillin plus gentamicin.

In patients allergic to ampicillin, erythromycin is a possible alternative treatment and urinary infections can also be treated with nitrofurantoin. In endocarditis, i.v. vancomycin is a good alternative when the organism has been shown to be sensitive. 30–55% of enterococci are resistant to tetracyclines.

References

PETER, G., A. SMITH: Group A streptococcal infections of skin and pharynx. New Engl. J. Med. *297:* 311 (1977).

SIMON, C.: D-Streptokokken und Cephalosporinempfindlichkeit. Med. Welt *34:* 1353 (1983).

WARD, J., H. KOORNHOF: Antibiotic-Resistant Pneumococci. In: J. REMINGTON, M. SWARTZ: Current Clinical Topics in Infectious Diseases. I. McGraw Hill, New York 1980.

f) Anaerobic Infections

Frequency: The anaerobic gram-positive *sporing bacilli* such as Clostridium perfringens, which causes gas gangrene, should be differentiated from the *non-sporing anaerobes*, the most important of which are listed in Table 37.

Bacteroides species are the most common anaerobic pathogens (80–90%, of which Bacteroides fragilis is found in more than half of all anaerobic infections).

Table 37. The important non-sporing anaerobes (facultative pathogens).

Gram stain	Cocci	Bacilli
Positive	Veillonella	Bacteroides fragilis Bacteroides melaninogenicus Fusobacterium necrophorum
Negative	Peptococcus Peptostreptococcus	Actinomyces israeli Propionibacterium acnes

Other pathogens include Peptostreptococcus species (anaerobic streptococci), and Peptococcus species (anaerobic staphylococci). Infections with fusobacteria, Veillonella, Propionibacterium, Campylobacter and Actinomyces are less common. The frequency of organisms in particular clinical infections often depends on the proximity of the infected organ to the mouth, intestinal or vaginal mucosa, where these anaerobes are regularly found in large numbers (300–2000 anaerobes to 1 aerobe in the colon). Bacteroides fragilis, which is normally found in the intestine, is a more common pathogen in abdominal and genital infections than in the lower respiratory tract. Where anaerobes cause lung infection, Bacteroides melaninogenicus is the commonest species involved.

Half of all infections with gram-negative anaerobic rods are mixed with facultatively anaerobic bacteria such as Escherichia coli and Klebsiella pneumoniae, and some 35% are multiple infections caused by 2–7 different anaerobes, including clostridia. These frequencies should be borne in mind, in view of the difficulties of culture and differentiation of anaerobes in the average clinical laboratory. Full bacteriological reports may require at least 2–3 days, and the clinician who suspects anaerobic infection on clinical grounds generally has to start treatment much earlier, based on his »best guess« of the most effective antibiotic combination to cover the likely aerobic and anaerobic bacteria involved. Certain clinical features such as pus with a foul, offensive odour, and spreading cellulitis, strongly suggest the presence of anaerobic infection, and some laboratories offer the rapid confirmation of the presence of anaerobes by the demonstration of typical volatile fatty acid peaks by direct gas-chromatographic examination of pus.

Illnesses: As well as gas gangrene (see p. 306, 444), tetanus (see p. 443), and botulism (see p. 364), anaerobes cause infection in the upper and lower respiratory tracts, the gastrointestinal and female genital tract. They can also cause endocarditis, septicaemia, and abscesses in organs such as the brain and liver. Anaerobes colonise areas where the oxidation/reduction potential is reduced as in parts of the body remote from active capillary perfusion such as the intestinal lumen, the vagina, tonsillar crypts and nasal sinuses. Aerobic bacteria use up oxygen and so improve the environment for anaerobes. Tissue injury can predispose to anaerobic infection by interrupting the capillary blood circulation, as occurs in surgical operations, arteriosclerosis and malignant tumours with chemical necrosis. The oxidation-reduction potential is reduced, a process often aided by multiple infection with O_2-consuming bacteria (e.g. Escherichia coli), which encourages the multiplication of anaerobic species with varying oxygen sensitivity. Some clostridia, for example, are much more sensitive to oxygen than Campylobacter. Anaerobic infection is often associated with localised thrombosis and thrombophlebitis, particularly in the pelvis. The exact cause is unknown, but could be the production of a bacterial heparinase or possibly an endotoxic effect. Infected emboli can give rise to small or large metastatic infarcts in the liver, lungs, brain and other organs, forming anaerobic abscesses. Severe cases of septicaemia due to gram-negative anaerobes often develop disseminated intravascular coagulation (consumption coagulopathy). Infections with non-sporing anaerobes are most often found in:

1. *The upper respiratory tract:* In chronic maxillary, frontal or sphenoidal sinusitis, peptostreptococci, Bacteroides fragilis, and Bacteroides melaninogenicus may be found alone or in combination with other facultatively anaerobic bacteria and/or other anaerobes. The same bacteria (plus Bacteroides oralis and fusobacteria) are found in dental caries and gingivitis.

2. *Lower respiratory tract:* Single or multiple lung abscesses, diffuse pulmonary infiltrates or necrotising pneumonia with cavitation can develop as a consequence of either inhalation of oro-pharyngeal secretions or of embolism from anaerobic infections in the abdomen or pelvis. The anaerobes usually found are Bacteroides melaninogenicus, fusobacteria, peptococci, peptostreptococci and Veillonella (often in association with staphylococci). Empyema may develop as a complication.

3. *Gastrointestinal tract:* Ulcers and tumours in the gastrointestinal tract form the portals of entry for aerobic and anaerobic bacteria, which can cause local or diffuse peritonitis, intra-abdominal abscesses and liver abscesses, sometimes with septicaemia. The commonest anaerobic causes are Bacteroides fragilis and Clostridium perfringens.

4. *Female genital tract:* Anaerobic septicaemia is a not uncommon complication of septic abortion and chorioamnionitis. Anaerobic salpingitis can also develop in the non-pregnant patient, for example as a complication of gynaecological operations. The anaerobes most frequently isolated are peptostreptococci, peptococci, Bacteroides species and clostridia. Mixed infections are common. Gonorrhoea must be excluded.

5. *Endocarditis:* Endocarditis caused by anaerobes is probably commoner than realised so far, and can often occur without underlying cardiac disease. Embolic complications are frequent. The primary focus is generally inflammation of the oropharynx or gastrointestinal tract. Acute and subacute endocarditis can be caused by Bacteroides fragilis, fusobacteria and Clostridium perfringens. Propionibacterium acnes, a normal skin resident, has been shown to cause endocarditis in a number of patients after the insertion of a prosthetic aortic valve.

6. *Central nervous system:* Cerebral abscesses due to anaerobes can arise from sinusitis or mastoiditis and generally lead to an epidural abscess and meningitis; they may also be metastatic, caused by infected emboli from a lung infection or endocarditis. Because of the reduced O_2 saturation of the arterial blood, anaerobic cerebral abscesses have a greater association with congenital cardiac defects with a right-left shunt than with any other heart defect.

Anaerobic culture and antibiotic sensitivity determination: Successful anaerobic culture depends on rapid transport of the specimen under anaerobic conditions to the laboratory and appropriate culture thereafter. A large specimen of pus is much more useful than a small swab. Once anaerobes have been isolated, differentiation of subspecies (other than Clostridia) is normally only undertaken by a reference laboratory. Slow growth and difficulties in evaluating anaerobic culture can delay the final result. Where the clinical features suggest mixed or anaerobic infection, the culture of a single anaerobe or of aerobic bacteria only does not exclude the possibility that further anaerobes are present. A gram-stained smear of the material submitted should always be examined thoroughly, because anaerobic bacteria may be seen microscopically even if they fail to grow. Direct gas chromatography of pus is also a useful, rapid indicator of the presence of anaerobic organisms.

Antibiotic sensitivity testing by the conventional disc method may give erroneous results when used for slow-growing anaerobes. Measurement of the minimal inhibitory concentration by tube dilution also gives variable results according to the technique used. Culture medium, pH, thickness of culture medium, bacterial inoculum and incubation period must be strictly standardised to achieve valid results. Bacteroides fragilis in particular can only be regarded as sensitive when the antibiotic concerned is completely stable to the β-lactamases of Bacteroides fragilis. In practice, cases where there is clinical suspicion of mixed or anaerobic infection are started on a combination of antibiotics which reliably covers Bacteroides fragilis as well as coexistent flora, such as a broad-spectrum bactericidal antibiotic + clindamycin or metronidazole.

Choice of antibiotic: Since most anaerobic infections involve *Bacteroides,* reliable activity against Bacteroides species is essential. Benzyl penicillin is well tolerated, can be safely given in high doses, and is an effective treatment for most anaerobic infections in the upper half of the body particularly those caused by Bacteroides melaninogenicus. Penicillin is active against most other anaerobes, including clostridia. The commonest cause of anaerobic infections in the lower half of the body, however, is Bacteroides fragilis, against which penicillin is ineffective. The most effective antibiotics in such cases are clindamycin and metronidazole, and both are active against the whole range of anaerobic species (see Table 38). Clindamycin used to be the antibiotic of choice against anaerobes and has the other advantage of excellent tissue penetration (including bone) and activity against gram-positive aerobes such as staphylococci and streptococci. The association of clindamycin with pseudomembranous enterocolitis, however, has led to its replacement by metronidazole as the antibiotic of choice against anaerobic infections in Great Britain, though not yet in the USA. Metronidazole is well tolerated, has excellent pharmacokinetic properties, and is conveniently given by the oral, rectal or intravenous routes. Resistance of Bacteroides fragilis and other obligate anaerobes to metronidazole has not yet been reported.

Other nitroimidazoles, cefoxitin, latamoxef and chloramphenicol are effective alternatives in most cases. Azlocillin, mezlocillin, piperacillin and cefotaxime have variable activity against anaerobes and are not sufficiently stable to the β-lactamase of Bacteroides fragilis.

Table 38. Minimal inhibitory concentrations (mg/l, or units/ml for penicillin) of various antibiotics in 50% of strains of non-sporing anaerobes (based on published reports).

Antibiotic	MIC in 50% of strains of				
	Bacteroides fragilis	Other Bacteroides species	Fusobacterium species	Peptococcus	Peptostreptococcus
Clindamycin	≤0.4	≤0.05	≤0.1	≤0.05	≤0.025
Metronidazole	≤1.6	≤0.4	≤0.1	≤0.4	≤0.2
Chloramphenicol	≤6.4	≤0.8	≤0.8	≤0.8	≤0.8
Erythromycin	≤6.4	≤0.4	≤6.4	≤1.6	≤0.1
Cefoxitin	≤8	≤0.4	≤0.4	≤0.4	≤0.4
Latamoxef	≤1.6	≤1.6	≤0.4	≤1.6	≤3.2
Cefotaxime	≤1.6	≤1.6	≤0.4	≤0.4	≤3.2
Azlocillin, mezlocillin	≤8	≤0.8	≤0.4	≤0.1	≤0.1
Carbenicillin	≤16	≤0.8	≤0.4	≤0.4	≤0.4
Tetracycline	≤12.5	≤0.8	≤0.8	≤0.8	≤0.8
Benzyl penicillin	≤25	≤0.4	≤0.1	≤0.1	≤0.1

Tetracyclines and erythromycin are not usually effective against Bacteroides fragilis, nor erythromycin in infections with fusobacteria. The frequency of resistance in Bacteroides fragilis is less than 3% with clindamycin and chloramphenicol, more than 60% with tetracyclines and more than 90% with penicillin.

Of the *other anaerobic gram-negative bacilli,* fusobacteria are the most sensitive to penicillin and are usually sensitive also to metronidazole, chloramphenicol, the tetracyclines and clindamycin, although occasional strains can be completely resistant to all these agents. Erythromycin has little activity against fusobacteria.

Anaerobic gram-positive cocci (Peptococcus, Peptostreptococcus) are almost always sensitive to clindamycin, penicillin and cephalothin but are often resistant to tetracycline (30–40%) and erythromycin (10–20%). With a few exceptions, metronidazole is also effective.

Of the *anaerobic gram-positive bacilli,* Actinomyces israeli is the most sensitive to penicillin but less sensitive to other agents and generally resistant to metronidazole. The most active antibiotic against Clostridium perfringens is benzyl penicillin followed in decreasing order of sensitivity by clindamycin, metronidazole, vancomycin, erythromycin and chloramphenicol. 20–30% of strains are resistant to the tetracyclines. Other Clostridium species (e. g. Clostridium ramosum) have variable resistance to penicillin, the tetracyclines, erythromycin and clindamycin, while metronidazole, vancomycin and chloramphenicol are always active. For Clostridium difficile, see p. 363.

References

BUSCH, D. F., V. L. SUTTER, S. M. FINEGOLD: Activity of combination of antimicrobial agents against bacteroides fragilis. J. infect. Dis. *133:* 321 (1979).
DORNBUSCH, K., C.-E. NORD, A. DAHLBÄCK: Antibiotic susceptibility of clostridium species isolated from human infections. Scand. J. infect. Dis. *7:* 127 (1975).
FERGUSON, I. R., L. L. SMITH: Bacteroides fragilis and nitroimidazoles. J. Antimicrob. Chemother. *2:* 220 (1976).
FINEGOLD, S. M., J. G. BARTLETT, A. W. CHOW et al.: Management of anaerobic infections. Ann. intern. Med. *83:* 375 (1975).
FINEGOLD, S.: Anaerobic Bacteria in Human Disease. Academic Press, New York 1977.
SUTTER, V. L., S. M. FINEGOLD: Susceptibility of anaerobic bacteria to 23 antimicrobial agents. Antimicrob. Ag. Chemother. *10:* 736 (1976).
TALLY, F. P., G. J. CUCHURAL, N. V. JACOBUS: Susceptibility of the Bacteroides fragilis Group in the United States in 1981. Antimicrob. Ag. Chemother. *3:* 536 (1983).
WEINRICH, A. E., V. E. DELBENE: Characterization of β-lactamase activity in anaerobic bacteria. Clin. Res *24:* 27 A (1976).

2. Septicaemia

Definition of septicaemia: Septicaemia is a generalised bacterial infection in which bacteria are released continuously or intermittently from a primary focus of infection into the blood stream, giving rise to a severe illness, including the formation of infected metastases in other organs. The portal of entry of the infective agent, e. g. an infected wound, can itself be the initial septic focus from which bacteria repeatedly enter the blood stream; once this site has closed or resolved, the septicaemia can continue to arise from a metastatic focus which may be difficult to find. Transient bacteraemia associated with minor, localised infections or after tonsillectomy or dental extraction does not cause severe symptoms and foci of infection do not develop in other organs except in particular abnormal situations (e. g. rheumatic damage to heart valves; prosthetic implants in the vascular or central nervous systems).

Septicaemias can be **classified** according to the species of causative organism, or to the portal of entry or initial septicaemic focus (e. g. tonsillitis, urinary infection, cholangitis, cholecystitis, septic abortion, umbilical infection etc.). The initial focus of cryptogenic septicaemia is, by definition, unknown. Septicaemia associated with foreign bodies and bacterial endocarditis are special forms.

The **clinical diagnosis** of septicaemia (based on intermittent fever, rigors, splenomegaly, demonstration of the initial and metastatic septic foci) is sometimes difficult because specific symptoms may be lacking in patients with impaired resistance (leukaemia, carcinomatosis, premature and newborn babies). Blood cultures should always be obtained where septicaemia is suspected to enable a bacteriological diagnosis to be made and specific chemotherapy to be given.

Important investigations:
1. *Blood cultures* as often as necessary, if possible before antibiotics are given. Blood is best cultured during a rigor but should not only be taken during peaks of temperature, since septicaemia can be afebrile under some circumstances, e. g. in the newborn and elderly. Each bottle of a set of two bottles containing suitable liquid media for aerobic and anaerobic culture is inoculated aseptically at the bedside without ventilation and sent to the laboratory. Blood should not be sent in plain specimen tubes because sensitive organisms can die in transit and time may be lost while the specimen is awaiting culture in the laboratory. Blood should be taken by venepuncture after careful skin disinfecton with tincture of iodine or 70% isopropyl alcohol. Blood should be cultured routinely under both aerobic and anaerobic conditions.

2. The *latex agglutination test* for the demonstration of antigen in serum, urine and possibly also CSF is sometimes positive when septicaemia is suspected with meningococci, pneumococci, group B streptococci, Haemophilus influenzae (type b), Candida albicans and Cryptococcus neoformans; false positive and false negative results sometimes occur. This test can also detect the cause of the septicaemia several days after treatment has begun.

3. *Bacteriological culture* of pus, cerebrospinal fluid, sputum, urine or aspiration of the septic focus or its metastases. If there is likely to be a delay before the specimens reach the bacteriological laboratory, purulent CSF or aspirated pus can also be inoculated into 2 broth culture bottles and precultured overnight in the hospital, if transport to the laboratory has to wait until the following day. Part of the specimen is sent in a sterile container or on a swab in transport medium for microscopic examination and the inoculation of special culture media.

4. *Sensitivity testing* of possible pathogens provides a basis for the choice of antibiotic and the dosage required.

5. *Treatment should, where necessary, be monitored* by further blood cultures, particularly if there is any clinical suggestion of relapse, a change in mixed infection or re-infection with a different organism.

General rules for the treatment of septicaemia:

1. If treatment is to be successful, the *initial septic focus must be cleared,* if necessary by drainage of pus or by operation.

2. Antibiotics must *be given for a sufficient period at adequate dosage,* since relapse is commoner when treatment is too short or the dose is too small. Bactericidal antibiotics are generally preferable although even they cannot completely protect against relapse. Bacteriostatic antibiotics can, however, be useful for later treatment, as prophylaxis against subsequent relapse. If a relapse occurs despite good therapy, the possibility of intercurrent resistance should be considered. Relapses are mostly caused by reinfection with a different pathogen or persistence of sensitive organisms in inaccessible sites such as large collections of pus.

3. The *choice of antibiotic* should be guided by the causative organism, the clinical picture and the antibiotic sensitivity pattern. Penicillins and cephalosporins are usually the most suitable antibiotics since they can be given in large doses without particular risk. Benzyl penicillin in large doses is the antibiotic of choice in septicaemia due to streptococci, pneumococci and meningococci (Table 39). *Antibiotic combinations* which increase bactericidal activity are recommended

Table 39. Daily dose in septicaemia.

Antibiotic	Adults	Children	Preferred route and dose-interval
Benzyl penicillin	20–40 mega-units	0.5 megaunits/kg, infants: 1 megaunit/kg	I. v. injection or short i. v. infusion every 6 hours
Ampicillin Flucloxacillin	6–10 (–20) g	150 (–400) mg/kg	Short i. v. infusion or slow injection every 6–8 hours, or i. m.
Azlocillin Mezlocillin Piperacillin Apalcillin	6–15 (–20) g	200–300 mg/kg	Short i. v. infusion or slow i. v. injection every 6–8 h, or i. m.
Ticarcillin	15–20 g	200–300 mg/kg	Short i. v. infusion or slow i. v. injection every 6–8 h, or i. m.
Cefazolin Cefoxitin Cefamandole	6 g	150 mg/kg	Short i. v. infusion or slow i. v. injection every 6–8 h, or i. m.
Cefuroxime Cefotaxime Ceftazidime	4.5 g 6 g 6 g	100 mg/kg 150 mg/kg 150 mg/kg	As cefazolin As cefazolin As cefazolin
Gentamicin Tobramycin Netilmicin	240–320 mg	3–5 mg/kg	Every 8–12 h i. m. or i. v.
Amikacin	1 g	10–15 mg/kg	Every 8–12 h i. m. or i. v.
Vancomycin	2 g	40 mg/kg	Short i. v. infusion every 12 h
Clindamycin	1.2 g	20–30 mg/kg	Short i. v. infusion every 6 h
Rolitetracycline	0.5 g	10 mg/kg	Slow i. v. injection every 12 h
Chloramphenicol	3 (–4) g	50–80 mg/kg	Oral or i. v. injection every 6–8 h
Metronidazole	1.5–2 g	20–30 mg/kg	Short i. v. infusion every 6–8 h

for infections with less sensitive or poorly accessible bacteria. Very broad spectrum combinations are useful for "best-guess" initial therapy. The combinations of cefoxitin + azlocillin, cefuroxime + azlocillin, and cefotaxime + azlocillin have been successful in clinical practice. Combinations of azlocillin or piperacillin with another cephalosporin are also useful. These combinations can be enhanced by an aminoglycoside, metronidazole or clindamycin. Penicillins or cephalosporins should not be given at the same time as a bacteriostatic antibiotic (chloramphenicol, tetracycline, erythromycin) because the bactericidal effect of the penicillin or the cephalosporin, which only occurs during active bacterial growth, is prevented. Doubt has recently be cast over whether such antagonism is significant in clinical practice. It is also important to avoid the addition of similar side effects of two components of a combination. Finally, the choice of antibiotic must take account of tissue diffusion or concentration in the CSF, bile, or urine, so that antibiotics are given which reach the site of infection in satisfactory concentrations.

4. Patients treated with large doses of antibiotics should be carefully observed for *side effects*, since generalised septicaemia can impair renal function and hence delay the excretion of the antibiotic. High doses of the disodium salt of carbenicillin can cause hypernatraemia and hypokalaemia. Neurotoxicity (convulsions) can occur after daily doses of more than 20 megaunits of benzyl penicillin, particularly when excretion is impaired, or with meningitis, when the permeability of the blood-CSF barrier is increased.

5. *Supplementary measures:* Treatment of shock, blood transfusion, correction of acidosis, fluid therapy, restoration of electrolyte balance and surgical measures.

6. *Failure of treatment may be* attributed to inadequate dosage, a change in infecting organism, an increase in bacterial resistance, relapse due to persistent forms, failure to eradicate the initial focus of infection, anatomical inaccessibility of the organisms (e.g. in an abscess cavity), or an incorrect choice of antibiotics.

Frequency of causes of septicaemia: At one time, streptococci and pneumococci were the commonest causes of septicaemia, but staphylococci and gram-negative intestinal bacteria such as Escherichia coli, Klebsiella, Enterobacter, Proteus, Pseudomonas aeruginosa and Bacteroides now predominate. Meningococci occur either sporadically or in small epidemics. Other organisms, such as Haemophilus influenzae, clostridia, Salmonella, Pasteurella multocida, gonococci, Aeromonas, Campylobacter and Serratia marcescens etc. are uncommon. Saprophytic bacteria (coagulase-negative staphylococci, Acinetobacter species, diphtheroids, aerobic spore-bearing bacilli) and yeasts can give rise to septicaemia under certain conditions such as the implantation of synthetic prostheses in cardiac operations, or after shunt operations (Spitz-Holter valve, Scribner shunt).

a) Treatment when the Cause of Infection Is Known

Staphylococcus aureus septicaemia: The bacteraemia is usually continuous and originates from skin infections (sometimes with lymphangitis), wound or umbilical infections, thrombophlebitis, mastoiditis, parotitis or pneumonia. Relatively common in heroin addicts and in intravascular foreign body infections. Septic metastatic foci commonly occur in the kidneys, bone marrow, joints, brain and meninges, lungs, endocardium etc.

The tendency to abscess formation and to inadequate treatment is associated with a considerable relapse rate; a prolonged course of antibiotics, preferably as a combination of a β-lactam antibiotic with fusidic acid, should be given.

Treatment: Benzyl penicillin may be given for sensitive staphylococci in a dose of 20–40 megaunits daily for adults and older children and 3–10 megaunits for the newborn and infants, in several short i. v. infusions. Combination with fusidic acid is advisable.

For penicillin-resistant staphylococci, use flucloxacillin, 6–12 g a day in 3–4 short i. v. infusions or slow i. v. injections for adults and 150–400 mg/kg for children; cefazolin (6 g a day for adults) is an alternative. 3 g of fusidic acid a day may be added.

In cases of penicillin allergy, use cefazolin, cefazedone, cefuroxime or cefamandole, 6–8 g a day for adults, 200 mg/kg for children, in 3–4 short i. v. infusions or slow i. v. injections. Erythromycin or clindamycin should be considered where cross-hypersensitivity between penicillins and cephalosporins is suspected.

In patients with cephalosporin allergy or with methicillin-resistant staphylococci, consider vancomycin as a daily dose of 2 g in adults or 40 mg/kg in children, divided into two short i. v. infusions. Avoid vancomycin in renal failure because of the increased risk of ototoxicity.

Length of treatment: 4–6 weeks, or even longer, may be necessary. Reduce dosage when improvement is established, but continue parenteral administration. Avoid combinations with bacteriostatic antibiotics if possible. Because of its good penetration, fusidic acid (in combination with flucloxacillin) is recommended for deep abscesses, and surgical drainage and the removal of infected foreign bodies is also necessary.

Fosfomycin and rifampicin should be kept in reserve for staphylococcal septicaemia resistant to the above antibiotics.

Staphylococcus epidermidis septicaemia: Septicaemia with coagulase-negative staphylococci has recently become more common. Intravenous foreign bodies (intravenous catheters, dialysis shunts etc.) have been the main portals of entry. Occasional cases develop endocarditis. The diagnosis can only be made when the same strain is isolated on a number of occasions from blood culture. Multi-resistant strains which include resistance to methicillin are quite frequent.

Treatment must be based on antibiotic sensitivities, e. g. with flucloxacillin or a parenteral cephalosporin + gentamicin. Methicillin-resistant strains are not treatable with penicillins or cephalosporins, even if apparently sensitive *in vitro*. The infected foreign body should, if possible, be removed.

Group A streptococcal septicaemia is relatively uncommon nowadays, but can still be fulminating and must always be treated very seriously. Portals of entry are provided by infections of the skin, wounds, the female reproductive tract or the upper respiratory tract. Fulminant infections which progress rapidly and affect a number of sites in the body occur regularly.

Treatment: Benzyl penicillin, 5–10 (–20) megaunits/day for adults in several short i. v. infusions or injections; 1–3–5 megaunits/day over 1–2 weeks in small children and the newborn. When clinical recovery is well established, treatment may be changed to phenoxymethyl penicillin, 0.75–1.5 g a day for 2 weeks. Alternatives (in cases of penicillin allergy) are a parenteral cephalosporin (see Table 39), clindamycin (0.9–1.2 g a day) or vancomycin.

Pneumococcal septicaemia may be a complication of pneumonia but is sometimes seen in patients with impaired resistance (splenectomy) as a complication of sinusitis, or with no recognisable portal of entry. The disease can progress rapidly with septic shock and occasionally meningitis.

Treatment: Large doses of benzyl penicillin, as for Group A streptococcal septicaemia.

Group B streptococcal septicaemia is particularly a disease of the newborn where it is seen in two forms, one of early onset acquired in utero and manifest in the first 24–48 hours of life, and one of late onset, presumably acquired at birth or soon after but presenting after an interval of a few weeks. The disease can be fulminating and the prognosis is often poor. It is occasionally found in adults with impaired resistance.

Prompt *treatment* with benzyl penicillin gives the best results, though parenteral cephalosporins and broad-spectrum penicillins also eliminate group B streptococci effectively.

Septicaemia with other streptococci: Viridans or non-haemolytic streptococci of other groups are not uncommonly isolated in blood cultures from patients without endocarditis.

They can be a sign of bacteraemia without septicaemia, and can also arise from colonic carcinoma or mixed anaerobic infection. Apart from the enterococci, such streptococci are almost always sensitive to penicillin but treatment should often take the possible presence of other organisms into account, as part of a gut-related mixed infection from which streptococci have been the only component to be isolated.

Treatment with benzyl penicillin + metroindazole is often, therefore, better than penicillin alone.

Enterococcal septicaemia caused by Streptococcus faecalis is relatively common, but that due to S. faecium or S. durans is rare. The portal of entry is usually through the intestinal or urogenital tract, occasionally through extensive burns. Septicaemic metastases are uncommon. Often associated with bacterial endocarditis (see p. 315), and sometimes as part of a mixed infection with enterobacteria and Bacteroides. Infections with other group D streptococci (e.g. S. bovis, S. equinus) are usually sensitive to cefazolin and cefazedone.

Treatment: Ampicillin, 6–10 (–20) g a day for adults and older children; 150–400 mg/kg for young children, divided into 4 short i.v. infusions or slow i.v. injections. The bactericidal activity of ampicillin is greatly enhanced by combination with gentamicin.

Tetracycline i.v. or vancomycin i.v. are alternatives in patients who are allergic to penicillin. The cephalosporins as a group have very poor activity against enterococci; even cefazedone, which is the most active representative, is much inferior to ampicillin.

Meningococcal septicaemia: The portal of entry is the nasopharynx and the septicaemia is usually accompanied by meningitis or arthritis and rarely by endocarditis; the most severe (the Waterhouse-Friderichsen syndrome) is commonest in children and was almost always fatal. Meningococci can occasionally be demonstrated in stained blood smears as gram-negative kidney-shaped diplococci.

Treatment: Benzyl penicillin in a daily dose of 20–30 megaunits in adults, 0.5 megaunits/kg in younger children and 1 megaunit/kg in the newborn, in 4–6 short i.v. infusions or slow i.v. injections. Combination with other antibiotics is not necessary. Treatment should continue until the patients's clinical improvement is well established and the ESR has returned to normal. The initial high doses of penicillin may be reduced once improvement has started. Meningococci are nowadays often resistant to sulphonamides, which are therefore no longer reliable.

Chloramphenicol should be given to patients with penicillin allergy, or a strong history of epileptiform convulsions, in an adult dose of 3 (−4) g a day (50–80 mg/ kg for children) orally or i.v. Prophylaxis is sometimes advisable for close (usually household) contacts and the choice of agent should be based on the antibiotic sensitivities of the index strain. If sensitive to sulphonamides, give sulphadiazine twice daily for two days in the following doses: 250 mg (babies aged 3 m. – 1 y.), 500 mg (children aged 1–12 y.) or 1 g (adults). If resistant to sulphonamides, give rifampicin 5 mg/kg (babies aged 3 mo.–1 y.), 10 mg/kg (children aged 1–12 y.) or 600 mg (adults). Primary rifampicin resistance has been reported. Minocycline is an alternative to rifampicin (see p. 122).

The **Waterhouse-Friderichsen syndrome** occurs in meningococcal and other forms of septicaemia and is expressed as profound shock, loss of water and electrolytes, internal and external bleeding and a consumption coagulopathy with thrombocytopenia and a deficiency of fibrinogen, prothrombin and factors V and VII.

Treatment consists not only of large doses of penicillin but also of expanding the plasma volume, correcting the electrolyte imbalance, heparin (to prevent further clotting abnormalities), the possible administration of antithrombin III or streptokinase to activate fibrinolysis, and fresh blood transfusions to replace the lack of clotting factors. The role of prednisone is controversial since it may favour the development of a consumption coagulopathy.

Escherichia coli septicaemia is the commonest form in the newborn and young infant. It is also found as a complication of urinary infection or cholangitis in children and adults and often gives rise to septic shock, which carries a high mortality rate.

Treatment: Cefotaxime, gentamicin and amikacin are likely to be effective against almost all infections caused by Escherichia coli. Other antibiotics should only be given when the results of sensitivity tests are available. For sensitive isolates, ampicillin i. v. 6–10 (−20) g daily for adults, 200–400 mg/kg for children, given as 4 short i. v. infusions or slow i. v. injections per day may be used. Mezlocillin or piperacillin may also be considered and are often more active against sensitive strains.

In cases of ampicillin resistance, a cephalosporin stable to β-lactamase (e. g. cefotaxime) may be used (dosage: see Table 39); gentamicin, tobramycin and amikacin are alternatives, and can usefully be combined with a cephalosporin to treat multi-resistant strains. Duration of therapy: usually at least 2–3 weeks.

In **septic shock,** broad-spectrum bactericidal antibiotics should be started at once in high doses. Either an aminoglycoside, a β-lactam agent, or both in combination may be necessary until a bacterial isolate is obtained and sensitivities tested. Because renal function can be acutely impaired in septicaemia, frequent and careful monitoring of aminoglycoside concentrations is essential when these antibiotics are used. The view that bactericidal antibiotics can exacerbate septic shock is obviously incorrect. Other measures include prednisone, 50–100 (−1000) mg for adults, 5–8 mg/kg for children, replacement of volume, correction of acidosis, digitalis, oxygen and haemodialysis in cases of renal failure.

Treatment: Shock lung must be adequately treated with positive pressure ventilation if necessary. The fluid balance should be carefully controlled by monitoring central venous and pulmonary wedge pressure and urinary output. Adrenaline, noradrenaline and drugs which cause peripheral vasoconstriction are contraindicated. Prednisone can be useful. In disseminated intravascular coagulation, treatment with antithrombin III etc. is necessary at the appropriate stage.

Klebsiella and Enterobacter septicaemia occur not uncommonly in hospitals. Initial foci include otitis media, pneumonia, infections of wounds, the urinary tract or venous catheter sites, and cholangitis. Septic shock is common and antibiotic treatment must be guided by sensitivity testing because antibiotic resistance is usually present.

Treatment: Cefotaxime and other antibiotics in the cefotaxime group have the greatest activity against Klebsiella. Enterobacter aerogenes is regularly inhibited by the newer cephalosporins. Most strains of Enterobacter cloacae, however, are resistant to all penicillins and most cephalosporins, although they are sometimes sensitive to tetracycline, chloramphenicol and co-trimoxazole. A few klebsiellas and enterobacters are resistant to the aminoglycosides. Klebsiella or Enterobacter septicaemia is best treated with a combination of a newer cephalosporin and an aminoglycoside, which is often synergistic. Chloramphenicol, tetracyclines, or co-trimoxazole can also be used against sensitive strains. Most penicillins (ampicillin, carbenicillin) are inactive against Klebsiella, though mezlocillin and piperacillin have some activity against a few strains of Klebsiella pneumoniae.

Serratia marcescens septicaemia is increasingly found in intensive care units and usually arises from infections of the urinary or respiratory tracts or of venous catheter sites.

Treatment is difficult because strains are commonly resistant. Cefotaxime or ceftazidime are usually the best, alone or in combination with an aminoglycoside such as amikacin. Mezlocillin or piperacillin also act on most strains of Serratia. Sensitive strains may respond to other antibiotics.

Dosage: see Table 39.

Proteus septicaemia: Common foci are infections of the urinary, intestinal or biliary tracts or the middle ear. Often gives rise to septic shock. Treatment may vary with the type of Proteus and the antibiotic sensitivity pattern.

Treatment: Ampicillin (Proteus mirabilis and sensitive strains): 10–20 g a day for adults and 200–400 mg/kg for children in 3–6 short infusions or i. v. injections. A parenteral cephalosporin is an alternative in patients with ampicillin allergy. Mezlocillin and piperacillin are more active than ampicillin. The best agents against Proteus vulgaris and other indole-positive strains are cefotaxime and ceftazidime. Gentamicin and amikacin are effective against most species of Proteus and are generally combined with β-lactam antibiotics. The eradication of indole-positive strains is often difficult and other drugs such as mezlocillin, piperacillin or chloramphenicol may be expected from sensitivity testing to be effective.

Dosage: see Table 39.

Pseudomonas septicaemia usually originates from infections of the urinary tract, burns or wounds and is a life-threatening septic complication of leukaemia. Septic shock is frequent and treatment is difficult because of the limited range of sensitivities of the organism. The *treatment* of choice is a combination of azlocillin (15 g a day) or ceftazidime (6 g a day) with tobramycin (160–320 mg a day); piperacillin, cefsulodin or apalcillin are possible alternatives.

Haemophilus septicaemia: The initial focus is usually the nasopharynx or respiratory tract and septicaemia with this organism is often associated with meningitis, septic arthritis, endocarditis (generally subacute) and acute epiglottitis in young children.

Treatment: The treatment of choice used to be intravenous ampicillin in high dosage, and this is still effective where the strain is sensitive. However, strains which produce β-lactamase and hence are resistant to ampicillin are becoming commoner and ampicillin can no longer be relied on before sensitivities are available. Intravenous chloramphenicol is an effective alternative, although resistance to chloramphenicol is also occasionally found. Cefotaxime is much more active than ampicillin and is stable to β-lactamase. Other alternatives are cefuroxime or cefamandole (dosage: see Table 39).

Clostridium septicaemia is caused by Clostridium perfringens (the causative organism of gas gangrene) or other clostridia and arises from wound, intestinal or puerperal infections, particularly after abdominal operations, abortions and in patients with bone-marrow insufficiency. Acute haemolysis with jaundice and disseminated intravascular coagulation are frequent complications.

Treatment: Benzyl penicillin, 10–20 megaunits a day, parenterally is the treatment of choice, and other antibiotics such as cephalosporins, tetracyclines, chloramphenicol and metronidazole are possible, though less satisfactory, alternatives. Treatment with hyperbaric oxygen in a special chamber is an important, though still somewhat controversial, adjunct to treatment, but is only available in a few specialized clinics. The value of antitoxin against Clostridium perfringens is doubtful.

Bacteroides septicaemia may be acute or chronic, with a primary focus in the genital tract, nasopharynx or intestinal tract. Subacute endocarditis is uncommon, but abscesses with foul smelling pus are characteristic. Often associated with anaerobic streptococci, enterococci or Escherichia coli.

Treatment: Since sensitivity testing of Bacteroides is technically difficult and time-consuming, initial treatment should be with clindamycin i.v., metronidazole i.v. or cefoxitin. These agents are reliably effective against all species of Bacteroides including B. fragilis, which is not susceptible to penicillin although other species of Bacteroides and anaerobic streptococci, which are often associated, generally are. Chloramphenicol, azlo- and mezlocillin, piperacillin and other nitroimidazoles are often effective alternatives, but other penicillins, cephalosporins or aminoglycosides are not indicated in infections caused by Bacteroides.

Melioidosis is caused by Pseudomonas pseudomallei and presents acutely as septicaemia with profuse diarrhoea or subacutely and chronically with abscesses, particularly of the skin and bones. High mortality rate.

Treatment: Tetracyclines or chloramphenicol in high dosage. Initial treatment should always be combined with gentamicin or co-trimoxazole, and abscesses should be drained where necessary.

Occasional bacterial causes of septicaemia: Gonococci (treat with penicillin or cefotaxime if resistant), Listeria (ampicillin), Pasteurella multocida (penicillin or tetracycline), Campylobacter (chloramphenicol, erythromycin, tetracycline), Aeromonas (penicillin or tetracycline), Salmonella (see p. 449).

Fungal septicaemia occurs not infrequently in patients whose resistance to infection is impaired by immunological deficiencies, malignancies, cortisone treatment or venous catheter infections. Important causes of disseminated fungal sepsis are Candida species, Aspergillus, Coccidioides immitis, Torulopsis glabrata and Histoplasma capsulatum.

Treatment: Amphotericin B i.v., with the addition of flucytosine if in vitro sensitivity can be shown. Flucytosine is always inactive against histoplasmosis and coccidioidomycosis.

b) Treatment when the Cause of Infection Is Unknown

If the patient has a severe infection and the causative organism is not yet known, initial treatment must be guided by the clinical features. The choice of antibiotic must be based on the possible portals of entry, septic foci, the presence of underlying diseases which impair resistance and the development of septic shock or renal failure. *Bactericidal antibiotics are preferable.* Combinations of antibiotics are generally needed to extend the spectrum of activity and increase the likelihood of clinical efficacy. The best initial treatments available currently are based on β-lactamase-stable cephalosporins such as cefoxitin, cefotaxime or ceftazidime. They can be supplemented by an aminoglycoside and/or by metronidazole if necessary. If, in addition to enterobacteria, Pseudomonas aeruginosa is a likely pathogen, ceftazidime is a good first choice. A combination of cefoxitin or cefotaxime with azlocillin or piperacillin is a sound alternative, possibly with tobramycin also. Antibiotic combinations of this sort have a spectrum broad enough to include almost all the bacterial causes of septicaemia, including Bacteroides fragilis, when cefoxitin, azlocillin or metronidazole are included. The principal bacterial exception is Streptococcus faecalis which is resistant to cephalosporins and aminoglycosides and, if suspected, should be treated with ampicillin or azlocillin. Fungal infection is also unaffected by very broad spectrum combinations and, indeed, colonisation and sometimes infection by fungi such as Candida is actively encouraged by their use, particularly if given for long periods and/or in intensive care units. Many clinical forms of septicaemia are associated with a typical range of organisms, which should be covered by any initial treatment.

Septicaemia associated with infections of the normal **urinary tract** is commonly caused by Escherichia coli and other enterobacteria and may be treated with β-lactamase-stable cephalosporins, piperacillin, mezlocillin or an aminoglycoside. More resistant gram-negative rods (Proteus, Pseudomonas, Serratia, Klebsiella and Enterobacter) are often found after urological operations in patients with chronic indwelling catheters and where there are congenital, neurological or other urinary abnormalities. *Initial treatment* is best performed with combinations of a β-lactam such as cefoxitin, cefuroxime, cefotaxime, mezlocillin, azlocillin or piperacillin, with an aminoglycoside such as gentamicin, tobramycin or netilmicin. This initial treatment should be reviewed as soon as antibiotic sensitivities are available.

The causative organisms of **biliary septicaemia** cannot be reliably obtained by culture of the duodenal contents; blood culture should always be performed. Escherichia coli, other enterobacteria, micro-aerophilic and anaerobic streptococci are the commonest causes. Bacteroides, clostridia and Pseudomonas are found less frequently.

Mezlocillin, piperacillin and cefotaxime are probably the most suitable agents for *initial treatment* since they have an adequate spectrum of activity, high serum, tissue and biliary concentrations, no loss of activity in bile, and their use is well supported by clinical trials. The tetracyclines were once the drugs of choice, but should no longer be given in severe biliary infections because of the widespread resistance amongst enterobacteria. Mechanical factors sustaining cholangitis or cholecystitis, such as gall stones, must be removed by operation. Septic complications after endoscopic retrograde cannulation of the pancreatic duct (ERCP) are often caused by Pseudomonas. Cefazolin, cefazedone or ampicillin are useful in infections of the bile ducts without cholestasis. Co-trimoxazole by intravenous infusion is a satisfactory alternative, followed by oral treatment later. The combination of a β-lactam antibiotic with an aminoglycoside is often valuable.

Postoperative septicaemia, which often originates in infected wounds, is commonly caused by penicillin-resistant staphylococci. Mixed infections with gram-negative bacteria are not uncommon, particularly in abdominal wounds. A cephalosporin with good activity against staphylococci (e.g. cefazolin, cefazedone) may be given as *initial treatment,* but when the patient is seriously ill, flucloxacillin or a cephalosporin can be given in combination with an aminoglycoside such as gentamicin.

Wound infections after intestinal or gynaecological operations are generally mixed, due to enterobacteria, Bacteroides fragilis and anaerobic streptococci. Initial treatment must be effective against enterobacteria and anaerobes such as Bacteroides. This spectrum of pathogens is usually covered by a combination of cefotaxime + metronidazole, or cefoxitin + azlocillin. In severe infections where an aminoglycoside is used, a combination of ampicillin or an acylamino penicillin, gentamicin and metronidazole is generally effective.

Septicaemia after minor skin lesions (with lymphangitis): Mainly caused by staphylococci and sometimes streptococci as well. *Treatment* with flucloxacillin or cefazolin i.v.

Septicaemia in patients with bone-marrow suppression (e.g. leukaemia) may be caused by a number of microorganisms, including Pseudomonas aeruginosa, Escherichia coli, Klebsiella, Proteus and staphylococci. But many other pathogens and opportunistic organisms also have to be considered.

When the cause of the septicaemia is not known, previous antibiotic treatment, the clinical picture and any likely portals of entry should be considered. Broad-spectrum bactericidal combinations such as cefoxitin + azlocillin + gentamicin, or cefotaxime + azlocillin + amikacin, or piperacillin plus gentamicin, should be given. *Treatment* may be needed for a considerable time.

Septic abortion and puerperal sepsis (see p. 402): The commonest causes are Bacteroides, followed by Escherichia coli, staphylococci, aerobic and anaerobic streptococci, clostridia etc., often in mixed infections. A cervical swab for gram stain and culture (aerobic and anaerobic) and blood cultures should be taken before starting treatment; a vaginal swab is adequate if the infecting organism is Streptococcus pyogenes, but in other cases may give misleading results either because the infecting agent is not isolated, or because the organisms isolated are so frequently present in the vagina of apparently healthy women that their pathogenic significance is uncertain.

Treatment with high doses of antibiotics should cover the expected range of causative bacteria. A cephalosporin such as cefoxitin or cefotaxime, or amoxycillin combined with metronidazole should be given to patients who are not seriously ill.

In patients with more severe illnesses, combinations which include mezlocillin, piperacillin, cefotaxime, metronidazole, latamoxef or clindamycin with an aminoglycoside may be necessary. If β-haemolytic streptococci or clostridia are isolated, benzyl penicillin in high doses is the treatment of choice. Where necessary, retained products of conception should be removed by curettage, and in extreme cases emergency hysterectomy may be needed. Active measures should be taken to treat shock.

Septicaemia complicating severe tonsillitis or tonsillar abscess is generally caused by Bacteroides, staphylococci or haemolytic streptococci and very rarely by gram-negative bacteria.

Treatment: A parenteral cephalosporin such as cefoxitin or cefuroxime i. v., if necessary combined with intravenous clindamycin; benzyl penicillin or flucloxacillin may also be used. If septic thrombosis develops in the jugular vein, ligature may be necessary.

Foreign body septicaemia originates from an infected foreign body such as a prosthetic heart valve, a Spitz-Holter valve, a Scribner shunt or an indwelling venous catheter. Bacteraemia is considerably more frequently associated with central venous catheters than with peripheral lines. The risk of septicaemia is much greater in neutropenic patients, when veins are inflamed or thrombosed, and when the same venous catheter is used for a long period without being changed. Other complications are also associated with venous catheters, such as thrombophlebitis, cellulitis, endocarditis, infection of prosthetic implants and septic embolism and infarction (e. g. pulmonary infarction).

The causative agents are mainly saprophytic skin organisms, the commonest being staphylococci (70–80%) with gram-negative bacilli (10–20%) and fungi (1–5%) occurring less frequently. These organisms can originate from the skin of the patient or attendant staff. The contamination of total parenteral nutrition fluids by Candida is a particularly serious risk, and other fungi such as Aspergillus, Torulopsis glabrata and Mucor are occasionally found. Aqueous infusion fluids are not uncommonly contaminated by Klebsiella, Enterobacter, Serratia, Pseudomonas cepacia and Citrobacter freundii.

The diagnosis of venous catheter septicaemia can be difficult. Culture of blood from the venous catheter and the peripheral circulation both qualitatively and quantitatively is of value since blood from the venous catheter usually contains at least 10 times as many bacteria as that obtained by peripheral venepuncture (>2000 organisms/ml). Quantitative blood culture is best performed by the pour-plate method in which 1 ml of blood is thoroughly mixed with 9 ml of molten agar in a sterile petri dish. The identical organisms can sometimes be recovered from the infusion container, and from the site of entry and the tip of the venous catheter. When fungal septicaemia is suspected, it is better to culture arterial blood since venous blood often contains no fungi.

Treatment may be attempted with flucloxacillin or cefazolin in high dosage (as for staphylococcal septicaemia, p. 300). Clindamycin or vancomycin are possible alternatives staphylococci resistant to flucloxacillin. Very resistant strains sometimes respond to synergistic combinations such as rifampicin plus trimethoprim. When other infecting organisms are isolated, antibiotic sensitivity testing must be used to guide treatment with β-lactamase-stable cephalosporins, aminoglycosides, azlocillin, mezlocillin, piperacillin etc. Fungal infections (usually candida) are treated with amphotericin B + flucytosine. If possible, the foreign body should be removed. When a Spitz-Holter valve with a Rickham reservoir appears infected, the injection or perfusion of gentamicin into the system (see p. 329) is sometimes effective.

There is some dispute about whether venous catheter septicaemia should be treated first by antibiotics alone, without removal of the catheter. The prospects of success are much reduced when thrombophlebitis has developed or when fungal or pseudomonal infection is present. In some cases, however, treatment with effective antibiotics eliminates the bacteria from the blood either temporarily or permanently. Antibiotic treatment should be assumed to have failed if the temperature does not return to normal within 2 to 3 days.

Bacteraemia arising from contaminated intravenous infusion solutions is usually transient and treatment with antibiotics without a change of catheter is normally sufficient.

Treatment with a cephalosporin alone or in combination with an aminoglycoside is advisable, even when the infection resolves spontaneously. Severe reactions and septicaemias have been associated with bacterial contamination of stored blood.

Neonatal septicaemia can vary greatly in its presentation and clinical features. It can develop *in utero* (e. g. Listeria), during birth (Escherichia coli, Pseudomonas, group B streptococci etc.) and post-partum (staphylococci and other organisms).

Prompt, early *treatment* is essential when infection is first suspected (once blood and CSF have been collected for culture). Because of the serious prognosis, a combination of antibiotics is usually given, based on the likely causes of infection but modified to take account of the physiological impairment of drug metabolism and excretion at this age (see p. 502).

Treatment should be well tolerated, cover a broad spectrum of bacteria, and include resistant staphylococci. Some useful combinations for initial treatment are a cephalosporin together with an acylamino penicillin, e. g. cefuroxime + azlocillin, cefotaxime + azlocillin, cefuroxime + piperacillin or cefotaxime + piperacillin. These combinations can be complemented by an aminoglycoside (gentamicin, tobramycin or amikacin) and should now replace the combination of penicillin or ampicillin with an aminoglycoside.

References

BALTCH, A. L., P. E. GRIFIN: *Pseudomonas aeruginosa* bacteremia: A clinical study of 75 patients. Amer. J. med. Sci. *274:* 119 (1977).

BEATTY, H.: Staphylococcus aureus Bacteremia. In: REMINGTON, J., M. SWARTZ: Current Clinical Topics in Infectious Diseases. I. McGraw Hill, New York 1980.

GENTRY, L. O., I. D. WILKINSON, A. S. LEA, M. F. PRICE: Latex agglutination test for detection of candida antigen in patients with disseminated disease. Eur. J. clin. Microbiol. *2:* 122 (1983).

GOPAL, V., A. BISNO: Fulminant pneumococcal infections in "normal" asplenic hosts. Arch. intern. Med. *137:* 1526 (1977).

MONTGOMERIE, J. Z., J. E. EDWARDS, Jr.: Association of infection due to *Candida albicans* with intravenous hyperalimentation. J. infect. Dis. *137:* 197 (1978).

PHILLIPS, I., P. D. MEERS, P. F. D'ARCY: Microbiological Hazards of Infusion Therapy. MTP Press, Lancaster, England 1977.

PROBER, C. G., B. TUNE, L. HODEN: *Y. pseudotuberculosis* septicemia. Amer. J. Dis. Child. *133:* 623 (1979).

REINICKE, V., B. KORNER: Fulminant septicemia caused by *Y. enterocolitica*. Scand. J. infect. Dis. *9:* 249 (1977).

SIMON, C., M. ENGFER: Erregerspektrum und Therapie der Septikämien im Kindesalter. Klin. Pädiat. *190:* 175 (1978).

SIMON, C., U. LINDNER, J. H. HARTLAPP: Therapie und Prophylaxe der Venenkathetersepsis. Fortschr. antimikrob. Chemother. *3–6:* 28 (1984).

SIMON, C., A. BAHR, G. KRELLER, D. KIOSZ: Untersuchungen über eine optimale Blutkulturtechnik. Mschr. Kinderheilk. *132:* 168 (1984).

SIMON, C., G. KRELLER, A. BAHR, D. KIOSZ: In vitro comparison of fluid blood culture media. Infection *12:* 64 (1984).

STILLE, W.: Klinik septikämischer Erkrankungen. Infection *4:* 185 (1976).

ZIMMERMAN, J. E.: Acute septicemic melioidosis. Successful treatment with gentamicin. JAMA *213:* 2266 (1970).

3. Infective Endocarditis

Frequency of bacterial causes: Viridans and non-haemolytic streptococci 65–85%, enterococci 5–10%, non-bacteraemic forms 10–20%, staphylococci 5–15% and gram-negative intestinal bacteria 2–6%. Staphylococci and gram-negative intestinal bacteria are usually associated with acute endocarditis and streptococci with subacute endocarditis (the classical endocarditis lenta). Almost all microbial species can occasionally cause endocarditis (Haemophilus influenzae, H. aphrophilus, gonococci, pneumococci, Campylobacter, Erysipelothrix rhusiopathiae, Brucella, Bacteroides species, Candida species, Coxiella burneti etc.). Endocarditis in heroin addicts is often caused by staphylococci, gram-negative bacilli and fungi. Endocarditis can also occur in immunocompromised patients as a result of bacteraemia or fungaemia arising from an indwelling venous catheter.

Acute ulcerative endocarditis (septic endocarditis), which is generally caused by Staphylococcus aureus, can attack and rapidly destroy normal heart valves. Septic metastases may develop in the brain, meninges, kidneys or on the skin. *Endocarditis after open heart surgery* can occur in the first two months or later after the operation. Staphylococcus aureus or epidermidis, Pseudomonas aeruginosa and fungi (Candida) are usually found in the early forms and are particularly serious when they infect prosthetic valves or teflon patches. Late forms are generally caused by staphylococci and streptococci. The characteristic symptoms of endocarditis may be absent. Because skin organisms are often involved, several positive blood cultures may be necessary to be sure of the diagnosis.

Subacute bacterial endocarditis classically described as endocarditis lenta, is usually caused by viridans or non-haemolytic streptococci or enterococci and occasionally by staphylococci or fungi. It virtually always affects a diseased or congenitally abnormal valve, usually after old rheumatic heart disease. The mitral and aortic valves are the most commonly involved. Cases of pure mitral stenosis are rarely affected. The clinical features are changing heart murmurs, fever, high ESR (except for polycythaemia in cyanotic heart disease), symptoms of focal nephritis, splenomegaly and small skin haemorrhages. There is often a recent history of dental extraction, tonsillectomy, abdominal surgery or intestinal disease. If there is a thick fibrinous exudate on the infected valves or if the causative organisms are very fastidious and difficult to grow in liquid media, cultures can sometimes fail to yield an isolate. It can then be difficult to differentiate the condition from rheumatic endocarditis or lupus erythematosus. Culture-negative endocarditis is uncommon with good blood culture technique, and when it occurs, coxiella infections should be excluded by serological tests.

Echocardiograms are very useful for the localisation of valvular or mural vegetations and for the diagnosis of valve perforation.

Bacteriological diagnosis: Antibiotic treatment of acute septic endocarditis should not begin until at least 2 sets of blood cultures have been taken at short intervals; if subacute endocarditis is suspected 3–5 blood cultures should be taken at intervals of 4–6 hours. When good culture techniques are used, further cultures are seldom contributory. The prognosis depends on the availability of an isolate, together with quantitative sensitivity testing and, where necessary, testing for synergy and bactericidal activity. Because a number of causative organisms of endocarditis are difficult to culture, a reliable general blood culture technique is essential, using liquid or biphasic media which support aerobic and anaerobic bacteria as well as fungi. A suitable blood culture technique is described on p. 296.

The treatment of endocarditis is governed *by rules* similar to those for the treatment of septicaemia (see p. 297), but with different doses and varying duration of treatment. While bacteriostatic drugs can be effective in other forms of septicaemia, bacterial endocarditis can only be eradicated by a bactericidal agent. Corticosteroids and anticoagulants are contraindicated because of the risk of valve perforation or embolic disease.

The *efficacy of antibiotic treatment* may be *predicted* by determining (a) the minimal inhibitory concentration (MIC) and minimal bactericidal concentration (MBC) of the antibiotics used against the patient's isolate; (b) the presence or absence of synergy in the antibiotic combination used against the patient's isolate, or (c) the bactericidal activity of the patient's serum during treatment against his own isolate.

Treatment can be considered *satisfactory* when dilutions of at least 1 in 4 are completely bactericidal to the patient's isolate and this index, which is easily determined in a hospital bacteriology laboratory, correlates well with the clinical outcome of treatment.

Criteria of successful treatment: Defervescence, return to normal ESR, resolution of clinical symptoms, absence of fever after discontinuation of antibiotics and subsequent negative blood cultures. Treatment at full antibiotic dosage should continue for 4–6 weeks or until the ESR returns to normal. Longer courses of treatment are necessary for endocarditis after the insertion of a prosthetic heart valve, and the prognosis is poor. Blood concentrations should be carefully monitored when potentially ototoxic antibiotics (e. g. gentamicin etc.) are used and when renal failure is suspected. Blood should be taken immediately prior to an injection, when the serum concentrations should be less than 1 mg/l if no accumulation of the aminoglycoside has occurred.

Surgical replacement of the diseased valve should be considered early if the causative organism is resistant to bactericidal therapy, or if signs of valve perforation develop.

Treatment

Streptococcal endocarditis is mostly subacute *(endocarditis lenta)* and due to viridans and non-haemolytic streptococci or pneumococci. Benzyl penicillin is the drug of choice at a dosage related to the sensitivity of the isolate, in combination with gentamicin at standard dosage (240 mg daily in patients with normal renal function).

Standard treatment (also applicable to less sensitive strains of streptococci with minimal inhibitory concentrations *in vitro* of 1–2 units of penicillin/ml):

20–30 megaunits of benzyl penicillin sodium in 3–4 short i. v. infusions, and possibly as a large dose of procaine penicillin i. m. at night. The addition of an aminoglycoside (formerly streptomycin, now gentamicin, 80 mg i. m. 2–3 times a day) is of proven value with the lower doses of penicillin used formerly, and is essential when the sensitivity to penicillin is poor. Treatment should last for (3–) 4–6 weeks, if possible until the ESR has returned completely to normal. Blood cultures taken at intervals during treatment should be negative.

Where the *streptococci* are very sensitive to penicillin (MIC less than 0.1 units/ ml), the dose of penicillin can be reduced to 5(−10) megaunits per day though it is advisable to combine with probenecid (500 mg by mouth 4 times a day) to increase the penicillin blood concentration. In patients allergic to penicillin, combine cefazolin i. v. in high dosage with gentamicin, having excluded cross-allergy. Vancomycin and clindamycin are alternative treatments.

Enterococcal endocarditis is generally subacute but occasionally acute and is difficult to treat because of antibiotic resistance. Occurrence in women is usually after febrile abortion or during a urinary infection.

Treatment: Benzyl penicillin, 30–60 megaunits a day or ampicillin or amoxy-cillin, 10–20 g a day in 2–3 short infusions or slow i. v. injections (for 6–8 weeks); combination with gentamicin (80 mg i. m. or i. v. 3 times a day) is essential to overcome the Eagle effect (see p. 267) and to achieve bactericidal activity through synergy. The failure to treat with this synergistic combination amounts to clinical malpractice.

Vancomycin may be used as an alternative to ampicillin in cases of *allergy,* but should not be combined with other ototoxic antibiotics. Mezlocillin is the most active penicillin *in vitro* against enterococci, but clinical experience of this agent is still limited. Like all β-lactam antibiotics in enterococcal endocarditis, mezlocillin should only be given in combination with gentamicin.

If treatment with bactericidal antibiotics fails, a long-term treatment with doxycycline can be palliative.

Endocarditis caused by Streptococcus bovis (also in Lancefield group D but not a true enterococcus) is often associated with carcinoma of the colon and is more responsive to antibiotics than enterococcal endocarditis.

Treatment: Benzyl penicillin (30–40 megaunits a day) + gentamicin.

Endocarditis with Staphylococcus aureus or S. epidermidis: If the organism is *sensitive to penicillin,* give benzyl penicillin, 20–40 megaunits a day, as 4–6 short infusions, or slow i. v. injections.

Against *penicillin-resistant* organisms, give flucloxacillin, 12–15 g in 4–6 short infusions or slow i. v. injections combined with gentamicin (80 mg i. m. 3 times). The addition of fusidic acid is also effective.

In cases *resistant to flucloxacillin,* give vancomycin 1 g i. v. twice a day (see p. 167), or lincomycin i. v., 1.2 g twice a day. *Allergy to penicillin:* treat with cefazolin i. v. in high dosage (exclude cross-allergy).

Long-term treatment is necessary; when improvement is sufficient for oral antibiotics to be given, continue with flucloxacillin or phenoxymethyl penicillin by mouth, according to sensitivities. If antibiotic treatment of post-cardiotomy endocarditis fails, a further operation should be considered which should remove residual foci of infection, particularly if mycotic vegetations are still present.

Endocarditis due to gram-negative bacteria carries a poor prognosis, is little affected by antibiotics and maximum dosage is always necessary (see Table 39). In general, a combination of a β-lactam antibiotic with an aminoglycoside should be given, according to antibiotic sensitivities.

Escherichia coli: Cefotaxime (or possibly cefuroxime or mezlocillin) + gentamicin.

Klebsiella pneumoniae: Cefotaxime (or cefoxitin) + gentamicin.

Enterobacter species: According to antibiotic sensitivity testing, cefotaxime or latamoxef + gentamicin.

Pseudomonas aeruginosa: Azlocillin + tobramycin, possibly also piperacillin, cefsulodin or ceftazidime in combination with amikacin.

Proteus mirabilis: Cefotaxime + gentamicin, or alternatively ampicillin + gentamicin.

Other Proteus species: Cefoxitin (or cefotaxime) + an aminoglycoside, or alternatively mezlocillin or piperacillin in combination with amikacin.

Salmonellae: Ampicillin (or mezlocillin) + an aminoglycoside, or alternatively cefotaxime.

Serratia: Cefotaxime (or ceftazidime) + an aminoglycoside, or alternatively mezlocillin or piperacillin, in combination with amikacin.

Haemophilus species: Cefotaxime + an aminoglycoside should replace the former treatment with ampicillin + an aminoglycoside.

Campylobacter endocarditis: Occurs in both healthy and damaged heart valves. The organism is isolated from anaerobic blood culture and treatment should be with gentamicin i. m. + clindamycin i. v. for at least 4 weeks.

Fungal endocarditis: Occurs in heroin addicts, after cardiac operations and in patients with prolonged indwelling catheters. Candida or aspergillus may be involved and can sometimes only be cultured from arterial blood.

In Candida endocarditis: Give amphotericin B, in increasing dosage up to 1 mg/ kg/day (see p. 175), in combination with flucytosine (*if in vitro* activity has been proven). Surgical removal of the infected valve, with prosthetic replacement, is usually essential. Large septic emboli should also be treated surgically.

Q-fever endocarditis: Coxiella burneti cannot be isolated from blood culture. A provisional diagnosis is made in the absence of other bacterial causes of the endocarditis, but with a positive C. burneti CFT and a supporting clinical picture. *Treatment* may be attempted with doxycycline (200 mg per day) for ½–1 year, or another tetracycline for 1–2 years, but often fails to sterilise the valve. Prosthetic valve replacement is almost always necessary.

Culture-negative endocarditis: If cultures of several blood samples using satisfactory culture methods remain sterile in a patient not pre-treated with antibiotics and with a typical clinical picture of subacute endocarditis, a diagnosis of culture-negative endocarditis must be made and the patient should be treated with benzyl penicillin, 40 megaunits a day, + gentamicin, 240 mg a day. If a clinical response fails to occur within 48–72 hours, a causative organism resistant to penicillin and gentamicin (Q-fever, chlamydiae, Haemophilus) should be suspected and the patient treated with doxycycline. Endocarditis due to Bacteroides fragilis (anaerobes) is best treated with clindamycin, cefoxitin or metronidazole i. v., alone or in combination.

Initial treatment before culture results are available: Endocarditis cannot be satisfactorily treated without the culture of the organism from the blood and the determination of quantitative sensitivities. If antibiotics are started before a bacterial diagnosis is made, subsequent attempts to isolate the causative organism may be worthwhile by stopping antibiotics and taking blood cultures after

2–3 days. If a bacterial cause is still lacking, continue treatment according to the clinical picture either with benzyl penicillin (40 megaunits a day) + gentamicin, as for subacute streptococcal endocarditis, or treat as acute staphylococcal endocarditis. In cases resistant to therapy, use a combination of a β-lactamase-stable cephalosporin with gentamicin.

Endocarditis in heroin addicts: Staphylococci cause the majority (approx. 50%) of infections and enterobacteria about 20%. Pseudomonas, streptococci, enterococci, Candida and mixed infections are less common. The endocarditis is usually acute and often affects the right side of the heart with multiple pulmonary infiltrates. Heart murmurs are sometimes absent. Left heart involvement suggests a poor prognosis. Severe neurological signs frequently develop, caused by metastatic foci of infection. Because of the poor prognosis, *antibiotic treatment* should be started as soon as possible after taking the initial blood cultures, with combinations such as: cefoxitin + azlocillin + gentamicin, or cefotaxime + azlocillin + gentamicin. The antibiotic regime should be modified according to the results of sensitivity testing. Candida endocarditis requires surgical removal of the valve and treatment with amphotericin B + flucytosine (if the isolate is sensitive to the latter).

All forms of bacterial endocarditis can extensively **damage the affected heart valves** and give rise to uncontrollable heart failure, correctable only by urgent valve replacement. When endocarditis follows open heart surgery, the infected prosthetic valve may itself need replacement but a trial of intensive bactericidal antibiotic therapy may be worthwhile before operative removal.

Prevention of endocarditis: The development of bacterial endocarditis can be prevented in certain circumstances by prophylactic antibiotics. Patients with rheumatic heart disease or congenital heart defects or who have had cardiac surgery or a previous attack of bacterial endocarditis are at particular risk when they undergo dental extractions, tonsillectomy, urogenital or intestinal surgery or open heart surgery and these procedures should be covered by antibiotic prophylaxis.

Choice of antibiotic and dosage:

For tonsillectomy, adenoidectomy or dental extraction, give benzyl penicillin 1–2 megaunits 2 hours before the operation (not earlier because of the risk of selection of penicillin-resistant bacteria) followed by 1 megaunit 6 hours later. Alternatively, the same total dose of procaine penicillin may be given 2 hours before the procedure. If oral prophylaxis is required, adult patients not allergic to penicillins should take amoxycillin 3 grams by mouth 1 hour before the procedure;

children aged 5–10 should take half the adult dose and children under 5 one quarter the adult dose.

Amoxycillin is preferred to phenoxymethyl penicillin in the recommendations of the British Society of Antimicrobial Chemotherapy (1982) on the grounds of improved absorption. For patients in hospital, this working party recommended the following prophylaxis for dental, genitourinary, obstetric, gynaecological and gastrointestinal procedures:

a) Patients to be given a general anaesthetic who are *not allergic to penicillins* but who have received penicillin in the previous month or who have a prosthetic heart valve should receive amoxycillin 1 g i. m. in 2.5 ml of 1% lignocaine plus gentamicin 120 mg i. m. immediately before induction of anaesthesia or 15 min before the dental procedure. A further 500 mg of amoxycillin should be given by mouth 6 hours later. Children under 10 should receive half the adult dose of amoxycillin and 2 mg/kg body weight of gentamicin.

b) Patients *allergic to penicillin* who are to be given a general anaesthetic should receive a single dose of vancomycin 1 g by slow i. v. infusion over 20–30 min followed by gentamicin 120 mg i. v. before induction of anaesthesia. Children under 10 should receive vancomycin 20 mg/kg and gentamicin 2 mg/kg body weight in the same way.

There is a risk of staphylococcal endocarditis, particularly with Staphylococcus epidermidis, in heart surgery and diagnostic procedures in the heart and great vessels, for which prophylaxis with flucloxacillin or cefazolin i. v. should be given, possibly supplemented with gentamicin.

References

American Heart Association, Committee on Prevention of Rheumatic Fever and Bacterial Endocarditis: Prevention of Rheumatic Fever. Circulation *55:* 1 (1977).

American Heart Association, Committee on Prevention of Rheumatic Fever and Bacterial Endocarditis: Prevention of Bacterial Endocarditis. Circulation *56:* 139A (1977).

BISNO, A.: Treatment of infective endocarditis. Grune & Stratton, New York 1981.

DAVIS, W. A., II, J. G. KANE, V. F. GARAGUSI: Human aeromonas infections. A review of the literature and a case report of endocarditis. Medicine *57:* 267 (1978).

DICK, D. C., C. G. A. McGREGOR, K. G. MITCHELL, R. G. SOMMERVILLE, D. J. WHEATLEY: Endocarditis as a manifestation of Chlamydia B infection (psittacosis). Brit. Heart. J. *39:* 914 (1977).

DUMA, R. J.: Infections of Prosthetic Heart Valves and Vascular Grafts. University Park Press, Baltimore 1977.

ELSTER, A. K., L. M. MATTES: Haemophilus aphrophilus endocarditis: Review of 23 cases. Amer. J. Cardiol. *35:* 72 (1975).

EVERETT, E. D., J. V. HIRSCHMANN: Transient bacteremia and endocarditis prophylaxis. A review. Medicine *56:* 61 (1977).

JULANDER, I.: Haemophilus parainfluenzae: An uncommon cause of septicemia and endocarditis. Scand. J. infect. Dis. *12:* 85 (1980).

KAMMER, R. B., J. P. UTZ: Aspergillus species endocarditis. Amer. J. Med. *56:* 506 (1974).

KARCHMER, A. W., E. B. STINSON: The Role of Surgery in Infective Endocarditis. In: J. REMINGTON, M. SWARTZ: Current Clinical Topics in Infectious Diseases. I. McGraw Hill, New York 1980.

KIMBROUGH, R. C. III, R. A. ORMSBEE, M. PEACOCK: Q fever endocarditis in the United States. Ann. intern. Med. *91:* 400 (1979).

LYNN, D. J., J. G. KANE: Haemophilus parainfluenzae and influenzae endocarditis: A review of forty cases. Medicine *56:* 115 (1977).

MYEROWITZ, P. D., P. GARDNER, C. CAMPBELL, J. LAMBERTI, R. L. REPLOGLE, C. E. ANAGNOSTOPOULOS: Early operation for left-sided Pseudomonas endocarditis in drug addicts. J. thorac. cardiovasc. Surg. *77:* 577 (1979).

NASTRO, L. J., S. M. FINEGOLD: Endocarditis due to anaerobic gram-negative bacilli. Amer. J. Med. *54:* 482 (1973).

O'MEARA, J. B.: Brucella melitensis endocarditis: successful treatment of an infected prosthetic mitral valve. Thorax *29:* 377 (1974).

RAHIMTOOLA, S. H.: Infective Endocarditis. Grune & Stratton, New York 1978.

SAFFLE, J. R., P. GARDNER, S. C. SCHOENBAUM: Prosthetic valve endocarditis. The case for prompt valve replacement. J. thorac. cardiovasc. Surg. *73:* 416 (1977).

SHANSON D. C., R. F. U. ASHFORD, J. SINGH: High dose oral amoxycillin for preventing endocarditis. Brit. med. J. *280:* 446 (1980).

SKLAVER, A. R., T. A. HOFFMAN, R. L. GREENMAN: Staphylococcal endocarditis in adults. South. Med. J. *71:* 638 (1978).

VAN DER BEL-KAHN, J. M., C. WATANAKUNAKORN, M. G. MENEFEE, H. D. LONG, R. DICTER: Chlamydia trachomatis endocarditis. Amer. Heart J. *95:* 627 (1978).

WEIR, E. K., H. S. JOFFE: Purulent pericarditis in children: An analysis of 28 cases. Thorax *32:* 438 (1977).

Working Party Report: The antibiotic prophylaxis of infective endocarditis. Lancet *II:* 1323 (1982).

4. Bacterial Pericarditis

Bacterial pericarditis arises either by *haematogenous spread* of organisms (Staphylococcus, Haemophilus, Neisseria) or by *direct* spread from an adjacent focus (pneumonia, mediastinitis, hilar tuberculosis). The exudate is generally purulent in septic pericarditis, serous in viral pericarditis, scanty and serofibrinous in rheumatic and uraemic pericarditis and often haemorrhagic with multiple often loculated, serous effusions in tuberculous pericarditis (pleural effusions, constrictive pericarditis). Pathogenic bacteria are absent in the post-cardiotomy syndrome, an important feature in the differential diagnosis.

Treatment: In suppurative pericarditis, antibiotics should be active against the causative organism (staphylococci, streptococci etc.), and appropriate for the underlying infection, whether septicaemia (see p. 300), pneumonia (p. 347) or tuberculosis (p. 464). In cases of previously treated purulent pericarditis in which no pathogen has been isolated a cephalosporin + gentamicin should be given. Large effusions should be tapped and constrictive pericarditis treated by pericardectomy. The postpericardiotomy syndrome responds well to anti-inflammatory therapy with aspirin or corticosteroids.

Reference

GERSONY, W. M., A. H. HORDORF: Infective endocarditis and disease of the pericardium. Pediatr. Clin. North Amer. *25:* 831 (1978).

5. Meningitis

Meningitis is best **classified** according to its cause, whether viral, bacterial, fungal or protozoal. Although the distinction between lymphocytic and purulent meningitis is important, it is not invariably related to aetiology, because not all cases of lymphocytic meningitis are caused by viruses (tuberculous, cryptococcal and leptospiral meningitis, and the phase of resolution of purulent meningitis); not all cases of purulent meningitis are bacterial (a polymorphonuclear leucocytic exudate can predominate at the beginning of an echo or coxsackie virus meningitis). The distinction between serous meningitis, with a clear CSF and a cell count of less than 300/μl, and purulent meningitis with cloudy CSF and a cell count greater than 300/μl is also not an entirely reliable guide to the cause.

Viruses are frequently associated with serous meningitis but so, on occasion, are bacteria and fungi (tubercle bacilli, Treponema pallidum, Campylobacter, Leptospira, Listeria). On the other hand, cloudy CSF is not always an index of bacterial meningitis, since quite high cell counts of around 300/μl are found in certain viral infections (e. g. mumps meningitis, echovirus meningitis), making the CSF slightly opaque. At the onset of bacterial meningitis, the cell counts can still be low and may not rise until later in the course of the infection, sometimes despite treatment. In purulent bacterial meningitis, the lactate dehydrogenase (LDH) and lactic acid content of the CSF are greatly increased. Non-infectious causes such as leukaemia, irritation from adjacent lesions (sympathetic meningitis in sinusitis, otitis, mastoiditis, brain abscess), brain tumour etc. should also be considered. When clinical signs of meningitis are present, other causes such as a subarachnoid haemorrhage, cervical spine syndrome and encephalitis have to be excluded.

A lumbar puncture should be performed whenever meningitis is suspected, and before beginning antibiotic treatment. The cell count should if possible be performed within 30 min of CSF collection, at which time methylene blue, gram, and giemsa preparations are made for the differentiation of cells. The rapid identification of meningococcal, pneumococcal and haemophilus antigen in CSF is now possible using a simple latex agglutination technique which can readily be performed in every hospital laboratory. A negative result does not, however, exclude a bacterial cause.

When pneumococci are present in the CSF smear they are often very numerous. They are lanceolate gram-positive diplococci, often extracellular and surrounded by a mucous capsule. Meningococci are predominantly intracellular in the cytoplasm of polymorphonuclear leucocytes; they are gram-negative, kidney-shaped diplococci and are often only present in small numbers in the CSF. Haemophilus influenzae is a fine gram-negative extracellular rod of varying size (pleomorphism); in some cases it resembles a cocco-bacillus, and in others it is a very long and spindly gram-negative bacillus. Other causes of meningitis are only broadly classifiable as gram-negative or gram-positive rods or cocci by microscopic examination.

Regardless of the microscopical findings, a bacterial culture should always be made. Where the CSF cell count is below 1000/μl, a Ziehl-Neelsen stain of the centrifuged deposit should be made and acid-fast bacilli sought. The CSF from serous meningitis should be refrigerated overnight and examined for a spider web clot of suspected tuberculosis the next day. If found, the clot is examined for acid-fast bacilli microscopically after heat-fixation and staining by the Ziehl-Neelsen method.

Where gram-positive or gram-negative cocci or bacilli are seen, a rapid direct sensitivity test with the appropriate antibiotics can be performed with an inoculum from the spun deposit and read within 8–12 hours. A blood culture before treatment should always be taken since it is often positive in haematogenous meningitis, sometimes when the CSF is still negative. The patient should be examined for the likely focus of infection, such as sinusitis, otitis media, lobar pneumonia, skull fracture etc., if necessary in consultation with an ophthalmologist, an otorhinolaryngologist or a chest physician. A chest x-ray is useful in pneumococcal meningitis (concomitant lobar pneumonia or bronchiectasis) and in tuberculous meningitis. A low CSF sugar with a predominantly lymphocytic picture is very suggestive of tuberculous meningitis. Where the CSF is serous but the cell count increased, viral culture should be performed on CSF, a throat swab and faeces, and serum samples taken in the acute phase and 10–14 days later may be usefully tested for a rise in specific antibody titres.

Antibiotic treatment should be started as a matter of **urgency,** since any delay may prejudice the chance of a complete cure. Early fatalities during the first 24 hours of treatment are generally due not to failure of antibiotics but to the effects of an already well-established meningitis or to a fulminant infection with particularly virulent organisms. The clinical outcome may well depend on the rapidity with which the patient can be admitted to hospital, the CSF examined and treatment commenced. Where possible, the patient should not be given an antibiotic before the lumbar puncture has been performed because of the danger of failure to culture the causative organism and test antibiotic sensitivities. If the transport of the patient to hospital is likely to take more than 2 hours, however, an antibiotic may be given as immediate treatment before lumbar puncture, such as cefotaxime 2 g slowly i. v. or i. m. for adults and 100 mg/kg for small children. This course may be life-saving in fulminant meningococcal septicaemia and meningitis, which is readily recognisable by a spreading purpuric rash in a shocked patient with worsening meningism and a deteriorating level of consciousness.

The CSF usually becomes sterile after 24 hours of successful treatment, and a further lumbar puncture is useful at this time.

The **frequency** with which different organisms cause meningitis depends to some extend on the patient's age. While meningococci are the commonest single bacterial cause of meningitis in adults and older children (about 40–50%, or 25% overall), pneumococci are twice as common as causes of meningitis in adults (about 40%) as in children. Meningitis due to Haemophilus influenzae, on the other hand, accounts for about 20% of cases in children and only 1% in adults. Meningitis due to enterobacteria (Escherichia coli, Klebsiella etc.) and group B streptococci predominates in the newborn and young infants. Other bacterial causes of meningitis (salmonellae, staphylococci, streptococci, Listeria, Pseudomonas aeruginosa, Klebsiella pneumoniae, Enterobacter aerogenes, Proteus etc.) are rare in younger adults. In the elderly, pneumococci commonly cause meningitis, Listeria and Enterobacteria occasionally, while meningococci are rare.

The culture of skin organisms such as Staphylococcus epidermidis, Corynebacteria and aerobic spore-bearing bacilli must be evaluated critically, since they may well be contaminants unless the patient has an indwelling Spitz-Holter valve or a CSF rhinorrhoea. Mixed infections sometimes occur in otogenic meningitis.

The **CSF penetration** of the antibiotics given is a key factor in successful treatment. The percentage of the serum concentration of various antimicrobials to enter the CSF of normal individuals is about 50% for certain sulphonamides, 30–50% for chloramphenicol, 30% for minocycline, about 10% for the other tetracyclines and less than 1% for penicillins and cephalosporins. Some antibiotics diffuse better through infected meninges into the CSF than they do in healthy persons. Effective CSF concentrations are obtained more rapidly after i. v. injection than after oral or i. m. administration. In meningitis, high doses of benzyl penicillin (10–20 megaunits/day) produce effective concentrations against meningo- and pneumococci in the CSF. If the CSF is not sterile after one day of systemic treatment, an additional intrathecal antibiotic may be administered if there is any likelihood that the meningitis is caused by enterobacteria, which is extremely rare in adults. The dosage recommendations (see Table 41, p. 329) must be meticulously followed with intrathecal antibiotics in order to avoid dangerous side effects; correct technique (slow injection of 1 ml in 1 min once a day only, for no longer than 2–3 days) must be followed. The intraventricular route is preferable to the lumbar intrathecal in infants with an open fontanelle. When benzyl penicillin is given by the lumbar intrathecal route, the dosage of penicillin given systemically should be reduced from 20 to 5–10 megaunits/day in order to avoid the neurotoxicity associated with CSF concentrations that are too high. Adequate tissue concentrations are as important as the CSF levels. The choice of antibiotic and its proper dosage are, therefore, more important for successful treatment than intrathecal administration, the effect of which may be unreliable.

Meningitis is not suitable for the clinical trial of a new antibiotic. It is unethical to use inadequately tested antibiotics in bacterial meningitis until animal experiments have clearly shown adequate CSF penetration and efficacy in experimental meningitis, and the clinical effectiveness of the agent in less serious infections in man is well established.

Other aspects of treatment: Intensive care, treatment of respiratory distress, tracheotomy in cases with prolonged unconsciousness, mechanical ventilation and regular aspiration of respiratory secretions, treatment of shock, maintenance of fluid and electrolyte balance, parenteral or nasogastric nutrition etc. Unconscious patients should receive antacids through a nasogastric tube to prevent stress ulcers. Cerebral oedema should be treated with dexamethasone i. v. (10 mg initially, then 4 mg every 6 h), and with frusemide. Repeated lumbar puncture may be needed to relieve pressure, and is useful to monitor treatment, since an increase in the CSF cell count may indicate failure of treatment or a change of infection. Epileptiform convulsions may arise as a result of penicillin overdosage and a maximum of 20 megaunits of benzyl penicillin a day in adults or 12 megaunits a day in children should be given in the acute phase of meningitis, when the permeability of the blood-CSF barrier is increased. Convulsions caused by penicillin overdosage can be controlled with diazepam (Valium) or barbiturate, and the penicillin may have to be discontinued temporarily. If a brain abscess is suspected, a computerized axial tomogram (CT scan) should be obtained as soon as possible, in order to guide any neurosurgical intervention. Once antibiotic treatment has started, antrotomy may be performed in cases of definite otogenic meningitis, and sinus irrigation where sinusitis is the initial focus.

Failure of antibiotic treatment where the CSF continues to yield positive cultures, the cell count increases or fever continues, can have a number of causes, including choice of the wrong antibiotic, underdosage, re-infection with a new microorganism, persistence of a local focus of infection (cervical abscess, subdural abscess, cranial osteomyelitis, sinusitis, mastoiditis, otitis etc.), purulent meta-stases in the brain, subdural haemorrhage, loculated residual foci of meningitis, relapse after premature cessation of antibiotics, metastatic abscesses in other organs (e. g. endocarditis) etc. Persisting fever is sometimes caused by an allergy to drugs (drug fever) and may be associated with eosinophilia and a skin rash. A rise in temperature and vomiting in the newborn and children are often caused by a developing hydrocephalus, which should be treated by the insertion of a shunt. Symptoms of blockage of CSF circulation due to fibrin clots are particularly associated with pneumococcal or staphylococcal meningitis and can be treated by intralumbar instillation of streptokinase (50000 units), and also by small quantities of prednisone: 10–20(–50) mg once a day for adults and 2 to 10 mg for children. Purulent meningitis can cause subdural effusion in children, especially with pneumococcal infection, which can be detected by echoencephalography and computerized axial tomography.

The appropriate antibiotic, given in the correct **dosage** (see Table 40) by the best route (always parenteral to begin with, and i. v. if possible) for a sufficiently long period are all important in obtaining optimal blood, tissue and CSF concentrations, which should be bactericidal where possible. When penicillins are used, they should be continued in high dosage even when the meningitis is healing, because decreasing CSF penetration in a resolving meningitis may otherwise lead to relapse. Chloramphenicol, which penetrates into CSF better, can be used as an alternative to penicillin, as can a sulphonamide or co-trimoxazole, provided the bacterial isolate is sensitive. These alternatives also have the advantage of being well absorbed by mouth, at a late stage of treatment in children.

The value of *cephalosporins* in meningitis varies according to the individual preparations. The earlier cephalosporins and some of the newer ones are unsuitable for the treatment of meningitis. Only cefuroxime, cefotaxime, ceftriaxone and latamoxef have been shown to be clinically effective in meningitis to date. They are active in many infections by otherwise resistant enterobacteria and Haemophilus influenzae. The newer cephalosporins and other β-lactam antibiotics soon to be introduced should only be used to treat meningitis when careful clinical trials have established their effectiveness for this indication.

a) Initial Therapy (Pathogen Unknown)

When pneumococci or meningococci are *seen by direct microscopy* and the latex agglutination test with CSF, serum or urine is positive, benzyl penicillin is the drug

Table 40. Dosage of parenteral agents used to treat meningitis.

Antibiotic	Daily dose for children	Daily dose for adults
Benzyl penicillin	(Maximum dose 12.0 megaunits) 1.0 megaunits/kg (newborn) 1.0 megaunits/kg (infant) 0.5 megaunits/kg (older children)	10–20 (–30) megaunits
Ampicillin Flucloxacillin	100 mg/kg (newborn) 300 mg/kg (infants up to 3 months) At least 2 g (children 1/4–2 yrs) At least 4 g (children 2-6 yrs) At least 6 g (children older than 6 years)	6–10 (–20) g
Azlocillin Mezlocillin Piperacillin	100 mg/kg (newborn) 300 mg/kg (older children)	15–20 g
Cefotaxime	100 mg/kg (newborn) 150 mg/kg (older children)	6–8 g
Latamoxef	60 mg/kg (newborn) 100 mg/kg (infants)	4–6 g
Chloramphenicol	25 mg/kg (the newborn in the 1st and 2nd week) 50 mg/kg (3rd–4th week) 80–100 mg/kg (infants) 50–80 mg/kg (older children)	3 (–4) g

of choice. If no organisms are seen or if, in a young child, gram-negative bacilli are detected microscopically, the cause may be Haemophilus influenzae; the specific latex agglutination test is usually positive. Cefotaxime is now the treatment of first choice and preferable to chloramphenicol or ampicillin.

Where direct microscopy fails to show organisms in adults, Listeria is occasionally a cause, though it is commoner in the newborn; ampicillin, which is also effective against meningococci, is then the best initial therapy though chloramphenicol may also be used.

Many organisms can cause meningitis in *the first two months of life* and a combination of cefotaxime, piperacillin and gentamicin in adequate dosage (see Table 40) has generally proved to be satisfactory initial treatment.

b) Therapy (Pathogen Known)

Meningococcal meningitis is almost always haematogenous in origin. Meningococcal antigen of serogroups A, B and C can now be demonstrated rapidly using the latex agglutination test which is also positive in patients in whom treatment has already been started. CSF should be cultured in the usual manner; where there is no diagnostic bacteriological laboratory on site and delay in transit may occur, the CSF may be inoculated into a commercial kit consisting of a dip slide within a blood culture bottle (Roche Diagnostics) and incubated pending transmission.

Benzyl penicillin in large doses is the antibiotic of choice (20 megaunits a day for adults, 0.5 megaunits/kg/day for children and 1 megaunit/kg/day for the newborn) in short i.v. infusions every 6–8 hours until improvement (at least 3 days after defervescence) followed by a reduced dose (5–10 megaunits) for a total of 2 weeks.

In patients *allergic to penicillin* give chloramphenicol in the dosage shown in Table 40. Treatment with a sulphonamide alone is no longer reliable because of the prevalence of sulphonamide-resistant strains of meningococci. Treatment of the *Waterhouse-Friderichsen syndrome* is described on p. 303. Minocycline may be used for prophylaxis in close (household) contacts in a dose of 100 mg twice a day for adults and 2 mg/kg twice a day for children for 2–5 days in epidemics with sulphonamide-resistant meningococci (see p. 303 also).

An alternative used because of minocycline-associated giddiness is rifampicin 600 mg in adults, 10 mg/kg in children aged 1–2 years, and 5 mg/kg in children under one year old, all twice a day for 2 days. Rifampicin resistance has, however, been reported in meningococci.

Pneumococcal meningitis is haematogenous in origin or spreads directly from the paranasal sinuses, mastoid, a cerebral abscess or skull fracture; examination by an otorhinolaryngologist may be helpful, as may surgery after antibiotic treatment.

Treatment: Benzyl penicillin in large dosage (20 megaunits a day for adults, 0.5 megaunits/kg for children and 1 megaunit/kg for the newborn) given as a short i. v. infusion every 6 hours. Duration of treatment: at least 10 days on full dosage. Meningitis caused by penicillin-resistant pneumococci has been reported in South Africa; the only reliably effective antimicrobial in many cases was rifampicin.

Because of the relatively high mortality of pneumococcal meningitis despite antibiotic treatment, the risk of relapse and the possibility of persistent, inaccessible infection in the paranasal sinuses, which formed the initial focus of meningitis, high-dose penicillin treatment should be continued for several weeks. Chloramphenicol is the best alternative in patients allergic to penicillin; it also penetrates CSF well, even if the meninges are not inflamed. Additional intrathecal penicillin is not necessary.

Haemophilus influenzae meningitis is of haematogenous, otogenic or rhinogenic origin, is much commoner in children than in adults, and can carry a poor prognosis. It is mainly caused by serotype b, in which case the rapid latex agglutination test for the demonstration of antigen in CSF, serum or urine is usually positive, even after treatment has begun.

Treatment: Chloramphenicol or ampicillin have until recently been the drugs of choice. The testing of ampicillin sensitivity is unreliable since not all resistant strains produce β-lactamase *in vitro* and some resistant strains can appear sensitive. The number of strains resistant to chloramphenicol, and sometimes to both antibiotics, has increased and cefotaxime has therefore become the most reliable treatment of Haemophilus meningitis. Latamoxef is used as an alternative to cefotaxime in the U.S.A. Haemophilus prophylaxis is now advised for children under 4 years who have been in close contact with the patient. Oral rifampicin 20 mg/kg per day up to a maximum dose of 600 mg should be given for 4 days. This is based on a secondary attack rate of approximately 5% in contacts aged 2 years or less in comparison with an overall rate of 0.4%.

Escherichia coli meningitis may have few, ill-defined signs in infants, which are easily overlooked. The prognosis is poor. It is rare in adults, in whom it is usually found after head injuries or neurosurgical operations, and occasionally found after urogenital surgery.

Treatment: When plump gram-negative rods are seen on direct microscopy of the CSF deposit, an antibiotic combination in high dosage should be given before culture and antibiotic sensitivities are available because the disease is life-threatening.

Cefotaxime is now more successful than traditional treatment with chloramphenicol, mezlocillin or ampicillin in combination with gentamicin (for dosage, see Table 40). Intrathecal instillation of gentamicin or another antibiotic once a day is only necessary if bacteria are still present in the CSF after 24 hours.

Where the organisms are sensitive, the high-dosage treatment is continued for 3–4 weeks. Treatment must be guided by antibiotic sensitivity testing, since enterobacteria vary considerably in their sensitivity to different antibiotics.

Listeria meningitis is generally intrauterine in origin in premature and full-term neonates, although it can occur in later childhood and occasionally in adults, usually when resistance is lowered by some underlying disease. It is always haematogenous and develops into a purulent or serous meningitis.

Treatment: Ampicillin i. v., 6–10 g a day for adults (200–400 mg/kg for children) in 3–4 single doses.

Minocycline may be used in cases of allergy to penicillin (200 mg a day for adults, 4 mg/kg a day for children).

Large doses of benzyl penicillin (20 megaunits), piperacillin and chloramphenicol have also been given successfully. Duration of treatment: until the CSF has returned to normal, and generally for at least 3 weeks. A sequential course of minocycline (which penetrates CSF quite well) or ampicillin derivatives at intervals of 2–3 weeks is strongly recommended because of the high risk of relapse. Cephalosporins are ineffective.

Staphylococcal meningitis: Occurs during staphylococcal septicaemia or endocarditis of otogenic, rhinogenic or post-traumatic origin. Staphylococcal meningitis may accompany a septic focal encephalitis or a brain abscess, and the initial focus should always be sought. Staphylococci are the usual causes of septicaemia and meningitis associated with shunts (after hydrocephalus operations) and are sometimes combined with ventriculitis. If the shunt is the only part of the system to be infected, it can be rendered sterile by injecting 0.5–1 mg of gentamicin intrathecally into the cranial or distal arm. In most cases, however, the infected shunt has to be removed for the infection to be eradicated.

Treatment: Benzyl penicillin + flucloxacillin i. v. initially (dosage: see Table 40), until antibiotic sensitivities are available. Benzyl penicillin i. v. may be given for sensitive staphylococci, and flucloxacillin i. v. for penicillin-resistant staphylococci (dosage: see Table 40).

Cefuroxime i. v. is an alternative in patients allergic to penicillin, since it achieves better CSF concentrations than many other cephalosporins. The dose is 6 g a day for adults and 100 mg/kg for children in 3–4 short infusions. Other antibiotics should only be used if they are found to be sensitive on testing, and are

Table 41. Dosage for intrathecal administration (once a day).

Antibiotic	Children	Adults
Benzyl penicillin	Not indicated	Not indicated
Ampicillin	5–10 mg	10–20 (–40) mg
Cloxacillin	5–10 mg	10–20 mg
Cephaloridine	20 mg	30–50 mg
Polymyxin B	2 mg	5 mg
Gentamicin[1]	0.5–1 mg	5 mg

[1] for intrathecal administration.

known to achieve satisfactory CSF concentrations. Cloxacillin may be given once a day for 2–3 days by the intrathecal route (for dosage, see Table 41).

High-dose antibiotic therapy should be maintained for 3–4 weeks, and followed by a further 3–4 weeks of flucloxacillin, cephradine, clindamycin or erythromycin (according to sensitivity testing) to prevent relapse.

Group B streptococcal meningitis has become the second commonest cause of meningitis in Britain and Western Europe in the newborn and young infant (Escherichia coli still being the commonest). Non-capsulated gram-positive diplococci are seen in the CSF deposit. The latex agglutination test is positive in CSF and serum.

Treatment is as for pneumococcal meningitis.

Enterococcal meningitis is rare, and is an occasional complication of enterococcal endocarditis. The initial focus must be eradicated.

Treatment: Ampicillin i. v. (dosage: Table 40). Minocycline i. v. in cases allergic to penicillin, 0.2 g a day for adults, and 4 mg/kg for children.

Duration of treatment: 2–4 weeks, followed by minocycline for 2–3 weeks to prevent relapse.

Pseudomonas aeruginosa meningitis generally arises by direct inoculation, not uncommonly after diagnostic, therapeutic or surgical procedures. Spread is sometimes direct from the ear and sometimes haematogenous as part of a Pseudomonas septicaemia.

Treatment: Azlocillin or piperacillin i. v. in combination with tobramycin (dosage: Table 40); cefsulodin, ceftazidime or amikacin in case of resistance to other agents.

An additional intrathecal instillation of polymyxin B (dosage: Table 41) may be necessary for at least 2–3 days. Alternatively, tobramycin may be given intrathecally as well as parenterally.

Duration of treatment: until the CSF returns to normal.

Salmonella meningitis is a rare complication of typhoid or paratyphoid fever or salmonella gastro-enteritis, particularly in children.

Treatment of choice: Chloramphenicol (dosage: Table 40, p. 325). Because of the risk of relapse, treatment should be followed with a further course of oral chloramphenicol or, if the total recommended dose has been exceeded or early signs of marrow depression are seen, with amoxycillin, cefotaxime or co-trimoxazole. Combination initially with gentamicin is advisable, since salmonella meningitis is difficult to eradicate effectively. Duration of treatment: at least 3 weeks, preferably longer.

Meningitis due to Klebsiella or Enterobacter is rare (except in the newborn and young infant), and difficult to treat effectively because of the frequent and variable antibiotic resistance of these organisms.

Treatment: Because of the poor prognosis, combined treatment with effective drugs on the basis of tested antibiotic sensitivities is essential, preferably with a combination of a β-lactamase-stable cephalosporin (e. g. cefotaxime against Klebsiella, latamoxef in high dosage against Enterobacter) with gentamicin or amikacin. Sensitive strains may be treated with mezlocillin, piperacillin, chloramphenicol or co-trimoxazole in combination with an aminoglycoside, which may need to be given intrathecally once a day (dosage: Table 41) until the CSF becomes sterile.

Proteus meningitis: *Treatment* according to the species of Proteus and the antibiotic sensitivity pattern. Cefotaxime, latamoxef, ampicillin or mezlocillin in combination with gentamicin are recommended. Chloramphenicol may be used if the isolate is sensitive.

Campylobacter meningitis is rare, occurring generally in the newborn, occasionally crossing the placenta. The clinical picture is of septicaemia, sometimes accompanied by mucous and blood-stained diarrhoea and associated with encephalitis, generally in the newborn. The CSF may be grossly clear, but with a moderate increase in cells and gram-negative curved rods in a stained smear. Culture should be performed anaerobically on special culture media, incubated for several days.

Treatment: Parenteral chloramphenicol at a dosage related to age (Table 40) for 1–2 weeks or alternatively with gentamicin i. m. + clindamycin i. v.

Fungal meningitis (Candida albicans, Cryptococcus neoformans, and very occasionally Aspergillus fumigatus): CSF culture on Sabouraud's agar is often only positive after prolonged incubation (up to 10 days). Cryptococcus can only be seen microscopically after staining with India ink. A latex agglutination test is available for the detection of antigen in CSF or serum, and an ELISA method for Aspergillus fumigatus. *Treatment* should be attempted with amphotericin B i. v. in combination with flucytosine (dosage: p. 175 and p. 182), supplemented by intrathecal instillation of amphotericin B. Prednisone (10 mg) is first instilled by the intralumbar (or in young infants the intraventricular route) and followed by slow instillation of amphotericin B (0.5 mg) diluted with CSF in the syringe. This dose is repeated after 2–3 days. Candida albicans and Cryptococcus neoformans should always be tested against flucytosine in vitro since resistant strains occur. If the meningitis is associated with a Spitz-Holter or other valve implant, this foreign body must be removed.

Amoebic meningo-encephalitis: *Naegleria fowleri* is transmitted by water from ponds, lakes, unchlorinated swimming baths and occasionally tap water and penetrates the nasal mucosa, probably through the cribriform plate. The meningitis is acute and often fatal and motile amoebae may be seen microscopically in uncentrifuged purulent CSF which has not been cooled. The organism may be cultured and treatment is with amphotericin B, possibly in combination with rifampicin.

Acanthamoeba species is spread by the blood stream in immunosuppressed patients and gives rise to a granulomatous encephalitis with a low-grade accompanying lymphocytic meningitis. The causative organism may be shown in brain biopsy but not in the CSF. Treatment with sulphonamide and flucytosine may be tried.

Serous meningitis: For the treatment of tuberculosis, see p. 471; for syphilis, p. 434; for leptospirosis, p. 457. Tuberculosis is suspected in a meningitis of insidious onset, with progressive clinical deterioration, decreasing CSF sugar and cranial nerve palsies. Diagnosis and antibiotic sensitivities must be confirmed by bacteriological culture. The diagnosis of syphilis and leptospirosis is made serologically. Viral meningitis is *not* treated with antibiotics.

Partially treated purulent meningitis in which no pathogen has been seen or cultured but which shows signs of improvement should be treated further with the same antibiotic, i. e. benzyl penicillin, ampicillin, cefotaxime or chloramphenicol. Treatment should otherwise be continued with chloramphenicol as when clinical progress is unsatisfactory. Despite treatment, the latex agglutination test for meningococci, pneumococci and Haemophilus influenzae often remains positive in the CSF for several days.

Culture-negative purulent meningitis: An acute meningitis which has not already been treated, where there is no indication of an otogenic or rhinogenic origin and from which no bacterial pathogen has been isolated, has, in adults, most probably been caused by meningococci, which may not survive transport to the laboratory. Such cases should be treated with large doses of benzyl penicillin. Metastatic foci on the skin and a purpuric rash suggest meningococcal infection. Chloramphenicol or cefotaxime in combination with gentamicin are preferable in cases of suspected otogenic or rhinogenic meningitis. Meningococcal infections are rare in the newborn and chloramphenicol or cefotaxime are preferable in infants because of the relatively greater incidence of meningitis with Haemophilus influenzae at this age.

Cerebral abscess: See p. 391.

References

BAYER, A. S., J. E. EDWARDS, Jr., J. S. SEIDEL: Candida meningitis. Medicine 55: 477 (1976).

BELOHRADSKY, B. H., R. ROOS, S. DÄUMLING, W. MARGET: Cephalosporine im Vergleich bei der Behandlung der bakteriellen Meningitis im Neugeborenen- und Kindesalter. FAC 1: 207 (1982).

BENNETT, J. E., W. E. DISMUKES, R. J. DUMA: A comparison of amphotericin B alone and combined with flucytosine in the treatment of cryptococcal meningitis. New Engl. J. Med. 301: 126 (1979).

BERMAN, B. W., F. H. KING, D. S. RUBINSTEIN, S. S. LONG: Bacteroides fragilis meningitis in a neonate successfully treated with metronidazole. J. Pediat. 93: 793 (1978).

EICKHOFF, T. C.: In-vitro and in-vivo studies of resistance to rifampin in meningococci. J. infect. Dis. 123: 414 (1971).

GUTTLER, R. B., H. N. BEATY: Minocycline in the chemoprophylaxis of meningococcal disease. Antimicrob. Ag. Chemother. 1: 397 (1972).

HEIMANN, G., H. SKOPNIK, U. BERGT, H.-T. TRAN: Liquorkinetik von Chloramphenicol und Cefotaxim bei Kindern. FAC 2–1: 99 (1983).

HELWIG, H., F. DASCHNER: Cefotaxim – eine Alternative zur Behandlung der eitrigen Meningitis im Kindesalter? Dtsch. med. Wschr. 107: 1343 (1982).

PAISLEY, J. W., J. A. WASHINGTON: II Susceptibility of Escherichia coli K 1 to four combinations of antimicrobial agents potentially useful for treatment of neonatal meningitis. J. infect. Dis. 140: 183 (1979).

RAHAL, J. J. Jr.: Diagnosis and Management of Meningitis Due to Gram-Negative Bacilli in Adults. In: J. REMINGTON, M. SWARTZ: Current Clinical Topics in Infectious Diseases I. McGraw Hill, New York 1980.

SANDYK, R., M. J. W. BRENNAN: Unusual presentation of primary klebsiella meningitis: successful treatment with cefotaxime. Postgrad. med. J. 59: 256 (1983).

STEINBERG, E. A., G. D. OVERTURF, J. WILKINS, L. J. BARAFF, J. M. STRENG, J. M. LEEDOM: Failure of cefamandole in treatment of meningitis due to *H. influenzae* type b. J. infect. Dis. *137* [Suppl.]: 180 (1978).

VAN DER WAARDE, K., M. VAN DER WIEL-KORSTANJE: Treatment of ventriculitis with gentamicin in an infant born with spina bifida. Scand. J. infect. Dis. *4:* 165 (1972).

WARD, J. I., T. F. TSAI, G. A. FILICE, D. W. FRASER: Prevalence of ampicillin- and chloramphenicol-resistant strains of *Haemophilus influenzae* causing meningitis and bacteremia: National survey of hospital laboratories. J. infect. Dis. *138:* 421 (1978).

6. Respiratory Infections

Upper respiratory infections are viral in origin in more than 90% of cases. Antibiotics are only indicated if a bacterial cause has been found, the illness is severe, or if a primary viral infection has given rise to bacterial superinfection. Antibiotics are also useful for the prevention of bacterial complications of influenza in patients with severe underlying chest disease.

Bacterial infection is suggested by:
1. purulent secretions from an inflamed mucosa,
2. peripheral granulocytosis,
3. predominance of a potential pathogen in cultures taken from a patient who is not receiving antibiotics,
4. painful regional lymphadenitis,
5. no connection with a known viral epidemic.

Viral infections are generally characterised by serous rhinitis, bilateral catarrhal conjunctivitis, non-suppurative pharyngitis, vesiculation, swelling of lymphoid follicles, herpangina, tracheitis with a dry cough (particularly with influenza), generalised lymphadenopathy, a non-specific rash, myalgia, a normal peripheral white cell count, or an epidemiological connection with a known outbreak of viral infection. Respiratory infections of bacterial and viral origin cannot reliably be distinguished by clinical or haematological findings.

Bacterial infections of the lower respiratory tract are almost always associated with some disorder of the normal mechanisms of resistance (ciliary activity, mucous secretion, alveolar phagocytosis, cough reflex, IgA, IgG, IgE, lysozyme, white cell function etc.). This protective system can be disrupted by viral infection, chemical or physical damage, aspiration, pressure of a foreign body etc. The lower respiratory mucosa is normally sterile. Pathogens must be distinguished from commensal mouth bacteria when expectorated sputum is examined, which is often difficult and can give rise to misinterpretation of culture results. Once antibiotics have been given, considerable changes can occur in the mouth and pharyngeal flora which may further complicate the picture. If the sputum is macroscopically purulent, microscopic examination of a gram-stained fleck of pus may help the interpretation of culture results, although there are pitfalls for the overconfident here, in that pneumococci are often indistinguishable from heavy oral contamination with commensal viridans streptococci in direct microscopic examination.

a) Rhinitis

If purulent rhinitis persists for more than 2–3 weeks, the possibility of paranasal sinusitis should be investigated. Although rhinitis of the newborn is often caused by staphylococci, the possibility of gonorrhoea and congenital syphilis must be excluded. Purulent rhinitis in infants is occasionally caused by group A streptococci.

Treatment of nasal diphtheria is as for pharyngeal diphtheria (p. 336). Antibacterial therapy of purulent rhinitis is necessary when complications such as purulent sinusitis arise and antibiotic treatment depends on the pathogen isolated. Treatment with phenoxymethyl penicillin (active against pneumococci and Streptococcus pyogenes) may be given or, if that fails, with flucloxacillin, which is active against penicillin-resistant staphylococci.

b) Tonsillitis, Pharyngitis

Lacunar, follicular and catarrhal tonsillitis are generally caused by β-haemolytic streptococci of Lancefield group A. A tonsillar exudate is not pathognomonic and may be absent, so a throat swab should always be cultured on media selective for haemolytic streptococci. A high peripheral blood white cell count is very suggestive of streptococcal pharyngitis, as is tenderness of the posterior cervical lymph nodes and the absence of rhinitis.

Treatment: Phenoxymethyl penicillin in normal dosage for 10–14 days, and a minimum of 7 days; this is important not only to prevent complications, particularly rheumatic fever and post-streptococcal glomerulonephritis, but also to eradicate streptococci from the throat, for a proportion will still have positive cultures after ten days of therapy and require a further course. In the USA benzathine penicillin (0.9 megaunits) in combination with procaine penicillin (0.3 megaunits) is given as a single intramuscular injection which is effective for 10 days. Sulphonamides and co-trimoxazole are inferior to penicillin nowadays because some streptococci are resistant and activity is lower. Tetracyclines should not be given because they are not bactericidal, they carry a much greater risk of side effects, and many streptococcal strains (30–40%) are resistant. Ampicillin should also be avoided because it is less active than benzyl penicillin, and is associated with a cutaneous allergy, particularly in patients with glandular fever and similar disorders. Penicillin lozenges (not available in Britain) should never be given because of the risk of allergy and topical treatment with antiseptics is ineffective and does not prevent the serious complications of streptococcal infection. Infectious mononucleosis should be suspected in younger patients who do not respond to penicillin within 48 hours.

Penicillin allergy: Erythromycin by mouth, 1 g a day for adults, 30 mg/kg a day for children; cephalexin or cephradine, 2 g a day for adults and 50 mg/kg for children may also be given.

Vincent's angina is uncommon nowadays, and classically presents as a greasy ulcer, usually on the tip of the tonsil and often unilateral with no fever. It is more commonly associated with gingival sepsis. Fusospirochaetosis is probably not a disease in itself, but possible underlying diseases should be considered. Treatment with benzyl penicillin is normally adequate.

Chronic tonsillitis: The tonsils are inflamed, fissured and difficult to move, with a purulent exudate and pain on peritonsillar pressure. Some patients have an increased antistreptolysin 0 titre. Where clinically indicated, tonsillectomy should be performed under antibiotic cover with penicillin in normal dosage orally or i. m. from a few hours before surgery to 48–72 hours afterwards.

Pharyngitis is usually viral in origin, so antibiotics are not required. Phenoxymethyl penicillin should be given on suspicion of streptococcal pharyngitis, which is not uncommon, and treatment is as for lacunar tonsillitis (see above). Gonococcal pharyngitis is only cured with large doses of benzyl penicillin or, when resistant, by cefuroxime or cefotaxime.

c) Peritonsillar or Retropharyngeal Abscess, Ludwig's Angina

Causative organisms: Aerobic and anaerobic streptococci, staphylococci, Bacteroides etc.

Treatment: Clindamycin orally or i. v., 1.2 g a day, or flucloxacillin 6 g a day. Benzyl penicillin is a less suitable alternative since not all the bacteria involved are susceptible. Cefoxitin may also be used in severe infections. Needle aspiration and drainage of the pus or superficial incision is necessary; tonsillectomy may be necessary for peritonsillar abscess to remove the risk of recurrence. The pus should be examined microscopically and cultured both aerobically and anaerobically. A rare complication is jugular vein thrombosis with septicaemia and the vein may require ligation.

d) Diphtheria

Tonsillar and pharyngeal diphtheria are characterised by a grey, adherent membrane on the throat and tonsils which may spread to the soft palate. Fever is moderate and may be absent and some patients develop shock and a peripheral leucocytosis. At least three swabs should be taken from beneath the pseudomembrane, examined microscopically for suspicious gram-positive bacilli and stained to show metachromatic granules. Culture should include a medium containing potassium tellurite. The nose, ear, conjunctiva, larynx and wounds can also be affected. Because of childhood immunisation, diphtheria is now very uncommon in Western Europe and the USA but should be considered in patients from countries where routine immunisation is not practised. Glandular fever should always be excluded (blood film, Paul Bunnell test etc.).

Treatment: When diphtheria is suspected, give diphtheria antitoxin, 10,000–20,000 units i. m. Benzyl penicillin 1.2–2.4 megaunits is given simultaneously and continued for 10 days. Give further antitoxin on the next 2 days; steroids may be used in severe cases. The patient may require intubation or even tracheotomy. Patients allergic to penicillin should receive erythromycin for 10 days. Strict bed rest is essential because of the risk of myocarditis and an electrocardiogram should be regularly checked. Three nasal and throat swabs should be negative three days after completion of treatment. Carriers and excretors should be treated with erythromycin in doses up to 2 g a day for adults and 40 mg/kg/day for children for 2 weeks.

Reference

ZAMIRI, I., M. G. MCENTEGART: The sensitivity of diphteria bacilli to eight antibiotics. J. clin. Path. *25:* 716 (1972).

e) Infectious Mononucleosis (Glandular Fever)

This condition is characterised by a moderate or high, usually prolonged fever, sometimes accompanied by a whitish, removable membrane on the swollen tonsils. There is generalised lymphadenopathy and splenomegaly. The peripheral blood count is characteristic with more than 50% mononuclear cells of which more than 10% are atypical lymphocytes. The monospot (modified Paul-Bunnell) test is usually positive in the acute phase of the infection, though it may be negative from the outset. IgM antibodies to the Epstein-Barr virus can be demonstrated in the serum although they disappear soon after recovery, whereas IgG antibodies persist.

Treatment: Because glandular fever is a viral infection, *antibiotics are contra-indicated* unless group A streptococci are cultured. The use of antibiotics, particularly ampicillin, in glandular fever is associated with allergic skin rashes (p. 46). Corticosteroids may be useful if severe pharyngotonsillar oedema threatens to obstruct the airway. Bed rest is desirable during the acute phase of the illness.

f) Candida Stomatitis (Thrush)

A whitish, removable membrane is present on the oral mucosa in the absence of fever. Thrush is usually secondary to an underlying disease (e. g. diabetes mellitus), immunodeficiency or broad-spectrum antibiotic treatment. Yeasts may be seen microscopically in a smear of material stained with methylene blue or gram, and cultured.

Treatment is generally *topical*, with nystatin, miconazole, clotrimazole or amphotericin B as lozenges, a mouthwash or an oral gel, and may need to be prolonged because of the risk of relapse. *Systemic* treatment is now available with ketoconazole, 200–400 mg in adults and 3 mg/kg in children, once a day with food until at least one week after symptoms have resolved and cultures have become negative. The maximum daily dose in adults should not exceed 600 mg.

g) Secondary Throat Infections

Throat infections may arise as a consequence of bone marrow suppression, e. g. leukaemia, agranulocytosis, when they are usually mixed (aerobic and anaerobic streptococci, Bacteroides, enterobacteria, Pseudomonas etc.). The causative organism can change rapidly. The important measure is to treat the underlying disease effectively. Where agranulocytosis is drug-induced, stop the likely causative agent forthwith. Very broad-spectrum antibiotic therapy, where possible in bactericidal combinations (p. 514) is recommended until the bone marrow recovers.

h) Laryngitis and Acute Epiglottitis

Laryngitis is usually associated with acute tracheitis in adults (hoarseness and a barking cough), generally as a result of viral infections (measles, influenza or parainfluenza) and very rarely as a primary or secondary bacterial infection (Haemophilus influenzae, streptococci, pneumococci or staphylococci). The presentation in children is more commonly as an *acute epiglottitis*, with a rapid onset, marked inspiratory stridor but no barking cough; these infections are usually due to Haemophilus influenzae and may be fatal unless intubation or tracheotomy can be performed. The organism is readily cultured from the blood and may also be detected by latex agglutination of the serum. Subglottic laryngitis in children is generally viral in origin, with a gradual onset and no pain on swallowing. The symptoms are less severe and the illness usually responds to conservative treatment. Expiratory and inspiratory stridor is characteristic of acute laryngotracheobronchitis in the newborn and small infants. The laryngitis is usually caused by viruses but other causes of croup, especially acute epiglottitis and diphtheria, must always be considered since they demand urgent treatment, including antibiotics. Symptoms of laryngeal diphtheria include hoarseness, a barking cough, inspiratory stridor where there is marked membrane development, dyspnoea, and jugular retraction. Chronic hoarseness can be caused by tuberculosis, syphilis or a carcinoma, and all require special treatment.

Treatment of acute laryngitis: Inhalation of steam and mucolytic agents, antitussives, and mild sedation. An attempt may be made to relieve swelling with calcium i.v. and prednisone. Acute epiglottitis in children demands urgent hospital admission for intubation or tracheotomy, and immediate antibacterial treatment with cefotaxime or cefuroxime.

Treatment of laryngeal diphtheria: See. p. 336.

i) Acute Bronchitis

Almost always viral (influenza, parainfluenza and other viruses), which often lead to secondary bacterial infections, particularly with pneumococci or Haemophilus influenzae. Superinfection with staphylococci, streptococci, Bacteroides, meningococci, Klebsiella and Pseudomonas occasionally follows. Viral infections are likely when there is a dry cough (tracheitis), hoarseness, pharyngitis and a watery nasal discharge. Purulent sputum is suggestive of secondary bacterial infection.

A primary bacterial bronchitis can be caused by Bordetella pertussis (see p. 455), Branhamella catarrhalis, Mycoplasma pneumoniae (which does not necessarily cause pneumonia) and Chlamydia trachomatis, often with a pertussis-like cough, as well as Haemophilus influenzae in pre-school children. Any cough which persists for longer than 2 weeks in older children and young adults is suggestive of Mycoplasma pneumoniae infection.

Antibiotic treatment for patients at high risk (infants, the elderly, and patients with lowered resistance because of underlying systemic or lung disease): Erythromycin, azidocillin, amoxycillin or cefaclor, all of which are active against pneumococci, Haemophilus influenzae and Branhamella catarrhalis. When pneumococci are cultured, give phenoxymethyl penicillin; other pathogens are treated according to the bacterial isolate and its antibiotic sensitivity pattern. Unlike cephalexin and cephradine, cefaclor has good activity against Haemophilus influenzae, even when resistant to ampicillin and erythromycin. Erythromycin is effective in bronchitis due to Mycoplasma pneumoniae and Chlamydia trachomatis. If the cough and purulent sputum persist and the sputum quantity is not reduced, further cultures and chest x-rays should be taken. For the technique of sputum examination, see below.

j) Chronic Bronchitis

This disease is commonest in the elderly and smokers. Chronic bronchitis is a non-specific condition, characterised by chronic, recurrent cough with sputum production and very often combined with emphysema and bronchial obstruction. Acute exacerbations are due to bacterial superinfection. The long-term sequelae can be severe respiratory insufficiency and cor pulmonale. Recurrent broncho-pneumonia and lung abscesses are much less common. Haemophilus influenzae and pneumococci are the commonest causes of acute exacerbations of chronic bronchitis. Staphylococci, Klebsiella, and Pseudomonas aeruginosa are relatively rare.

Chronic bronchial irritation and epithelial damage impair the mechanism of bacterial elimination from the bronchial tree, so the bronchi are constantly colonised with bacteria. Special causes in children are immunodeficiency, α_1-antitrypsin deficiency, chronic granulomatosis, Kartagener's syndrome, cystic fibrosis (mucoviscidosis) and foreign body aspiration.

Technique of sputum examination:

Sputum should be examined microscopically and by culture and, where necessary, cytologically as well. The antibiotic sensitivities of potential pathogens are determined. A fresh, deeply expectorated sputum collected after rising in the morning and cleaning the teeth, but before breakfast, is the best material for routine examination. Sputum may also be obtained at any time in the hospital patient by deep expectoration with the aid of physiotherapy, and transtracheal aspiration or even direct lung puncture have been used in some centres. Fibre-optic bronchoscopy for uncontaminated sputum collection is less traumatic and is especially useful in treatment failures.

The object of sputum culture is to isolate potential pathogens present in the secretions of the lower respiratory tract but ignore commensal mouth bacteria.

With experience, this can be achieved by careful selection of purulent material for direct microscopic examination and culture. MAY (1968), however, showed that sputum is heterogeneous and there were considerable differences between individual purulent portions, even in the same specimen. To remove contaminant mouth flora, some advocate washing the sputum with physiological saline before inoculation on to solid media; others then recommend liquefaction with, for example, 1% pancreatin or n-acetyl cysteine, mixed in equal proportions and shaken for 15 min before inoculation. A further refinement is to dilute the digested sputum 1:1000 to obtain a semi-quantitative selection based on numbers of organisms present, though such techniques are arbitrary and reliable only in fresh specimens. Where delay in transport to the laboratory may occur, commercial culture media are available for direct inoculation at the bedside, hence avoid death of some organisms and overgrowth of others in transit. Whatever method is chosen to suit local circumstances, sputum culture is one of the least satisfactory of bacteriological investigations and should be supplemented in patients with pneumonia by culture of the blood, which will often yield pneumococci and confirm a diagnosis of lobar pneumonia when sputum culture is equivocal.

Antibiotics are of limited value because the functional and anatomical abnormalities are already present, but they are sometimes effective in suppressing acute exacerbations. Long-term treatment during the winter may reduce the frequency of exacerbations and is based on tetracycline, amoxycillin and co-trimoxazole, which act against Haemophilus influenzae and pneumococci and can be given for long periods. However 10–30% of pneumococci and 5–10% of Haemophilus influenzae strains are resistant to tetracycline; strains resistant to ampicillin and erythromycin are also found. The penicillins penetrate relatively poorly into sputum, so large doses have to be given. Relatively high sputum concentrations are obtained with minocycline, erythromycin, cefaclor and co-trimoxazole. Because of the risk of bone-marrow suppression, chloramphenicol, which used to be given frequently, is no longer recommended.

Two methods of treatment are in use:
1. *Intermittent therapy:* Acute exacerbations with purulent sputum, increasing cough and fever are treated with oral amoxycillin (1.5 g a day) for 1–3 weeks, or with an ampicillin ester such as talampicillin, pivampicillin or bacampicillin (2.4 g a day), a tetracycline derivative or co-trimoxazole. The prompt commencement of treatment is very important. Cooperative patients should keep a suitable antibiotic at home in order to start treatment as soon as purulent sputum reappears. Other pathogens such as staphylococci, Klebsiella or

Pseudomonas are uncommon, and a different drug must then be used according to antibiotic sensitivity results.

2. *Long-term treatment:* In certain cases, long-term treatment is useful, particularly during the winter months when exacerbations are more frequent, to prevent acute attacks and control the progression of obstructive bronchitis. Antibiotics used in this way are doxycycline (100 mg daily), minocycline (200 mg daily), co-trimoxazole (2 tablets twice daily), amoxycillin by mouth (1.5 g daily), and the ampicillin esters. Phenoxymethyl penicillin and sulphonamides are less active against Haemophilus influenzae and are therefore inferior to the amino penicillins.

Treatment is successful when the sputum loses its purulence and diminishes in quantity, and breathing and lung function improve. Because the causes of infection change frequently, bacteriological examination of the sputum is necessary before and during therapy.

The clinical picture can be improved considerably by supportive therapy including drugs which reduce bronchospasm or secretion, postural drainage of the bronchi (Trendelenburg's position), respiratory physiotherapy, inhalation of antibiotics through a modern nebuliser, digitalisation in cardiac insufficiency, climatic changes etc. In severe acute exacerbations, aspiration drainage of the respiratory tract, intubation, mechanical ventilation, rehydration, aminophylline i.v. may be necessary. Persistent atelectasis may require bronchoscopy, treatment of pneumonia etc. Improvement can also be achieved with aerosols of broncholytics, secretolytics, detergents, saline and other means. Treatment of paranasal sinusitis (see p. 419) is also sometimes helpful. At the beginning of winter, the patient should be vaccinated against the current or anticipated strain of influenza because of his increased risk.

k) Bronchiolitis

Only occurs in infants and small children. *Pathogens:* Respiratory syncytial and other viruses, sometimes with bacterial superinfection (Haemophilus, staphylococci). Specific chemotherapy is not available. Secondary infection is treated with cefuroxime or cefamandole i.v. or oral cefaclor. Supportive treatment with oxygen, humidification of respired air, digitalisation, prednisone, controlled fluid and electrolyte treatment and mechanical ventilation are all important.

l) Bronchiectasis

Usually mixed bacterial infection with pneumococci and Haemophilus influenzae. Other organisms (staphylococci, gram-negative rods, Pseudomonas, anaerobes) and mixed infections are commoner than in chronic bronchitis.

The initial *antibiotic treatment* of acute exacerbations is directed against the main organisms (pneumococci, Haemophilus). Ampicillin, amoxycillin, azidocillin, co-trimoxazole, mino- or doxycycline or erythromycin are given for at least 5–7 days. Antibiotics are then directed against the bacteria isolated, if considered significant. The infecting agents change frequently, so the sputum should be regularly examined bacteriologically. As antibiotics often penetrate bronchiectatic pus poorly, systemic treatment can be supplemented by antibiotic inhalations such as neomycin (200 mg/ml), polymyxin B or gentamicin (10 mg/ml), thiamphenicol (see p. 129), bacitracin (250 units/ml) or tyrothricin (1 mg/ml) 2–3 times a day. As with chronic bronchitis, long-term treatment with doxy- or minocycline or co-trimoxazole is useful in severe cases. Antibiotics are only of limited value in bronchiectasis and other measures such as mucolytics, postural drainage and possibly lobectomy, when the bronchiectasis is localised, also play a part.

m) Cystic Fibrosis (Mucoviscidosis)

Patients with cystic fibrosis are threatened by severe, recurrent chest infections which are caused by Haemophilus influenzae, staphylococci, Pseudomonas aeruginosa, P. cepacia, P. maltophilia and other bacteria. Antibiotics can generally be given intermittently as required, alternating between tobramycin or amikacin, azlo- or mezlocillin, ceftazidime or cefamandole, co-trimoxazole or clindamycin. Staphylococcal infection is effectively treated with flucloxacillin plus fusidic acid. Long-term treatment is sometimes necessary in severe cases. Chronic infection with Pseudomonas is often not eradicable. Cystic fibrosis with lung involvement can be alleviated by intensive inhalation therapy as well as by bronchial drainage. After inhalation of a mucolytic drug, the patient inhales a topical antibiotic using an inhaler of good quality (see above). Many inhalers are heavily contaminated with Pseudomonas and re-usable ones should be carefully cleaned and sterilised regularly. Cystic fibrotics are now often reaching adult life. Many have chronic Pseudomonas chest infections and extensive changes in their chest x-rays. The infection with Pseudomonas cannot be eradicated, even with otherwise effective drugs, but clinical improvement often follows antipseudomonal treatment with intermittent parenteral antibiotics, e. g. ceftazidime + tobramycin for 10–14 days.

n) Pneumonia

The **main forms** are *bronchopneumonia* (especially in babies and the elderly), *lobar pneumonia* and *interstitial pneumonia* (pneumonia of viral type, in mycoplasma infections, ornithosis and Q-fever). *Genuine viral pneumonia* without bacterial involvement is rare and associated usually with influenza, parainfluenza, adenoviruses, respiratory syncytial viruses and with varicella. Correlation between a particular form of pneumonia and a given pathogen is closest in primary pneumonias. The clinical picture of the more frequent secondary pneumonias is changed considerably by the primary disease and factors which lower resistance (e. g. cystic fibrosis, mitral valve disease, heart failure, pulmonary oedema, caustic gas inhalation and prolonged mechanical ventilation, aspiration, alcoholism, pulmonary infarction etc.).

Particular forms of pneumonia:
Pneumonia with abscess formation (due to staphylococci, Klebsiella pneumoniae, anaerobes);
haematogenous pneumonia (septic pulmonary metastases);
pneumonia complicating infectious diseases (whooping cough, measles, chickenpox, influenza, actinomycosis, nocardiosis, brucellosis, tularaemia, plague, anthrax, typhoid fever etc.);
chronic or recurrent pneumonia (often superimposed on a bronchial carcinoma);
caseous pneumonia (tuberculosis);
fungal pneumonia (Candidasis, aspergillosis, cryptococcosis, histoplasmosis);
postoperative pneumonia (see p. 352, 390);
perinatal pneumonia (due to aspiration of infected amniotic fluid or atelectasis);
Pneumocystis carinii pneumonia (in babies from the second to the sixth month of life, but commoner in adults and older children with extreme impairment of bodily defences or malnutrition), sometimes occurring simultaneously with pulmonary cytomegalovirus infection. These infections often complicate the acquired immunodeficiency syndrome *(AIDS)*.

Diagnosis: Wherever possible, a sputum sample should be carefully examined and cultured, preferably obtained by deep expectoration with physiotherapy, by fibre-optic bronchoscopy or by transtracheal aspiration (TTA), so that material is reliably obtained from the lower respiratory tract. Culture of mycoplasma, chlamydia and rickettsia is usually only available in certain laboratories and requires special transport media. If tuberculosis is suspected, a Ziehl-Neelsen stain of a sputum smear or laryngeal swab should be examined; if carcinoma is suspected, perform a cytological examination of the sputum and bronchoscopy. In

30% of cases of pneumococcal pneumoniae, a blood culture also yields the organism, but this is rarely the case in other types of pneumonia.

For pneumococcal, haemophilus, candida and aspergillus pneumonia, antigen can be detected in the serum and urine by rapid latex agglutination, as in infections with streptococci of group B and meningococci. Secretions obtained by deep aspiration using fibre-optic bronchoscopy can also be cultured for Legionella, anaerobes, Pneumocystis carinii and fungi. Chlamydia trachomatis causes pneumonitis in young infants and oncological patients and can be demonstrated in pharyngeal secretions by immunofluorescence or cell culture.

Frequent **bacterial causes** of pneumonia are pneumococci, staphylococci and Klebsiella pneumoniae. Other streptococci, Haemophilus influenzae, meningococci, Pseudomonas aeruginosa and Bacteroides are less common (Table 42). The range of pathogens varies considerably according to the clinical situation. Gram-

Table 42. Causes of different clinical forms of pneumonia.

Clinical form	Common causes	Occasional causes
Lobar pneumonia, segmental pneumonia	Pneumococci	Klebsiella, streptococci, Legionella
Post-influenzal pneumonia	Staphylococci, pneumococci	Haemophilus, streptococci
Suppurative broncho-pneumonia	Staphylococci, Bacteroides	Klebsiella, Pseudomonas
Aspiration pneumonia	Bacteroides, anaerobic streptococci	Staphylococci, pneumococci etc.
Postoperative pneumonia	Staphylococci	Pneumococci, streptococci, Klebsiella
Primary interstitial pneumonia	Mycoplasma	Psittacosis (ornithosis), Q-fever, Legionella
Pneumonia during prolonged mechanical ventilation	Pseudomonas, Klebsiella	Proteus, staphylococci, Candida
Secondary pneumonia in immunodeficient patients without prior antibiotic treatment	Staphylococci, Klebsiella, pneumococci, Bacteroides	Esch. coli, Serratia etc.
Secondary pneumonia during antibiotic therapy	Any facultative pathogen, particularly those affected by standard antibiotic therapy, often including multiresistant strains of Pseudomonas, Klebsiella, Staphylococcus, and Serratia	

negative rods (Pseudomonas, Klebsiella) are commoner in patients with a tracheotomy or on mechanical ventilation; these organisms also colonise tracheostomy sites and endotracheal tubes, particularly if the patient is receiving antibiotics; they should only be regarded as causes of pneumonia in such patients if the tracheal secretion is clearly purulent and there are supportive radiological changes. Pseudomonas and enterobacteria also cause pneumonia in leukaemics and the newborn, mostly generated in the latter by the aspiration of infected amniotic fluid.

Because gram-negative rods are often part of the oral flora, particularly when the patient has received certain antibiotics, the diagnosis of gram-negative pneumonia from sputum culture is difficult. Viridans streptococci, non-pathogenic neisseriae and Bacteroides species are normally found in the mouth and therefore also in the sputum, as occasionally are pneumococci, staphylococci, Haemophilus influenzae and Candida species, though generally in smaller quantities. Klebsiella, Escherichia coli and Pseudomonas are rarely present in the sputum of the normal patient. Treatment with ampicillin, certain other broad-spectrum antibiotics and also with large doses of benzyl penicillin causes selection of gram-negative bacilli in the oral cavity which has no relevance in patients not suffering from a serious underlying disease. The selection of gram-negative bacilli can, however, play an important epidemiological role as a reservoir of potential pathogens in a group of severely ill patients, for example in an intensive care unit.

A **serological diagnosis** by the demonstration of a rising titre of specific antibodies in the patient's blood is possible for some causes of pneumonia, including the following:

Psittacosis and ornithosis:	CFT (sometimes WR positive)
Mycoplasma pneumoniae:	CFT, cold agglutinins
Chlamydia trachomatis:	immunofluorescence
Coxiella burneti (Q-fever):	CFT
Influenza, parainfluenza virus:	immunofluorescence
Respiratory syncytial virus:	immunofluorescence
Cytomegalovirus:	CFT, immunofluorescence (IgM antibodies)
Pneumocystis carinii:	immunofluorescence
Toxoplasma gondi:	immunofluorescence (IgM antibodies)
Staphylococci:	antistaphylolysin titre
Group A streptococci:	ASO titre, antistreptococcal DNAse b etc.
Legionellosis:	immunofluorescence

Other serological methods such as the enzyme-linked immunosorbent assay (ELISA) and specific microscopical immunofluorescence are now superceding the complement fixation test (CFT) in many centres since they are more specific, more economical of expensive reagents and readily automated when performed in batches of larger numbers of tests.

The blood count in bacterial pneumonias usually shows a polymorph neutrophilia with a marked left shift; viral pneumonias tend to show a left shift without a neutrophilia. The ESR is raised in almost all types of pneumonia. When there are characteristic radiological findings, a specific history such as contact with birds, tuberculin conversion, contact with cases of influenza together with relevant associated signs (e.g. conjunctivitis, skin rash, myalgia etc.) may suggest a particular pathogen for which specific tests can be carried out. If, for technical reasons, the clinical diagnosis is not confirmed by bacteriological, virological or serological tests, the response to a given treatment can sometimes confirm a working diagnosis. In certain forms of viral pneumonia (e.g. influenza, parainfluenza, RSV, CMV), the virus may be cultured from a throat swab or other specimen. The delay before results are available makes this procedure retrospective in the individual patient, though often valuable in identifying causes of epidemics.

Principles of treatment: Antibiotic treatment should always be as appropriate as possible and based on relevant culture results and antibiotic sensitivities. A direct gram stain of the sputum or the result of a latex agglutination test on serum may give a guide for initial treatment in primary pneumonias. In secondary pneumonia, a bacterial diagnosis from culture of expectorated sputum is almost impossible because many pathogens of pneumonia are found in the mouth flora of hospital patients. Endobronchial aspirates through a fibre-optic bronchoscope, and transtracheal aspirates (TTA) are more reliable, and direct microscopy gives a better guide to the likely cause in urgent cases. In patients with a tracheotomy or on long-term mechanical ventilation, the trachea is usually colonised by gram-negative bacilli. This is not necessarily a sign of pneumonia or the risk of pneumonia.

A suitable antibiotic is initially given parenterally in relatively large doses, which may be reduced and, where appropriate, given orally when the patient becomes convalescent. Bactericidal antibiotics are theoretically better, but are not essential. Pneumonias due to gram-negative bacilli should if possible be treated with a combination of an aminoglycoside and a β-lactam antibiotic (e.g. cefotaxime or ceftazidime). The duration of treatment depends on the clinical and radiological findings and should be of adequate length, particularly where there is evidence of abscess formation.

Table 43. Treatment of pneumonia of known bacterial cause (subject to sensitivity test).

Bacterial cause	Treatment of choice	Alternatives
Pneumococci, streptococci, staphylococci (non-penicillin-ase-producers), meningococci	Benzyl penicillin	Cefazolin, erythromycin
Staphylococci (penicillinase-producers)	Flucloxacillin + fusidic acid	Cefamandole, cefazolin, clin-damycin
Klebsiella pneumoniae	Cefotaxime + gentamicin	Mezlocillin + amikacin (or gentamicin)
Pseudomonas aeruginosa	Azlocillin + tobramycin	Cefsulodin, piperacillin, ceftazidime, amikacin
Haemophilus influenzae	Ampicillin, cefotaxime	Mezlocillin, piperacillin, tetracycline
Bacteroides species	Metronidazole	Cefoxitin, clindamycin, chloramphenicol
Mycoplasma pneumoniae, Chlamydia psittaci, Coxiella burneti	Doxycycline	Erythromycin (mycoplasma only)
Legionella pneumophila	Erythromycin	Minocycline, rifampicin
Chlamydia trachomatis	Erythromycin	Doxycycline

Good general care, digitalis, fluid balance, oxygen treatment, fresh air for children, drainage in bronchial obstruction, sedation, inhalations etc. are also important. Severe pneumonias are best managed in hospital and cases of respiratory failure should be treated in a well equipped intensive care unit. Pooled normal human immunoglobulin should only be given to patients with hypogammaglobulinaemia. Corticosteroids are only justified in exceptional cases (septic shock). The choice of antibiotics in pneumonia may be based on rules given in Table 43.

α) Treatment of Pneumonia (Pathogen Known)

Pneumococcal pneumonia: The pneumococcus is still the commonest cause of primary pneumonia, which can be lobar or segmental. Pneumococci are found in the sputum and blood culture and the latex agglutination test in serum and urine is often positive, even after treatment has begun. A secondary pneumococcal pneumonia may occur in the compromised host.

Treatment: The drug of choice is still benzyl penicillin, since resistant pneumococci remain extremely uncommon. 4–10 megaunits of benzyl penicillin are given parenterally as an i. v. infusion or i. m. for the first 2 days of the illness or until defervescence (usually within 48 hrs), followed by 600 mg–1.2 g of phenoxy-methyl penicillin a day for at least 2 weeks. Cefazolin or erythromycin may be used in penicillin-allergic patients. Tetracyclines are unreliable because resistant pneumococci are often found. Infections with penicillin-resistant strains, which are extremely rare in Europe, should be treated with rifampicin.

Pneumonia due to other streptococci: Group A streptococci are rare causes of pneumonia although they are then associated with abscess formation and pleural empyema. Group B streptococci are relatively common causes of congenital pneumonia. Rapid latex agglutination with serum, urine or pleural pus is positive.

Treatment: Benzyl penicillin, cefazolin or cefuroxime in patients with penicillin allergy (dosage as for pneumococcal pneumonia).

Staphylococcal pneumonia commonly causes multiple abscesses of the lungs and often pyothorax, pneumothorax or septicaemia. Occurs particularly in young infants (often with pneumatoceles), in patients with impaired immunity or underlying diseases such as cystic fibrosis, thrombophlebitis associated with venous catheters, heroin addiction and after operations and influenza.

Penicillin-resistant staphylococcal infections should be treated with a penicillin-ase-stable penicillin, preferably flucloxacillin i. v. (5–10 g a day for adults, 100–200 mg/kg for children), possibly in combination with fusidic acid. After defervescence and clinical improvement, continue flucloxacillin or dicloxacillin by mouth (2–3 g a day for adults, 100 mg/kg for children) for several weeks if necessary, until the lung changes have completely resolved (high risk of relapse). Treat alternatively with lincomycin i. v. (1.8 g daily) or with oral clindamycin (900 mg daily).

Penicillin-sensitive staphylococcal pneumonia should be treated in the same way as pneumococcal pneumonia, but for a longer period.

In patients *allergic to penicillin* give cefuroxime, cefamandole or cefazolin, 4–6 g a day for adults, or clindamycin, vancomycin or fusidic acid; the last mentioned can also be used for methicillin-resistant strains or in the rare cases of allergy to cephalosporins.

Klebsiella pneumonia (Friedländer's pneumonia) is a rare cause of primary, lobar pneumonia, but commoner as a secondary infection in patients with severe underlying disease. Often found in alcoholics, producing a viscous, bloodstained mucopurulent sputum. The infection usually becomes chronic and has a high mortality.

Treatment is difficult and antibiotics should always be given in combination, such as cefotaxime (6 g a day) + gentamicin (240–480 mg a day), or cefoxitin + gentamicin (amikacin for gentamicin-resistant strains).

Fever subsides slowly during treatment, which should be continued for several weeks because of the risk of relapse.

Pseudomonas pneumonia is always secondary, particularly in cystic fibrosis, leukaemia, and mechanical ventilation. The prognosis is poor and frequently associated with pulmonary microabscesses.

Treatment: Azlocillin (6–15 g a day in 3 divided doses) + tobramycin (240 mg daily). Alternatives are piperacillin, cefsulodin or ceftazidime.

Difficult to cure, and long courses of treatment are often necessary. The simultaneous intratracheal instillation of an aminoglycoside may be useful in intubated or tracheotomised patients.

Serratia pneumonia is rare, and may arise from contaminated ventilators or humidifiers. Patients affected almost always have impaired resistance or severe underlying disease.

Treatment: According to antibiotic sensitivity testing, preferably ceftazidime or cefotaxime i.v. (6 g daily), in combination with gentamicin or amikacin. Mezlocillin or piperacillin may be used if sensitive.

Haemophilus influenzae pneumonia: Rare. Found most commonly in elderly patients with chronic bronchitis and in children under 5 years of age. Lobar or bronchopneumonia. Latex agglutination positive (serum or pleural fluid) only in infections with type b strains.

Treatment: Initially with cefotaxime i.v., 4–6 g in adults in 3 divided doses following oral cefaclor, 2 g a day for adults, for 3–4 weeks. Sensitive strains may be treated with ampicillin or amoxycillin. Tetracyclines or co-trimoxazole are suitable for follow-up treatment of sensitive strains.

Whooping cough pneumonia: Particularly dangerous in young infants and generally associated with superinfection by staphylococci or other bacteria. A combination of ampicillin and cloxacillin was commonly used in the past but a β-lactamase stable cephalosporin such as cefuroxime, 60 mg/kg a day, is now preferred; it is also active against Bordetella pertussis.

Fungal pneumonia: Associated with Candida albicans, invasive aspergillosis, mucormycosis or cryptococcosis. The diagnosis is difficult because of its chronic course and frequent occurrence in patients with agranulocytosis, leukaemia, or tumors. The presence of fungi in the sputum is not evidence in itself of a pulmonary mycosis, nor justification for treatment with amphotericin B, which has severe side effects. The demonstration of fungi in tracheal or bronchial secretions obtained by transtracheal aspiration or bronchoscopy, in pleural pus or in blood culture is more convincing, particularly when accompanied by radiological evidence of infiltration or cavitation. A rapid latex test for fungal infections is under development.

Treatment: Amphotericin B (see p. 175 for dosage) in combination with flucytosine (see p. 180) for several weeks, supplemented by inhalation of nystatin or amphotericin B with a modern inhaler. Alternatives: miconazole i.v. or ketoconazole orally (see p. 184, 187). Discontinue other antibiotics. Aspergilloma will not respond to chemotherapy and must be removed surgically.

Histoplasmosis occurs mainly in the USA as a fairly innocuous primary pulmonary infection. Chronic cavitating pulmonary histoplasmosis or disseminated histoplasmosis in immunosuppressed patients, which often begins in the lungs, should be treated with amphotericin B for 2–4 weeks and treated surgically where necessary.

Pneumonia due to rare pathogens (Pseudomonas pseudomallei, see p. 251), Achromobacter, Escherichia coli, Proteus etc.): *Treatment* according to antibiotic sensitivities as for septicaemia with the same organism. For anthrax, see p. 446; actinomycosis: see p. 460; typhoid fever: see p. 449.

Primary interstitial pneumonia may be caused by Chlamydia psittaci or trachomatis, Coxiella burneti (Q-fever), or Mycoplasma pneumoniae. These organisms were formerly classified with the viruses because of their small size, but can be grown on inanimate media (except for chlamydias) and inhibited by antibiotics and so are biologically classified as bacteria. *Diagnosis* is made on clinical and serological grounds. Tetracycline is the drug of choice if interstitial pneumonia is suspected on the grounds of severe headache, high fever, relative bradycardia, perihilar opacities with fan-shaped striations or opacities on the x-ray, and leucocytosis. Rolitetracycline i.v. can be given in the beginning (0.5 g a day for adults, 10 mg/kg for children), followed by an oral tetracycline after defervescence.

Oral doxycycline (200 mg a day) is an alternative. Duration of treatment: 14 days. If there is no response to tetracycline, other causes should be sought. Erythromycin is also effective against Mycoplasma pneumoniae and Chlamydia trachomatis.

Pneumocystis-carinii pneumonia is an interstitial pneumonia which may produce a plasma cell response and occurs particularly with leukaemia (often in the terminal stage) and other causes of immunosuppression, both iatrogenic, e.g. after renal transplantation, and acquired, e.g. the acquired immunodeficiency syndrome (AIDS). It also occurs in premature and newborn babies and malnourished children often together with cytomegalovirus chest infection. Symptoms are progressive tachypnoea and dry cough, but no chest signs on auscultation. X-ray changes, where present, are mostly bilateral and sometimes focal. There is a high mortality rate, though spontaneous resolution occasionally occurs.

Diagnosis is based on lung biopsy or bronchial lavage, stained by silver impregnation. Pneumocystis cannot be cultured routinely and sputum examination is unhelpful. Serum antibody can be detected by immunofluorescence.

Treatment is with co-trimoxazole in large doses (20 mg/kg of trimethoprim and 100 mg/kg of sulphamethoxazole per day, i.e. almost 4 times the normal dose). When other causes have been excluded, patients at high risk are often treated with co-trimoxazole on clinical suspicion (without lung biopsy). The earlier treatment with pentamidine, 4 mg/kg i.m. once a day for 7–10 days, causes serious side effects (such as uraemia and megaloblastic changes in the bone marrow).

β) Treatment When the Pathogen is Not Known (Table 44)

When bacteriological results are not available, or sputum cannot be obtained, proceed as follows:

1. **Primary pneumonia in non-immunocompromised patients** is usually caused (if bacterial) by pneumococci or staphylococci; the latter are no longer always sensitive to penicillin.
   Initial treatment should be with benzyl penicillin in a large dose (e.g. 4–10 megaunits twice a day) for a day or two until defervescence, followed by 1.2–2.4 g of phenoxymethyl penicillin per day. Flucloxacillin or cefazolin, which are also effective against penicillin-resistant staphylococci may now be preferable. If the fever persists for more than 48 hours, infection with mycoplasma, psittacosis or Q-fever should be suspected and a tetracycline given (e.g. rolitetracycline i.v., 250 mg twice a day). Once improvement is established, change to oral doxycycline. If this treatment is also ineffective and the temperature remains high after 48 hrs, the cause may be penicillin-resistant staphylococci, Klebsiella or another gram-negative bacillus. The treatment has to be guided by bacteriological results (see above).
   The failure of β-lactam antibiotics in pneumonias in infants in the first year of life is likely to be due to Chlamydia trachomatis infection which should be treated with erythromycin (50 mg/kg per day). In adults with unresponsive pneumonias, legionellosis should be considered (see p. 354).

2. **Primary interstitial pneumonia:** Mucopurulent sputum, no leucocytosis, high fever and relative bradycardia, widespread opacities on x-ray and a suspicion of mycoplasma pneumonia, psittacosis or Q-fever. *Treat* with doxycycline.

Table 44. Treatment of pneumonia of unknown cause.

Clinical presentation	Treatment of choice	Alternatives
Lobar pneumonia, segmental pneumonia	Benzyl penicillin	Cefazolin, erythromycin
Post-influenza pneumonia	Flucloxacillin + fusidic acid	Cefuroxime, cefamandole, doxycycline + clindamycin, cefazolin
Primary interstitial pneumonia	Doxycycline	Erythromycin
Suppurative pneumonia	Cefoxitin + gentamicin	Ceftazidime or cefotaxime + metronidazole, clindamycin + gentamicin
Aspiration pneumonia	Cefoxitin + gentamicin	Clindamycin + cefotaxime, cefotaxime + metronidazole
Post-operative pneumonia	Cefotaxime + gentamicin	Cefoxitin + azlocillin
Pneumonia in prolonged mechanical ventilation	Azlocillin + gentamicin; ceftazidime + gentamicin	Cephalosporin + azlocillin or piperacillin
Secondary pneumonia (in hospital without previous treatment)	Cefotaxime, possibly with gentamicin	Cefoxitin
Secondary pneumonia (under antibiotic treatment)	Cefoxitin + azlocillin + gentamicin, cefotaxime + aminoglycoside	Doxycycline + erythromycin

Measles or chicken pox can cause primary pneumonia in immunosuppressed children; the latter may now be treated with acyclovir (see p. 536).

3. **Secondary pneumonia, often arising in hospital** (e. g. postoperatively, in immunocompromised patients or pulmonary infarction) is often caused by resistant organisms (staphylococci, Klebsiella etc.) and is often mixed with Haemophilus influenzae, pneumococci, Bacteroides, and very occasionally Legionella.
   Treatment is either with large doses of a cephalosporin (cefoxitin, cefamandole, cefotaxime), 6 g a day for adults, 100 mg/kg for children, or with a penicillin plus an aminoglycoside. If a tetracycline is used, clindamycin should be added for its activity against anaerobes and staphylococci, because many hospital staphylococci are resistant to tetracycline. The bronchial tree is rapidly colonised by gram-negative bacilli in patients receiving mechanical ventilation. It is always difficult to decide whether bacteria isolated from the trachea are the

causes of pneumonia; if this is clinically likely, treatment must also be active against Pseudomonas, e.g. azlocillin (15 g a day) + gentamicin (120–240 mg a day) + flucloxacillin (3 g a day). If antibiotic treatment fails, consider fungal or pneumocystis pneumonia or tuberculosis.

4. **Bronchopneumonia in chronic bronchitis** is usually a mixed infection with pneumococci, Haemophilus influenzae, staphylococci or gram-negative bacteria. When bacteriological results are not available, treat with a broad-spectrum antibiotic which has not been used recently for long-term treatment (e.g. tetracycline, a cephalosporin, ampicillin + cloxacillin) initially, and change on the basis of antibiotic sensitivity testing when available.

5. **Aspiration pneumonia** can occur in patients who are unconscious, have disorders of swallowing, intoxication (alcohol etc.), post-operatively, in obstructions due to neoplasms etc. Abscess formation, possibly with pleural empyema, can also occur. The infections are almost always mixed with anaerobes (fusobacteria, Bacteroides, peptostreptococci, and peptococci), sometimes with aerobic organisms (staphylococci, Pseudomonas and enterobacteria). The sputum is foul and offensive.
Bacteriological culture of sputum is unhelpful because of contamination with oral flora and transtracheal aspiration is advisable.
Treatment: Cefoxitin, which is also effective against anaerobes, possibly in combination with gentamicin, which is particularly useful in mixed infections with enterobacteria and Pseudomonas. Suitable alternatives are clindamycin i.v. or metronidazole i.v. + cefotaxime i.v.

6. **Influenza pneumonia** can appear in epidemics of influenza and tracheobronchitis and in severe cases is usually a superinfection with staphylococci, pneumococci etc.
Initial treatment should be with flucloxacillin plus fusidic acid. Alternatives are cefazolin, cefamandole, cefuroxime, or clindamycin + doxycycline.

7. **Pneumonia of the newborn** often originates in areas of atelectasis or after aspiration of infected amniotic fluid (gram-negative bacilli, group B streptococci, mixed infections). Young infants are also predisposed to staphylococcal pneumonia.
Treatment: Parenteral cefuroxime + azlocillin, cefotaxime + piperacillin, cefoxitin (also active against anaerobes) + gentamicin, or piperacillin + gentamicin.

8. **Pneumonia in the first 6 months of life** accompanied by an eosinophilia is usually due to *Chlamydia trachomatis. Drug of choice:* erythromycin.

o) Legionellosis

In 1976, there was an epidemic of an unusual form of severe pneumonia in Philadelphia (USA). A number of isolated cases and small epidemics have since been seen in many countries.

The *causative agent,* Legionella pneumophila, was unknown until then. It is a gram-negative bacillus, difficult to culture and is common in the inanimate environment (water, soil), where it may coexist with other forms of life such as free-living amoebae. It can spread by a number of ways including contaminated air-conditioning systems and tap water.

Several hospital outbreaks of legionellosis have been described, which have particularly affected elderly patients with extensive underlying disease, as well as patients with lowered resistance, e.g. after renal transplantation. The disease presents as a severe pneumonia which does not respond to the usual treatment with penicillins or cephalosporins. Extrapulmonary symptoms are disturbances of consciousness (encephalopathy), watery diarrhoea, vomiting and disorders of renal function. Milder illnesses with high fever, headaches and muscle pain are also reported (Pontiac fever). Demonstration of the causative organism is difficult in culture, although selective media containing L-cysteine are now available.

The *diagnosis* is still generally based on the demonstration of a rising titre of serum antibody using a specific immunofluorescence test.

Treatment: Penicillins, cephalosporins and aminoglycosides are all ineffective in Legionella infection, but erythromycin, rifampicin and minocycline are clinically active. The relatively *poor prognosis* of inadequately treated legionellosis justifies a trial of treatment with erythromycin in high dosage (up to 1.2 g every 6 h i.v. for at least 3 weeks) which can be supplemented with rifampicin in standard dosage if necessary.

p) Lung Abscess

Primary lung abscesses develop in the course of a pneumonia or septicaemia (when metastatic abscesses may also develop at other sites). The most common bacterial causes are staphylococci, anaerobic streptococci, Bacteroides species and occasionally Klebsiella pneumoniae and Pseudomonas aeruginosa. *Secondary abscesses* often develop in the lung as a result of bronchial obstruction due to a bronchogenic carcinoma or the aspiration of a foreign body. An abscess or necrotising lung infection can also develop in a pulmonary infarct or an infected lung cyst. These infections are usually mixed, with both aerobic and anaerobic bacteria. Sputum culture is often unhelpful because the pathogens of lung abscesses are also found in the mouth flora of healthy persons. A transtracheal aspiration or bronchoscopy should be performed early to obtain pus for bacteriological examination. If the abscess drains into a bronchus, large amounts of pus are coughed up with a fetid offensive smell in anaerobic infections. Other cavitating lesions such as tuberculosis, melioidosis, actinomycosis, nocardiosis, mycoplasma infections, amoebiasis and fungal infections (histoplasmosis, coccidioidomycosis) should be excluded in the differential diagnosis. Pneumatoceles arising from infantile staphylococcal pneumonia should not be confused with lung abscesses.

Treatment: Because the abscesses are almost always due to mixed infection, treatment should cover all the common causative agents of lung abscess (staphylococci, anaerobic streptococci, Bacteroides, enterobacteria), even if only one species has been isolated. Clindamycin i.v. (1.2 g a day) + gentamicin i.m. (320 mg a day) have been commonly used and include all the likely components of a mixed infection. Cefoxitin (6 g a day) with gentamicin is a suitable alternative with the same range of action. Benzyl penicillin in large doses (20 megaunits a day) is active against anaerobic streptococci as well as non-penicillinase-producing staphylococci and sensitive strains of Bacteroides. When penicillin-resistant staphylococci have been isolated, flucloxacillin, cefazolin or cefamandole are also indicated. For anaerobic infections, metronidazole may be added. Any antibiotics must be given in large doses because of the difficulty of achieving adequate concentrations in lung abscesses. Prolonged treatment (6–8 weeks) is usually necessary to achieve a cure.

Improvement is shown by defervescence, reduction in sputum volume, disappearance of pathogens from the sputum and radiological decrease of the abscess cavity. Drainage of the abscess into a bronchus is an important prerequisite for cure. Aspirated foreign bodies underlying an abscess-forming pneumonia have to be removed by endoscopy. Recurrent abscess-forming pneumonia in the same segment may be a sign of bronchial carcinoma. If conservative treatment for at least 8 weeks has resulted in no improvement, surgery should be considered (resection of a segment, or lobectomy).

q) Empyema

Usually develops at the same time as, or following, pneumonia, and associated often with pneumothorax. Nearly always due to rupture of a lung abscess in infants, when pleural drainage is essential. In adults, generally associated with an aspiration pneumonia, or as a continuation of the infection. Sometimes associated with a subphrenic abscess or amoebic liver abscess. Pulmonary tuberculosis is nowadays a rare cause of empyema.

When empyema is clinically suspected, try to obtain a sample for bacteriological testing by needle aspiration of the pus; the prognosis is much better when a known cause can be treated. Foul smelling pus is a sign of mixed anaerobic infection. As well as staphylococci, pneumococci, aerobic and anaerobic streptococci, Bacteroides, Pseudomonas aeruginosa, Klebsiella pneumoniae and other organisms are sometimes isolated. Latex agglutination for pneumococci, group B streptococci and Haemophilus in serum or pleural pus remains positive for several days after antibiotic treatment has started.

Since the causative organisms are easily seen and cultured in the pus, *antibiotic treatment* can be given, as for pneumonia where the pathogen is known (see p. 347). In less serious cases, antibiotic treatment can be supplemented by local measures such as drainage, irrigation, or instillation of substances into the cavity. In pyopneumothorax, viscous pus or loculated empyema, prompt drainage is essential if serious atelectasis or a residual empyema are to be prevented. Drainage bottles used nowadays can be attached to the patient's body, permit more freedom of movement and thus improve pulmonary ventilation. The following antibiotics may be instilled in the concentrations below into the pleural cavity although such instillation is not usually necessary with systemic therapy:

gentamicin[1])	1%	rolitetracycline	0.2–1%
amikacin[1])	0.2–1%	oxacillin	1%
polymyxin B[1])	0.1%	streptomycin[1])	2.5%

In some cases, surgical measures such as rib resection or decortication are necessary.

References

ATKINSON, G. W., H. L. ISRAEL: 5-Fluorocytosine treatment of meningeal and pulmonary aspergillosis. Amer. J. Med. *55:* 496 (1973).

BARKER, G. A.: Current management of croup and epiglottitis. Pediat. Clin. North Amer. *26:* 565 (1979).

BEEM, M. O., E. SAXON, M. A. TRIPPLE: Treatment of chlamydial pneumonia of infancy. Pediat. *63:* 198 (1979).

BROOK, I., S. M. FINEGOLD: Bacteriology and therapy of lung abscess in children. J. Pediat. *94:* 10 (1979).

---

[1]) Because of the possibility of absorption, the prescribed daily dosage should not be exceeded.

CORDES, L. G., H. W. WILKINSON, G. W. GORMAN: Atypical legionella-like organisms: Fastidious water-associated bacteria pathogenic for man. Lancet *2:* 927 (1979).

FADEN, H. S.: Treatment of Hemophilus influence type b epiglottitis. Pediatrics *63:* 402 (1979).

FINEGOLD, S. M., R. D. MEYER: Legionnaire's Disease. In: J. REMINGTON, M. SWARTZ: Current Clinical Topics in Infectious Diseases I. McGraw Hill, New York 1980.

FINLAND, M., M. W. BARNES: Changing ecology of acute bacterial empyema: Occurence and mortality at Boston City Hospital during 12 selected years from 1935 to 1972. J. infect. Dis. *137 (13):* 274 (1978).

FOY, H. M., C. BROOME, P. HAYES: Legionnaire's disease in a medical care group in Seattle 1963–75. Lancet *1:* 767 (1979).

FRASER, D. W., T. TSAI, W. ORENSTEIN: Field Investigative Team. Legionnaire's disease. Description of an epidemic. New Engl. J. Med. *297:* 1189 (1977).

FROMMELL, G. T., F. W. BRUHN, J. D. SCHWARTZMAN: Isolation of Chlamydia trachomatis from infant lung tissue. New Engl. J. Med. *296:* 1150 (1977).

GECKLER, R. W., D. H. GREMILLION, C. K. MCALLISTER: Microscopic and bacteriological comparison of paired sputa and transtracheal aspirates. J. Microbiol. *6:* 396 (1977).

HARMONY, B., M. SANDE, A. SYDNOR: Etiology and antimicrobial therapy of acute maxillary sinusitis. J. infect. Dis. *139:* 197 (1979).

HARRISON, H. R., M. G. ENGLISH, C. K. LEE, E. R. ALEXANDER: Chlamydia trachomatis infant pneumonitis. New Engl. J. Med. *298:* 702 (1978).

HARRISON, H. R., M. G. ENGLISH, C. K. LEE, E. R. ALEXANDER: Chlamydia trachomatis infant pneumonitis: Comparison with matched controls and other infant pneumonitis. New Engl. J. Med. *298:* 702 (1978).

HØIBY, N., P. O. SCHIØTZ: Pulmonary infections in cystic fibrosis. Acta pediat. scand. *Suppl. 301* (1982).

HUGHES, W. T., S. FELDMAN, S. CHAUDHARY, M. J. OSSI, S. K. SANYAL: Comparison of trimethoprimsulfamethoxazole and pentamidine in the treatment of Pneumocystic carinii pneumonitis. J. Pediat. *92:* 285 (1978).

HUGHES, W. T., S. KUHN, S. CHANDHARY, S. FELDMAN, M. VERZOSA, R. J. A. AUR, C. PRATT, S. L. GEORGE: Successful chemoprophylaxis for Pneumocystis carinii pneumonitis. New Engl. J. Med. *297:* 1419 (1977).

JOHN, J. F., Jr.: Trimethoprim-sulfamethoxazole therapy of pulmonary melioidosis. Amer. Rev. resp. Dis. *114:* 1021 (1976).

JONES, R., J. I. SANTOS, J. C. OVERALL: Bacterial tracheitis. JAMA *242:* 721 (1979).

KIRBY, B. D., K. M. SNYDER, R. D. MEYER: Legionnaire's disease: Report of sixty-five nosocomially acquired cases and review of the literature. Medicine *59:* 188 (1980).

KLASTERSKY, J., C. HENSGENS, J. NOTERMAN: Endotracheal antibiotics for the prevention of tracheobronchial infections in tracheostomized unconscious patients. A comparative study of gentamicin and aminosidin-polymyxin B combination. Chest *68:* 302 (1975).

KULCZYCKI, L. L., T. M. MURPHY, J. A. BELLANTI: Pseudomonas colonization in cystic fibrosis. A study of 160 patients. JAMA *240:* 30 (1978).

LAU, W. K., L. S. YOUNG: Trimethoprimsulfamethoxazole treatment of Pneumocystis carinii in adults. New Engl. J. Med. *295:* 716 (1976).

MAY, J. R.: Chemotherapy of chronic bronchitis. English University Press Ltd., London 1968.

MCCURDY, J. A., Jr.: Peritonsillar abscess. Arch. Otol. *103:* 414–415 (1977).

MOLTENI, R. A.: Group A β-hemolytic streptococcal pneumonia. Amer. J. Dis. Child. *131:* 1366 (1977).

POTTER, M. E., A. F. KAUFMANN: Psittacosis in humans in the United States, 1975–1977; from Center for Disease Control: J. infect. Dis. *140* 131 (1979).

SIMON, C., D. SOMMERWERCK, J. FRIEHOFF: Der Wert von Doxycyclin bei Atemwegsinfektionen (Serum-, Speichel-, Sputum-, Lungen- und Pleuraexsudatspiegel). Prax. Pneumol. *32:* 266 (1978).

SIMON, C., A. WANASUKA, D. KIOSZ: Der Latex- und Koagglutinations-Test in Serum und Urin bei kindlichen Pneumonien. Mschr. Kinderheilk. in press (1984).

SIMPSON, R. M., J. J. COGSWELL, E. R. MITCHELL: Legionnaire's disease in an infant. Lancet *2:* 740 (1980).

SOMMERWERCK, D., C. SIMON, J. FRIEHOFF: Minocyclin zur Therapie von Atemwegsinfektionen. Sputum-, Pleuraexsudat- und Lungenspiegel. Dtsch. med. Wschr. *103:* 822 (1978).

WILKINSON, P. J., A. J. BALL, J. DORAN, W. A. GILLESPIE, V. S. ORTON: Routine laboratory assessment of postoperative chest infection: a prospective study. J. clin. Path. *30:* 417 (1977).

7. Infections of the Gastrointestinal Tract

a) Enteric Infections

General remarks: The development of a bacterial gastroenteritis is dependent on a number of factors such as the dose of infecting bacteria, their virulence and the patient's resistance. The only enteropathogenic bacteria virulent enough to give rise to infection after a small infecting dose are Shigella, Vibrio cholerae and enteropathogenic Escherichia coli. Salmonella infection, on the other hand, generally only develops after a massive infecting dose of many millions of organisms. Bacteria usually multiply in the contaminated food (minced meat, mayonnaise etc.). Other factors can increase the susceptibility of the patient, such as age (in enteropathogenic Escherichia coli infection), malnutrition (in cholera), lack of gastric acidity, impaired host defences and severe systemic disease.

There are two main types of severe enteric infection. In the *cholera type* secretion and reabsorption in the small intestine is disrupted; there is not usually any fever. In *dysentery,* organisms invade the colonic wall and the mucosa subsequently ulcerates again, usually with fever. Both forms are fairly readily distinguished by demonstrating pus cells in the faeces, which are only found in large numbers in invasive enteritis.

Many factors related to the causes of enteric infections are still not clear. A recognised bacterial or viral cause is still only found in half of all cases of acute diarrhoea. Possible causes of non-specific diarrhoea, where no cause is found, include infections with micro-organisms not yet recognised as causes of diarrhoea, dietary abnormalities, inadequate digestion due to enzyme deficiencies and other gastro-intestinal disorders.

Demonstration of enteric pathogens: Direct microscopy of a gram-stained smear of faeces may show the organism in post-antibiotic staphylococcal and clostridial enterocolitis. If amoebic dysentery is suspected, a wet preparation is examined microscopically for vegetative parasites and cysts; if specialist examination is not available locally, several stools collected in a period following the use of a saline laxative should be preserved with polyvinyl alcohol or 3.5% formalin and sent to a parasitological laboratory. The stool should also be cultured for salmonellae, shigellae, Yersinia enterocolitica and Campylobacter. Cases of severe diarrhoea following antibiotics should have a note to this effect on the request form because selective culture for Clostridium difficile and the inoculation of tissue cultures for toxin detection can be performed. Bacteria (salmonellae, Clostridium botulinum, Bacillus cereus, staphylococci etc.) and toxins should also be sought in food remnants and vomit after cases of food poisoning.

Acute enteric infections can be caused by viruses (rota-, adeno- and enteroviruses). Rotaviruses can now be detected rapidly in the stool by ELISA. Conventional virus culture is usually of retrospective value only, to shed light on the epidemiology of an outbreak.

When the cause of diarrhoea is not obvious, a number of non-infective conditions such as ulcerative colitis, Crohn's disease, food allergy, irritable colon, malabsorption, pancreatic insufficiency, lactose intolerance, laxative abuse, fructose intolerance, Addison's disease, hyperthyroidism, pheochromocytoma and poisoning should be considered.

α) Treatment of Enteric Infections

Systemic treatment: Enteric infections tend to be self-limiting and heal spontaneously. Chemotherapy is superfluous in mild, non-invasive infections. Severe cases of enteric infection with fever, bloodstained or purulent diarrhoea resembling dysentery, and enteric infections complicating primary diseases such as leukaemia, hepatic cirrhosis and immunosuppression should be treated with systemic antibiotics, which should be given by mouth. Co-trimoxazole and ampicillin are the drugs of choice for the treatment of severe bacterial dysentery when the cause is not confirmed. Tetracyclines are useful in cases of suspected Yersinia infection and cholera. Non-absorbed antibiotics such as neomycin, polymyxin and poorly absorbable sulphonamides are active but rarely used. Parenteral antibiotics should only be given to patients with enteric infections in exceptional circumstances. The role of new β-lactam antibiotics such as cefoperazone, ceftriaxone and mezlocillin which achieve high intestinal concentrations is still uncertain. Fluid and electrolyte replacement can be more important in severe enteric infections than chemotherapy.

Shigella dysentery: Acute febrile diarrhoea (bacillary dysentery) with tenesmus and mucous, often bloodstained, stools. The resistance of shigellae to sulphonamides and antibiotics, particularly ampicillin, has been increasing, especially among strains of Shigella sonnei. Where antibiotics are given, therefore, they should be chosen on the basis of tested sensitivities, particularly during an epidemic. Severe infections may be treated with co-trimoxazole (960 mg twice a day for adults, 10–15 mg/kg twice a day for children) or ampicillin (3 g orally a day for adults, 100 mg/kg for children), both by mouth for 5 days. The poorly absorbed sulphonamides are unsatisfactory, as are antibiotics with a local effect only and which produce no tissue concentrations. Amoxycillin is unreliable in bacterial dysentery.

Salmonella enteritis is an acute, sometimes febrile gastroenteritis of variable intensity which usually occurs 8–24 hours after a meal contaminated with salmonellae. It often occurs in outbreaks. Typhoid and paratyphoid fevers, which are septicaemic illnesses, should not be confused with salmonella enteritis as they are treated quite differently.

Mild, transient infections resolve spontaneously and are self-limiting, so antibiotics are unnecessary. More severe infections with fever and bloody diarrhoea, or in the first year of life may require systemic antibiotics, particularly in patients with a high fever, septicaemia or immunological impairment, because of the risk of metastatic infection of other organs (e.g. osteomyelitis, septic arthritis). Use ampicillin (3–5 g a day for adults, 100–150 mg/kg for children), or co-trimoxazole (960 mg twice a day). Despite its good clinical effect, chloramphenicol should not be used for the treatment of mild salmonella enteritis because of its haematoxicity. There is strong evidence that unnecessary antibiotic treatment of salmonella enteritis actually prolongs the subsequent carrier state (p. 452).

Salmonella gastroenteritis in patients with severe underlying diseases (leukaemia, immunosuppression, organ transplantation, cirrhosis etc.) carries a considerable risk of septicaemia and metastatic infection. Treatment with ampicillin, co-trimoxazole, mezlocillin or cefotaxime (parenteral) should always be given to such patients.

Yersiniosis: An infection due to Yersinia pseudotuberculosis or Yersinia enterocolitica usually presents as enteritis or rarely septicaemia but may mimic appendicitis as a result of the associated mesenteric lymphadenitis. A not uncommon disease, although the cause is often not demonstrated by culture of Yersinia from mesenteric lymph nodes excised at laparotomy for suspected appendicitis. Faecal cultures may be positive. Serological diagnosis is available, detecting specific antibodies by a rising titre. Most cases recover spontaneously. Tetracyclines and co-trimoxazole are effective.

Campylobacter gastroenteritis is currently the commonest bacterial form of gastroenteritis in Britain. It is generally a mild infection, particularly in children and adolescents. The causative organism, Campylobacter jejuni, is widely distributed in animals and infections are often caused by food (meat, milk, dairy products). Outbreaks sometimes occur, associated with failures of pasteurisation of milk, contaminated water supplies etc. The disease follow a course similar to that of Salmonella gastroenteritis. Culture requires special methods. Curved bacilli can be demonstrated in the stool by phase-contrast microscopy. Erythromycin shortens the period of excretion of the organism, but its efficacy in reducing the severity and duration of symptoms is not yet established.

Cholera and cholera-like illnesses present as acute enteritis with persistent watery stools, fluid and electrolyte loss due to toxin, hypovolaemic shock, metabolic acidosis, muscle cramps, and aphonia. Severe cases show a characteristic clinical picture. The causative bacteria can be demonstrated by microscopy and culture. Cholera is not encountered in Northern, Central or Western Europe, but can still be acquired in the Mediterranean area. A cholera-like illness is sometimes found in other forms of gastroenteritis due, for example, to salmonella and enterotoxigenic strains of Escherichia coli.

Treatment is primarily by fluid and electrolyte replacement with infusions containing glucose, and correction of the metabolic acidosis. If the infusion is continued (maintenance therapy), the fluid loss must be carefully monitored by clinical and laboratory tests to prevent relapse into shock. If parenteral fluids are not available or cannot be given, oral replacement is recommended (20 g glucose, 4 g NaCl, 4 g $NaHCO_3$, 1 g KCl in 1 litre of water).

Antibiotic treatment with tetracycline for at least 5 days is effective in rapidly eliminating Vibrio cholerae from the bowel, so reducing stool volume and the i.v. fluid requirement.

Tetracycline may be given in a dose of 1 g per day to adults and 50 mg/kg to children, both orally. Co-trimoxazole and ampicillin are also effective, particularly where tetracycline-resistant cholera vibrios are found during an epidemic.

Prophylaxis: Vaccination is not fully effective and careful hygiene in endemic areas is very important.

Escherichia coli gastroenteritis: Escherichia coli can cause different forms of enteritis. Enterotoxin-forming strains cause severe intestinal infection in infants. Hospital infections have often occured in the past. This type of enteritis is particularly serious in the newborn. Diarrhoea is associated with loss of weight, anorexia and vomiting. Leucocytes cannot be demonstrated microscopically in the stool. The mortality rate in premature babies is more than 10%. The second form, which resembles a dysentery, is caused by infection with strains of Escherichia coli which have invasive properties and can lead to a dysentery-like clinical picture, especially in older children. The stool contains numerous leucocytes.

Treatment: Infections with enterotoxigenic Escherichia coli should be treated primarily by fluid and electrolyte replacement. Antibiotics have been used but there is much uncertainty about their value. Non-absorbable agents such as neomycin, colistin, polymyxin B and paromomycin may be given by mouth for a week, and nystatin (1 ml of suspension by mouth 3 times a day to prevent fungal overgrowth) added. Dysentery-like infections should be treated with poorly absorbable sulphonamides, ampicillin or co-trimoxazole.

Travellers' diarrhoea: Travellers to Southern Europe and other warm climates often suffer acute, usually afebrile diarrhoea. There is no clear cause. Enterotoxigenic strains of Escherichia coli are apparently the cause in many cases, although other agents such as salmonellae, shigellae, enteroinvasive Escherichia coli, Vibrio parahaemolyticus, Giardia lamblia and viruses can also be involved.

Treatment: Rapid spontaneous resolution occurs in mild forms without fever or systemic features. Severe cases may respond to co-trimoxazole in the usual dosage. The value of prophylaxis is disputed but careful hygiene is important. Quinoline derivatives, e. g. iodochlorhydroxyquinoline (Enterovioform) can have dangerous side effects (e. g. subacute myelooptic neuropathy) when used prophylactically or for treatment and in some countries (e. g. Britain) have been withdrawn.

If simple treatment fails, the stool should be examined microscopically for ova, cysts and parasites. If protozoa are found, give metronidazole; helminths or their eggs should be treated with mebendazole or thiabendazole. An oral balanced sugar and electrolyte solution is useful as are simple preparations to relieve diarrhoea. Anti-diarrhoeal agents containing antibiotics should be avoided. Loperamide has some value but should be avoided in small infants because of the danger of toxic megacolon and only one or two doses should be given.

Necrotising enterocolitis is a life threatening disease of the newborn with severe abdominal distention and blood stained stools in 25% of cases, often accompanied by perforation of ulcers, peritonitis and ileus. The course is rapid and often fatal.

The cause is unknown, but ischaemia or damage to the intestinal mucosa by local toxin is assumed to facilitate the penetration of bacteria. The associated peritonitis is always a mixed infection.

Treatment in cases with peritonitis and septicaemia is with gentamicin + cefotaxime parenterally, dosing with care because of the impaired renal function at this age. An alternative is cefotaxime + piperacillin + clindamycin (i.v.). Intestinal perforation (free air in the abdomen) requires immediate operation. Other measures include fluid replacement, the treatment of shock, possible mechanical ventilation, a nasogastric tube and peritoneal dialysis.

Viral gastroenteritis: Often occurs in younger children, usually as a mild intestinal illness due to rotaviruses, coronaviruses, enteroviruses, echo, coxsackie, polioviruses, and adenoviruses. Virus can be detected in the stool by the ELISA technique, by latex agglutination and by electron microscopy. There is no specific treatment, although mixtures of chalk and kaolin are sometimes given.

Antibiotic-associated colitis: Antibiotic treatment can disrupt the normal intestinal flora and lead to the overgrowth of certain potentially pathogenic bacteria such as staphylococci, Bacteroides fragilis, Pseudomonas aeruginosa and other resistant organisms. One serious form of enterocolitis is caused by the selection of Clostridium difficile, and is particularly associated with clindamycin, lincomycin and ampicillin, and less frequently with tetracyclines, the newer penicillins and cephalosporins and co-trimoxazole. It is expressed by profuse diarrhoea, vomiting, collapse and circulatory failure (see p. 160).

The fully developed syndrome of pseudomembranous enterocolitis is chronic, sometimes fatal, and has a course similar to that of ulcerative colitis. In both diseases numerous leucocytes can be demonstrated microscopically in the stool. Clostridium difficile toxin can be detected in the stool by its cytopathic effect in tissue culture. The diagnosis can be confirmed by demonstrating typical changes on colonoscopy.

Treatment must be started on clinical suspicion. Severe cases of pseudomembraneous enterocolitis with a sudden onset of profuse diarrhoea and systemic symptoms carry a poor prognosis, and treatment of shock by fluid and electrolyte replacement is very important. All antibiotics should be discontinued immediately and vancomycin given by mouth (250–500 mg every 4–6 hours for 7–10 days). Higher doses are not necessary. Metronidazole is also effective against Clostridium difficile.

Bacterial food poisoning: The most important bacterial causes are salmonellae (incubation period 8–25 h) and exotoxin-producing staphylococci (incubation period 1–6 h). Other bacteria can also cause mild or severe diarrhoea when present in food in large amounts (e. g. Pseudomonas aeruginosa, Bacillus cereus, Aeromonas hydrophila, Plesiomonas shigelloides, Clostridium perfringens, Proteus etc.). The causative agents are more easily detected in the food than in the stool.

In mild cases, *symptomatic treatment* is sufficient, e. g. with chalk or kaolin mixtures, electrolyte infusions, antispasmodics etc., because the symptoms are often due purely to the toxins present in the food. Antibiotic treatment of salmonella food poisoning is only required in exceptionally severe cases; the disease is normally mild and self-limiting, and antibiotics have been clearly shown to prolong the duration of bacterial excretion in the stool.

Botulism: Diarrhoea and vomiting with symmetrical cranial nerve paralysis in a fully conscious patient. Risk of respiratory arrest. Toxin may be detected by animal inoculation in the serum and in food remnants. Intestinal botulism has occasionally been described in infants who develop the typical neurological features and disturbances of cardiac rhythm but no diarrhoea despite the presence of toxin-producing clostridia in the intestine. Wound botulism is very rare.

Treatment: Immediate administration of trivalent botulinum antitoxin, corticosteroids, treatment of shock, intensive care, mechanical ventilation if necessary, and a cardiac pacemaker. Unabsorbed toxin is removed with magnesium sulphate, active charcoal tablets or an enema. Benzyl penicillin is recommended to interrupt the formation of toxin in the intestine, in a dose of 4 megaunits a day for adults and 50,000 units/kg in children i. v.; it is not, however, effective in infantile intestinal botulism.

Enteritis caused by Vibrio parahaemolyticus: Halophile vibrios have frequently caused food infections in Japan and the U.S.A., associated mainly with mussels, raw fish or contaminated meals. Vibrio parahaemolyticus has only occasionally been described in Europe. The disease follows a similar course to that of salmonella enteritis with diarrhoea (sometimes bloodstained), gastric discomfort, nausea, vomiting, headache and moderate fever. Spontaneous resolution usually occurs within 2–5 days. Co-trimoxazole can be useful in severe cases.

Amoebic dysentery: Acute or chronic form. Many patients are asymptomatic cyst passers, carrying the cysts only in the lumen of the bowel. Diagnosis is made by the microscopical demonstration of cysts and minutae forms of amoebae in the faeces, if necessary by sending a preserved stool to a reference laboratory (see p. 359). Intestinal mucosal involvement is confirmed by the presence of tissue (magna) forms which only occur in the fresh stool. The presence of an amoebic liver abscess can be confirmed by a CT scan or an ultrasound investigation. Antibodies are detectable in the serum in tissue infections by latex agglutination, an indirect haemagglutination antibody test, by indirect immunofluoroscence and by CFT.

Asymptomatic infestation of the bowel lumen must be distinguished from tissue infection. Metronidazole is the drug of choice, given by mouth in a dose of 750 mg 3 times a day (10–15 mg/kg 3 times a day for children) for 5 days in mild infections and for 10 days in severe infections. It is active against all forms of the disease (including liver abscess), and, because of the risk of tissue invasion, should also be used for asymptomatic infections of the bowel lumen, and for carriers. To avoid relapse luminal cysts can be eradicated by a sequential course of diloxanide furoate, 500 mg 3 times a day for ten days. In liver abscess, which is usually solitary, admit to hospital and give bed rest, restrict food or give a liquid diet and treat fluid and electrolyte imbalance. Signs of rupture into the pleura, pericardium or peritoneum should be carefully sought. Chloroquine in combination with emetine or dihydro-emetine can be used in metronidazole intolerance or occasional failures of treatment. Large liver abscesses may need aspiration on one or more occasions. Further complications are secondary infections and hepatic vein thrombosis. Relapses can occur in the first 6 weeks of treatment and patients should be observed carefully during this period.

The *treatment* and *prophylaxis of infections of the lumen* of the bowels can also be achieved with quinoline derivatives (short-term), ornidazole, tinidazole, or diloxanide furoate.

Balantidial dysentery: Acute or protracted colitis with bloodstained stools. Infection is often symptom-free. Balantidia can easily be seen under the microscope. Pigs and other animals are the sources of infection.

Treatment: Oral metronidazole, 75–100 mg for 5 days, or tetracycline, particularly oxytetracycline, 2 g per day by mouth.

Giardiasis: Acute or chronic infestation with Giardia lamblia affecting the small intestine and transferred by drinking water, food, or direct contact (humans or domestic animals). Commoner in children and immunosuppressed patients. The parasites are demonstrated microscopically in duodenal contents and less reliably in the stool because of intermittent excretion. Direct demonstration of antigen in the stool using an ELISA technique is now possible.

Treatment: Metronidazole, 750 mg a day for adults (in three single oral doses), 250 mg a day for children of 4–8 years and 125 mg a day for children under 4 years. A single dose of tinidazole (2 g for adults and 1 g for children from 6–12 years) is also effective provided asymptomatic carriers are treated at the same time.

Cryptosporidiosis is caused by the protozoon Cryptosporidium and occurs in man and animals including domestic animals. The disease can occur at any age but is particularly associated with immune deficiency (e. g. AIDS) and gives rise to a cholera-like diarrhoea, usually with fever and colic, often with a protracted course, sometimes with a malabsorption syndrome (sub-total villous atrophy in the small intestine). The parasite can be shown microscopically in a small intestinal biopsy after alcohol fixation and staining with Giemsa, and oocysts can be shown in the stool after Giemsa staining.

Treatment: No effective treatment yet known.

Whipworm infections: The large intestine is infested with Trichuris trichiura. The disease is variable. The diarrhoea may be mucous and sometimes blood-stained, with colic and occasionally rectal prolapse. Commoner in tropical countries. The characteristic yellowish ova may be demonstrated in the stool.

Treatment: Mebendazole (200 mg twice a day for 3 days) or thiabendazole (25 mg/kg twice a day for 3 days).

Ulcerative colitis: Non-infectious, ulcerative inflammation of the large intestine of uncertain aetiology; bacterial infections play a secondary role. The antibacterial treatment does not therefore eliminate the cause.

The following drugs are recommended: sulfasalazine, 4–8 g initially, then 1.5–3 g/day as a maintenance dose for long-term treatment once improvement occurs. Its effect depends on the release and absorption of 5-amino salicylic acid in the intestine, and not on antibacterial activity. Close monitoring is required because of frequent side effects (allergic rashes, fever etc.). If sulphonamides fail, treatment with metronidazole may be attempted.

Antibiotic combinations effective against anaerobes and enterobacteria are indicated in acute toxic colitis or severe exacerbation of a secondary bacterial infection (e. g. cefotaxime + metronidazole, or cefoxitin + azlocillin). The chances of success are not high, however. Can also be treated with prednisone, sedatives, diet, blood transfusions (in emergencies), and psychotherapy. Surgical measures (colectomy) are required in 15–20%.

Crohn's disease: Non-infectious granulomatous inflammation of the distal small intestine and less often of the colon. Aetiology unknown. Bacterial infections may play a secondary role in the development of fistula. As with ulcerative colitis, long-term treatment with sulfasalazine is recommended. Fever, fistula and local collections of pus often require additional antibiotic therapy. Benzyl penicillin, metronidazole or combinations with activity against anaerobes and enterobacteria (e. g. gentamicin + clindamycin, cefoxitin + piperacillin, cefotaxime + metronidazole) can be used.

b) Appendicitis

Uncomplicated appendicitis should not be treated with antibiotics alone; prompt appendicectomy is the treatment of choice. Antibiotics should be given in complicated cases (perforation, peritonitis, portal vein phlebitis, intra-abdominal abscess). Chemotherapy is also required if surgery cannot be performed immediately. This treatment (including metronidazole) is also necessary when appendicitis is suspected but an amoeboma cannot be excluded, as in the tropics. Severe systemic reactions such as a poor general condition and high fever are also indications for preoperative antibiotic treatment. The *chemotherapy of appendicitis* should cover the common agents found in mixed infections (Bacteroides fragilis, anaerobic streptococci and enterobacteria). Treat with combinations such as cefoxitin + piperacillin, or cefotaxime + metronidazole.

c) Peritonitis

There are many causes of perforating peritonitis, and the resultant infections are usually mixed, including Bacteroides, anaerobic streptococci and enterobacteria. Primary peritonitis is uncommon, and usually caused by streptococci or pneumococci, particularly in the nephrotic syndrome and cirrhosis. Meconium peritonitis occurs in newborn babies with cystic fibrosis and is not bacterial. Peritonitis can follow peritoneal dialysis (e. g. with Candida) or be caused by gonococci.

Therapy: Surgery is almost always essential, usually with drainage as well as removal of the cause of the infection. The peritoneal exudate should always be cultured, and antibiotic therapy should always be started before the operation. Because intestinal perforation gives rise to a mixed bacterial infection, an apparently pure culture should never be accepted as showing the sole pathogen; anaerobes die easily during transport. Thus culture of Escherichia coli, for example, does not show this to be the sole causative agent. Antibiotic treatment must always cover the whole range of potential pathogens. Recommended combinations: cefotaxime + metronidazole, cefoxitin + piperacillin or mezlocillin + gentamicin + metronidazole. The combination of chloramphenicol + clindamycin + gentamicin which used to be popular is now rarely recommended. Acute renal failure often occurs at the same time and should be taken into account. The intraperitoneal instillation of an aminoglycoside or polymyxin is not as well distributed or as effective as parenteral therapy, and can give rise to a dangerous neuromuscular blockade with respiratory arrest (antidote: prostigmine and calcium gluconate i.v.). The intraperitoneal use of tetracyclines is often very irritant. Chloramphenicol in the injectable form (as the succinate) is not active when instilled directly. Most antibiotics and particularly the penicillins and cephalosporins are so rapidly absorbed when given intraperitoneally that local treatment has no advantage. Peritoneal irrigation with povidone iodine is of questionable value (low activity, absorption of iodine and povidone).

Benzyl penicillin i.v., 5–10 megaunits a day, is the drug of choice in streptococcal, pneumococcal and gonococcal peritonitis.

d) Pancreatitis

Pancreatitis is usually due to autodigestion. Bacterial infection, which is usually mixed, only plays a secondary role in the late stages of the disease. Treatment consists of the management of shock, analgesics, aspiration of the gastric contents, fasting, parenteral nutrition, atropine, calcium gluconate i.v. (in hypocalcaemia), and the treatment of any known cause, e.g. gall stones, by surgery if necessary. If antibiotic treatment is required, rolitetracycline i.v. (250 mg twice daily, 10 mg/kg for children), or mezlocillin i.v. (3–6 g a day for adults, 150 mg/kg for children in 3–4 divided doses) may be tried. Cefotaxime or cefoperazone may also be considered.

e) Liver Abscess

Occurs as a complication of biliary sepsis, after infected portal vein thrombosis and in amoebic liver abscess.

Bacterial causes include Bacteroides species, anaerobic and microaerophilic streptococci, and less frequently enterobacteria and staphylococci. The diagnosis is difficult: liver tenderness on percussion, ultrasound studies, CT scanning, hepatic scintigraphy, liver angiography, and amoebic antibody studies in the serum, and possibly the demonstration of amoebae in the stool. Large abscesses may need aspiration under antibiotic cover.

The *treatment* has to cover all the likely causes including Entamoeba histolytica; antibiotic combinations are therefore necessary, such as mezlocillin + metronidazole, cefotaxime + metronidazole, or ampicillin + gentamicin + metronidazole. Other possible combinations include clindamycin, cefoxitin, piperacillin or another aminoglycoside. Treatment of amoebic abscess is described on p. 365.

f) Infections of the Biliary Tract

There is no clear correlation between particular agents and the clinical picture. Bile duct infections are nearly always secondary to a mechanical obstruction such as a stone, tumour, papillary stenosis etc. Primary bacterial cholangitis with no mechanical cause occurs only in Southeast Asia. Cholecystitis and empyema of the gall bladder are also nearly always due to obstruction.

The *causative organisms* include Escherichia coli, aerobic and anaerobic streptococci, Bacteroides species, and occasionally other enterobacteria, salmonellae, Clostridium perfringens etc., often in mixed infections. Culture of the causative agents is difficult, because not all patients have positive blood cultures. Culture of the duodenal contents is not helpful. Bile should always be sent for a cultural examination after operation or ERCP. An *antibiotic* used for treating biliary infections should fulfil the following *criteria:*
1. Activity against organisms associated with biliary infection.
2. High blood and tissue levels.
3. Effective concentrations in the hepatic bile (not only as inactive metabolites).
4. Adequate biliary concentrations in cholestasis.
5. No antagonistic effect of bile on the activity of the antibiotic.

The antibiotic treatments of cholecystitis and cholangitis are broadly similar. Tetracyclines used to be the drugs of choice and they are excreted in the bile in high concentrations. Their spectrum of activity includes most of the causes of bile duct infections. Treatment with tetracyclines has often been disappointing, however, and the high failure rate may be explained by an antagonism of the bile to the activity of the tetracyclines. Tetracyclines are not active at the normal slightly alkaline pH of the bile. The inactivation of tetracyclines in the bile is also reflected by the failure to eliminate bacteria. β-Lactam antibiotics, on the other hand, rapidly clear the bile of bacteria. Mezlocillin and cephalosporins which achieve satisfactory biliary concentrations (e. g. cefotaxime, cefoperazone) are generally suitable for the treatment of biliary infections. β-Lactam antibiotics such as ampicillin, cefazolin, cefazedone, and cefoxitin, are concentrated in the bile when there is no cholestasis, so are not always suitable for biliary sepsis. Aminoglycosides can also be used in combination therapy; the concentrations in bile are lower than in blood, but aminoglycosides are more active in the bile than in the serum. Co-trimoxazole achieves good biliary concentrations and, when given by i. v. infusion, is a good choice for the treatment of acute cholecystitis and cholangitis.

In severe biliary infections, use a combination of a β-lactam antibiotic with an aminoglycoside. The importance of adequate biliary concentrations in the treatment of biliary infections should not be overestimated, for tissue concentrations also play a major role. Recommended treatment for uncomplicated biliary infections: cefotaxime or cefoperazone (4–6 g a day) or mezlocillin (6–15 g), alone or with gentamicin (160–240 mg a day). If there is no cholestasis, amoxycillin (6–15 g a day), cefazolin (4–6 g a day), cefazedone (4–6 g a day), cefoxitin (6 g a day), or co-trimoxazole may also be used.

Mild biliary infections may be treated orally with amoxycillin (3 g a day), co-trimoxazole (1.92 g a day) or doxycycline (200 mg a day).

Further treatment: The most important measure for the effective treatment of cholangitis is the removal of the obstruction by operation or papillotomy. Without these measures, the biliary infections will recur.

When there is an *empyema of the gallbladder,* cholecystectomy under antibiotic cover is necessary either as an acute operation or at an interval after the acute infection has been brought under control by antibiotics. The temporary improvement brought about by chemotherapy does not remove the necessity of a subsequent definitive operation. Antibiotic treatment of biliary infections is of limited value.

Because bacterial infections (fever, septicaemia, cholangitis, pancreatitis) often complicate endoscopic surgery of the bile ducts (e.g. ERCP), such procedures may be carried out under antibiotic *prophylaxis.* Mezlocillin, cefazedone or cefotaxime are suitable for this purpose, and should be started shortly before the procedure and only continued for a short period afterwards.

References

ARNON, S. S., F. F. MIDURA, K. DAMUS: Honey and other environmental risk factors for infant botulism. J. Pediat. *94:* 331 (1979).

BLAKE, P. A.: Cholera: A possible endemic focus in the United States. New Engl. J. Med. *302:* 305 (1980).

BLASER, M. J., I. D. BERKOWITZ, F. M. LaFORCE: Campylobacter enteritis: Clinical and epidemiological features. Amer. J. intern. Med. *91:* 179 (1979).

CHANG, M. J., L. M. DUNKLE, D. VAN REKEN: Trimethoprim-sulfamethoxazole compared to ampicillin in the treatment of shigellosis. Pediatrics *59:* 726 (1977).

CHERUBIN, C. E., J. F. TIMONEY, M. F. SIERRA, P. MA, J. MARR, S. SHIN: A sudden decline in ampicillin resistance in Salmonella typhimurium. JAMA *243:* 439 (1980).

DE BAKEY, M., G. JORDAN: Hepatic abscesses. Surg. Clin. North Amer. *57:* 325 (1977).

DE, S., A. CHAUDHURI, P. DUTTA, D. DUTTA, S. P. DE, S. C. PAL: Doxycycline in the treatment of cholera. Bull WHO *54:* 3505 (1976).

ECKERT, P., H. P. EICHFUSS: Peritonitis. Thieme, Stuttgart 1978.

ENAT, R., SR. POLLACK, S. LIN: Treatment of Salmonella typhimurium salmonellosis. Lancet *2:* 638 (1978).

FORMAL, S. B., R. B. HORNICK: Invasive *Escherichia coli.* J. infect. Dis. *137:* 641 (1978).

GUERRANT, R. L., R. G. LAHITA, W. C. WINN: Campylobacterosis in man: Pathogenic mechanisms and review of 91 bloodstream infections. Amer. J. Med. *65:* 584 (1978).

HELM, E., W. STILLE: Akute Enteritis durch Aeromonas hydrophila. Dtsch. med. Wschr. *95:* 18 (1970).

HELM, E. B., I. PAULUS, P. M. SHAH, W. STILLE: Antibakterielle Aktivität von Antibiotika in menschlicher Galle. Infection *4:* 94 (1976).

HYAMS, J. S., W. A. DURBIN, R. J. GRAND, D. A. GOLDMANN: Salmonella bacteremia in the first year of life. J. Pediat. *96:* 57 (1980).

International Conference on Diarrhea of Travelers: New directions in research: A summary. J. infect. Dis. *137:* 355 (1978).

JOHNSON, R. O., S. A. CLAY, S. S. ARNON: Diagnosis and management of infant botulism. Amer. J. Dis. Child. *133:* 586 (1979).

KARMALI, M. A., P. C. FLEMING: *Campylobacter* enteritis in children. J. Pediat. *94:* 527 (1979).

KOHL, S.: *Yersinia enterocolitica* infection in children. Pediat. Clin. North Amer. *26:* 433 (1979).

KROGSTAD, D. J., H. C. SPENCER, G. R. HEALY: Amebiasis. New Engl. J. Med. *297:* 1329 (1977).

LAMBERT, H. (Ed.): Infections of the GI-tract in clinics in gastroenterology. Saunders. London 1979.

LAUWERS, S., M. DeBOECK, J. P. BUTZLER: *Campylobacter* enteritis in Brussels, letter. Lancet *1:* 604 (1978).

MARKS, M. I., C. H. PAI, L. LAFLEUR: Yersinia entercolitica gastroenteritis: A prospective study of clinical, bacteriologic, and epidemiologic features. J. Pediat. *96:* 26 (1980).

METZGER, J. F., G. E. LEWIS, Jr.: Human-derived immune globulins for the treatment of botulism. Rev. infect. Dis. *1:* 689 (1979).

NELSON, J. D.: Comparison of trimethoprim-sulfamethoxazole and ampicillin therapy for shigellosis in ambulatory patients. J. Pediat. *89:* 491 (1976).

NELSON, J. D., H. KUSMIESZ, L. H. JACKSON, E. WOODMAN: Treatment of Salmonella gastroenteritis with ampicillin, amoxicillin or placebo. Pediatrics *65:* 1125 (1980).

RETTIG, P. J.: Campylobacter infections in human beings. J. Pediat. *94:* 855 (1979).

RODRIGUEZ, W. J., C. CONTRINI, C. J. COHEN: *Yersinia enterocolitica* enteritis in children. JAMA *242:* 1978 (1979).

SACK, R. B., J. L. FROEHLICH, A. W. ZULICH: Prophylactic doxycycline for travelers' diarrhea: Results of a prospective double-blind study of Peace Corps volunteers in Morocco. Gastroenterology *76:* 1368 (1979).

SAEBO, A.: Liver affection associated with *Yersinia enterocolitica* infection. Acta chir. scand. *143:* 445 (1977).

SACK, D. A., D. C. KAMINSKY, B. SACK, J. N. INOTIA, A. R. RAY, A. Z. ZAPIKIAN, F. ØRSKOV, I. ØRSKOV: Prophylactic doxycycline for traveler's diarrhea. New Engl. J. Med. *298:* 758 (1978).

STILLE, W., R. TIMMLER (Eds.): Gallenweg-Infektionen. Steinkopff, Darmstadt 1977.

TEDESCO, F., R. MARKHAM, M. GURWITH, D. CHRISTIE, J. G. BARTLETT: Oral vancomycin for antibiotic-associated pseudomembranous colitis. Lancet *2:* 226 (1978).

TERRANOVA, W., P. A. BLAKE: Bacillus cereus food poisoning. New Engl. J. Med. *298:* 143 (1978).

WOLFE, M. S.: Giardiasis. Pediat. Clin. North Amer. *26:* 295 (1979).

8. Infections of the Urogenital Tract

a) Urinary Infections (Including Pyelonephritis)

Introduction: The division of infections of the urinary tract into pyelonephritis and cystitis, i.e. upper and lower urinary tract infections, gives rise to certain difficulties. There are a number of infections which cannot be clearly classified into one or other group and which should simply be called urinary infections. Cystitis can, of course, be the first stage of a pyelonephritis, but the likelihood of a lower urinary infection developing into chronic pyelonephritis has apparently been overrated in the past. This risk seems to be higher in children than in adults because replacement of damaged renal tissue by scar tissue has a more severe effect in the growing kidneys. Any cause of obstruction such as outflow obstruction, stones, ureteric valves, ureterocele and prostatic hypertrophy is an important factor in the development of urinary infection. Appropriate investigations such as a micturating urogram and ultrasound should be carried out at the first sign of relapse of the urinary infection, if not before.

A practical *classification of urinary infections* is into *obstructive* and *non-obstructive* forms. Congenital malformations such as hydronephrosis, megaureter, urethral valves and other anomalies are the cause of 10–20% of recurrent urinary infections in children, particularly in boys.

Urinary infections are common in diabetes mellitus and pregnancy, in both of which regular urine tests are necessary. Repeated urinary infections are virtually inevitable in patients with a paraplegic bladder, and often lead to chronic renal failure. Infections of an obstructed urinary tract carry a considerable risk of septicaemia, the prognosis of which is often poor.

Chronic pyelonephritis is sometimes asymptomatic in life and first becomes apparent at post-mortem examination. Every relapse of an acute pyelonephritis which has not been eradicated can, even if occurring after a symptom-free interval, be an acute exacerbation of chronic pyelonephritis. It is often difficult to decide at what stage chronic pyelonephritis develops, with its subsequent progression to the end-stage, small, contracted kidney. The signs of chronic pyelonephritis develop insidiously, although eventually the diagnosis becomes clear; they comprise polyuria, anaemia, attacks of fever, bacteriuria sometimes without leucocyturia, hypertension and severe electrolyte imbalance due to tubular insufficiency.

Microbiological examination of the urine: Reliable methods of examination and culture of urine, and the correct evaluation of the results, are essential for rational treatment. Unnecessary treatment may be given on the basis of results from urine culture which has been performed incorrectly (e. g. unsterile container, incorrect method of collection, delay in transit to the laboratory, misinterpretation of vaginal flora in dip-slide cultures). On the other hand, failure to examine the urine appropriately may lead to an acute infection being missed.

Collection of urine for microbiological examination: Mid-stream urine is normally used for urine microscopy and culture. The procedure for collection of a mid-stream urine is as follows: First clean the urethral meatus or vulva with physiological saline or a weak disinfectant such as 2% hydrogen peroxide solution. Urine is best collected from the woman in the position for gynaecological examination. Use a special sterile urine collection bag in infants which should be briefly attached to the vulva or over the penis. The urine is collected from adults into a sterile container and should be cultured within 30 min or cooled at once to 4° C and sent as soon as possible to the laboratory. In small children and in emergencies, a catheter specimen may be necessary, particularly if the leucocyte count in a spontaneously voided urine is raised. Suprapubic aspiration of a full bladder is a safe and reliable method of urine collection even in infants and the newborn. If there is no local bacteriological laboratory, a dip-slide culture can be used (see below), and supplemented by a cell count and a methylene-blue stain of a voided sample. Another alternative is to use 1% boric acid as a urine preservative.

Examination for cells: The fresh, uncentrifuged mid-stream urine is examined microscopically in a counting chamber for white cells (counts above $20/mm^3$ are abnormal) and red cells, and the sediment is examined on a cover-slip for casts, particularly granular casts. The white cell count in a urine deposit can be misleading, since large variations can occur, due to mechanical causes.

Granulocytes can now be detected in the urine by the use of test strips (e. g. Cytur, Chemstrip). The method estimates the chloroacetate esterase content of both intact and lysed granulocytes and has a 90–95% correlation with quantitative cell counts. False positive and false negative results can occur. Provided the urine is collected correctly, this method can be readily used by the physician in his consulting room or when making domiciliary visits, as well as by the patient herself.

Bacteria can also be detected microscopically in a fresh, uncentrifuged mid-stream urine, particularly if stained with methylene blue. Bacteria are not normally present and, if seen in large numbers in a fresh specimen, are suggestive of significant bacteriuria; in such cases, a direct disc sensitivity test (see below) can often give a readable result the next day.

Quantitative bacterial count: A bacterial count of more than 100000/ml of urine indicates a significant bacteriuria. Contaminants or bacteria from the urethral flora occur in smaller numbers, usually less than 10000/ml, and a count between 10000 and 100000 bacteria/ml is borderline. In untreated pyelonephritis, the bacterial and cell counts rise in parallel. A high urinary bacterial count in the presence of a normal leucocyte count can be due to incorrect specimen collection, though it can also constitute an asymptomatic bacteriuria which may be an early phase of pyelonephritis. Equivocal findings without clinical symptoms are best checked before starting any antibiotic treatment. Dip-slide cultures are nowadays easily performed in any general practice or clinical laboratory. The interpretation of a 24 h culture is quite straightforward and can even be done by trained ancillary staff. The absence of demonstrable bacteriuria usually excludes the possibility of a urinary tract infection, except in occasional cases of infections due to anaerobes, and other fastidious organisms which do not grow on the dip-slide culture media. A full antibiotic sensitivity test is not always necessary in uncomplicated urinary infections diagnosed by dip-slide in general practice. However, the identification of bacteria and performance of antibiotic sensitivity tests always requires a well-equipped bacteriological laboratory. In complicated urinary infections, therefore, the incubated dip-slide and not the urine should be sent to the bacteriological laboratory if it is very remote from the patient. The nitrite test is unreliable.

Antibiotic sensitivity testing. Because of the high urine concentrations of antibiotics *in vivo*, bacteria disappear rapidly from the urine during treatment. This may seem to render *in vitro* testing superfluous, but the antibiotic sensitivity profile enables the drug with the highest activity in concentrations corresponding to blood and tissue levels to be selected. Because bacterial causes of urinary infections may respond in different ways to antibiotics, and because antibiotic resistance is becoming common, particularly in hospital, antibiotic sensitivity testing has become a necessity.

Frequency of different pathogens in acute, uncomplicated urinary infection: Escherichia coli 60–80%, enterococci, Proteus (mainly Proteus mirabilis), Klebsiella, Enterobacter and Pseudomonas aeruginosa about 5% each. Staphylococcus epidermidis and S. saprophyticus, group B streptococci, anaerobes, Providencia, Alcaligenes, Serratia and Candida are less common in uncomplicated cases. Changes of infecting organism, mixed infections and infections with multi-resistant organisms occur more frequently in chronic pyelonephritis and after urological operations. The culture of diphtheroids, enterococci or staphylococci in scanty numbers is evidence of contamination of the urine by genital flora. Urine obtained through a freshly inserted catheter or by suprapubic aspiration often contains the causative organisms in pure culture and is normally sterile.

Principles of treatment of urinary infections: Urinary infections used to be treated by antibiotics or chemotherapeutic agents for 10 to 14 days to produce effective tissue and urine levels. Urinary antiseptics or chemotherapeutic agents which act mainly by high urinary concentrations were thought to be inferior to chemotherapeutic agents which produce high blood and tissue levels. Cystitis without renal parenchymal involvement can safely be treated as with a urinary chemotherapeutic agent. In recent years, however, it has become apparent that almost all uncomplicated infections of the lower urinary tract and some of the upper urinary tract can successfully be treated with one dose of the agent. It has become practical to divide urinary infections into those responsive to single dose treatment and those which do not respond. Single dose therapy should not be given in the presence of obstruction (e.g. stenosis), recent urological operations or clinical evidence of pyelonephritis. The earlier recommendation of 10–14 days of treatment for chronic pyelonephritis is probably too short and longer courses should be given at least in males.

All urinary infections should be followed up by urine culture after completing the antibiotic treatment in order to detect any relapse (by the same agent) or reinfection (by a different agent). In either case, a further course of an appropriate agent should be given. Long-term treatment should be considered for urinary tract obstructions which cannot be removed (e.g. infected renal calculi), and also used for the prophylaxis of ascending infection in recurrent urinary infections of young females.

Table 45. Concentration of solutions for intravesicular instillation.

Drug	Concentration for intravesicular instillation
Amphotericin B	100 µg/ml
Miconazole	100 mg undiluted intravenous solution
Nitrofurantoin for instillation*	0.05–0.1%
Nitrofurazone	0.2%
Neomycin	0.5% and 1.0%
Neomycin + sulphaurea	9.0% (sulphaurea)
Noxythiolin	1.0–2.5%
Sulphonamide, e.g. sulphasomidine	5.0%
Polymyxin B sulphate	0.1%
Polymyxin B sulphate (75,000 units) + neomycin (20,000 units) and bacitracin (1000 units)	Powder for reconstitution

* not available in Britain.

Intravesicular instillation of an antibiotic is not an adequate treatment of a urinary tract infection. Disinfectants should be used for bladder washouts in patients at particular risk, following the recommended dosage (Table 45) to avoid irritation.

If continuous catheterisation is necessary a closed system for collection of the urine is essential to prevent bacteria ascending into the bladder. Urinary infection is difficult to prevent, either by washouts or chemoprophylaxis. Suprapubic bladder drainage causes far fewer complications than an indwelling urethral catheter.

Criteria of effective treatment: Sterilisation of the urine after 48 hours, with the disappearance of urinary leucocytes, defervescence, resolution of dysuria and loin pain and the return of the peripheral white cell count, ESR and blood urea to normal. Regular microscopy and culture of the urine during and after treatment are advisable and a persistent bacteriuria, irrespective of the bacterial count, suggests a failure of treatment or change of infecting agent. An acute pyelonephritis can only be regarded as cured if the culture is negative two weeks after the completion of treatment.

Change of infecting agent: The antibacterial treatment of mixed infections not infrequently selects strains of resistant bacteria. Treatment with ampicillin frequently selects ampicillin-resistant klebsiellae, in which case the antibiotic should be changed or another agent added, based on the sensitivities of the bacteria involved.

There are various reasons for *antibiotic therapy* to *fail*, including mixed infection, a change of infecting organism, secondary resistance, mechanical factors (obstruction, calculus, anatomical abnormalities), prostatitis, a wrong diagnosis (renal tuberculosis, trichomoniasis), or inadequate treatment (underdosage, too short a course, wrong choice of drug).

α) Treatment of Acute Urinary Infections (Tables 46, 47)

Treatment when the pathogen is known:
The most effective drug tested against the bacterial isolate (usually amoxycillin or co-trimoxazole) should be given. 10–14 days used to be considered the necessary duration of treatment, but this has now largely been superceded by a single dose which is less expensive, associated with fewer side effects, and carries no problems of patient compliance. Amoxycillin, bacampicillin and co-trimoxazole are effective orally in a single dose, as are injectable antibiotics such as cefotaxime, gentamicin and other aminoglycosides. Signs of acute pyelonephritis or obstruction are contraindications to one-dose treatment. If relapse or reinfec-

Table 46. Antibiotic treatment of urinary infection, based on sensitivity testing.

Causative organism	Oral antibiotic	Parenteral antibiotic	Second-line antibiotic	Urinary antiseptic
Escherichia coli	Ampicillins, co-trimoxazole, gyrase inhibitors[1]	Cefazolin, mezlocillin	Cefotaxime, gentamicin	Nitrofurantoin
Klebsiella	Gyrase inhibitors[1], co-trimoxazole, amoxycillin + clavulanate	Gentamicin, cefotaxime	Mezlocillin, amikacin, oral cephalo-sporins	Nitrofurantoin
Enterobacter spp.	Gyrase, inhibitors[1], co-trimoxazole	Cefotaxime, gentamicin	Ceftazidime, amikacin	Nitrofurantoin
Serratia marcescens	Gyrase inhibitors[1], co-trimoxazole	Ceftazidime, gentamicin	Amikacin, mezlocillin	Nitrofurantoin
Proteus mirabilis	Ampicillins, co-trimoxazole, gyrase inhibitors[1]	Cefazolin, gentamicin	Amikacin, mezlocillin	
Proteus vul-garis, morganii, rettgeri	Gyrase inhibitors[1], possibly co-trimoxazole	Cefotaxime, piperacillin, gentamicin	Amoxycillin + clavulanate, amikacin, mezlocillin	
Pseudomonas aeruginosa	Gyrase inhibitors[1], carfecillin, carindacillin	Azlocillin, piperacillin, tobramycin, gentamicin	Ceftazidime, cefsulodin, amikacin	
Enterococci	Ampicillin, gyrase inhibitors[1]	Mezlocillin	Erythromycin, tetracycline, co-trimoxazole	Nitrofurantoin
Staphylococci	Flucloxacillin	Benzyl penicillin, cefazolin, oral cephalo-sporin	Phenoxymethyl penicillin, co-trimoxazole	Nitrofurantoin

[1] Norfloxacin, ofloxacin, ciprofloxacin etc.

Table 47. Dosage for chemotherapy of urinary infections.

	Drug	Average daily dose on continuous therapy		Dose-interval (hours)	Reduce dose in renal failure	Dose for single-dose treatment (g)
		Children (mg/kg)	Adults (g)			
oral	Amoxy-cillin	50	1.5	6–8	No	1.5–3.0
	Bacampi-cillin	60	2.4	6–8	No	1.6–3.2
	Cepha-lexin	100	4.0	6–8	No	–
	Co-trimox-azole	40	1.9	12	Slightly	1.92
	Doxy-cycline	2	0.1	24	No	–
	Tetra-cycline	20	1.0	8–12	Yes	–
	Nalidixic acid	Contra-indicated	4.0	6	Slightly	Unsuitable
	Nitro-furantoin	5	0.15–0.3	8	Yes	Unsuitable
	Pipemidic acid	Contra-indicated	0.8	12	?	Unsuitable
	Nor-floxacin	Contra-indicated	0.8	8	?	0.8
parenteral	Cefurox-ime	60	1.5–4.5	6–8	Slightly	1.5–3
	Cefo-taxime	60	3.0–6.0	6–8	Slightly	1.0–2.0
	Azlocillin, mezlocillin	100	6.0	6–8	Slightly	?
	Pipera-cillin	100	6.0	6–8	Slightly	?
	Amikacin	15	0.5–1.0	12	Yes	0.5
	Genta-micin	2–3	0.16–0.24	8–12	Yes	0.12
	Tobra-mycin	2–3	0.16–0.24	8–12	Yes	0.12

tion are found at regular follow-up, treatment has to start again. In single-dose treatment, the urine should be checked at 48 hours, 5 and 10 days. Women with recurrent urinary infections may need subsequent prophylaxis of ascending infection with a urinary chemotherapeutic agent.

Treatment when the pathogen is not known: Patients with severe symptoms of acute urinary infection may need to start treatment before bacteriological results are available. The history is important in such cases. Resistant bacteria (Pseudomonas, Enterobacter) rarely cause the first urinary infection in a patient unles there is preceding urological surgery. Treatment may be started with amoxycillin, bacampicillin or co-trimoxazole. A single dose of cefotaxime or an aminoglycoside may also be effective. When the bacteriological results become available, treatment may be continued or changed according to sensitivity testing. Follow-up cultures are particularly important after single-dose treatment. Multi-resistant organisms are more common in urinary infections after urological surgery, bladder catheterisation or the relapse of pyelonephritis. An antibiotic such as gentamicin, a cephalosporin or piperacillin should then be used for initial treatment, continuing or changing when antibiotic sensitivities are known. Single-dose treatment is not suitable for complicated urinary infections. If a parenteral agent cannot be given initially, co-trimoxazole would seem to be more effective in complicated urinary infections than ampicillin derivatives. The urine should be cultured before treatment begins and, where possible, 2–3 days after treatment has started to confirm the clearance of bacteria. A persistent significant bacteriuria is a sign of inadequate treatment due to a change of pathogen, resistance, incorrect intake of the drug etc.

β) Treatment of Pyelonephritis

Acute pyelonephritis with fever, loin pain on percussion, peripheral leucocytosis and a high ESR puts the patient at risk of septicaemia and necrotising pyelonephritis with permanent damage.

The causes of acute pyelonephritis are often mechanical (stones, obstruction, malformations) which can be relieved surgically. Like other urinary infections, mild diseases can be treated with ampicillin derivatives or co-trimoxazole. Complicated forms and pyelonephritis after urological surgery require bactericidal antibiotics such as one of the newer cephalosporins or an acylamino penicillin in high dosage and possibly combined with an aminoglycoside.

Chronic pyelonephritis has not been adequately defined as an entity in the past. The term includes recurrent pyelonephritis, chronic obstructive urinary infections (e. g. infected renal calculi, nephrocalcinosis) and super-infected interstitial nephritis of other causes (e.g. phenacetin kidney). Exacerbations of chronic pyelonephritis should be treated in the same way as the acute disease, once the urine has been microbiologically investigated. Regular urine cultures are particularly important in chronic pyelonephritis because of the high rate of relapse, reinfection, secondary resistance and change or persistence of the infecting agent. Every recurrence and reinfection should be treated with a further course of the appropriate antibiotic.

Since bacteria can persist for long periods in the renal medulla in chronic pyelonephritis, treatment for several months is justifiable. Long-term suppression with an agent such as co-trimoxazole may become necessary in chronic pyelonephritis when there are marked anatomical or functional changes. Cases of chronic pyelonephritis which are resistant to treatment may require intermittent high doses of a penicillin or cephalosporin, possibly in combination with an aminoglycoside.

Suppressive treatment of chronic pyelonephritis should not be confused with the **prophylaxis of ascending infection in females.** The cause of recurrent urinary infections in women is much more likely to be due to a failure of the mechanisms which prevent the ascension of bacteria through the urethra. Poor genital hygiene, sexual activity and infrequent micturition may play a part. If such patients take a chemotherapeutic agent for long periods in small doses, the risk of recurrent urinary infections can be reduced. The most suitable agents for this purpose are co-trimoxazole (240–480 mg per day) or cephalexin (250 mg).

Pyelonephritis in pregnancy: Pyelonephritis is more likely to occur in pregnancy, which can precipitate an acute attack of a pre-existing but asymptomatic chronic pyelonephritis. Simple urinary infection in pregnancy is treated in the same way as acute pyelonephritis, except that many antibiotics (gentamicin, tobramycin, kanamycin, streptomycin, colistin, polymyxin B, tetracycline, co-trimoxazole, nitrofurantoin and gyrase inhibitors such as nalidixic acid, norfloxacin etc.) are best avoided because of the risk of fetal toxicity. Sulphonamides are contraindicated in the two weeks before the expected date of delivery because of the risk of neonatal jaundice and, in severe cases, kernicterus. Urinary infections in pregnancy are in practice treated with ampicillins, oral cephalosporins or sulphonamides. Suitable alternatives are cefazolin, cefotaxime, piperacillin, azlocillin and mezlocillin. Regular bacteriological monitoring is very important after treatment for the remainder of pregnancy, and definitive investigation of the urinary tract may be indicated after delivery.

Acute pyelonephritis of pregnancy is often preceded by asymptomatic bacteriuria, and can be prevented by screening all pregnant women at the end of the first trimester, and treating those who are positive. If a simple screening test such as microscopy for white cells or a dip-slide is positive, a full urine culture of a spontaneous mid-stream urine should be performed. Amoxycillin is generally suitable for asymptomatic bacteriuria. If regular semiquantitative urine cultures show persistence of the bacteriuria, an appropriate antibiotic may be needed long-term, possibly throughout the pregnancy.

b) Cystitis

Clinical symptoms do not always distinguish clearly between simple cystitis and pyelonephritis. Dysuria and frequency are not solely caused by acute cystitis; they can also be due to urethritis (e. g. in gonorrhoea or a trichomonas infection). Simple cystitis is not accompanied by fever, leucocytosis, a high ESR or loin pain on percussion. Cystitis can, however, be part of the picture of pyelonephritis. Recurrent cystitis resistant to standard antibiotic therapy is occasionally due to renal tuberculosis. Every case of cystitis must, therefore, be properly investigated by urinary microscopy and culture. Enterobacteria are the commonest causes of both cystitis and pyelonephritis. An acute haemorrhagic cystitis can also be caused by adenoviruses or, in oncological patients, by cyclophosphamide.

Simple cystitis tends to resolve spontaneously. *Treatment* should be based on the common bacterial isolates. A single high dose of co-trimoxazole or amoxycillin is usually adequate; an alternative is a single parenteral dose of a cephalosporin or an aminoglycoside. Failure of single-dose therapy when the causative organism remains sensitive frequently suggests occult renal involvement.

Cystitis is often treated with urinary chemotherapeutic agents such as pipemidic acid, cinoxacin or nalidixic acid for 7–10 days. When cystitis is treated effectively, the symptoms resolve promptly. Persistence of symptoms is a sign of inadequate treatment and gonorrhoea or an infection due to trichomonas or chlamydia should be excluded.

c) Urethritis

Non-gonococcal urethritis can be caused by Chlamydia trachomatis (see below), Ureaplasma urealyticum, Gardnerella, Escherichia coli, Proteus, enterococci or staphylococci, which can be detected in men in the urethral secretions. The white cell count of the forestream urine is higher than in the remainder. Urethritis can be due to meatal stenosis, foreign bodies, a tumour, a periurethral abscess or a diverticulum. Juvenile urethritis can be due to thread-worms or to the vulvovaginitis which results from poor hygiene. Herpes simplex viral infection in the patient may be associated with Herpes genitalis in the sexual partner.

As with acute pyelonephritis, bacterial urethritis should be treated with a long course of an effective antibiotic in order to prevent periurethral abscesses, urethral stricture, ascending infection or epididymitis. In severe cases, local treatment with a disinfectant irrigation of potassium permanganate 1:5000, silver nitrate 1:5000 or an instillation of zinc sulphate (0.25–1%) or mercurochrome (0.5–2%) may also be given. Oral tetracycline is an effective treatment for mycoplasma infections (Ureaplasma urealyticum). Systemic acyclovir (see p. 536), 5 mg/kg three times a day for 5 days, is useful in Herpes simplex urethritis.

Gonorrhoea is shown by the presence of gram-negative intracellular diplococci in the urethral secretion, confirmed where possible by culture. The treatment of choice is benzyl penicillin or, when the strain is resistant, cefuroxime, cefotaxime, cefoxitin or spectinomycin (see p. 435).

Chlamydia trachomatis urethritis (inclusion body urethritis) is now one of the commonest sexually transmitted diseases in Western Europe, and is a common cause of post-gonococcal urethritis. Inclusion bodies appear in the affected urethral epithelial cells and are seen as red cytoplasmic granules in a Giemsa stain of a urethral smear; they are often crescent-shaped around the nucleolus. The agent can also be shown by direct immunofluorescence using a test kit with monoclonal antibodies. It can also be grown in cell culture on a cover slip, but this requires 2–3 days.

Treatment: Tetracyclines, erythromycin or a sulphonamide for at least 2 weeks, with appropriate antibiotic treatment of any underlying secondary bacterial infection. Tetracycline is also effective against simultaneous infection with ureaplasmas.

Candida urethritis: Irrigation with nystatin is the treatment of choice, when Candida albicans is shown by microscopy or culture in the urethra. Cutaneous candidiasis on the external genitalia may be treated with a suitable cream (e.g. clotrimazole, miconazole). Endogenous reinfection may occur. Where candidiasis is confirmed, resistant cases can often be successfully treated with oral ketoconazole, miconazole i.v. or nifuratel.

Trichomonas urethritis: Trichomonas vaginalis is a frequent cause of urethritis in women and men in whom it may also be latent; the partner of a woman with trichomonal vaginitis should therefore also be treated. Milky, sometimes frothy, mucopurulent or even frankly purulent secretion is discharged from the urethra sometimes with prostatic involvement also. Typical flagellates are seen in a wet preparation or in a gram- or Pappenheim-stained smear of the urinary deposit.

Like trichomonal vaginitis (see p. 400), *treatment* is with metronidazole or a single dose of tinidazole or ornidazole, 4 tablets of 500 mg each in a single dose, preferably after meals. The infected sexual partner should also be treated.

d) Prostatitis, Epididymitis, Orchitis

There are *various causes,* including gram-negative bacilli, gonococci, staphylococci, streptococci, anaerobes, Chlamydia trachomatis and tubercle bacilli. Prostatitis is often accompanied by cystitis and urethritis with dysuria and bacteriuria.

Causal treatment is often not possible because the bacterial cause is difficult to demonstrate. Where possible, prostatic secretion should be obtained for culture by massage. Acute prostatitis may be treated at first with a tetracycline (e. g. minocycline or rolitetracycline i. v.), possibly in combination with gentamicin (240 mg per day). If parenteral administration is effective, change to the oral route after 1 week and continue for at least 4 weeks to reduce the risk of recurrence. Co-trimoxazole diffuses better into the prostatic tissue than any other antibiotic and is thus the oral treatment of choice. Large doses of benzyl penicillin (20 megaunits a day) or cefotaxime (6 g a day) are also often effective, especially if gonorrhoea is suspected. Surgical treatment may be unavoidable, particularly if abscesses form.

Antibiotics are less effective in *chronic infection,* particularly in chronic prostatitis. Pathogens are difficult to isolate, though comparative quantitative cultures of prostatic secretion, bladder urine, obtained by needle aspiration, and a forestream urine for urethral flora may be worthwile. Possible bacterial causes include enterobacteria, Pseudomonas, enterococci etc. Treatment can be attempted with co-trimoxazole, 2 tablets per day for 1–3 months, provided the peripheral blood count is regularly checked.

References

BAILEY, R. R., G. D. ABOTT: Treatment of urinary tract infection with a single dose of trimethoprim-sulfamethoxazole. Canad. med. Assoc. J. *118:* 551 (1978).

BARTLETT, J., W. WEINSTEIN, S. GORBACH: Prostatic abscesses involving anaerobic bacteria. Arch. intern. Med. *138:* 1369 (1978).

BERGER, R. E., E. R. ALEXANDER, G. D. MONDA, J. AMSELL, G. MCCORMICK, K. K. HOLMES: Chlamydia trachomatis as a cause of acute "idiopathic" epididymitis. New Engl. J. Med. *298:* 301 (1978).

CAESAR, M., W. STILLE: Die Chemotherapeutika der Nalidixin-Gruppe. Zuckschwerdt, München 1984.

FANG, L. S. T., N. E. TOLKOFF-RUBIN, R. H. RUBIN: Efficacy of single-dose and conventional amoxicillin therapy in urinary tract infection localized by the antibody-coated bacteria technique. New Engl. J. Med. 298: 413 (1978).
HARNISCH, J. P., R. E. BERGER, E. R. ALEXANDER, G. MONDA, K. K. HOLMES: Etiology of acute epididymitis. Lancet 1: 819 (1977).
JACOBS, N. F., jr., E. S. ARUM, S. J. KRAUS: Nongonococcal urethritis: The role of Chlamydia trachomatis. Ann. intern. Med. 86: 313 (1977).
SCHACTER, J.: Chlamydial infections. New Engl. J. Med. 298: 428, 490, 540 (1978).
SIMON, C., J. HALIM: Zur bakteriologischen Diagnose einer Harnwegsinfektion. Pädiatr. Praxis 29: 427 and 433 (1984).
STAMM, W. E., K. F. WAGNER, R. AMSEL, E. R. ALEXANDER, M. TURCK, G. W. COUNTS, K. K. HOLMES: Causes of the acute urethral syndrome in women. New Engl. J. Med. 303: 409 (1980).

9. Surgical Infections

a) Wound Infections

Wound infections commonly occur postoperatively in hospital and after trauma. Local antibiotics are only effective if the wound is extremely superficial. Systemic antibiotics are essential for the treatment of deep wounds once signs of local inflammation or involvement of the draining lymphatics (lymphangitis) are seen.

Wound infections, in particular abscesses, tend to heal spontaneously, though often with considerable local scarring. The aim of chemotherapy as an adjunct to surgical measures is to accelerate the process of healing and to prevent complications such as lymphangitis, septicaemia and metastatic abscess formation.

Causative organisms: Predominantly staphylococci, although resistant gram-negative bacilli such as Pseudomonas aeruginosa, Proteus vulgaris, Enterobacter cloacae and Bacteroides spp. are becoming increasingly common. Streptococci and clostridia are infrequent nowadays, though potentially much more serious. Mixed infections are the rule.

Diagnosis: A provisional diagnosis can often be made from a gram-stained smear of pus from the wound, but culture and sensitivity testing of significant bacterial isolates should always be performed. In principle, any suppurating wound should be examined bacteriologically. Where the infection fails to resolve, further cultures should be performed during treatment to exclude the possibility of superinfection with resistant organisms.

Antibiotic therapy should be directed against the bacterial isolate (Table 48). In mild wound infections, an oral antibiotic at normal dosage may be sufficient. Severe infections require higher doses of a parenteral agent. Systemic antibiotics should usually be continued until the wound has completely healed.

The treatment of postoperative wound infections where the **pathogen is unknown** must cover staphylococcal infection, for which the best treatment is a penicillinase-stable penicillin such as oral flucloxacillin (2–3 g a day for adults in 3–4 divided doses or 1 g for children aged 2–6 and 80 mg/kg for children aged 0–2). Severe infections may respond better to cefazolin or cefazedone (3–6 g a day).

Less severe wound infections following trauma outside hospital may be adequately treated with phenoxymethyl penicillin. *Severe wound infections,* which are often mixed, require a broad-spectrum combination such as cefoxitin + azlocillin, cefoxitin + piperacillin, cefotaxime + clindamycin, or ampicillin + gentamicin + metronidazole. Any of these combinations should cover nearly all the important pathogens. Cephalosporins of the cefotaxime group are not suitable as single agents for the treatment of severe wound infections because of their poor

Table 48. Antibiotic treatment of wound infections.

Causative organism	Antibiotic of choice	Second-line antibiotics
Staphylococci	Penicillinase-stable penicillins, cefazolin	Clindamycin, fusidic acid, vancomycin
Streptococci	Benzyl penicillin, an oral penicillin	A cephalosporin, erythromycin
Pseudomonas aeruginosa, Proteus vulgaris	Azlocillin + tobramycin, ceftazidime, cefoxitin, gentamicin, cefotaxime, ceftazidime	Gentamicin, amikacin, cefsulodin, piperacillin, mezlocillin, amikacin, piperacillin
Klebsiella	Cefoxitin, gentamicin, cefotaxime	Amikacin, mezlocillin, piperacillin, latamoxef
Escherichia coli	An ampicillin or cephalosporin	Gentamicin, co-trimoxazole, mezlocillin
Enterococci	An ampicillin	Erythromycin, tetracycline, mezlocillin
Pasteurella multocida	Benzyl penicillin	A tetracycline
Bacteroides fragilis	Clindamycin, cefoxitin	Metronidazole
Clostridium perfringens	Benzyl penicillin	Tetracycline, a cephalosporin, metronidazole

Table 49. Indications for chemoprophylaxis in surgery.

Indication	Antibiotics	Reason
Heavily contaminated wounds and delay in initial wound closure	Benzyl or phenoxymethyl penicillin	Prevention of tetanus, gas gangrene and streptococcal infection
Compound fractures, traumatic penetration of joints or body cavities	Cefoxitin or cefuroxime, possibly with an amino-glycoside	Mixed infections are common and often include anaerobes; risk of gas gangrene
Gunshot and stab wounds	Benzyl penicillin; in thoracic or abdominal injuries, broad-spectrum combinations	Infection inevitable; risk of gas gangrene
Severe burns	Benzyl penicillin (20–30 megaunits a day) for the first week	Prevention of streptococcal infection
Animal or human bites	Benzyl or phenoxymethyl penicillin	High risk of infection with streptococci or Pasteurella multocida
Implantation of plastics and metals	Flucloxacillin, cefaman-dole, cefazolin	Foreign bodies predispose to post-operative wound infec-tions (mainly staphylococcal)
Open heart surgery	Flucloxacillin, cefazolin, cefamandole	Prevention of post-operative endocarditis (usually staphy-lococcal)
Transplants	Flucloxacillin, cefazolin	Prevention of infections with staphylococci and streptococci
Neurosurgical operations	Cefotaxime, chloramphenicol	Increased risk of infection
Operations in heavily contaminated areas (oeso-phagus, rectum, colon)	Cefoxitin + azlocillin, cefotaxime +piperacillin +metronidazole	Mixed infections with aerobic and anaerobic organisms are unavoidable
Operations of patients with lowered resistance (e. g. bone marrow suppression)	Cefotaxime + azlocillin, ceftazidime	Increased risk of infection
Amputation of ischaemic lower limb	Benzyl penicillin	Prevention of gas gangrene

activity against Bacteroides, staphylococci and Pseudomonas. Tetracyclines are also unsuitable for wound infections because many staphylococci and almost all strains of Pseudomonas are resistant. Ampicillin and co-trimoxazole are only effective against a few of the possible causes of wound infection, and aminoglycosides given alone have poor clinical efficacy. Aminoglycosides may, however, be combined with β-lactam antibiotics to good effect.

Prophylaxis of wound infections: The routine use of antibiotics after aseptic operations should be discouraged because it is unlikely to be of benefit, yet it exposes the patient to possibly harmful side effects and increases the risk of selection of resistant strains which may be disseminated in the hospital environment. Strict asepsis during the operation, in débridement and drainage is still the best means of prevention of wound infections; even in trivial injuries, antibiotic therapy is no substitute for meticulous wound dressing technique. Antibiotic prophylaxis should only be given in exceptional cases where the risk of infection is particularly high (Table 49). Most of these indications may justifiably be regarded as early treatment of infections which are already present.

Prophylaxis must be given promptly if it is to be effective, and is usually started at the induction of anaesthesia. If circumstances arise during the course of an operation which make antibiotic prophylaxis necessary, such as the opening of a viscus, a suitable agent should be given immediately. The administration of antibiotic prophylaxis in surgery is thus largely the task of the anaesthetist. Such prophylaxis should be brief, although opinions about the optimal length vary between one dose and 3 days of treatment.

Although still not uncommon in some units, 10–14 days of routine antibiotics are unnecessary and may be harmful. General caution in the prophylactic use of antibiotics in surgery should never lead to the omission of prophylaxis of gas gangrene which is essential in some circumstances (see p. 444).

b) Burns

Minor burns are treated as other skin injuries. The outcome with extensive, third degree burns depends on the severity of any complicating infection. While antibiotic therapy can be life-saving in severe burns, prophylactic antibiotics in minor burns are undesirable because of the risk of selection of resistant microorganisms. The main *causative organisms* are Pseudomonas aeruginosa and resistant staphylococci, though Proteus, Klebsiella, Enterobacter, enterococci and fungi (Aspergillus, Mucor, Candida) occur occasionally. Infections with group A streptococci are particularly dangerous though infrequent. Such infections can prevent the adherence of skin grafts and destroy residual epithelial tissue. Septicaemia is most commonly caused by Pseudomonas aeruginosa, Staphylococcus aureus, Enterobacter and Proteus, all of which carry a high mortality.

Diagnosis: Wound swabs before starting treatment and then once or twice a week are helpful, since the wound flora can quickly change. Complete eradication of bacteria is not usually possible. If septicaemia ensues, blood cultures should be taken. Other infectious complications such as pneumonia and thrombophlebitis should be carefully looked for.

Suggested treatment regime for extensive burns:

Week 1: Benzyl penicillin in high dosage (20–30 megaunits a day for adults, or 0.5 megaunits/kg/day for children, in 2–3 short intravenous infusions).

Week 2: A combination such as azlocillin (6 g a day i.v.) + flucloxacillin (3 g a day i.v.) + tobramycin (80–100 mg a day i.m.).

This treatment covers the risk of severe streptococcal infection during the first week and prevents generalised infection in the second week, though it does not prevent the colonisation of wound surfaces with Pseudomonas, staphylococci etc. The regimen may need to be modified in the light of bacteriological results. *Renal insufficiency,* which commonly complicates severe burns, must be taken into account in the antibiotic dosage (see p. 508).

Local antibiotic treatment can be very useful in severe burns but is often impaired by tissue necrosis. During the first few days after injury, moist compresses with 0.5% silver nitrate solution have proved effective, not only because of their bactericidal effect on Pseudomonas aeruginosa, but also because of their healing effect on the wound surface. The following antibiotics may be used locally in a concentration of 0.1%: neomycin, gentamicin, polymyxin B, bacitracin (1000 units/ml). Silver sulphadiazine (Flammazine), povidone iodine and mafenide (see p. 194) are also used locally on burns. When the burns are extensive, however, there is a risk of percutaneous absorption with possible systemic side effects. The risk of skin sensitization makes penicillins and cephalosporins unsuitable for local treatment.

General measures play a very important part in the course of the illness, particularly the treatment of shock by infusions, the maintenance of fluid, electrolyte and protein balance, treatment of acidosis, analgesia, oxygen, tetanus immunisation, treatment of renal failure and protection from hospital infection. Where smoke has been inhaled, pneumonia may also develop, often with gramnegative bacilli. The burn must be thoroughly cleaned, debrided as widely as possible and grafted. Severe burns are best managed in a sterile environment with regular bacteriological monitoring, conditions which are best provided in a proper burns unit.

c) Hand Infections

Common causes are staphylococci, and occasionally streptococci or gram-negative bacteria (e. g. Pseudomonas). Infections of the nails are sometimes due to Candida albicans. Treatment depends on the site of infection.

Cutaneous paronychia: Incision, drainage and fixation. Antibiotics are not absolutely necessary for staphylococcal infections, but even superficial whitlows should be treated with antibiotics if the infection is streptococcal (risk of tenovaginitis) or there are complications or lowered host resistance (e.g. leukaemia).

Subcutaneous, osseous or articular paronychia, and purulent tenovaginitis: Surgical treatment here is just as important as antibiotics, which are only effective if given very early, before the formation of pus. In general, antibiotics serve only to reduce the rate of complications (lymphangitis, septicaemia, chronic osteo-myelitis, palmar cellulitis). The choice of antibiotic is determined by the microscopic and cultural findings from the pus.

When *clusters of cocci* are seen in the direct smear of pus or when no organisms are seen (although the likelihood is still of staphylococcal infection), flucloxacillin, which is penicillinase-stable, should be given in an oral daily dose of 2–3 g to adults and children of school age, and 100 mg/kg to infants. In cases of penicillin allergy, give clindamycin (900 mg a day by mouth). Because of the risk of relapse, treatment should be continued for an adequate length of time.

When *gram-positive cocci are seen in chains* (streptococci), phenoxymethyl penicillin should be given in a dose of 1.5–3 megaunits (approx. 1–2 g) a day in three divided doses.

Gram-negative organisms are treated according to their antibiotic sensitivity pattern; if their sensitivity has not been tested, a cephalosporin is a good first choice.

d) Postoperative Septicaemia

The general recommendations for antibiotic therapy of septicaemia (see p. 297) apply to postoperative septicaemia as well. Since these infections are often acquired in hospital, the causative organisms (e. g. staphylococci, Pseudomonas aeruginosa, Bacteroides fragilis, Proteus, Escherichia coli, Klebsiella or Enterobacter) often display *antibiotic resistance*. A bacteriological diagnosis is therefore very important. Successful treatment depends upon the detection and removal or treatment of the initial septic focus, such as an infected wound, venous catheter, foreign body, indwelling urethral catheter, or septic thrombophlebitis. Blood cultures and wound swabs (or free pus if present) should always be taken for microbiological examination before starting antibiotics.

Where the **pathogen is known,** treatment should be as described in the chapter on septicaemia (see p. 300).

Where the **pathogen is not known,** treatment is based on the likely range of pathogens. When the patient is severely ill, very broad spectrum combinations are indicated, such as cefoxitin + piperacillin or cefotaxime + azlocillin. Following operations with a high risk of anaerobic infection, metronidazole or clindamycin should be added to any of these combinations. The addition of gentamicin, which enhances the bactericidal effect, can be useful. The combination of ampicillin, gentamicin and metronidazole is still often used in postoperative abdominal sepsis. The initial treatment may need modification in the light of bacteriological results and clinical progress.

e) Postoperative Pneumonia

Factors which predispose to postoperative pneumonia include hypoventilation, atelectasis, inhalation anaesthesia, aspiration, lengthy and difficult operations, pre-existing chronic lung diseases, and chest or upper abdominal operations where coughing is painful. The use of bacterially contaminated anaesthetic or ventilatory equipment can give rise to severe pneumonias in the immediate postoperative period, the *causes* of which include resistant staphylococci, Klebsiella, Enterobacter or Pseudomonas. Endogenous infections with pneumococci, Haemophilus influenzae and anaerobes are also common, particularly in patients with pre-existing lung disease. Every effort should be made to find the cause of postoperative pneumonia, including chest physiotherapy to obtain deeply expectorated sputum, blood culture and transtracheal aspiration where available (see p. 343).

Treatment: See p. 353.

f) Infected Gangrene

Primary cause: Impaired arterial perfusion of the leg. *Secondary infection* occurs with staphylococci, aerobic and anaerobic streptococci, Clostridia and gram-negative bacteria (Pseudomonas aeruginosa, Proteus, Bacteroides etc.); such infections are almost always mixed. Relief of the vascular obstruction is essential, or amputation may be necessary. Secondary infection (wet gangrene) may be treated with benzyl penicillin, 10–40 megaunits i. v. a day (anaerobic streptococci are only slightly sensitive), flucloxacillin, 6–10 g i. v. a day (for staphylococci resistant to penicillin), gentamicin, 240 mg i. m. a day and/or azlocillin, 15–20 g i. v. a day (effective against Pseudomonas aeruginosa and other gram-negative bacteria), if necessary also with clindamycin, cefoxitin or metronidazole i. v. This infection can be life-threatening and combinations of two or three antibiotics to reinforce the antibacterial effect and broaden the spectrum are desirable. Severe infected gangrene can in some circumstances give rise to disseminated clostridial infection (see p. 444).

g) Cerebral Abscess

Cerebral abscesses are usually of otogenic, traumatic or haematogenous origin. Typical sources are mastoiditis, the paranasal sinuses (sinusitis), a boil on the nose or lip (with septic thrombophlebitis) or a skull fracture. Haematogenous spread can occur from infected bronchiectatic foci, lung abscesses, skin infections, bacterial endocarditis and congenital heart defects with a right-to-left shunt. They occasionally also occur as a complication of purulent meningitis. The abscess is localised by computerized tomography (CT scan). Rupture of a cerebral abscess into a ventricle or the subarachnoid space is a dangerous complication.

Causes: Staphylococcus aureus, Bacteroides, anaerobic streptococci; otogenic cerebral abscesses are often due to Escherichia coli, Proteus or Klebsiella etc.

Rare causes include Nocardia asteroides (sometimes associated with pulmonary nocardiosis), Entamoeba histolytica (often with simultaneous lung and liver involvement, see p. 364), Toxoplasma gondi (mainly in AIDS), and fungi.

Treatment: Neurosurgical drainage at the optimal time, together with high doses of antibiotics, as for pyogenic meningitis (see p. 325).

In most cases, the initial treatment of a brain abscess must be undirected. Benzyl penicillin is the most effective agent against anaerobic streptococci and sensitive staphylococci; a high dose of 20–40 megaunits is necessary because of the poor diffusion into the abscess. Metronidazole has also been used with good effect in cerebral abscess. The advantages are good penetration into the brain and abscess cavity and high activity against anaerobes. The combination of benzyl penicillin (20–40 megaunits a day) + metronidazole (1.5–2 g i. v. a day) is rational. When penicillin-resistant staphylococci are isolated, flucloxacillin is indicated (10 g a day for adults and 300–400 mg/kg for children) or clindamycin, cefazolin or fusidic acid as alternatives. Otogenic cerebral abscesses may alternatively be treated with chloramphenicol, cefotaxime or latamoxef. Mixed anaerobic infection is common, so a combination with metronidazole is advisable. Increased intracranial pressure due to cerebral oedema should be treated with i. v. diuretics (e. g. frusemide or mannitol) and steroids (e. g. dexamethasone).

h) Subdural Empyema

Whenever apparent pyogenic meningitis is associated with a sterile CSF, frontal sinusitis, hemiparesis, hemiplegia or aphasia, a subdural empyema should be considered. The diagnosis is made by computer-assisted tomography and the treatment is primarily by drainage. Antibiotic therapy is as for cerebral abscess, namely benzyl penicillin + metronidazole or cefotaxime + metronidazole when the pathogen is not known.

In the rare cases of *extradural abscess,* antibiotics can lead to resolution without surgical intervention.

References

BASKIN, T. W., A. ROSENTHAL, B. A. PRUITT, Jr.: Acute bacterial endocarditis: A silent source of sepsis in the burn patient. Ann. Surg. *184:* 618 (1976).

BERG, B., G. FRANKLIN, R. CUNEO, E. BOLDREY, B. STRIMLING: Nonsurgical cure of brain abscess: Early diagnosis and follow-up with computerized tomography. Ann. Neurol. *3:* 474 (1978).

CROCKER, E. F., J. LEICESTER: Cerebral abscess due to *Listeria monocytogenes.* Med. J. Aust. *1:* 90 (1976).

DeLouvois, J., P. GORTVAI, R. HURLEY: Bacteriology of abscesses of the central nervous system: A multicentre prospective study. Brit. med. J. *2:* 981 (1977).

DeLouvois, J., P. GORTVAI, R. HURLEY: Antibiotic treatment of abscesses of the central nervous system. Brit. med. J. *2:* 985 (1977).

DOMINGUE, J. N., C. B. WILSON: Pituitary abscesses: Report of seven cases and review of the literature. J. Neurosurg. *46:* 601 (1977).

FARMER, T. W., G. R. WISE: Subdural empyema in infants, children and adults. Neurology *23:* 254 (1973).

GOLDSTEIN, E. J., D. M. CITRON, B. WIELD, J. BLACHMAN, V. L. SUTTER, T. A. MILLER, S. M. FINEGOLD: Bacteriology of human and animal bite wounds. J. clin. Microbiol. *8:* 667 (1978).

INGHAM, H. R., J. B. SELKON, C. M. ROXBY: Bacteriological study of otogenic cerebral abscesses: Chemotherapeutic role of metronidazole. Brit. med. J. *2:* 991 (1977).

KLASTERSKY, J., M. HUSSON, D. WEERTS-RUHL, D. DANEAU: Anaerobic wound infections in cancer patients: comparative trial of clindamycin, tinidazole, and doxycycline. Antimicrob. Ag. Chemother. *12:* 563 (1977).

KLEIN, D. M., M. E. COHEN: *Pasteurella multocida* brain abscess following perforating cranial dog bite. J. Pediat. *92:* 588 (1978).

KOLB, R., I. JASCHEK, G. HITZENBERGER, H. PICHLER: Gegenüberstellung von Blutspiegel-
verläufen und Konzentrationskurven im Wundsekret nach Penicillin-Infusion. Infection
4: 113 (1976).
LAU, W. Y., S. T. FAN, T. F. YIU, G. P. POON, S. H. WONG: Prophylaxis of
postappendicectomy sepsis by metronidazole and cefotaxime; a randomized, prospective
and double blind trial. Brit. J. Surg. 70: 670 (1983).
LINDBERG, R. B., B. A. PRUITT, jr., A. D. MASON, jr.: Topical chemotherapy and
prophylaxis in thermal injury. Chemotherapy, 3: 351 (1976).
MIDDLETON, F. G., P. F. JURGENSON, J. P. UTZ, S. SHADOMY, H. J. SHADOMY: Brain abscess
caused by Cladosporium trichoides. Arch. intern. Med. 136: 444 (1976).
WATSON, G. W., T. J. FULLER, J. ELMS, R. M. KLUGE: Listeria cerebritis. Relapse of
infection in renal transplant patients. Arch. intern. Med. 138: 83 (1988).
WHITENER, D. R.: Tuberculous brain abscess: Report of a case and review of the literature.
Arch. Neurol. 35: 148 (1978).

10. Osteomyelitis and Septic Arthritis

a) Osteomyelitis

Osteomyelitis can occur in *four forms*, each of which requires a different mode
of treatment:
1. acute haematogenous osteomyelitis (mainly in children),
2. acute postoperative or post-traumatic osteomyelitis,
3. osteomyelitis by direct spread from a local focus,
4. chronic osteomyelitis.

Acute haematogenous osteomyelitis is usually *caused* by staphylococci, and
occasionally by streptococci, Bacteroides, Pseudomonas, salmonellae or Brucella.
In young children and the elderly, Haemophilus influenzae is also an occasional
cause. Posttraumatic osteomyelitis is also often caused by staphylococci, but other
organisms such as Proteus, Pseudomonas aeruginosa, Escherichia coli and others
are relatively commoner; these infections are often mixed. A special form of
chronic osteomyelitis is Brodie's abscess, which is usually staphylococcal.

Diagnosis: Treatment is much more likely to be effective when the causative
organisms have been cultured and their antibiotic sensitivities determined. The
pathogens of post-traumatic osteomyelitis are much more readily isolated by
culture of a wound swab, than those of acute haematogenous osteomyelitis, where
culture of the blood or of the initial septic focus (frequently pyoderma) must be
relied on. When a subperiosteal abscess has formed, pus may be obtained by
needle or drill biopsy. In osteomyelitis due to Staphylococcus aureus, the

antistaphylolysin titre usually rises from its normal value of 1–2 units/ml in adults to 5–10 units/ml or more; this does not occur with Staphylococcus epidermidis. Osteomyelitis with group A streptococci, salmonellae or brucellae can also be diagnosed serologically. Haemophilus type b and group B streptococcal infections can be rapidly detected by latex agglutination of the serum and urine. Radiological alterations usually occur only after the third week of the disease. An early diagnosis can be made by a skeletal scintiscan.

The **treatment of acute haematogenous osteomyelitis** is based on the same principles as that of septicaemia. Bactericidal antibiotics should generally be given at maximal dosage. Because many antibiotics diffuse poorly into bone, there is a considerable risk of relapse if the course of treatment is too short. An adequate period of treatment and careful follow-up are therefore essential. Infections with penicillin-sensitive staphylococci are best treated with *benzyl penicillin* (10–40 megaunits a day in 2–3 short i. v. infusions) whose activity is greater than that of other penicillins against sensitive strains. When the staphylococci are resistant to penicillin, a penicillinase-stable penicillin should be given i. v. or clindamycin parenterally, as follows:

Flucloxacillin i. v.: Adults 6–10 g and children 200–300 mg/kg a day.

Clindamycin: Adults 300–600 mg i. v. or i. m. and children 20–40 mg/kg each three times a day. Parenteral therapy can be followed with oral clindamycin, 900–1200 mg a day for adults and 20 mg/kg/day for children in 4 divided doses.

Fusidic acid has also been used successfully to treat osteomyelitis. The pharmacokinetics of this agent are very good, but resistance may develop rapidly during treatment, so combination with a second antistaphylococcal agent is advisable. The daily dosage for adults is 2 g, and for children 30 mg/kg in 3–4 divided doses after meals.

The *cephalosporins* are similar in their antibacterial activity against staphylococci to the penicillinase-stable penicillins, and show extensive cross-resistance to flu- and dicloxacillin. The cephalosporins should only be considered in patients with penicillin allergy.

When a *large subperiosteal abscess* has formed, pus should be aspirated and an antibiotic instilled if necessary (see septic arthritis, p. 396).

Osteomyelitis caused by other agents is treated according to the antibiotic sensitivity. When the causative organisms are penicillin sensitive (e. g. streptococci), benzyl penicillin in high dosage is the treatment of choice. Infections caused by Haemophilus influenzae are treated with ampicillin i. v. or, if ampicillin-resistant, with cefuroxime or cefotaxime. Pseudomonas infections should be treated with a combination of tobramycin and azlocillin.

When the *cause of acute haematogenous osteomyelitis is unknown* antibiotics should be started at high dosage as soon as a clinical diagnosis has been made and blood cultures and a swab from any initial focus have been taken. A combination of benzyl penicillin (40 megaunits a day i. v.) and flucloxacillin (6–10 g a day for adults and 40–100 mg/kg a day for children) covers more than 90% of the likely bacterial causes (staphylococci, streptococci). Haemophilus is a relatively common cause in small children aged 1–6 years, in whom a combination of flucloxacillin and cefotaxime (or ampicillin) is the most appropriate initial therapy. Pseudomonas and other gram-negative bacilli should be considered in the newborn or patients with severe immunological deficiencies, for which broad-spectrum combinations such as cefotaxime, piperacillin and gentamicin are the most suitable. Once the antibiotic sensitivity pattern is known, the most suitable agent is continued. Staphylococcal osteomyelitis is best treated with a combination of either benzyl penicillin or flucloxacillin with fusidic acid. When blood cultures remain negative, flucloxacillin should be continued. If there is no clinical improvement, further bacteriological investigations may be necessary.

Duration of therapy: Clinical improvement is usually rapid after the initial high-dose intravenous therapy, following which antibiotics may be continued orally. Staphylococcal osteomyelitis is treated with flucloxacillin or benzyl penicillin intravenously for 2–3 weeks, followed by oral flu- or dicloxacillin (3 g a day for adults, 100 mg/kg for children) or phenoxymethyl penicillin (2 megaunits a day for adults, and 1 megaunit for children) or clindamycin.

Osteomyelitis by direct spread: Osteomyelitis of the jaw, which can arise by direct spread from a dental root infection or maxillary sinusitis, has several causes. This infection is usually due either to staphylococci or to mixed anaerobes.

High doses of antibiotics are indicated in addition to operative drainage. If staphylococcal infection can be excluded, initial treatment with high doses of benzyl penicillin is rational with i. v. clindamycin as an alternative in cases of failure.

Chronic osteomyelitis has now become rare, and is most likely to occur when the acute infection has not been treated promptly or for long enough. Chronic staphylococcal osteomyelitis was common in the pre-antibiotic era and frequently required surgical intervention for the removal of sequestra, osteoplasty etc. When the cause is unclear, tuberculosis and brucellosis should be excluded. Local treatment with intra- or periosseous instillation of antibiotics or irrigation and drainage of the osteomyelitic cavity are possible, supplemented nowadays by the insertion of gentamicin polymethylmethacrylate (PMMA) beads (see p. 138).

Wherever possible, antibiotic *treatment* should be guided by the bacterial isolate and its antibiotic sensitivity pattern. High doses of systemic antibiotics have little chance of success when given alone, but are useful adjuncts to other forms of treatment and should be continued for a considerable period after healing becomes established. Chronic staphylococcal infections are usually treated with flucloxacillin, fusidic acid or clindamycin. Infections with enterobacteria should be treated with cefotaxime, piperacillin or mezlocillin in combination with gentamicin. Osteomyelitis caused by Pseudomonas is best treated with azlocillin + tobramycin. Anaerobic infections are best treated with benzyl penicillin (except where caused by Bacteroides fragilis), clindamycin or metronidazole.

b) Septic Arthritis

Suppurative arthritis arises after trauma, haematogenous or direct spread from an infected focus of osteomyelitis or soft-tissue infection. It is occasionally iatrogenic following the intra-articular injection of corticosteroids.

Common causes: Staphylococci, and occasionally streptococci, pneumococci, gonococci, meningococci, salmonellae, enterobacteria or anaerobes etc., and in children, Haemophilus influenzae.

Treatment: After aspiration of the pus and collection of blood cultures, antibiotic treatment is based on the likely origin of the arthritis and the result of the culture of the pus. The dosage and duration of treatment are similar to that given for acute osteomyelitis and septicaemia. Joint irrigations with antibiotics are not generally necessary. Systemic antibiotic therapy may be supplemented in infections resistant to treatment by intra-articular infections in the following concentrations:

oxacillin	1%	gentamicin	0.5%
ampicillin	1%	amikacin	0.25%
piperacillin	1%	polymyxin B	0.1%
		amphotericin B	5 (−20) mg/ml

References

CHATER, E. H., J. FLYNN, A. L. WILSON: Fucidin levels in osteomyelitis. J. Irish med. Ass. *65:* 506 (1972).

GOLDENBERG, D. L., A. S. COHEN: Acute infectious arthritis. A review of patients with nongonococcal joint infections. Amer. J. Med. *60:* 369 (1976).

RAFF, M. J., J. C. MELO: Anaerobic osteomyelitis. Medicine *57:* 83 (1978).

SEPTIMUS, E. J., D. M. MUZLER: Osteomyelitis. Recent clinical and laboratory aspects. Orth. Clin. North. Amer. *10:* 347 (1979).

TETZLAFF, T. R., J. B. HOWARD, G. H. MCCRACKEN, JR., E. CALDERON, J. LORRONDO: Antibiotic concentration of pus and bone of children with osteomyelitis. J. Pediat *92:* 135 (1978).

THIRUMOOTRHI, M. C., A. S. DAJANI: Y. enterocolitica osteomyelitis in a child. Amer. J. Dis. Child. *132:* 578 (1978).

WAHLIG, H., E. DINGELDEIN: Gentamycin bei alloarthroplastischen Operationen. Klinische und experimentelle Ergebnisse. Chemotherapie *1:* 189 (1976).

11. Gynaecological Infections

The general rules of antibacterial chemotherapy also apply to gynaecological and obstetric infections. During pregnancy, however, some antibiotics are potentially toxic to the fetus and others should only be used with caution (see p. 494). Deep infections of the female genital tract are potentially serious and are best treated with high doses of systemic antibiotics. Superficial genital infections can usually be cleared with local antibiotic therapy. It is unusual for the pathogen to be known at the start of treatment because the causative organisms in pelvic infections may only be isolated after special procedures such as curettage, or from material obtained at operation or blood culture. The more accessible superficial genital infections are often due to a mixture of facultative pathogens and material for culture frequently fails to clarify which organism is the primary cause. The doctor often has to base his initial choice of antibiotic on the frequency with which potential pathogens are found.

a) Bartholinitis

The commonest *causes* are Staphylococcus aureus or gonococci, with occasional mixed anaerobic infections. Where possible, treatment should be according to the isolate. When staphylococci are cultured or when no pathogen is found, a penicillinase-stable penicillin such as flucloxacillin, 2–3 g a day by mouth, is indicated, and continued until the local symptoms resolve. Gonococcal bartholinitis should be *treated* with benzyl penicillin (4 megaunits a day for at least 1 week) or cefuroxime which is also effective against penicillin-resistant strains (see p. 436). Incision and drainage may be necessary.

b) Vulvitis

Local treatment with topical antibiotics on the basis of the culture results is generally sufficient, and systemic antibiotic therapy is usually necessary only for deep infections such as abscesses, cellulitis or gangrene.

Infections with Candida albicans are common and may be *treated* with antifungal agents, either imidazole derivatives such as clotrimazole, miconazole, econazole, isoconazole or ketoeonazole, or other antifungals such as nystatin, amphotericin B, pimaricin or ciclopiroxolamine. Possible underlying diseases such as diabetes mellitus, skin diseases, allergies and venereal disease should be considered, as well as other predisposing factors such as oral contraceptives and broad-spectrum antibiotics.

c) Vulvovaginitis in Children

The *causative organisms* are rarely gonococci, but much more commonly streptococci, pneumococci, staphylococci, Haemophilus, gram-negative rods, Trichomonas and Candida albicans. Culture often yields intestinal bacteria (usually contaminants) and microscopic examination of the smear or slide preparation is more reliable (see vaginitis). Herpetic vulvovaginitis is also not uncommon and is generally due to herpes virus type 1 in children. Small blisters or ulcerations are present on the labia minora, sometimes associated with painful inguinal lymphadenitis on both sides (treatment: p. 537).

Treatment is given according to the bacterial isolate. Culture-proven gonococcal infection should be treated with 1 megaunit of benzyl penicillin a day for 5 days, combined if necessary with an oestrogen (caution: risk of haemorrhage). Infections with Haemophilus, pneumococci or streptococci may be treated with systemic antibiotics such as amoxycillin, an ampicillin ester or cefaclor etc., supplemented with twice daily baths using a mild soap, and education about personal hygiene. Overanxious mothers should be reassured. The presence of a foreign body should be excluded. When threadworms are the cause of the vulvovaginitis, the patient should be treated with mebendazole or pyrvinium (see p. 486) and advised on hygienic measures, e.g. changing underwear, cutting fingernails short etc. Infections with Trichomonas vaginalis are treated with metronidazole or ornidazole (for dosage, see vaginitis). A congenital or acquired rectovaginal fistula should be excluded.

d) Vaginitis in Adults

Vaginitis is often combined with vulvitis and vulvovaginitis with urethritis. Vaginal infections giving rise to a discharge are often secondary to an underlying disease such as carcinoma, diabetes or hormonal imbalance. Thus the investigation of any infection should include a search for the underlying cause. When the cause of a vaginal discharge is not immediately apparent, syphilis, gonorrhoea and tuberculosis should be excluded. The lack of oestrogens after the menopause predisposes to vaginitis, as do some deodorant sprays and foreign bodies (tampons, pessaries). Disruption of the normal vaginal flora (Lactobacillus acidophilus) allows potentially pathogenic organisms to invade.

The *commonest causes of* non-specific vaginitis are Gardnerella vaginalis (formerly known as Corynebacterium vaginale or Haemophilus vaginalis), chlamydiae, Bacteroides and streptococci, often occurring as mixed infections. Gonococci occur after the menopause. Candida and Trichomonas vaginitis are specific entities and can be recognised by direct microscopy of the discharge.

Bacterial vaginitis: When douches or instillations of antibacterial and antifungal antiseptics (e. g. povidone iodine) are used, the risk of secondary fungal infections is less than when purely antibacterial agents are used. Tetracyclines are often taken for the local treatment of non-specific vaginitis. Metronidazole is effective against Gardnerella vaginalis and Trichomonas. Once the symptoms have resolved, the normal vaginal flora can be restored with the aid of lactose and oestrogens. In senile vaginitis, a local oestrogen cream is a useful supplement to antibiotic therapy.

Candida vaginitis gives rise to a white, sometimes friable vaginal discharge, often accompanied by severe pruritus vulvae. Vaginal thrush is a typical complication of antibiotic treatment. The yeasts can be shown microscopically with a methylene blue stain as budding cells and pseudomycelia. Culture on Sabouraud's or malt agar.

Treatment: Local treatment with nystatin pessaries or ointment: 1 pessary into the vagina 1–3 times a day for 1–2 weeks, treating the vulva simultaneously with ointment. Miconazole vaginal cream is introduced every evening high into the vagina with an applicator. Alternatives are clotrimazole, econazole, ciclopiroxolamine, nifuratel, or povidone iodine. Relapses are frequent. The partner should be treated at the same time if he has candida balanitis or urethritis. Predisposing factors such as diabetes, pregnancy, oral contraceptives and antibiotic therapy should be taken into account.

Trichomonas vaginitis may be acute or chronic, symptomatic or non-symptomatic. An offensive purulent vaginal discharge is common, sometimes associated with dysuria. The vigorous movement of the trichomonads is best shown microscopically on a pre-warmed slide using a fresh preparation, or one stained with methylene blue. Culture is possible in a special nutrient solution. Mixed infections with Candida albicans or Gardnerella are not uncommon.

Treatment: Metronidazole, 250 mg 3 times a day for adults, 125 mg for girls aged between 6 and 10 and 62.5 mg twice a day for girls aged between 2 and 5. Treat for 6 days and do not repeat before 4–6 weeks. Whenever possible, treat the infected partner as well, since trichomonas infection in the male can give rise to urethritis or be asymptomatic. Alternative treatments are tinidazole, ornidazole and nimorazole in a single dose of 2 g. The stronger trichomonocidal activity of these compounds permits single-dose therapy.

During the first few months of pregnancy, alternatives such as topical metronidazole or pimaricin as vaginal pessaries can be carried out twice a day for 10 days. Douching with povidone iodine is also effective. Systemic use of the nitroimidazoles should be avoided.

Herpes simplex vulvovaginitis may be acute or chronically recurrent and in adults is usually due to herpes virus type 2. An extensive vesicular eruption which may ulcerate is found in the vulva, vagina and on the cervix and perineum. It is very painful, especially during micturition, sometimes with urinary retention. During pregnancy, there is a risk of miscarriage, premature delivery, and neonatal death as a result of generalized herpes. When the initial infection occurs near term, delivery by caesarean section is advisable. A vaginal smear stained by the Papanicolaou method shows intranuclear inclusion bodies in multinucleate giant cells. Secondary infection with bacteria or fungi is common. Local treatment is with povidone iodine (vulval toilet, vaginal gel and pessaries), baths, compresses, or a trial of adenine arabinoside ointment (3%) or acyclovir cream (0.5%) 1–2 times a day for 2–3 weeks. In severe cases, systemic acyclovir can be given in a dose of 5 mg/kg 3 times a day for 5 days as short i.v. infusions.

e) Pelvic Inflammatory Disease

Adnexitis, endometritis, parametritis and pelveoperitonitis are often due to gonococci, Chlamydia trachomatis, anaerobic bacteria (streptococci, Bacteroides, Clostridia) and sometimes aerobes (staphylococci, enterococci, Escherichia coli, Enterobacter, Proteus, Pseudomonas aeruginosa and Gardnerella). Isolation of the causative organism is usually difficult but should be attempted from cervical secretion, pus, material obtained at operation or laparoscopy, or blood-culture). Anaerobes are usually only recovered when the specimen is put in a strictly anaerobic transport medium, or is inoculated immediately into an evacuated container.

The importance of chlamydiae in the pathogenesis of pelvic inflammatory disease has only recently been recognized. Cell culture of material obtained at operation or laparoscopy occasionally yields these organism if special transport medium is used. These agents can also be demonstrated microscopically in direct smears by immunofluorescence using monoclonal antibodies.

Gonococci may be demonstrated by immunofluorescence, by a methylene blue or gram stain of cervical, urethral or rectal pus, or by immediate culture of Thayer-Martin medium or transmission to the laboratory in Stuart's or Amies' transport medium.

When tuberculosis is suspected, menstrual blood should be cultured and if necessary inoculated into animals. When the cause of a cervical discharge is not obvious, carcinoma must be excluded.

Treatment of acute pelvic infections: High doses of antibiotics related as far as possible to culture and antibiotic sensitivities. Since the causative organisms often cannot be cultured, empirical treatment is necessary. High doses of benzyl penicillin (10 megaunits twice a day as a short i. v. infusion) will cover streptococci, gonococci, clostridia and many strains of Bacteroides and staphylococci. Severe infections should be treated with cephalosporins, preferably cefoxitin, which is also effective against Bacteroides fragilis. An alternative is a combination of clindamycin i. v. (1.2 g a day) and gentamicin i. m. (320 mg a day).

In *post-abortal adnexitis,* infection with penicillin-resistant staphylococci should be considered and i. v. clindamycin is often effective, as well as against Bacteroides.

Metronidazole will eradicate anaerobes as causes of adnexitis, particularly in mixed infections. Latamoxef, which is effective against most anaerobes and enterobacteria, is also useful. Treatment with tetracyclines is usually effective in chlamydial infection if given for at least two weeks.

When local suppuration has occurred (pyosalpinx, ovarian abscess, or pelvic abscess), the chances of success with antibiotics alone are less and operative drainage is necessary.

Treatment of a resolving adnexitis with corticosteroids accelerates the resolution of the infection but should only be given under full antibiotic cover.

Chronic adnexitis may be due to tuberculosis, which should be treated by triple antituberculous therapy for several months (see p. 463).

f) Febrile Abortion

These are mostly mixed aerobic and anaerobic infections with Bacteroides fragilis, various enteric bacteria, streptococci and enterococci. Clostridia, staphylococci and other organisms are less common. Culture of blood, cervical smear and placental tissue is important and the results must be interpreted carefully. Even where only one causative organism is found, the infection may be mixed.

Antibiotics in high dosage should be started early. Milder cases may be treated initially with high doses of benzyl penicillin (10–30 megaunits a day i. v.) which covers streptococci and Clostridia. In more severe cases, particularly with perforation of the uterus or signs of peritonitis, treatment should also cover non-sporing anaerobes such as Bacteroides and enterobacteria. Suitable treatment in such cases is cefoxitin + gentamicin or cefotaxime + metronidazole.

The development of *septic shock* suggests infection with gram-negative rods and should be treated with cefoxitin (6 g a day) + piperacillin (5–15 g a day) or cefotaxime + metronidazole, both of which cover the range of causative organisms.

Antibiotics should be continued for at least 6–8 days after the fever has settled and until all local signs of infection have resolved. Surgical measures such as curettage are often necessary. The control of shock and anuria and coagulation disorders is also very important. Tetanus hyperimmune globulin (250 I. U. i. m.) + active tetanus immunisation may be necessary after an artificially induced illegal abortion. In gas gangrene (treatment of choice: benzyl penicillin), hyperbaric oxygen in a high pressure chamber may also be used. Heparin should be given if diffuse intravascular coagulation arises (p. 303).

Septic thrombophlebitis of the pelvic veins can occur with infected abortion and post-partum, and is usually caused by a mixed infection of Bacteroides fragilis and anaerobic cocci. The treatment of choice is an effective anti-anaerobic agent such as cefoxitin, latamoxef or cefotaxime + metronidazole, together with additional anticoagulant therapy.

g) Postpartum Infections

The *causative organisms* are generally the same as for febrile abortion, with the addition of β-haemolytic streptococci and Clostridia (gas-gangrene). The portal of entry of these organisms is either the puerperal uterus or wounds of the perineum or caesarean section. Mixed infections are common.

Antibiotic treatment is largely that of septic abortion, but antibiotics should always be given at maximal dosage because of the risk of fatal puerperal sepsis.

Any fever in the puerperium is suspicious of a puerperal infection; a swab of the lochia and any purulent discharge and blood cultures should be taken, followed by high doses of antibiotics such as benzyl penicillin (10–20 megaunits a day i.v. in 2–3 divided doses). Obstetric intravaginal manipulations can give rise to an infection with anaerobes and resistant staphylococci, which should be treated with the addition of a penicillinase-stable penicillin such as flucloxacillin.

When puerperal sepsis is suspected, very broad spectrum treatment such as cefoxitin + azlocillin or cefotaxime + piperacillin should be given. Metronidazole may also be added. When renal function is normal, an aminoglycoside may be advantageous. General measures such as the maintenance of blood pressure and of diuresis are very important, as are the drainage of abscesses, curettage, and, in emergency, hysterectomy.

The *prophylactic use* of antibiotics after an uncomplicated delivery is *not* advisable since it can encourage postpartum uterine infection with multiresistant microorganisms.

h) Mastitis

The *causative organisms* of acute mastitis in the puerperium are almost invariably staphylococci. Streptococci and other pyogenic bacteria occur only in exceptional cases. The bacteria are initially found in the milk and later also in pus from the abscess. The portals of entry are usually cracks or fissures on the nipple.

Treatment should be started early with an antistaphylococcal agent, preferably a penicillinase-stable penicillin such as flucloxacillin 3 g a day by mouth. Should the organism be sensitive, however, benzyl penicillin is the treatment of choice.

In cases with *penicillin allergy* or methicillin-resistant staphylococci, suitable alternative antibiotics are clindamycin (1.2 g a day), fusidic acid (4 g a day), erythromycin (2 g a day) and possibly cefuroxime or cefamandole (cross-allergy is rare). Antibiotic treatment will only be effective if started as early as possible and continued at full dosage for a sufficient period of time. It is advisable, therefore, to give a high parenteral dose initially and to continue antibiotics orally once the local infection begins to improve. If an abscess has already formed, antibiotics should prevent further spread and metastatic foci. Other symptomatic measures are also important, such as suppression of lactation and cold compresses, as well as the incision and drainage of any abscess. The baby should not be fed from an infected breast because the milk contains bacteria and pus and can give rise to infection in the child.

Opinions vary as to the value of *local antibacterial applications* to the nipple as a preventive measure. Strict attention to *hygiene* in the delivery room and maternity ward is very important, however.

Mastitis of a non-lactating breast is less common, and is usually caused by mixed anaerobic organisms (Bacteroides, peptostreptococci), for which clindamycin, cefoxitin or metronidazole are usually the best choice.

i) Pyrexia during Labour

When signs of chorioamnionitis occur after the premature rupture of the membranes or where fever of uncertain origin develops during labour, antibiotics are indicated.

The *range of causative organisms* corresponds largely to these found in febrile abortion with the addition of group B streptococci and Listeria.

Antibiotics should be chosen which readily cross the placenta, enter the fetal circulation and pass through the fetal urine into the amniotic fluid. Penicillins and cephalosporins have this property, are often highly concentrated in the amniotic fluid and cause no side effects in the baby. When there is a risk of severe intrauterine infection in the fetus, high daily doses are needed. This treatment is not effective, however, against strains resistant to penicillins or cephalosporins. Blood cultures should be taken from the baby after birth, the blood picture monitored and prompt treatment given with a combination such as cefotaxime or cefuroxime + piperacillin or gentamicin. If the mother develops septicaemia, which is often accompanied by shock and disseminated intravascular coagulation, the same broad-spectrum therapy should be given as to the baby.

j) Pyelonephritis during Pregnancy

Urinary infections are common during pregnancy and the *causative organisms* are similar to those of uncomplicated urinary infections outside pregnancy. Escherichia coli is the commonest cause. Treatment is similar to that of other urinary infections (see p. 375), except that the possible toxicity to the fetus of the antibiotics used must be taken into account (see p. 494).

The ampicillins and cephalosporins are the mainstay of treatment. Co-trimoxazole, the aminoglycosides and tetracyclines should be avoided. If significant bacteriuria can be demonstrated repeatedly it should be treated with antimicrobials even if asymptomatic, since the patient may be developing acute pyelonephritis.

References

ADENIYI, J. C.: *Haemophilus vaginalis* bacteremia. Canad. med. Assoc. J. (1980).

ALY, R., H. I. MAIBACH, M. BRITZ: Quantitative microbiology of the human vulva. Brit. J. Dermatol. *101:* 445 (1979).

CHOW, A. W., J. R. MARSHALL, L. B. GUZE: A double-blind comparison of clindamycin with penicillin plus chloramphenicol in treatment of septic abortion. J. infect. Dis. (Suppl.) *5:* 35 (1977).

GIBBS, R. S., P. M. JONES, C. J. WILDER: Antibiotic therapy of endometritis following cesarean section, treatment successes and failures. Obstet. Gynec. *52:* 31 (1978).

LEDGER, W. J.: The surgical care of severe infections in obstetric and gynecologic patients. Surgery *136:* 753 (1973).

LEDGER, W. J.: Infection in the Female. Lea & Febiger, Philadelphia 1977.

MARDH, P. A., T. RIPA, L. SVENSSON, L. WESTROM: Chlamydia trachomatis infection in patients with acute salpingitis. New Engl. J. Med. *296:* 1377 (1977).

MULLER-SCHOOP, J. W., S. P. WANG, J. MUNZINGER, H. U. SCHLAPFER, M. KNOBLAUCH, R. W. AMMANN: Chlamydia trachomatis as possible cause of peritonitis and perihepatitis in young women. Brit. med. J. *1:* 1022 (1978).

PHEIFER, T. A., P. S. FORSYTH, M. A. DURFEE, H. M. POLLOCK, K. K. HOLMES: Nonspecific vaginitis: Role of Haemophilus vaginalis and treatment with metronidazole. New Engl. J. Med. *298:* 1429 (1978).

SPIEGEL, C. A., R. AMSEL: Anaerobic bacteria in nonspecific vaginitis. New Engl. J. Med. *303:* 601 (1980).

WOLNER-HANSSEN, P., L. WESTROM, P. A. MARDH: Perihepatitis and chlamydial salpingitis. Lancet *1:* 901 (1980).

DI ZEREGA, G., L. YONEKURA, S. ROY: A comparison of clindamycin-gentamicin and penicillin-gentamicin in the treatment of post cesarean section endomyometritis. Amer. J. Obstet. Gynecol. *134:* 238 (1979).

12. Eye Infections

The antibiotic treatment of eye infections requires detailed knowledge. Acute conjunctivitis is not the only cause of red eye; careful ophthalmological examination and accurate diagnosis of the causative agent are essential for safe and effective treatment.

Diagnosis and treatment, particularly by subconjunctival or retrobulbar injection of an antibiotic, remain the task of the experienced ophthalmologist.

Forms of chemotherapy:

Severe bacterial infections of the outer eye, such as gonoblennorrhea or corneal ulceration, and intraocular or orbital infections which are inaccessible to local treatment should be treated with **systemic antibiotics.** Antibiotics diffuse at different rates from the blood into the various parts of the eye with the poorest concentrations in the bradytrophic tissues of the cornea, the lens, and the vitreous body. Treatment of intraocular infections must overcome the barrier between blood and aqueous humor and between blood and the vitreous body. Chloramphenicol is suitable agent for this purpose, achieving 50% of serum concentrations at these sites. Sulphonamides vary according to the preparation but achieve 40–80% of serum concentrations, oxytetracycline and tetracycline approximately 15–20%, benzyl penicillin, ampicillin, streptomycin, rolitetracycline and demethylchlortetracycline about 10% and kanamycin only 4%. Thus higher doses of antibiotics than usual are necessary if an adequate intraocular concentration is required. Examples are 250 mg of rolitetracycline i.v. a day or 1.5–2 g of streptomycin i.m. The barrier between blood and aqueous humor may, however, be more permeable in the infected eye, so that higher concentrations of the antibiotic than usual may be achieved. Information about new antibiotics in this respect is scarce. Agents which achieve high CSF concentrations are probably of value in deep eye infections as well.

Local treatment may be given by external application, subconjunctival and retrobulbar injection and by direct injection into the chamber or vitreous body.

Conjunctival and corneal infections may be treated effectively by *antibacterial eye-drops* (Table 50). The ability of an antibiotic to penetrate the anterior parts of the eye depends on its solubility in both water and lipoids, since the corneal epithelium is rich in lipoids and presents a barrier to non-lipoid-soluble agents. Most sulphonamides and antibiotics penetrate the intact cornea in minimal quantities if at all, although corticosteroids and isoniazid penetrate more easily. Epithelial lesions and changes in the lipoid barrier, e.g. through iontophoresis, allow some drugs to penetrate more deeply but they never pass the ciliary body. When giving antibiotics externally, an isotonic solution or ointment in a suitable base is applied to the conjunctival sac. *Ointments* remain in the eye longer than solutions and are also more stable. They may impair vision, however, cause contact dermatitis more frequently than solutions and they may inhibit corneal epithelial mitosis which is not usually affected by eye drops. It may be practical to give eye drops by day and ointment overnight. The addition of hemicellulose to eye drops increases their viscosity and prolongs their retention time. The treatment will only be effective if the antibiotic is present in effective concentrations for a long period; it must, therefore, be given regularly at short intervals. Eye

Table 50. Concentration of antimicrobials in eye drops and ointments.

Agent	Eye drops	Eye ointment
Gentamicin, tobramycin	0.3%	0.3%
Kanamycin	0.5–1%	0.5%
Gramicidin	–	0.025%
Polymyxin B	0.1–0.2%	0.1–0.2%
Framycetin	0.5%	0.5%
Neomycin	0.5–1%	0.5%
Bacitracin	300 units/ml	300 units/g
Tyrothricin	0.06%	0.06%
Erythromycin	–	0.5%
Chlor-, Azidamphenicol	1%	1%
Tetracycline	0.5–1%	0.5–1%
Sulphonamide	4–10%	4–5%
Pimaricin	1%	1%
Nystatin	100,000 i. units/ml	100,000 i. units/g
Amphotericin B	0.5–1%	0.5–1%
Miconazole	1%	1%
Acyclovir	–	3%
Idoxuridine	0.1%	0.5%
Vidarabine	–	3%

drops should be given every 15 min initially, then every 2 hours, whereas an eye ointment could be initially used every 1–2 hours, then every 4 hours. Eye baths can be given several times a day for 10–30 min. When the cornea is infected or oedematous, the antibiotic may penetrate the aqueous humor.

Subconjunctival injection may be given by the ophthalmologist for certain corneal and anterior chamber infections and permits antibiotics to diffuse through the sclera into the anterior part of the eye. Thus a high antibiotic concentration can be achieved for several hours in the aqueous humor. This is especially useful in intraocular infections, keratitis, serpiginous keratitis and blennorrhoea. 0.3–0.5 ml of the antibiotic solution is injected once or twice a day, e.g. 300,000–500,000 units of benzyl penicillin or 20 mg of gentamicin. The longest tolerated course is usually 3 days.

The injection of benzyl penicillin once a day is tolerated but painful, and sometimes gives rise to an inflammatory reaction. The number of injections must therefore be limited. Pain associated with subconjunctival injection can be minimised by the prior injection (5 minutes before) of 0.1 to 0.2 ml of 2% lignocaine into the subconjunctival space. The subconjunctival injection of other antibiotics such as ampicillin (40–50 mg), carbenicillin (50 mg), methicillin (50 mg), cephaloridine (50 mg), cefazolin (50 mg), amikacin (25 mg), gentamicin or tobramycin (20 mg), amphotericin B (0.05–0.1 mg), miconazole (5 mg) or isoniazid (10–20 mg) may be necessary for certain infections. Experience with the new β-lactam antibiotics is limited. The subconjunctival injection of amphotericin B can cause persistant yellow discoloration of the conjunctiva; and red nodules develop at higher dosage (>5 mg), which gradually regress after treatment has been stopped.

The *retrobulbar injection* of an antibiotic in severe intraorbital infections is used to attain a sufficient antibiotic concentration in the retrobulbar space and around the optic nerve. Higher concentrations are attained in the inner eye than after subconjunctival injection. This form of treatment should always be complemented with high intravenous doses of the same antibiotic.

Direct injection into the *anterior chamber* of the eye not infrequently damages the lens or cornea, and is only used in exceptional circumstances.

Injections into the *vitreous body* can be indicated in endophthalmitis.

Choice of antibiotic for local treatment: Bacterial culture and sensitivity testing are not essential in most superficial ocular infections, such as mild conjunctivitis which tend to heal spontaneously. When a trial of treatment of conjunctivitis fails, however, cultures and sensitivity tests should be performed. In severe eye infections, such as ulceration or endophthalmitis, a bacteriological diagnosis should always be attempted at the outset. When the cause cannot be established, the clinical picture may be suggestive of certain organisms against which treatment should be directed. Thus central corneal ulcers are often due to pneumococci, other streptococci or Pseudomonas. If such initial treatment does not result in improvement after 2–3 days, treatment should be changed to another antibiotic.

For local treatment aminoglykosides usually have a rapid mode of action; they cover staphylococci, proteus and other enterobacteria. Gentamicin and tobramycin are well tolerated, have a broad spectrum of action and are available as drops and ointment. Neomycin gives rise not infrequently to allergic reactions. Polymyxin B is only active against Pseudomonas aeruginosa and other gram-negative bacilli and occasionally causes allergy. Some eye ointments and drops contain combinations of antibiotics such as polymyxin B, neomycin and bacitracin; polymyxin B and trimethoprim; polymyxin B and oxytetracycline; polymyxin B and neomycin; neomycin and gramicidin; or polymixin B, neomycin and gramicidin. Tyrothricin which is only active against gram-positive bacteria is available in eye ointment in some countries, but not in Britain. Preparations containing chloramphenicol for local use with the stable chloramphenicol derivative acid-amphenicol or with a tetracycline are only bacteriostatic, seldom sensitise and have proved effective in clinical practice. Local preparations with rifamipicin are available in some countries but carry the risk of secondary resistance. The antifungal agent pimaricin is available in an eye ointment and can be used to treat infections with Candida. Ocular preparations of miconazole and amphotericin B are only available in special centres. Of the sulphonamides, sulphisomidine and sulphafurazole are available as local preparations in some countries, but only sulphacetamide, the most water-soluble sulphonamide, is available in Britain. Because of the high risk of sensitisation, penicillin eye drops and ointment have been withdrawn. Preparations containing silver have a disinfectant action but should only be given for short periods because of the risk of silver toxicity.

Possible side effects of local antibiotic treatment:
1. Irritation of the eye may occur when the concentration in the solution is too high, when large crystals are present in an ointment, when there is a shift in pH or when the drops or ointment become contaminated with Pseudomonas, Proteus, other bacteria, fungi or viruses.
2. Allergic reactions may occur, particularly to treatment with penicillin, streptomycin and sulphonamides, and are shown as an eczema or oedema of the eyelid, conjunctivitis or, in the case of systemic treatment, a systemic response.
3. Post-antibiotic keratoconjunctivitis is sometimes caused by Pseudomonas aeruginosa, staphylococci or fungi (e.g. Candida albicans). Glucocorticoids in some antibiotic eye drops or eye ointments also predispose to infection with fungi (e.g. the development of a mycotic keratitis). An infection with Herpes simplex, which in its early stages can only be recognized with a slit lamp, may be activated. Since corticosteroids are contraindicated in a superficial keratitis caused by herpes simplex and in corneal epithelial defects, local ophthalmic preparations which combine antibiotics and steroids should only be prescribed by an ophthalmologist.

a) Infections of the Lid (and Lacrimal Apparatus)

Blepharitis: Ulcerating blepharitis is usually caused by staphylococci or streptococci. Secondary bacterial infections often occur in eczematous dermatitis of the lids and in chronic seborrhoeic blepharitis.

Local treatment: First remove any crusts with moist, warm compresses using physiological saline or olive oil; if ulceration has occurred, give gentamicin or neomycin with bacitracin eye ointment.

Systemic treatment: For severe infections, use flucloxacillin or benzyl penicillin.

External hordeolum (abscess of the sebaceous glands) and **internal hordeolum** (abscess of the Meibomian glands) are usually caused by Staphylococcus aureus. Orbital cellulitis occasionally occurs, with the risk of thrombophlebitis of the angular vein.

Local measures: Warm compresses or dry heat. If the abscess does not perforate spontaneously, incision may be necessary. Local preparations are usually ineffective since they fail to reach the site of infection.

Systemic treatment (for internal styes): Flucloxacillin or erythromycin.

Chalazion is a chronic infection of the Meibomian glands and is sometimes due to secondary infection.

Local treatment: When the infection has subsided, operative removal.

Abscess and cellulitis of the lid are usually due to infection with staphylococci. They occur after trauma, by direct spread from pyogenic infection of the paranasal sinuses or local osteomyelitis, or very occasionally as septic metastasis. There is a risk of orbital cellulitis or of septic thrombosis of the orbital veins.

Local treatment: Incision (ophthalmologist) if necessary.

Systemic treatment: Flucloxacillin, cefuroxime or cefamandole according to the causative organism and its antibiotic sensitivities. A systemic cephalosporin is preferable in cases of septicaemia.

Furuncle of the lid is caused by staphylococci and carries a risk of thrombophlebitis of the orbital veins and of meningitis.

Systemic treatment is as for a furuncle of the nose or lip (see p. 420), e. g. with flucloxacillin or cefamandole i. v.

Erysipelas of the lid: Caused by Streptococcus pyogenes.

Systemic treatment: Benzyl penicillin (see Erysipelas, p. 428).

Mycoses of the skin of the lid should be treated according to the fungal cause with local preparations which are tolerated by the eye (see p. 407, and Table 51, p. 426).

Herpes simplex virus infections of the lid give rise to small blisters with an umbilicated centre, which often occur on the lips as well. All cases should be examined by the ophthalmologist in order to localise the infection precisely and check whether there is corneal involvement.

Local treatment to protect the conjunctiva and cornea: acyclovir eye ointment every 4 hours. Secondary bacterial infection should be treated with neomycin, polymyxin and bacitracin eye ointment. Steroids are contraindicated.

Systemic treatment: Severe cases should be treated with acyclovir 5 mg/kg three times a day in short i. v. infusions for 5 days.

Vaccinia of the lids and/or the conjunctiva through vaccinia-virus infection (contact infection) carries a risk of corneal involvement and of loss of sight in 20–30% of cases.

Local treatment: Possibly gentamicin ointment if there is bacterial superinfection.

Systemic treatment: Give vaccinia hyperimmune globulin (0.3 ml/kg i. m. daily on 2–3 consecutive days), and possibly a trial of treatment with methisazone. Use a broad-spectrum antibiotic if there is evidence of bacterial superinfection.

Dacryoadenitis: Acute with infectious diseases such as mumps, or spreading from infections in the environment caused by staphylococci, streptococci, Klebsiella pneumoniae etc. Can be chronic in leukaemia, lymphogranulomatosis, tuberculosis, syphilis and trachoma.

Treatment: Moist or dry warmth and, in the case of bacterial infection, gentamicin eye ointment into the conjunctival sac, possibly with systemic treatment also with flucloxacillin for staphylococcal infection and according to the antibiotic sensitivities for other agents. Chronic infections should be treated according to their cause. When insufficient tears are formed, artificial tears may be used.

Dacryocystitis may be acute or chronic and is caused by obstruction to the flow of tears. Secondary causes are pneumococci, streptococci, staphylococci, Candida albicans etc. In the newborn, stenosis of the naso-lacrimal duct is a frequent underlying cause of dacryocystitis, and carries a risk of abscess formation or cellulitis of the lacrimal gland, which may discharge to the exterior and form a fistula. In chronic dacryocystitis, exclude tuberculosis, syphilis and trachoma.

Local treatment: Once the acute infection has subsided, the obstruction to flow should be removed by ophthalmologist, irrigating if necessary with an antibiotic solution according to the causative organism. When an abscess has formed, incision may be necessary, but carries the risk of fistula formation. Chronic dacryocystitis may be treated by dacryocystorhinostomy.

Systemic treatment: For the acute form, benzyl penicillin, cefazolin or gentamicin, according to the causative organism.

Orbital cellulitis: Spreading infection from a suppurative blepharitis, dacryocystitis, sinusitis, osteomyelitis of the jaw or dental root abscess. Haematogenous spread secondary to septicaemia also occurs. A wide range of organisms, including anaerobes, may be involved. Haemophilus influenzae (type b) and pneumococci are the commonest and often give a positive latex agglutination in serum and urine. A blood culture should always be performed.

Treatment: Operative drainage and removal of the cause may be necessary; initial treatment with high doses of antibiotics, e. g. cefotaxime i. v. + gentamicin or tobramycin should be given, but modified if necessary in the light of bacteriological results.

b) Conjunctival Infections

There are many infectious and non-infectious causes of conjunctivitis. Every case should if possible be examined with a slit-lamp to detect corneal changes such as a foreign body, injury or ulcer. A red eye may also be due to iridocyclitis or acute glaucoma. Antibiotic drops or ointment containing steroids should never be used before Herpes simplex infection has been excluded by examination with a slit-lamp.

The *commonest infective causes* of conjunctivitis are pneumococci, staphylococci, Haemophilus and adenoviruses. Isolates of Staphylococcus epidermidis, Sarcina sp., diphtheroids, viridans streptococci, Branhamella etc. are normal commensal flora.

Acute bacterial conjunctivitis is caused by pneumococci, staphylococci, Streptococcus pyogenes, Haemophilus, Proteus, Escherichia coli, Pseudomonas aeruginosa, gonococci, meningococci, Moraxella etc. and is often self-healing, though the course of the disease can be shortened by antibiotics effective against the causative organisms.

Local treatment: Gentamicin, neomycin and bacitracin or kanamycin eye ointment, polymyxin B + neomycin + gramicidin eye ointment or drops, and for Haemophilus, oxytetracycline + polymyxin B eye ointment.

Systemic treatment: Benzyl penicillin should be given for severe, purulent infections and those involving pneumococci, streptococci, gonococci and meningococci. Use flucloxacillin for staphylococci, amoxycillin, an ampicillin ester or cefaclor for Haemophilus, azlocillin or tobramycin for Pseudomonas and cefotaxime or cefuroxime for enterobacteria.

Conjunctival diphtheria: Diphtheria antitoxin and benzyl penicillin, as in other forms of diphtheria (see p. 336).
Local treatment: Eye ointment or drops (gentamicin, erythromycin).

Neonatal conjunctivitis (ophthalmia neonatorum) is catarrhal or purulent and occurs in the first two weeks of life as a result of infection before birth (premature rupture of the membranes), during or after delivery. *Causative organisms* include staphylococci, gonococci, pneumococci, Escherichia coli, streptococci, Pseudomonas aeruginosa and chlamydiae (inclusion conjunctivitis). Bacteriological examination will make the distinction from chemical conjunctivitis due to irritation by silver nitrate, in which the pus is sterile.
Local treatment: Bacterial infections should be treated with gentamicin, kanamycin or gentamicin + bacitracin eye ointment or polymyxin B + neomycin + gramicidin eye drops or ointment.
Systemic treatment is necessary in severe bacterial infections. The choice of antibiotics is based on sensitivity testing. Where culture is not available, use cefotaxime i. v. + azlocillin (effective also against Pseudomonas).

Gonoblenorrhea of the newborn or adult carries a risk of corneal involvement and blindness. Gonococci may be shown by a methylene blue or gram stain of the pus, or by immunofluorescence. Prophylaxis in neonates with 1% silver nitrate (1 drop in each conjunctival sac) has replaced prophylaxis with penicillin drops but fails in 0.1–0.2% of cases. Treatment should be started as soon as the condition is clinically suspected, since prompt therapy gives the best chance of full recovery.
Local measures: Irrigation, compresses, gentamicin or chloramphenicol eye drops. Protect the healthy eye.
Systemic treatment: Since strains resistant to benzyl penicillin occur cefuroxime i. v. should be given, 60 mg/kg a day to the newborn and 2 g a day for 3–6 days to adults. If gonococci are sensitive benzyl penicillin may be given, 0.4 megaunits a day for 3–6 days to the newborn and 1–4 megaunits a day to adults.

Inclusion blenorrhea in the newborn and adults is caused by Chlamydia trachomatis transferred from the genitalia or, in the newborn, from the birth canal and produces a mucopurulent exudate beginning 5–7 days after birth. Typical cytoplasmic inclusion bodies are seen microscopically in a Giemsa-stained smear or by immunofluorescence. The organism may be grown in cell culture in 2–3 days. Healing without permanent damage usually occurs spontaneously after a few weeks or months, and this period is shortened by chemotherapy. Late manifestations sometimes occur, however. Chlamydial pneumonitis can occur between 1 and 4 months in infants who have not received simultaneous systemic erythromycin.

Local treatment: Sulphonamide eye drops or ointment or tetracycline eye ointment for 1–2 weeks.

Systemic treatment: In severe cases, doxycycline. Erythromycin (50 mg/kg/day for at least 2 weeks) should always be given to the newborn with this condition.

Trachoma: Infection with Chlamydia trachomatis of a different serotype from that found in European countries. The different stages are acute catarrhal discharge, granular follicles on the conjunctiva, corneal lesions, pannus formation, blindness, deformation of the eye-lids and frequent secondary infection with staphylococci and other bacteria. Inclusion bodies can be shown in the epithelial cells by Giemsa staining. Sulphonamides are considered to be the prophylaxis and treatment of choice and are given both locally and systemically at the same time. Tetracyclines (e.g. doxycycline), erythromycin and chloramphenicol are also effective. Because of the danger of relapse, longer courses (3–4 weeks) are advisable, with sulphonamides repeated if necessary, with additional local measures such as expression of follicles.

Adenovirus conjunctivitis (epidemic keratoconjunctivitis) may occur alone or in association with pharyngo-conjunctival fever and is shown by follicular conjunctivitis with pre-auricular lymphadenopathy. Infections with adenovirus type 8 may produce pseudomembranes and subepithelial infiltration on the cornea. Adenovirus conjunctivitis gives rise to small intranuclear inclusion bodies and many mononuclear cells in a conjunctival smear. Healing is spontaneous in most cases after 3–4 weeks.

Local and systemic treatment: Antibiotics have no effect. Corneal infiltrates may be reduced by local steroids (an ophthalmological decision). Current trials of human fibroblast beta-interferon eye drops are promising, however.

c) Corneal Infections

Corneal ulcers and hypopyon: *Causative organisms:* Pneumococci, Pseudomonas, staphylococci, streptococci and enterobacteria. Mixed infections are common. Viruses (e.g. vaccinia virus) and fungi (e.g. Candida albicans) may also cause central ulceration. The causative organisms may be cultured from the ulcer exudate and antibiotic sensitivity testing is important for therapy. Severe complications (e.g. secondary glaucoma) may occur, and the condition should always be managed by an ophthalmologist who can determine what other measures are necessary.

Local treatment: Polymyxin B + neomycin + gramicidin, bacitracin + neomycin, gentamicin (except in pneumococcal or streptococcal infection), or oxytetracycline + polymyxin B. Deep ulcers with hypopyon may require subconjunctival injection of benzyl penicillin or other antibiotics by an ophthalmologist (see p. 407). Local amphotericin B, miconazole or pimaricin (natamycin) may be used for fungal infection.

Systemic treatment: Severe infections should be treated with high doses of benzyl penicillin if due to pneumococci, streptococci or some staphylococci, with flucloxacillin for penicillin-resistant staphylococci, with ceftazidime or azlocillin + tobramycin for Pseudomonas, or with other agents according to the bacterial isolate and its antibiotic sensitivities. A fungal infection can be treated with oral ketoconazole, i.v. miconazole or oral flucytosine.

Infections of the corneal margin: Usually spread from a conjunctivitis and are occasionally due to primary corneal infection (staphylococci, Haemophilus, or Moraxella); allergic, traumatic, trophic and toxic causes are also found, and some cases are drug-induced.

Antibiotic treatment is as for conjunctivitis and related to the cause.

Circumorbital abscesses frequently follow injury or operation or can be metastatic from septicaemia. The prognosis is poor because of the risk of panophthalmitis. The usual causes are pneumococci, Pseudomonas or other organisms.

Local treatment: According to the causative organism, with benzyl penicillin, gentamicin or polymyxin B by subconjunctival injection or polymyxin B, neomycin plus gramicidin eye ointment.

Systemic treatment should be started as soon as possible with benzyl penicillin (for pneumococcal infection), azlocillin + tobramycin (for Pseudomonas infection) or for other organisms on the basis of the results of culture and antibiotic sensitivities.

Herpetic keratitis is caused by Herpes simplex virus. Intranuclear inclusion bodies are found in a Giemsa or immunofluorescent preparation. Diagnosis and treatment should only be carried out by an ophthalmologist.

Systemic treatment: Acyclovir 5 mg/kg three times a day as a short i.v. infusion for 5 days.

Local treatment: Superficial (epithelial) infections may be treated with 3% acyclovir eye ointment or 0.1% idoxuridine drops or 0.5% ointment 4 times a day; the ointment should also be inserted overnight. Acyclovir eye ointment is a specific treatment for herpes infections (see 536). Steroids are strongly contraindicated. 3% vidarabine eye ointment (adenine arabinoside) is also sometimes effective. Disciform keratitis may be treated with local cortisone but not idoxuridine which should also be avoided in other forms with parenchymatous involvement, since this can damage the cornea particularly when used for long periods. Secondary bacterial infection may be treated with local gentamicin.

Ophthalmic zoster: Keratitis, iridocyclitis, hyperaemic conjunctivae, often with blisters on the lid. There is a risk of scleritis, secondary glaucoma, optic neuritis and ocular paralysis. Treatment should only be given by the ophthalmologist.

Acyclovir eliminates the virus rapidly and should be given in a dose of 10 mg/kg three times a day for ten days as a short i. v. infusion. Opinions are divided on the value of local or systemic steroid therapy, but this should not be given to patients with tumours. Secondary bacterial infection should be treated with local antibiotics or systemic antibiotics according to the bacterial isolate.

Parenchymatous keratitis: *Local treatment* with steroids under the guidance of an ophthalmologist while the underlying disease is treated simultaneously (see syphilis, p. 434, tuberculosis, p. 463).

Allergic keratoconjunctivitis: Secondary bacterial infection should be treated where it arises.

Local treatment: Tetracycline eye ointment with polymyxin B or gentamicin eye drops or ointment.

Keratomycosis: Caused by Candida albicans, Aspergillus, Fusarium or other fungi. Usually follows an injury or a primary bacterial or viral infection of the cornea, often after local steroid treatment. Corneal ulceration and involvement of the lid and conjunctiva may occur. The causative organism can be demonstrated by microscopy and culture.

Local treatment: An eye ointment of pimaricin in combination with chloramphenicol, econazole (1% solution) and possibly also amphotericin B or nystatin (see Table 50, p. 407).

Systemic treatment: Amphotericin B in severe cases (for dosage see p. 175) which is effective against candida, aspergillus and other organisms. Flucytosine may also be used if the fungus is sensitive.

Antibiotics and steroids are not effective against fungi and should not be used.

Bacterial endophthalmitis is rare and carries an unfavourable prognosis with impairment of visual acuity. Usually follows an operation or perforating injury and occasionally complicates a corneal ulcer or as a metastatic phenomenon in septicaemia in the immunosuppressed, in heroin addicts or endocarditis.

Causative organisms in postoperative endophthalmitis are mainly staphylococci, streptococci, anaerobes, enterobacteria, Haemophilus, Pseudomonas and occasionally fungi (Candida, Aspergillus etc.). Mixed infections occur. The causative organism may be isolated from an aspirate which is an important procedure because of the variety of possible causes and the need to differentiate from non-bacterial forms of endophthalmitis. The prognosis depends on the promptness of initial treatment and on the causative organism. Infections with staphylococci have a better prognosis than those with enterobacteria. Poor results of treatment are generally due to poor penetration of antibiotics into the vitreous body, and intravitreous injections are recommended in the following single doses: gentamicin 0.2 mg, benzyl penicillin 600 units, cephalosporins 0.25 mg.

Local treatment (topical and subconjunctival) must always be supplemented by *systemic treatment* at high dosage. In the past, benzyl penicillin or chloramphenicol were commonly used, generally in combination with an aminoglycoside. Although no great experience has been gained with other forms of therapy, combinations such as benzyl penicillin + metronidazole, benzyl penicillin + cefotaxime and cefotaxime + azlocillin seem more effective. Antibiotics which are strongly lipophilic and soluble in water (e. g. chloramphenicol) penetrate best into the vitreous body. A fungal infection can, if sensitive, be treated by systemic amphotericin B + flucytosine. Miconazole i. v. is the only effective agent against some fungi. Pimaricin (natamycin), amphotericin B or miconazole may be used locally (see Table 50 and p. 408).

References

BARZA, M.: Treatment of Bacterial Infections of the Eye. In: J. REMINGTON, M. SWARTZ: Current Clinical Topics in Infectious Diseases I. McGraw Hill, New York 1980.

BAUM, J.: Current concepts in ophthalmology: ocular infections. New Engl. J. Med. *299:* 28 (1978).

MEEK, E., B. GOLDEN: Ophthalmic infections. In: HOEPRICH, P.: Infectious Diseases. Harper & Row, New York 1977.

PEYMAN, G. A.: Antibiotic administration in the treatment of bacterial endophthalmitis, II. Intravitreal injections. Surv. Ophthalmol. *21:* 332 (1977).

RANDALL, R. W., J. P. RITCHEY: Medical therapy for aspergillus corneal ulcer. Arch. Ophthal. (N. Y.) *90:* 402 (1973).

RIEDER, J., B. ELLERHORST, D. E. SCHWARTZ: Übergang von Sulfamethoxazol und Trimethoprim in das Augenkammerwasser beim Menschen. Albrecht v. Graefes Arch. Ophthal. *190:* 51 (1974).

ROMANO, A., M. REVEL, D. GUARARI-ROTMAN, M. BLUMENTHAL, R. STEIN: Use of human fibroblast-derived (beta) interferon in the treatment of epidemic adenovirus keratoconjunctivitis. J. Interferon Res. *I:* 95–100 (1980).

SCHACTER, J.: Chlamydial infections. New Engl. J. Med. *298:* 428, 490, 540 (1978).

SCHLAEGEL, T. F., Jr. (ed.): Ocular histoplasmosis. Int. Ophthalmol. Clin. *15* (1975).

THIEL, R., F. HOLLWICH: Therapie der Augenkrankheiten. Thieme, Stuttgart 1981.

VASTINE, D. W., G. A. PEYMAN, S. B. GUTH: Visual prognosis in bacterial endophthalmitis treated with intravitreal antibiotics. Ophthal. Surg. *10:* 76 (1979).

VOIGT, G. J., W. BÖKE: Augeninfektionen des Neugeborenen. In: SIMON, C., V. v. LOEWENICH (eds.): Neugeboreneninfektionen. Enke. Stuttgart 1978.

WILSON, L. A.: External Diseases of the Eye. Harper & Row, London 1977.

13. Infections of the Ear, Nose, and Throat

The treatment of bacterial infections of the ear, nose and throat should be directed against the bacterial isolate and its antibiotic sensitivities; this requirement, though ideal, is difficult to fulfil in clinical practice. If sinusitis, laryngitis or tympanitis is not treated successfully, the consequences can be so severe that every attempt should be made to obtain a bacteriological diagnosis. The frequency of severe complications (otogenic meningitis, mastoiditis, jugular vein thrombosis and septicaemia) can only be reduced by the effective use of antibiotics.

To evaluate *bacteriological results* successfully, a knowledge of the normal bacterial flora of the mucous membranes of the nose, mouth and outer ear is very important. While viridans and non-haemolytic streptococci, commensal neisseriae and diphtheroids, Staphylococcus epidermidis, Sarcina and occasionally Staphylococcus aureus are normal nose and mouth flora, large numbers of coagulase-positive staphylococci, pneumococci, haemolytic streptococci, Pseudomonas aeruginosa, gonococci or Candida albicans are usually pathological. The assessment of the bacteriological findings is rendered more difficult by the fact that a number of pyogenic organisms (aerobic and anaerobic streptococci, Bacteroides and fusobacteria) occur as physiological flora in the mouth, nose and throat. Antibiotic therapy often selects Klebsiella and Escherichia coli in the mouth. The healthy external auditory canal normally only contains harmless skin organisms (staphylococci, Sarcina, gram-positive bacteria). Pneumococci, haemolytic streptococci, Pseudomonas aeruginosa, Escherichia coli, Klebsiella, Proteus and Mycoplasma pneumoniae do not occur and Staphylococcus aureus does not occur in large numbers.

Mixed infections with bacteria and viruses are not uncommon; the latter often predispose to harmful bacterial superinfections. When bacteriological findings are normal despite obvious clinical signs, a viral infection which would not respond to antibiotics should be considered. Failure to recognize anatomical abnormalities such as septal deviation or congenital malformations hinders effective antibiotic treatment since surgical corrections may be necessary before the infection will resolve. The difficult techniques of local insufflation, instillation or irrigation of antimicrobials should only be performed by the specialist who can best assess the chances for success of local treatment. Systemic antibiotic treatment is most effective in acute infections whereas chronic processes, especially in closed cavities, are less likely to respond to antibiotics alone.

Maxillary, ethmoidal, frontal or sphenoidal sinusitis usually originates in the nose. Maxillary sinusitis is less commonly related to dental infection (periostitis of a dental root, which is usually chronic with offensive pus). Haematogenous spread is possible. Catarrhal forms sometimes occur after acute rhinitis. Purulent infections are frequently unilateral and rarely bilateral or part of a pansinusitis; necrotizing infections occur in scarlet fever and influenza. Whereas acute sinusitis generally causes severe symptoms, fever, headache and a purulent nasal discharge are often lacking in chronic disease.

Chronic sinusitis is generally recognised by its consequences (pharyngolaryngitis, bronchitis, otitis media or anosmia) and a diagnosis is confirmed by rhinoscopy, aspiration, irrigation, ultrasound or x-ray examination. Any unilateral cold which lasts for more than 3 weeks is suggestive of sinusitis. Careful distinction between allergic and chronic polypoid sinusitis is essential. Nasal pus should be examined bacteriologically in every case, preferably of a specimen obtained by direct aspiration or sinus washout. A discharge can be provoked by releasing a compressed politzer bag. Common bacterial pathogens are staphylococci, group A streptococci, pneumococci, Haemophilus influenzae, Klebsiella pneumoniae, Branhamella catarrhalis, anaerobes, and other organisms.

Acute sinusitis is best treated with high doses of antibiotics to prevent serious complications as well as to treat the primary infection. The choice of antibiotic is based mainly on the severity of the infection and the bacterial isolate. Suppurative infections should be treated with cefuroxime or cefotaxime, which are active against pneumococci, other streptococci, haemophilus and staphylococci. Dental abscesses are treated with 5–10 megaunits of benzyl penicillin a day, once the tooth has been removed; this is effective against peptostreptococci and Bacteroides melaninogenicus. Severe cases with fever may also be treated with cefoxitin (active against anaerobes) or doxycycline i.v. + clindamycin i.v. Milder cases can be treated with an oral cephalosporin, doxycycline, erythromycin or amoxycillin. Other measures include aspiration of secretions, vasoconstrictive nose drops and, in suppurating infection, irrigation and instillation of a suitable antibiotic gel. Some cases (e.g. with mucous cysts which obstruct drainage) will require an operation. *Ethmoidal sinusitis* may be complicated by orbital cellulitis and *frontal sinusitis* by osteomyelitis, each demanding appropriate treatment. Meningitis, cerebral abscess and cavernous sinus thrombosis can all be complications of ethmoidal, sphenoidal or frontal sinusitis and are usually detectable by CT scan.

When antibiotics and local measures such as repeated drainage with washouts fail in subacute and chronic sinusitis, an operation may be necessary. Neomycin, neomycin with bacitracin, gentamicin and polymyxin may all be instilled locally, every fifth days for 2–3 weeks. A rare form of *chronic fungal sinusitis* normally caused by Aspergillus or Mucor is occasionally seen and should be treated by instillation of an antifungal agent.

Boils of the nose and lip are always caused by Staphylococcus aureus. Thrombophlebitis of the angular and ophthalmic veins can give rise to a life-threatening orbital cellulitis, cavernous sinus thrombosis, and meningitis. Nasal furuncles should therefore be treated promptly with flucloxacillin or an oral cephalosporin, 3–4 g a day in adults or 100 mg/kg in children. Sensitive infections may be treated with benzyl penicillin or phenoxymethyl penicillin, 3–5 megaunits a day. Patients allergic to penicillin should be given erythromycin 2 g a day (40 mg/kg in children) by mouth. Extensive incisions should be avoided wherever possible since they may encourage infection to spread into the veins or lymphatics. Patients with large furuncles with perifocal oedema should have bed rest, a fluid diet and be forbidden to speak.

Osteomyelitis of the upper or lower jaws is caused by staphylococci, streptococci or anaerobes and is often mixed. Any initial focus such as a tooth or sinusitis should first be treated. Benzyl penicillin should be tried; if it fails, alternatives are oral flucloxacillin or an oral cephalosporin; anaerobic infection should be treated with cefoxitin (6 g a day), clindamycin (1.2 g a day or 30 mg/kg in children) or metronidazole. Operative drainage is usually necessary.

Suppurative parotitis is usually caused by staphylococci, occasionally by streptococci. It occurs either in the presence of severe primary disease or after operation, mainly as an ascending infection but also secondary to salivary calculi or blockage of secretions. Suppurative parotitis should be distinguished from mumps, recurrent parotitis, tumours, tuberculosis, syphilis, sarcoidosis and Sjögren's syndrome. When pressure is applied to the parotid gland, pus pours out of the orifice and can be examined bacteriologically. Suppurative parotitis should be treated with flucloxacillin, an oral cephalosporin or erythromycin by mouth, and in severe cases with a cephalosporin i.v. (6 g a day). When there is liquefaction of pus, several stab incisions should be made parallel to the course of the facial nerve by an ENT surgeon.

Stomatitis has various causes and forms:

Ulcerating or gangrenous stomatitis: Occurs with underlying diseases and impaired resistance of various causes. The *causative agents* are generally anaerobes, and occasionally streptococci or staphylococci. Treatment is with benzyl penicillin in high dosage combined with metronidazole; if treatment fails or the disease is severe, cefoxitin i.v. may be used, possibly in combination with gentamicin.

Candida stomatitis (thrush): White plaques which can be wiped away. Yeasts can be shown microscopically in methylene blue preparations and in culture. Thrush generally occurs during antibiotic therapy and in the seriously ill.

Treatment: Nystatin or amphotericin B suspension by mouth, 1–2 ml 3–4 times a day, or pimaricin lozenges or miconazole gel.

Aphthous stomatitis: Caused by herpes or coxsackie viruses. Antibiotics are not indicated and local measures are available. Anaesthetic lozenges may be useful. Solitary aphthae are also unresponsive to antibiotic therapy.

Angular stomatitis (Perlèche): Usually due to secondary infection with Candida albicans, staphylococci or streptococci. *Local* treatment with nystatin cream (for Candida albicans) or neomycin cream (for bacterial pathogens).

Auricular perichondritis arises following injury with secondary infection (Pseudomonas aeruginosa, staphylococci etc.). *Systemic* and *local* antibiotic treatment should be guided by sensitivity testing; an associated abscess should be incised with debridement of the necrotic cartilage. A life-threatening necrotising otitis externa caused by Pseudomonas aeruginosa is described in diabetics and frequently develops into severe osteomyelitis. It must be treated parenterally with a combination such as azlocillin or piperacillin and tobramycin.

Erysipelas of the auricle spreads from lesions at the external auditory meatus or the skin of the head and is a group A streptococcal infection. Treat *systemically* with benzyl or phenoxymethyl penicillin (see p. 428).

Otitis externa, infectious eczema of the auditory canal and furuncle of the ear: Look for an underlying disease, e. g. diabetes. Bacterial, viral (herpes) and fungal infections (Candida, Aspergillus) can all occur. Infected eczema of the auditory canal can result from a chronic purulent cholesteatoma. Vesicles are found on the posterior wall of the auditory canal in otitic Herpes zoster. *Treatment* should be directed towards the organism concerned (Pseudomonas, staphylococci, Escherichia coli, Proteus etc.) and based on sensitivity testing. Treat locally with antibiotic paint or ointment using neomycin plus polymyxin B for infected eczema of the auditory canal or nitrofurazone drops or neomycin, polymyxin B and bacitracin ointment. Aspergillus otitis may be treated by the local application of 2% alcoholic salicylic acid or pimaricin. Furuncle of the ear with marked perifocal swelling and lymphadenitis should be treated with systemic antibiotics, e. g. flucloxacillin or an oral cephalosporin; incision is seldom necessary.

Otitis media is most commonly caused by pneumococci (>40%), group A streptococci, Haemophilus influenzae (especially in small children) and Staphylococcus aureus. Escherichia coli is sometimes the cause in infants. *Acute, serous otitis* media as part of a viral infection seldom requires antibiotics unless the patient has impaired immunity. Bacterial superinfection is relatively common.

Acute, purulent otitis media and necrotising otitis media should be treated with systemic antibiotics because of the risk of mastoid involvement. Local antibiotic ear drops (e. g. chloramphenicol, nitrofurazone) can only be effective in cases of purulent otitis media in which the ear-drum has perforated; neomycin and kanamycin should not be used in these circumstances, however, because of the risk of damage to the inner ear. A pulsating reflex on the secretion, or a protuberance on the mucous membrane is a sign that the drum has already perforated. If perforation has not occurred, repeated examination of the ear-drum is important in case specialist tympanocentesis is necessary. When otitis media is prolonged, the possibility of mastoiditis should be considered.

When the *cause is not known,* an ampicillin ester, amoxycillin or co-trimoxazole are effective against pneumococci, streptococci and Haemophilus influenzae, and oral cephalosporins would also be active against penicillinase-producing staphylococci. Cefaclor has good activity against Haemophilus, including ampicillin-resistant strains and should be given for 7–10 days. Phenoxymethyl penicillin is usually adequate for children over the age of 5, in whom Haemophilus infections are less common.

Erythromycin is effective against almost all the causes of acute bacterial otitis media, including Mycoplasma pneumoniae.

Doxycycline may be considered for older children and adults.

Specific treatment: When blind therapy fails, a diagnostic tap should be taken by a specialist using a fine cannula, so that exudate or pus from the middle ear can be cultured. *Otitis* caused by mucoid strains of *pneumococci* is often prolonged and associated with pale infiltration of the ear-drum and can develop insidiously with a mastoiditis; high doses of benzyl penicillin (5–10 megaunits a day) are recommended. Such pneumococcal infections can occur at any age, but are commoner in males than females, in the newborn and elderly. They are often accompanied by sudden hearing loss. Serum latex agglutination for pneumococcal antigen is usually positive.

Otitis media can accompany *scarlet fever* and should be treated with benzyl penicillin; it usually occurs late in the disease as a simple otitis media, though occasionally a severe necrotising otitis develops early, takes a severe course and leads to extensive perforation of the ear-drum, mastoiditis or labyrinthitis. Otitis media can accompany *measles* when it is usually bilateral, beginning a week or two after the rash and giving prolonged purulence and secondary bacterial infection. Blood blisters occur on the tympanic membrane in otitis or myringitis due to *Mycoplasma pneumoniae* or associated with *influenza*; a serosanguinous or purulent haemorrhagic secretion can also develop. The latter does not require antibiotics, although mycoplasma otitis is best treated with tetracycline or erythromycin. Otitis media associated with *diphtheria* can spread from the nose or throat and lead to a membranous infection (see p. 336).

When *acute otitis media relapses,* a predisposing cause should be sought. Myringotomy may be helpful, with the insertion of a ventilation tube to drain the middle ear, a procedure which is also used to relieve a chronic secretory otitis media.

In *chronic otitis media,* there is often persistent purulence of the mucous membrane, sometimes with bony destruction and secondary cholesteatoma formation. Intracranial complications such as cerebral abscess, meningitis or purulent labyrinthitis may develop. The ear-drum may be perforated centrally in mucosal infections or marginally when there is bone involvement, and foul pus may be discharged, containing bacteria such as Pseudomonas aeruginosa, Proteus, Klebsiella, Escherichia coli, Serratia or staphylococci. Mixed infections with aerobic and anaerobic bacteria (Bacteroides, peptococci, peptostreptococci) also occur. There is also a risk of hearing loss, so chronic otitis media should always be treated by an ENT specialist. Once the *bone* is involved, a drainage operation or tympanoplasty is usually inevitable, supported where necessary by local measures such as irrigation with disinfectant or antibiotic solutions, e.g. polymyxin B. The antibiotic sensitivities of the isolate should always be taken into account. Prolonged local neomycin or kanamycin can damage the inner ear. Systemic antibiotics are almost always ineffective.

Chronic middle ear effusions with a serous or mucous exudate should always be examined by an ENT specialist to determine the underlying cause (e.g. adenoids) and are often successfully treated by the insertion of ventilation tubes following myringotomy.

Mastoiditis develops in the second to fourth week of an acute suppurative otitis media and is accompanied by hearing loss, local pain and facial paralysis. Sometimes swelling or sagging of the posteriosuperior canal wall is present and the infection may form a fistula into the external auditory meatus. Since antibiotics do not penetrate into pus and necrotic tissue, antimicrobials alone are unlikely to be curative. The main value of antibiotics is to treat or suppress intracranial complications such as cerebral abscess, epidural or subdural empyema, or cavernous sinus thrombophlebitis which can all be localised by a CT scan. Most cases require an operation (mastoidectomy or antrotomy) under antibiotic cover (e.g. a cephalosporin). A longer course of antibiotics (3–6 weeks) is advisable after operation. Infections with mucoid pneumococci should be treated with high doses of benzyl penicillin.

Cervical lymphadenitis: When acute, the lymph nodes involved are painful and may form abscesses. When chronic, they are coarse and indolent. Their site depends on the initial focus: the submental and submandibular nodes drain to the lower jaw and teeth, while the superior cervical nodes drain the tonsils, nasopharynx and larynx. In systemic infections, cervical lymphadenitis can also be haematogenous. Non-specific lymphadenitis is usually staphylococcal or streptococcal, whereas specific infections may be due to tuberculosis, atypical mycobacteria, syphilis, toxoplasmosis, AIDS, cat scratch disease or infectious mononucleosis. Non-infectious causes such as leukaemia, lymphoma or tumours should also be considered.

Treatment of non-specific cervical lymphadenitis: If streptococcal, phenoxymethyl penicillin, if staphylococcal, an oral cephalosporin or flucloxacillin is advisable (also effective against streptococci) together with removal of the initial focus (tonsils, adenoids, teeth, gums etc.). When this treatment fails, exclude other causes of the disease by biopsy if necessary.

References

BARTLETT, J. G., S. L. GORBACH: Anaerobic infections of the head and neck. Otolaryngol. Clin. North Amer. *9:* 655 (1976).

BROOK, I.: Aerobic and anaerobic bacteriology of cervical adenitis in children. Clin. Pediat. *19:* 693 (1980).

CHAPNIK, J. S., M. C. BACH: Bacterial and fungal infections of the maxillary sinus. Otolaryngol. Clin. North Amer. *9:* 43 (1976).

CHORO, A. W., S. M. ROSER, F. A. BRADY: Orofacial odontogenic infections. Ann. intern. Med. *88:* 392 (1978).

FRASER, J. G., M. MEHTA, P. M. FRASER: The medical treatment of secretory otitis media: A clinical trial of three commonly used regimens. J. Laryngol. Otol. *91:* 757 (1977).

HAMORY, B. H., M. A. SANDE, A. SNYDER Jr., D. L. SEALE, J. M. GWALTNEY Jr.: Etiology and antimicrobial therapy of acute maxillary sinusitis. J. Infect. Dis. *139:* 197 (1979).

HERZ, G., J. GFELLER: Sinusitis in paediatrics. Chemotherapy *23:* 50 (1977).

LORENTZEN, P., P. HAUGSTEN: Treatment of acute suppurative otitis media. J. Laryngol. Otol. *91:* 331 (1977).

NELSON, J. D., C. M. GINSBURG, J. C. CLAHSEN: Treatment of acute otitis media of infancy with cefaclor. Amer. J. Dis. Child *132:* 992 (1978).

PANKEY, G. A.: Sinusitis, bronchitis and mycoplasmal pneumonia. Bull. N. Y. Acad. Med. *54:* 156 (1978).

PARADISE, J. L.: Otitis media in infants and children. Pediatrics *65:* 917 (1980).

RIDING, K. H., C. D. BLUESTONE, R. H. MICHAELS: Microbiology of recurrent and chronic otitis media with effusion. J. Pediat. *93:* 739 (1978).

SCHWARTZ, R. H., W. J. RODRIGUEZ, W. N. KHAN: TMP-SMX in the treatment of otitis media secondary to ampicillin-resistant strains of H. influenzae. Ann. Otol. Rhinol. Laryngol. *89 (Suppl. 68):* 281 (1980).

TETZLAFF, T. R., C. ASHWORTH, J. D. NELSON: Otitis media in children less than twelve weeks of age. Pediatrics *59:* 827 (1977).

WALD, E. R., G. J. MILMOE, A. BOWEN, J. LEDESMA-MEDINA, N. SALAMON, C. D. BLUESTONE: Acute maxillary sinusitis in children. New Engl. J. Med. *304:* 749 (1981).

14. Skin Infections

The initial question is whether the skin infection requires systemic antibiotic treatment. Mild infections can usually be managed with local treatment, whereas in extensive infections, whether superficial or deep, **systemic treatment** is always advisable.

Local antibiotic treatment is only justified when the infection is very superficial. Antibiotics do not diffuse through intact skin, so local antibiotics are unlikely to influence deep skin infections. Superficial infections susceptible to local treatment include superficial pyoderma, impetigo, some purulent wounds, 2nd and 3rd degree burns, secondarily infected leg ulcers and eczema. Local antibiotics are ineffective in cutaneous and subcutaneous infections such as erysipelas, boils, cellulitis, erysipeloid, anthrax, dermal tuberculosis etc.

Local antibiotics for skin infections should fulfil the following *criteria*:
1. slow development of bacterial resistance during treatment,
2. low risk of hypersensitivity,
3. no systemic use because of the risk of resistance or allergy.

As a general rule, where the causative organism is known, narrow-spectrum antibiotics should be given, whereas mixed infections should be treated with broader spectrum agents. Table 51 shows the agents used for local treatment of skin infections of which neomycin, gentamicin and kanamycin are broad-spectrum antibiotics, whereas polymyxin B is only effective against gram-negative bacteria. Bacitracin, tyrothricin and amphomycin* are effective against gram-positive bacteria and clotrimazole, miconazole, nystatin, pimaricin and ciclopirox-olamine are effective against certain fungi. Since superficial skin infections are often mixed or changing, proprietary preparations usually contain combinations of local broad spectrum antibiotics. Chemotherapeutic agents such as ethacridine lactate, clioquinol, chlorquinaldol, chlorhexidine, nitrofurazone and povidone iodine have all proved effective in the local treatment of superficial infections of the skin.

The advantages of local antibiotics for the treatment of skin infections are disputed because high, usually bactericidal concentrations can achieve a greater local effectiveness than can be obtained with systemic treatment. Antibiotic sensitivity testing has little or no application, therefore, to local treatment.

For local treatment of skin infections, the right *preparation* must be chosen (ointment, cream, spray, powder or solution). Sprays and solutions are generally more effective than creams or ointments; a cream (as an emulsion of oil in water)

---

* Amphomycin is no longer available in Britain, but is still marketed in the USA.

Table 51. Chemotherapeutic agents used for local treatment of the skin. The lower half are antifungals.

Agent	Combination with	Preparation
Neomycin (Framycetin)	– Bacitracin Polymyxin B	Ointment, powder Solution, ointment Powder, spray, styli
Gentamicin		Cream, powder, ointment, cream
Kanamycin		Ointment
Tetracycline		Ointment
Chloramphenicol		Ointment
Nitrofurazone		Ointment, powder
Polymyxin B	Oxytetracycline	Cream, ointment, powder, gel, spray
Tyrothricin		Powder
Fusidic acid		Ointment, gel, gauze, powder, solution
Erythromycin		Solution, emulsion
Amphomycin	Neomycin	Ointment
Povidone-iodine		Ointment, solution
Nystatin		Suspension, ointment, cream, powder, gel
Amphotericin B		Ointment, cream, lotion, solution
Pimaricin	With or without neomycin	Cream, powder, ointment, lotion
Variotin		Ointment, solution
Clotrimazole		Solution, cream, spray, powder
Miconazole		Lotion, solution, cream, powder
Econazole		Cream, powder, spray, lotion
Tolnaftate	– Nystatin	Cream, solution, powder Cream, ointment
Ciclopiroxolamine		Solution, cream, powder

is usually better than an ointment, which does not contain water. When the skin is dry, an ointment is preferable, especially for longer courses of treatment. The removal of exudate, crusts or areas of thick skin with a keratolytic ointment improves the conditions for local antibiotic treatment.

Local preparations of penicillins, cephalosporins or sulphonamides should be avoided because of the risk of hypersensitivity. On the other hand, tetracycline and chloramphenicol ointments which are widely used seldom cause allergy. Neomycin occasionally causes allergic reactions (contact dermatitis etc.), but such reactions are seldom seen with other local antibiotics. Other side effects of local antibiotic treatment are the disturbance of normal bacterial flora, fungal overgrowth (Candida albicans etc.) and systemic toxicity as a result of a partial cutaneous absorption.

Frequent causes of skin infection are staphylococci, streptococci, Pseudomonas aeruginosa, Escherichia coli, Proteus, Klebsiella and Candida albicans. Staphylococcus epidermidis, other micrococci, Sarcina, saprophytic corynebacteria and Bacillus species are normally found on the skin, as are other facultative pathogens on occasions (see above). The demonstration of the primary cause is often made difficult by subsequent superinfection.

a) Acute Bacterial Infections

Pyoderma (impetigo, follicular impetigo, sycosis barbae, pemphigus neonatorum, ecthyma simplex etc.): *Causative organisms* usually staphylococci, but occasionally streptococci and other bacteria.

Locally: Neomycin + bacitracin, kanamycin or gentamicin, amphomycin.

Systemically: In severe infections and patients with impaired resistance (e. g. the newborn), systemic spread is relatively common. Flucloxacillin should be given or an oral cephalosporin. Erythromycin is useful in cases of penicillin allergy. Streptococcal infections should be treated with benzyl or phenoxymethyl penicillin for at least 10 days to prevent nephritis.

Ecthyma gangrenosum is caused by Pseudomonas aeruginosa.

Local treatment: Polymyxin B, gentamicin or povidone-iodine.

Systemic treatment: When extensive, give azlocillin and tobramycin in high doses. Lesions which arise by haematogenous spread in leukaemia require long courses of therapy.

Abscess, cellulitis, sweat gland abscess, whitlow, gangrene: *Causative organisms* are staphylococci, streptococci and other bacteria. Therapy according to bacteriological results.

Local treatment: Incision if necessary.

Systemic treatment: Flucloxacillin orrally or i.v. (staphylococci), benzyl penicillin (streptococci), erythromycin or cefuroxime.

Erysipelas: *Causative organisms* are group A streptococci.

Systemic treatment: Benzyl or phenoxymethyl penicillin, 1.2 megaunits a day for 1–2 weeks. Patients allergic to penicillin receive erythromycin.

Recurrent erysipelas should be treated with benzyl penicillin i.v. or i.m., 10 megaunits a day for 10 days, possibly with subsequent long-term treatment with benzathine penicillin, 1.2 megaunits once a month for several months.

Boils (furuncles) are caused by staphylococci and have different forms.

Small solitary boil: Antibiotics not necessary (except for boils of the lip, nose or eyelid).

Large boils, or *carbuncle:* Incision if necessary. Flucloxacillin or an oral cephalosporin (only successful when treatment started early), erythromycin or fusidic acid in cases of penicillin allergy.

Furunculosis (multiple, recurring): Often occuring with primary diseases which lower resistance (diabetes etc.): Flucloxacillin or an oral cephalosporin.

Erysipeloid, caused by Erysipelothrix rhusiopathiae.

Systemic treatment: Phenoxymethyl penicillin 1–2 g a day for 10 days, or tetracycline in cases of penicillin allergy (see p. 447).

Anthrax boil, caused by Bacillus anthracis: see p. 446.

Tularaemia (cutaneo-glandular type), caused by Francisella tularensis.

Systemic treatment: Streptomycin i.m., for one week initially, usually combined with tetracycline (see p. 454).

Cutaneous diphtheria: A single i.m. dose of diphtheria antitoxin 10000 i.u. plus benzýl penicillin, 1.2–4 megaunits a day, or erythromycin, 40 mg/kg a day for 1 week.

Erythrasma: *Causative organism* is Corynebacterium minutissimum. Shown in a gram smear and by red fluorescence of the skin lesions under Wood's light. The organism may be cultured on special media.

Local treatment: Fusidic acid or tetracycline ointment; tolnaftate is also effective.

Systemic treatment: Oral erythromycin 2 g a day for 2 weeks. Alternative: Tetracycline.

b) Chronic Bacterial Infections

Cutaneous tuberculosis (Lupus vulgaris, tuberculosis cutis verrucosa, scrophuloderma) is very rare today and responds well to chemotherapy, especially isoniazid (adults 300 mg a day by mouth, and children 8–10 mg/kg). In order to prevent the development of bacterial resistance, combination with other anti-tuberculous agents (streptomycin, ethambutol, rifampicin etc.) is essential (see p. 463).

Swimming pool granuloma: Ulcerating nodes on the chin, elbows, lower leg and feet, caused by Mycobacterium marinum (also M. balnei).
Local treatment: Excision of subcutaneous nodes, *systemically* rifampicin + ethambutol if necessary.

Buruli ulcer: A chronic ulcerating infection, especially at the extremities. The *causative organism* is Mycobacterium ulcerans (which grows slowly and prefers 33° C). Common in tropical Africa, occurs in other tropical countries also. The ulcer is almost always solitary, not painful, and treatment is difficult. Streptomycin, rifampicin, clofazimide and co-trimoxazole may be effective. Wide surgical excision and local heat may be considered.

Actinomycosis (cervico-facial form) is caused by Actinomyces israeli (see p. 459).
Local treatment: Incision and drainage sometimes necessary.
Systemic treatment: Benzyl penicillin, 10 megaunits twice a day initially as a short i. v. infusion for 4–6 weeks, followed by phenoxymethyl penicillin, 1.2–3.0 g a day for 2–6 months, possibly longer.
In mixed infections with staphylococci, anaerobes etc., i. v. flucloxacillin or metronidazole may be given in addition. Tetracycline is an alternative to penicillin for the treatment of actinomycosis in cases of allergy. Sulphonamides are inferior to penicillin and are no longer used today, even in combination with other agents.

c) Bacterial Superinfections of Viral Infections

Bacterial superinfections, which are frequently mixed, were described with smallpox, smallpox vaccination and its complications, and still occur with Herpes simplex, herpes zoster, chicken pox and eczema herpeticum. Severe cases should be treated *systemically* with a penicillinase-stable penicillin (flucloxacillin) or with a broader spectrum agent such as a cephalosporin. *Local treatment*, e. g. with neomycin-bacitracin, amphomycin or kanamycin can be useful.

d) Secondary Infections in Dermatoses

Eczema, exudative neurodermatitis, blistering dermatosis, contact dermatitis, leg ulcers and acne can be secondarily infected with staphylococci, streptococci, and sometimes Proteus, Escherichia coli, Pseudomonas aeruginosa or Candida albicans. Chronic leg ulcers are always heavily colonised with bacteria, and should be treated with antimicrobials when there is clinical evidence of inflammation.

Local treatment with neomycin, gentamicin, kanamycin (see Table 51, p. 426), local disinfectants, polymyxin B for gram-negative bacteria, tyrothricin or amphomycin for gram-positive cocci and nystatin, miconazole or clotrimazole for Candida albicans. *Systemic therapy* is only necessary in severe cases or in the presence of dangerous pathogens (e. g. group A streptococci).

e) Acne and Rosacea

Acne: Systemic tetracyclines, e. g. minocycline, 50 mg a day by mouth, or doxycycline, 100 mg a day by mouth. Promote healing of the skin lesions which can be explained by suppression of the liberation of free fatty acids in the comedones by Propionibacterium acnes. A low daily dose of 100 mg of tetracycline is sometimes adequate when given for a long period. Erythromycin is equally effective. Local administration of erythromycin or clindamycin is inferior to systemic treatment but may be useful in mild disease. Other treatments such as alcohol soaks, expression of comedones, benzoyl peroxide, vitamin A acid and possibly hormonal treatment may be also useful.

The treatment often needs to be continued for long periods of time. Tetracyclines are not necessary for mild acne, but should be reserved for severe cases.

In **rosacea**, tetracycline or ampicillin suppresses papular lesions even though they are non-infective. When the changes resemble acne, give oral tetracycline (250 mg twice a day) for 4–6 months. Ampicillin may also help. The results of treatment are not as good as with acne.

f) Fungal Infections of the Skin

If fungal infection is suspected, the **diagnosis** should be confirmed microscopically by examination of a squash preparation with 1% KOH and also by culture, since certain dermatoses resemble fungal infection. Bacterial infections and allergic reactions can supervene.

The **imidazole derivatives** clotrimazole, miconazole and econazole have greatly improved the local treatment of cutaneous mycoses. As broad spectrum antimycotics, these are effective against dermatophytes and blastomycetes. Their local use is indicated in confirmed or suspected dermatophytosis, candida mycosis, erythrasma and pityriasis versicolor. Nystatin, pimaricin and povidone iodine are alternative local agents for superficial candida infections, such as Perlèche, interdigital infections, intertrigo and paronychia. Local application of ciclopirox-olamine is also effective and penetrates better than other agents into nails. For anal intertrigo due to candida, oral nystatin should be given at the same time to eradicate the colonic reservoir. Predisposing factors such as diabetes, local steroids and antibiotic applications should be excluded.

Griseofulvin is indicated in tinea (epidermophytosis and trichophytosis but not tinea versicolor), microsporum infections and favus. Resistance to griseofulvin has been found in some infections with Trichophyton rubrum, Microsporum canis and Epidermophyton floccosum. A failure of systemic griseofulvin is sometimes due to inadequate absorption and low serum concentrations. Since griseofulvin is more soluble in fat than in water, it is best taken with a fatty meal.

Infections of the toes do not usually respond well to griseofulvin. Since treatment is based on the incorporation of the antibiotic in the deeper layers of the skin from which it passes gradually to the surface, superficial areas and hairs must be treated with local antifungals such as tolnaftate from the outset. Removal of hair or nails and keratolytic treatment with 1–2% salicylic acid ointment improve the effectiveness of local measures.

Once improvement is seen, the initial dose of 500 mg of griseofulvin a day can be halved or the full daily dose be given on alternate days. Treatment may be required for 1–6 months, depending on the site and extent of the lesion. Improvement in skin lesions is seen at the earliest after 3–4 weeks, in the hair after 4–6 weeks, in the palms and soles after 6–8 weeks, in the fingernails after 3–6 months and in the toenails often only after 1–2 years.

A new alternative in severe fungal infections is systemic **ketoconazole,** which is sufficiently absorbed from the intestine. This drug is quite well tolerated but expensive and should be reserved for cases where local therapy has little chance of success. Serum transaminases should be checked during therapy.

Amphotericin B is indicated in generalized candidiasis, granulomatous candida infections and cryptococcosis, which are located in the deep layers of the skin. Prolonged therapy is almost always necessary, combined with flucytosine when the isolate is sensitive. The synergistic effect of this combination allows the dose of amphotericin B to be reduced. For the use and dosage of amphotericin B, see

p. 175; *contraindications:* pregnancy, severe hepatic and renal disease. An alternative in the treatment of generalized fungal infection is miconazole i. v. (see p. 184).

References

CUNLIFFE, W. J., R. A. FORSTER, N. D. GREENWOOD: Tetracycline and acne vulgaris: A clinical and laboratory investigation. Brit. med. J. *4:* 332 (1973).
MARKS, R., J. ELLIS: Comparative effectiveness of tetracycline and ampicillin in rosacea. A controlled trial. Lancet *2:* 1049 (1971).
NEEFE, L. I., C. U. TUAZON, T. A. CARDELLA: Staphylococcal scalded skin syndrome in adults: Case report and review of the literature. Amer. J. med. Sci. *277:* 99 (1979).
SULZBERGER, M. B.: Editorial. Systemic antibiotics in acne: A dermatologic viewpoint. JAMA *224:* 1184 (1973).

15. Sexually Transmitted Diseases

a) Syphilis

Penicillin is the drug of choice for the treatment of syphilis at every stage. In penicillin allergy, tetracycline or erythromycin (which are bacteriostatic only) or a cephalosporin may be used. Depot penicillins are preferred (procaine-, clemizole-, benzathine-penicillin); benzathine penicillin is usually given as a single dose. Acid-stable penicillins such as phenoxymethyl penicillin may not be taken reliably and are sometimes poorly absorbed, and benzyl penicillin requires frequent dosage. Because of the slow replication of the treponemes in the body, a treatment which give permanent penicillin concentrations for at least 14 days is recommended. Early treatment gives the best results because penicillin kills the actively dividing treponemes. Some authorities recommend supplementary steroid therapy at the start of penicillin treatment to avoid a Herxheimer reaction (fever, chills, systemic reaction, exacerbation of focal symptoms), and this regimen has also proven effective in the local treatment of the parenchymatous keratitis.

Diagnosis: Diagnostic tests should be completed before the first dose of penicillin is given. These include dark-ground microscopy of secretions from the primary lesion or a syphilitic condyloma. Blood and possibly CSF should also be collected for syphilitic serology. The Treponema pallidum haemagglutination (TPHA) test is the first to become positive since it also detects IgM antibodies which develop early. The cardiolipin reaction (as the VDRL slide test or cardiolipin CFT) becomes positive later in primary syphilis when regional lymphadenitis has developed. If these tests are positive, further serological tests will help determine the stage of infection, such as an indirect immunofluorescence test (FTA-ABS test) which detects specific treponemal IgM and increases sooner and falls more rapidly after treatment than specific treponemal IgG. Treponema-specific IgG antibodies are present in early secondary syphilis, in the latent period and in neurosyphilis.

Penicillin is so rapidly effective that reversion to seronegativity cannot be used as a criterion for successful treatment, since the titres decline slowly over many months. The cardiolipin titre usually falls to one third after adequate treatment. Specific trepomenal IgM antibodies are no longer detectable 3 to 24 months after the end of the treatment, while IgG antibodies usually persist longer. Serum IgM and IgG are within normal limits.

In the newborn of syphilitic mothers, it was once difficult to distinguish between maternal antibody and titres which had developed in the body because of active infection following transplacental spread of treponemes. If the mother has been adequately treated with penicillin, IgG antibodies transferred to the child fall steadily during the first year of life. A rise in titre in the baby and the appearance of specific syphilitic IgM show that the child has contracted the disease, since these antibodies are not transferred across the placenta.

Treatment: Clinically typical syphilis should be treated as soon as diagnostic specimens have been taken. There are several views about the *penicillin dosage* and *duration of treatment*. In the USA and certain other countries, a single injection of 2.4 megaunits of benzathine penicillin or a daily injection of 0.6 megaunits of procaine penicillin for 8 days are considered sufficient, whereas in Germany a daily i. m. injection of 1 megaunit of procaine penicillin for 15 days is preferred. The British practice is generally to treat early syphilis (of less than one year's duration) with the shorter course, but syphilis of more than one year's duration for the longer period.

Serological tests should be repeated 3, 6, and 12 months after treatment in order to detect relapse or reinfection. A fourth test should be performed in patients whose disease has persisted for more than one year. Patients with neurosyphilis should be followed up for at least 3 years with serological tests of blood and CSF. Declining titres can be demonstrated up to 1–2 years after penicillin therapy. A further course of penicillin should always be given if the serological titres rise or there is clinical deterioration, and usually also if the CSF remains positive. Reinfections are possible after successful treatment.

Acquired syphilis:

Adult syphilis either primary or secondary, of less than one year's duration is usually treated with a depot penicillin such as procaine or clemizole penicillin. A daily dose of 1 megaunit for 15 days is prefered in Germany, whereas 600,000 units a day for 8 days are acceptable in Britain and the USA. A single i. m. dose of 2.4 megaunits of benzathine penicillin is favoured as an alternative in the USA, given as two injections each of 1.2 megaunits in 4 ml at two different sites.

Syphilis of more than one year's duration should be treated with procaine penicillin, 600,000 units a day for 15 days, or with benzathine penicillin 2.4 megaunits i. m. weekly for three successive weeks. Benzathine penicillin should not be used for the treatment of neurosyphilis because CSF concentrations are variable and may be inadequate; most physicians would use benzyl penicillin in high dosage (up to 12 megaunits a day i. v.) for 14 days in such cases. The success of treatment should be monitored clinically and serologically for 1–2 years. A Herxheimer reaction may occur (fever, chills, increase in syphilitic lesions, due to the release of treponemal toxins) on the first day of treatment but generally requires no therapy; severe reactions, particularly in tertiary or neurosyphilis, may respond to prednisone 50 mg i. m. or i. v. In neurosyphilis, prednisone (60 mg a day) may be used prophylactically before and in the first 2 days after starting treatment. Patients with penicillin allergy should be given tetracycline or erythromycin, each 2 g a day for 3 weeks, or minocycline 100 mg twice a day for 2 weeks. In neurosyphilis, these antibiotics should be given for one month. These alternative treatments require long-term follow-up to detect possible relapse. Cephaloridine (1 g i. m. twice a day for 2 weeks) is more reliable than tetracycline and particularly suitable in pregnancy; cross-hypersensitivity with penicillin should first be excluded. Newer, less nephrotoxic cephalosporins may also be considered (e. g. cefuroxime, which achieves high fetal and amniotic fluid concentrations).

Congenital syphilis:

Infants: Give procaine penicillin i. m. or benzyl penicillin i. v. in a dose of 50,000 units/kg a day for 14 days up to a total dose of 700,000 u/kg. Prednisone (2 mg/kg) should be given at the same time because of the increased danger of a Herxheimer reaction in infants on the first day of treatment. Benzathine penicillin is not sufficiently reliable for use in congenital syphilis. This treatment normally leads to rapid improvement in the skin and mucosal changes and a gradual reduction in the hepatosplenomegaly and bone changes. The serological reactions do not usually revert to negative until after 3–6 months. The patient should be followed up serologically and clinically every 3 months at first, then at intervals of ½ and later 1 year; where necessary, the CSF should also be examined.

Oral treatment with phenoxymethyl penicillin, 200,000 units a day for 14 days up to a total dose of 2.8 megaunits is only possible in hospital where regular dosage can be ensured.

Pre-school children should receive procaine penicillin 500,000 units i. m. daily for two weeks. Children of school age may be given 1 megaunit a day for the same period.

Syphilis in pregnancy is treated with 1 megaunit of procaine penicillin a day for 15 days. For safety, this course may be repeated 1–2 months before the expected date of delivery, and should in any case be repeated if titres rise. Patients allergic to penicillin should receive erythromycin ethylsuccinate 2 g a day for 20 days.

Postnatal prophylaxis in the newborn is necessary if a seropositive mother has not, or has only inadequately been treated with penicillin. Since the newborn can be free of symptoms at first, and also seronegative during the latent period if infection occurred late in pregnancy, the child should be treated as soon as possible after birth in the same way as for manifest congenital syphilis. Regular serological follow-up is essential.

Postnatal prophylaxis is also necessary if the patient was treated with erythromycin during pregnancy because of penicillin allergy.

Prophylaxis can be given to contacts by a single injection of 2.4 megaunits of benzathine penicillin i. m., and reinfection should of course be avoided. A single dose of benzyl penicillin for gonorrhoea will not cure syphilis acquired on the same occasion, although the latter may be masked.

References

BUDELL, J. W.: Treatment of congenital syphilis. J. Amer. vener. Dis. Assoc. *3:* 168 (1976).
Center for Disease Control: Syphilis recommended treatment schedules. Amer. intern. Med. *85:* 94 (1976).
FIUMARA, N. J.: Syphilis in newborn child. Clin. Obstet. Gynecol. *18:* 183 (1975).
KAPLAN, J. M., G. H. McCRACKEN, Jr.: Clinical pharmacology of benzathine penicillin G in neonates with regard to its recommended use in congenital syphilis. J. Pediat. *82:* 1069 (1973).
SPARLING, P. F.: Diagnosis and treatment of syphilis. New Engl. J. Med. *284:* 642 (1971).

b) Gonorrhoea

This is the commonest sexually transmitted disease and is often unrecognised. The diagnosis should be confirmed bacteriologically. Gonococci can be seen microscopically with a methylene blue or gram stain or by immunofluorescence, and isolated on selective culture media (e. g. Thayer-Martin). The isolates must be identified by sugar fermentation reactions. Gonococci are best sought in cervical secretions in women; they may also be found in anal swabs (in women and homosexuals), urethral secretions, and in oro-pharyngeal swabs in gonococcal pharyngitis. The swab should be placed in a special transport medium (e. g. Amies' or Stuart's medium) immediately after collection, sent to the laboratory and cultured on selective media with CO_2 enrichment.

Asymptomatic carriers are common (up to 50% of infected women and 5% of infected men). The microscopic finding of gram-negative intra- or extracellular diplococci is not of itself sufficient evidence to make the diagnosis of gonorrhoea, since other Neisseriae (e. g. N. meningitidis) are occasionally cultured from the vagina, and other microorganisms (e. g. Mima etc.) can resemble neisseriae in gram smears. A *double infection* with gonococci and Treponema pallidum can occur and serological tests for syphilis should be followed up monthly for at least 4 months. A rise in temperature at the beginning of a course of penicillin for gonorrhoea is suspicious of undetected syphilis *(Herxheimer reaction)*.

Because of the possibility of failure, urethral smears in men and cervical and rectal swabs in women should be cultured after two weeks.

Treatment: Until recently, benzyl penicillin has been the antibiotic of choice. Penicillin-resistant gonococci have recently been isolated in many parts of the world and most have also been resistant to tetracycline and erythromycin. Where penicillin-resistant gonococci occur frequently, cefuroxime or cefotaxime should be used as the initial single dose treatment of gonorrhoea, and have a reliable effect. If benzyl penicillin is given in such areas, follow-up cultures are essential. Failure of treatment with cefuroxime or cefotaxime is usually due to diagnostic error or reinfection, particularly if both partners were not treated simultaneously. Postgonococcal urethritis with other bacteria sometimes occurs and is difficult to treat; tetracycline or, in severe cases, gentamicin i. m. may be tried. Apparent failures of treatment in cases where gonococci have not been cultured are often due to primary infections with penicillin-resistant organisms such as Chlamydia, Acinetobacter, Haemophilus, Candida, Trichomonas etc.

Recently acquired gonorrhoea: Should be treated with a single injection of 6 megaunits of clemizole or procaine penicillin i. m. given in several injection sites (single dose treatment); cases resistant to penicillin should receive a single injection of 1.5 g cefuroxime i. m. The addition of a single dose of 1 g of probenecid ½–1 hour before the penicillin or cefuroxime injection (see p. 34) reduces the failure rate. An i. v. infusion of 10 megaunits of benzyl penicillin over 60 min is also effective. Oral penicillins (e. g. phenoxymethyl penicillin) should not be used to treat gonorrhoea because their absorption is variable, giving a danger of underdosage. Benzathine penicillin is unreliable because of its low serum concentrations.

Resistant strains are particularly common in Southeast Asia and Africa. An alternative to cefuroxime is a single dose of cefotaxime (500 mg i.v. or i.m.) or cefoxitin (2 g i.v.).

Spectinomycin may also be used as single dose therapy, giving 2 g for urethral gonorrhoea in the heterosexual male and 4 g i.m. into two separate sites for gonorrhoea in the female or in proctitis and epididymitis. The failure rate is up to 10%. Ampicillin (3.5 g) or amoxycillin (3 g) + probenecid (1 g) are used as single dose treatment in the USA.

Patients allergic to penicillin used to be given tetracycline, 2 g a day for 1 week, or erythromycin, 2 g a day for 1 week, with a failure rate of up to 20%. An 8 day course of co-trimoxazole (1.92 g, i.e. 2 tablets, twice a day) may also be considered in patients allergic to penicillins and cephalosporins, though it is generally ineffective against penicillin-resistant strains.

Established gonorrhoea, proctitis or gonorrhoea with complications (salpingitis, endometritis, prostatitis, epididymitis etc.): When sensitive, give benzyl penicillin parenterally in a daily dose of 4 megaunit for 10 days, or cefuroxime, 6 g a day for 10 days. In pyosalpinx, ovarian abscess and similar conditions, consider surgery under antibiotic cover, preferably after the acute inflammation has settled.

Septicaemia, arthritis and meningitis: When sensitive, give aqueous benzyl penicillin (*not* in depot form) in a daily dose of 10–20 megaunits for 2–3 weeks (or 4 weeks in endocarditis); cefuroxime, 6 g a day for 10 days is an alternative. Systemic diseases of the newborn after amniotic infection following premature rupture of the membranes may be treated with cefuroxime, 100 mg/kg a day, or benzyl penicillin, 0.1 megaunits/kg a day.

Gonoblennorrhoea: Cefuroxime and cefotaxime are now more reliable than benzyl penicillin. Dosage of cefuroxime is 60 mg/kg a day for the newborn and 4.5 g a day for 7 days for adults. When gonococci are sensitive, treat with procaine or clemizole penicillin i.m., 0.4 megaunits/kg daily for the newborn and 4 megaunits a day for 7 days in adults; local treatment with gentamicin eye drops may also be given.

Vulvovaginitis in children: When sensitive, give procaine or clemizole penicillin, 0.5–1 megaunit a day for 5 days, or cefuroxime, 60 mg/kg a day for 5 days. A single dose of 0.1 megaunits/kg of procaine penicillin or 100 mg/kg of cefuroxime may be given as an alternative.

Gonococcal pharyngitis: Single dose treatment is less effective and bacteriological culture is essential. Patients should receive a longer course (5–10 days) of either procaine penicillin (1 megaunit a day) or cefuroxime (2 g a day). Spectinomycin and ampicillin are relatively ineffective.

References

BLANKENSHIP, R. M., R. K. HOLMES, J. P. SANFORD: Treatment of disseminated gonococcal infection. New Engl. J. Med. *290:* 267 (1974).

BAYTCH, H.: Minocycline in single dose therapy in the treatment of gonococcal urethritis in male patients. Med. J. Aust. *1:* 831 (1974).

Center for Disease Control, U. S. Public Health Service: Gonorrhea. CDC recommended treatment schedules, 1979. Morbidity and Mortality Weekly Report *28:* 13 (1979).

HART, G.: Penicillin resistance of gonococci in South Vietnam. Med. J. Aust. *2:* 638 (1973).

HOLMES, K. K., G. W. COUNTS, H. N. BEATY: Disseminated gonococcal infection. Ann. intern. Med. *74:* 979 (1971).

KARNEY, W. W., M. TURCK, K. K. HOLMES: Comparative therapeutic and pharmacological evaluation of amoxicillin and ampicillin plus probenecid for the treatment of gonorrhea. Antimicrob. Ag. Chemother. *5:* 114 (1974).

KAUFMAN, R. E., R. E. JOHNSON, H. W. JAFFE: Neonatal gonorrhea monitoring study: Treatment results. New Engl. J. Med. *294:* 1 (1976).

MÖHLENBECK, F., C. SIMON, U. TRAUB: Die hochdosierte Penicillin-G-Kurzinfusion zur Einmaltherapie der Gonorrhö. Med. Welt *27:* 935 (1976).

NELSON, J. M., E. MOHS, A. S. DAJANI: Gonorrhea in preschool and school aged children. JAMA *236:* 1359 (1976).

PEDERSEN, A. H. B., P. J. WIESNER, K. H. HOLMES, C. J. JOHNSON, M. TURCK: Spectinomycin and penicillin G in the treatment of gonorrhea. A comparative evaluation. JAMA *220:* 205 (1972).

PETZOLDT, D., K. GRÜNDER: Penicillinasebildende Neisseria gonorrhoeae. Hautarzt *28:* 507 (1977).

SAVAGE, G. M.: Spectinomycin related to the chemotherapy of gonorrhea. Infection *1:* 227 (1973).

SCHROETER, A. L., R. H. TURNER, J. B. LUCAS, W. J. BROWN: Therapy for incubating syphilis. Effectiveness of gonorrhea treatment. JAMA *218:* 711 (1971).

SPARLING, P. F., K. K. HOLMES, P. J. WIESNER: Summary of the conference on the problem of penicillin resistant gonococci. J. infect. Dis. *135:* 865 (1977).

THOMPSON, T. R., R. E. SWANSON, P. J. WEISNER: Gonococcal ophthalmia neonatorum. JAMA *228:* 186 (1974).

WIESNER, P. J., K. K. HOLMES, P. F. SPARLING: Single doses of methacycline and doxycycline for gonorrhea: A cooperative study of the frequency and cause of treatment failure. J. infect. Dis. *127:* 461 (1973).

c) Lymphogranuloma Venereum

Causative organism: Chlamydia trachomatis (certain serotypes). The initial stage is an isolated papule followed by a superficial painless ulcer with a sharp margin, swelling and suppuration of the inguinal lymph nodes; proctitis and genital elephantiasis are late sequelae. Primary infections of the vagina or intestine lead to marked swelling of the pelvic and perirectal lymph nodes; oropharyngeal infections are associated with cervical lymph node involvement.

The Frei test is positive (an intracutaneous test with 0.1 ml of antigen which is now no longer obtainable). Assay of antibodies (CFT) in serum is positive in more than 50% of cases, sometimes in chlamydial urethritis also. Cross-reactions occur in psittacosis-ornithosis and trachoma.

Treatment: Preferably 2 g of tetracycline a day or 200 mg of minocycline orally for 3 weeks, or longer in chronic disease. Relapse can occur. The buboes may be drained by aspiration if necessary. Rectal strictures may require dilatation and severe cases anoplasty. Sulphonamides and co-trimoxazole are generally effective (failure rate 7–10%).

References

BECKER, L. E.: Lymphogranuloma venereum. Int. J. Dermatol. *15:* 26 (1976).
McLELLAND, B. A., P. C. ANDERSON: Lymphogranuloma venereum. JAMA *235:* 56 (1976).

d) Chancroid

Causative organism: Haemophilus (Streptobacillus) ducreyi (now rare). Usually gives rise to multiple painful genital ulcers with a narrow margin of erythema; lymphangitis and inguinal lymphadenitis (bubo) are also found. The organism can be seen microscopically and cultured from secretions at the margin of the ulcer or from pus; dark ground microscopy for treponemes should also be performed. Double infections (chancroid + syphilis, chancroid + lymphogranuloma inguinale) can occur, and the condition may be confused with ulcerating herpes simplex blisters.

Treatment: 1–2 g of tetracycline a day or 200 mg of minocycline a day for 2–3 weeks (up to 4 weeks, if necessary) are usually effective. The addition of a short-acting sulphonamide (e.g. sulphafurazole, 1 g every 6 hours) to the tetracycline increases the chance of success. Cephalothin, erythromycin, streptomycin, co-trimoxazole and chloramphenicol have also been used to good effect, but penicillin is inactive. Aspiration and drainage of the buboes may be necessary.

References

FELTHAM, S., A. R. RONALD: A comparison of the in vitro activity of rosamicin, erythromycin, clindamycin, metronidazole, and ornidazole against Haemophilus ducreyi, including beta-lactamase producing strains. J. Antimicrob. Chemother. *5:* 731 (1979).

HAMMOND, G. W., C. J. LIAN: Antimicrobial susceptibility of Haemophilus ducreyi. Antimicrob. Ag. Chemother. *13:* 608 (1978).

HAMMOND, G. W., M. SLUTCHUK, C. J. LIAN: Ulcus molle. J. Antimicrob. Chemother. *5:* 261 (1979).

THOMSEN, J., B. FRIIS: The treatment of chancroid: Comparison of one week of sulfisoxazole with single doxycycline. J. Antimicrob. Chemother. *5 (3):* 257 (1979).

VOGEL, M. J.: Lymphogranuloma venereum. Med. J. Aust. *2:* 175 (1973).

16. Rheumatic Fever

Rheumatic fever occurs predominantly in children and young adults, usually 2–3 weeks after a group A streptococcal infection or later. The variability of the symptoms (fever, arthralgia, carditis, subcutaneous nodules, erythema) can make the distinction from other conditions with similar symptoms (Lupus erythematosus, polyarteritis nodosa etc.) difficult. Because of the therapeutic consequences of rheumatic fever, in particular the need for long-term penicillin to prevent recurrence, every effort to confirm this diagnosis should be made.

Treatment: Two weeks of penicillin should eliminate streptococci from the body, and phenoxymethyl penicillin, 250 mg, orally 3 times a day should suffice. If parenteral administration is required, use procaine or clemizole penicillin (0.6 megaunits a day); patients with penicillin allergy should receive erythromycin 1 g for 2 weeks. Salicylates may also be given for a longer period in a dose of 75–100 mg/kg for the first 3 days, then 50 mg/kg/day in 4 divided doses. Prednisone is given for rheumatic carditis in an initial dose of 50–100 mg a day for adults and 2 mg/kg for children. This treatment is normally given in hospital, and the dosage is progressively reduced until the patient is free of symptoms and the ESR has returned to normal.

Long-term penicillin prophylaxis is used to prevent further infection with group A streptococci which would cause the rheumatic fever to relapse in 30–50% of cases. Streptococcal reinfection can be suppressed with relatively low doses of penicillin given only twice a day. This prophylaxis should continue for 5 years after every episode of rheumatic fever.

After rheumatic carditis, particularly with permanent valvular damage, and when the rheumatic fever has relapsed more than once, penicillin must be given for life because of the increased danger with any intercurrent streptococcal

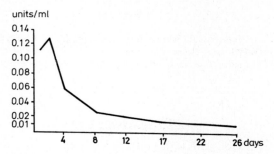

Fig. 33. Blood concentrations after a single i.m. injection of 1.2 megaunits of benzathine penicillin.

infection. If the disease started in childhood, such prophylaxis should be continued until at least the age of 25.

Three regimens are accepted for the prophylaxis of recurrent rheumatic fever:

1. Benzathine penicillin is injected i.m. once a month. This regimen gives adequate serum penicillin concentrations for 4 weeks and has the lowest failure rate (0.4%) but can cause local reactions with infiltration at the injection site and is strongly contraindicated in penicillin allergy. *Dosage:* 1.2 megaunits for adults and older children, and 0.8 megaunits for pre-school children, once a month (Fig. 33).

2. A low oral dose of 250 mg of phenoxymethyl penicillin twice a day. The failure rate of this regime is 3–5% because the patient may sometimes forget to take the drug.

3. In penicillin allergy, sulphonamides can be as effective as phenoxymethyl penicillin. Suitable preparations are sulfadiazine (1 g once a day for adults, 500 mg for pre-school children), or sulphamethoxydiazine 500 mg once a day. The failure rate is about 5%.

The long-term suppression of rheumatic fever must not be confused with the short-term prophylaxis of endocarditis with phenoxymethyl penicillin, amoxycillin, a cephalosporin or vancomycin to patients with old rheumatic heart disease who have to undergo an operation or dental extraction (see p. 317).

If long-term prophylaxis against rheumatic fever is not taken, a generous course of penicillin should be given every time the patient has symptoms which could even remotely be attributed to group A streptococcal infection, i.e. every sore throat or acute respiratory or wound infection.

The risk of recurrence of *acute glomerulonephritis* is small and does not require long-term penicillin.

References

DiSciascio, G., A. Taranta: Rheumatic fever in children. Amer. Heart J. *99:* 635 (1980).
Markowitz, M., L. Gordis: Rheumatic Fever. Ed. 2. Saunders, Philadelphia 1972.
Stillerman, G. H.: Rheumatic Fever and Streptococcal Infection. Grune and Stratton, New York 1975.

17. Scarlet Fever

Scarlet fever is a tonsillitis with a toxic rash caused by a toxigenic strain of *group A streptococcus* in a patient who has not developed antibodies to erythrogenic toxin from a previous infection with a similar strain. The infection is rapidly brought under control by prompt penicillin therapy which largely prevents the serious complications (nephritis, myocarditis). Scarlet fever should therefore be treated with penicillin for 10 days, after which a throat swab should be cultured for group A streptococci; if negative, and clinical symptoms have resolved, the patient can then return to school or community life. Urine examination and ECG are necessary in the course of scarlet fever to exclude the complications of nephritis or myocarditis. Differential diagnosis from toxic shock syndrome and drug exanthema may be difficult.

Treatment: Group A streptococci are sensitive to many antibiotics but benzyl penicillin has the strongest activity. Either phenoxymethyl penicillin for 10 days (250 mg a day in pre-school children, 300–500 mg for children of school age, and 600–750 mg for adults), or procaine penicillin i.m. (0.3 megaunits a day for pre-school children, 0.6 megaunits a day for children and adults) may be given. A single dose of benzathine penicillin i.m. of 0.6 megaunits (children) or 1.2 megaunits (adults) may be given as an alternative and produces adequate serum concentrations for at least 10 days.

In patients *allergic to penicillin*, give erythromycin in a daily dose of 2 g for adults and 50 mg/kg for children. The carrier rate is higher than after penicillin. Sulphonamides do not reliably prevent the complications of scarlet fever.

Contacts of streptococcal pharyngitis or scarlet fever can suppress the disease by taking therapeutic doses of penicillin.

References

Breese, B. B.: Streptococcal pharyngitis and scarlet fever. Amer. J. Dis. Child. *132:* 612 (1978).
Wannamaker, L. W., J. M. Matsen: Streptococci and Streptococcal Diseases. Academic Press, New York 1972.

18. Tetanus

Causative organism: Clostridium tetani. The clinical picture of toxic myoclonus in a patient with a normal level of consciousness is pathognomonic of tetanus.

Antibiotic treatment can limit further toxin production by eliminating bacteria from the site of primary infection. Benzyl penicillin is the most suitable agent, or an i.v. tetracycline in penicillin allergy. In deeply penetrating wounds, the organisms may be associated with foreign bodies and therefore only susceptible to antibiotics at high dosage. Antibiotic treatment of cases of tetanus should also cover the possibility of aspiration pneumonia and a mixed wound infection involving other bacteria. The treatment of choice is 10–20 (–40) megaunits of benzyl penicillin given as 2–3 i.v. short infusions, and 1 megaunit/kg/day for tetanus neonatorum. A tetracycline may be given i.v. in cases of penicillin allergy (250 mg twice a day for adults, 10 mg/kg for children) for at least 10 days.

Intensive care and the control of symptoms determine the outcome of the disease. This supportive treatment includes adequate sedation by diazepam and/or barbiturates, muscle relaxants, possibly propranolol, early tracheotomy and mechanical ventilation, aspiration of respiratory secretions, maintenance of fluid and electrolyte balance, parenteral feeding, control of hyperpyrexia by drugs and physical means, and surgical measures such as wound excision where necessary. Human tetanus hyperimmune globulin should always be given, even though only small quantities of circulating toxin may be neutralised. Dosage: 10000 units i.m. (never i.v.) at the start of the illness and 3000–5000 units on each subsequent day

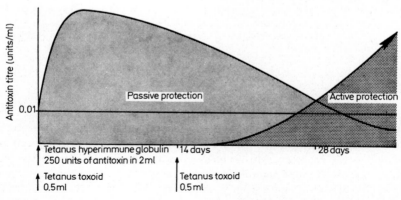

Fig. 34. Serum antitoxin titre after simultaneous vaccination with tetanus hyperimmune globulin and tetanus toxoid.

to a total of 30000 U or more. Because of the risk of late relapse or reinfection, active immunisation with two doses of 0.5 ml of tetanus toxoid four weeks apart should be started when the patient is discharged from hospital.

Tetanus prophylaxis after injury:

A booster dose of tetanus toxoid (0.5 ml i. m.) should be given to *fully immunised patients* whose last vaccination was more than 1 year previously. When the wound is contaminated, phenoxymethyl penicillin should also be given for 10 days, or tetracycline to patients allergic to penicillin.

Hyperimmune globulin (250 units) can also be given where the risk of tetanus is particularly high (extensive lacerations, delay in treatment, impaired blood supply etc.).

Non-immunised, or incompletely immunised patients should always be given tetanus hyperimmune globulin 250 units i. m. and 0.5 ml of tetanus toxoid i. m. at the same time in opposite sides of the body. Where the risk of tetanus is particularly high, 500 units of tetanus hyperimmune globulin should be given. Further doses of tetanus toxoid should be given after 2–3 weeks and 1 year (Fig. 34). Tetanus hyperimmune globulin alone can no longer be relied on to give full protection against tetanus. Animal antitoxins are no longer used because of sensitisation to foreign protein and their reduced half-life.

References

ARMITAGE, P., C. ROSEMARY: Prognosis in tetanus: use of data from therapeutic trials. J. infect. Dis. *138:* 1 (1978).

BENNETT, J. V.: Tetanus. In: HOEPRICH, P. D. (ed.): Infectious Diseases, p. 948. Harper & Row, Hagerstown 1977.

EDMONDSON, R. S., M. W. FLOWERS: Intensive care in tetanus: Management, complications and mortality in 100 cases. Brit. med. J. *1:* 1401 (1979).

Report of The Committee on Infectious Diseases: Tetanus p. 278. American Academy of Pediatrics, Evanston, Ill. 1977.

19. Gas Gangrene

Clostridium perfringens (welchii) is the *most important cause,* although other anaerobic clostridia such as Cl. novyi, Cl. septicum and Cl. histolyticum can also give rise to gas gangrene. Mixed infections with other anaerobes (peptostreptococci, Bacteroides) and enterobacteria are frequently found. These bacteria are almost ubiquitous and enter deep wounds through dirt or earth in road traffic accidents (particularly involving motorcycles), in injuries on farms or through gunshot wounds. They produce toxins under anaerobic conditions.

There are several clinical forms. **Clostridial cellulitis** develops slowly, does not involve muscular tissue, and carries a better prognosis than acute fulminating **clostridial myonecrosis,** which develops suddenly and progresses rapidly to severe systemic intoxication, intravascular haemolysis, septic metastatic foci and acute renal failure.

Postoperative gas gangrene can follow lower limb amputation for arteriosclerosis; the organisms apparently enter the stump wound through local lymphangitis. Other special forms are gas gangrene following criminal abortion, clostridial septicaemia in leukaemics which generally arises in the colon, and postoperative gas gangrene after operations on the gall bladder.

The **diagnosis** of gas gangrene is primarily clinical, but can rapidly be confirmed by the microscopic demonstration of typical gram-positive rods in material from the wound. Culture is not difficult but requires special media. Several other forms of cellulitis are associated with extensive subcutaneous gas and due to gram-negative bacilli, streptococci etc.

Treatment: When gas gangrene is suspected, high doses of benzyl penicillin (20–40 megaunits a day in 3–4 short i. v. infusions) should be started at once in an attempt to contain further spread of the infection. The clostridia of gas gangrene are always sensitive to penicillin. High doses are necessary to reach organisms in necrotic tissue. Metronidazole, cephalosporins or tetracycline are alternatives in penicillin allergy. Gangrenous myositis requires radical surgical excision of necrotic tissue and drainage of pus; the wound should be laid open. The value of hyperbaric oxygen is controversial; to be effective, this treatment has to be started early and the patient will need to be transported carefully to a chamber nearby. The disadvantages of such treatment are the lack of accessibility to the patient in a small chamber and the time restrictions on such treatment. Septic abortion requires thorough curettage or even hysterectomy. Clostridia are quite commonly found in the uterus, bile obtained at operation, and wounds after abdominal operations in the absence of clinical gas gangrene.

Benzyl penicillin should always be given to patients with such findings. Intravenous clindamycin or metronidazole should be given in addition to penicillin in mixed infections which include Bacteroides fragilis, and gentamicin when gram-negative bacilli are present.

Intensive treatment with blood or plasma transfusion, maintenance of fluid and electrolyte balance and haemodialysis in renal failure is very important. The administration of clostridial antiserum (horse) is controversial and dangerous; corticosteroids and gamma globulin are also of no value in the treatment of gas gangrene.

Prophylaxis: High doses of benzyl penicillin (5–20 megaunits a day) can prevent the development of gas gangrene in patients with contaminated wounds or severe tissue damage. Prophylaxis with moderate doses of penicillin should be given to any patient with a severely contaminated wound, or who is about to undergo lower limb amputation for ischaemia; the failure to do so may be regarded as medical negligence. Prophylactic antitoxin is not recommended.

References

CAPLAN E., R. KLUGE: Gas gangrene. Arch. intern. Med. *136:* 788 (1976).
DEVERIDGE, R. J., I. P. UNSWORTH: Gas gangrene. Med. J. Aust. *1:* 1106 (1973).
GOULON, M., A. BAREIS, PH. GAJDOS, S. GROSBUIS, P. BABINET, J.-C. RAPHAEL: La gangrène gazeuse. Traitement et prophylaxie. Nouv. Presse méd. *3:* 2539 (1974).
HITCHCOCK, C., F. DEMELLO, J. HAGLIN: Gangrene infection. Surg. Clin. North Amer. *55:* 1403 (1975).
RODING, B., P. H. GROENVELD, I. BOEREMA: Ten years' experience in the treatment of gas gangrene in hyperbaric oxygen. Surg. Gynec. Obstet. *134:* 579 (1972).
SCHMAUSS, A. K., E. BAHRMANN, W. FABIAN: Gasbrandbehandlung und hyperbare Oxygenisation. Zbl. Chir. *98:* 912 (1973).
WEINSTEIN, L., M. A. BARZA: Gas gangrene. New Engl. J. Med. *289:* 1129 (1973).

20. Anthrax

Causative organism: Bacillus anthracis. Nowadays uncommon, mainly affecting persons working with animals, or bone-meal fertiliser in agriculture. The typical malignant pustule of anthrax develops on the skin, and this is the commonest and least serious form which may heal spontaneously. Pulmonary and intestinal anthrax have a poor prognosis, as have anthrax septicaemia and haemorrhagic meningitis, which is generally fatal despite treatment. The large, gram-positive bacilli are clearly shown microscopically and readily cultured from pus or sputum and from the blood in systemic disease. Penicillin sensitivity is variable and high doses of benzyl penicillin should always be given.

Treatment: Benzyl penicillin i.v. (or i.m.). Cutaneous anthrax should be treated with at least 5 megaunits/day in adults or 0.1 megaunits/kg/day in children, and other forms with 20 megaunits a day in adults and 0.5 megaunits/kg/day in children.

Patients allergic to penicillin should receive a tetracycline such as rolitetracycline i.v. in a dose of 250 mg 2–3 times a day in adults and 10 mg/kg/day in children. An oral tetracycline may be given in a dose of 2 g a day in adults or 40 mg/kg/day in children. Cutaneous anthrax should be treated for 2 weeks and other forms for at least 4 weeks according to the severity of the disease.

References

CHRISTIE, A. B.: The clinical aspects of anthrax. Postgrad. med. J. *49:* 565 (1973).
LAMB, R.: Anthrax. Brit. med. J. *1:* 157 (1973).
NALIN, D. R., B. SULTANA, R. SAHUNJA: Survival of a patient with intestinal anthrax. Amer. J. Med. *62:* 130 (1977).
TAHERNIA, A. C., G. HASHEMI: Survival in anthrax meningitis. Pediatrics *50:* 329 (1972).

21. Erysipeloid

Causative organism: Erysipelothrix rhusiopathiae. This infection is particularly associated with butchers and meat handlers. Characteristic skin lesions occur on the hands and have a good prognosis; arthritis or septicaemia with endocarditis are rare complications. The organism can be cultured under anaerobic conditions from material taken from the skin.

Treatment of choice: Phenoxymethyl penicillin, 1.2 megaunits a day for 10 days, or benzyl penicillin, 5–20 megaunits a day for 4–6 weeks in septicaemia. Patients allergic to penicillin may be treated with tetracycline or erythromycin.

References

BAIRD, P. T., R. BENN: Erysipelothrix endocarditis. Med. J. Aust. *2:* 743 (1975).

22. Listeriosis

Neonatal listeriosis follows placental transfer of the organisms and frequently causes stillbirth, prematurity and inflammatory changes in the placenta. There are meconium staining of the amniotic fluid, septic jaundice, posterior pharyngeal granulomas, purulent conjunctivitis, bronchopneumonia, meningitis or encephalitis. Infections of late onset acquired during birth by contact with listerias in the vagina can cause meningitis or intestinal disease.

Early diagnosis is very important for successful treatment and can be made by bacteriological examination of the meconium (gram-positive rods in a gram-stained smear and in culture), nasal or conjunctival secretion, urine, CSF, blood, tracheal aspirate, placenta or lochia. The presence of gram-positive bacilli in the meconium, which is normally sterile, justifies immediate antibiotic treatment. The meconium should be cultured in all premature babies, regardless of whether they have signs of sepsis. Serological tests on maternal and cord blood are unreliable. When treated early, the chances of recovery increase to 50–80%. Even antibiotics with a good activity *in vitro* may be ineffective against organisms sequestered in deep granulomatous tissue, and long courses of treatment at high dosage are usually necessary.

Treatment of neonatal listeriosis: Treatment with ampicillin or piperacillin has proved superior to tetracyclines or chloramphenicol. Ampicillin is given at a dose of 200–400 mg/kg/day in 4 divided doses (i. v. or i. m.) for at least 3 weeks, and longer in meningitis. A further course of ampicillin for 14 days may be given after 2–3 weeks to prevent relapse. There is no need to treat the mother simultaneously if she is free of symptoms. Cephalosporins are unreliable.

Acquired meningoencephalitis: Listeria is unusual in that it gives rise to predominantly granulomatous meningitis. It affects mainly elderly patients whose resistance is lowered by underlying disease (immunosuppression, lymphoma, liver disease). Listeria generally only causes a moderate cerebrospinal pleocytosis (300–1000 cells/mm^3, many of which are mononuclear). Lower cell counts (less than 300/mm^3) or purulent CSF are occasionally found, similar to pyogenic meningitis. The *diagnosis* is readily made by CSF culture, although the organisms are sometimes missed by direct microscopy because of their small numbers. Serological methods are unreliable. Since listeria meningoencephalitis is always haematogenous in origin, there is no need to search for an initial nasal or otogenic focus.

Treatment: As in neonatal listeriosis, listeria meningitis is best treated with ampicillin. Adults should receive 6–12 g i. m. a day in 3–4 divided doses, and children 200–400 mg/kg/day. Tetracycline (1 g a day i. v., then orally) used to be preferred, but penetrates CSF poorly. Benzyl penicillin (20 megaunits a day) has been used with some success. Treatment should continue for at least 4 weeks because of the poor antibiotic penetration into the granulomatous tissue.

Septicaemia (acquired) should be treated in the same way as listeria meningitis.

Listeria infections in pregnancy are usually asymptomatic. They occasionally give rise to fever, pyelonephritis, endometritis, and very rarely meningitis.
Treatment: Ampicillin, 3–6 g a day, i. v. or orally for at least 2–3 weeks.

Oculoglandular or cutaneous forms: Ampicillin, 3–6 g or 100 mg/kg a day until clinical resolution. Tetracycline in penicillin-allergic patients.

References

Dykes, A., L. J. Baraff, P. Herzog: Listeria brain abscess in an immunosuppressed child. J. Pediatr. *94:* 72 (1979).

Halliday, H. L., T. Hirata: Perinatal listeriosis. Amer. J. Obstet. Gynecol. *133:* 405 (1979).

LARSSON, S., S. CRONBERG, S. WINBLAD: Listeriosis during pregnancy and neonatal period in Sweden 1958–1974. Acta paed. scand 68: 485 (1979).
RELIER, J. P.: Listeriosis. J. Antimicrob. Chemother. 5 (Suppl. A): 51 (1979).
SHACKELFORD, P. G., R. D. FEIGIN: Listeria revisited. Amer. J. Dis. Child 131: 391 (1977).
VISINTINE, A. M., J. K. OLESKE, A. J. NAHMIAS: Listeria monocytogenes infection in infants and children. Amer. J. Dis. Child 131: 393 (1977).

23. Salmonella Infections

Typhoid and paratyphoid fevers are caused by Salmonella typhi and S. paratyphi A or B. As septicaemiac diseases, they differ in pathogenesis, diagnosis and treatment from the less severe enteritis caused by S. typhi-murium and related food-poisoning strains which are generally limited to the intestinal tract. This separation is of practical use for the treatment of salmonella excretion, since excretors of Salmonella typhi and paratyphi are a greater danger to public health than those infected with food-poisoning strains, where excretion usually ceases spontaneously.

a) Typhoid and Paratyphoid Fever

Pathogens: Salmonella typhi, Salmonella paratyphi A and B, Salmonella sendai.

Clinical features: Septicaemic illness, which should not be confused with salmonella gastroenteritis.

Culture: The organisms can be cultured from the blood during the 1st week, and faeces and urine from the 2nd week onwards. The Widal test for specific serum agglutinins is useful in showing a rise in titre. Antibiotic sensitivity testing is important because multi-resistant strains of S. typhi resistant to chloramphenicol, co-trimoxazole, ampicillin and other agents are now found in some parts of the world.

Treatment: Chloramphenicol, for many years the standard treatment of typhoid, is now being superceded by co-trimoxazole. The risk of side effects is smaller and results are similar, although failures occasionally occur. Like chloramphenicol, co-trimoxazole produces a slow lysis of fever after an interval of 1–3 days, but complete defervescence does not occur before 5–6 days. Though they greatly improve the course of the disease, neither co-trimoxazole nor chloramphenicol can completely prevent complications such as intestinal bleeding, perforation, relapse (after completion of treatment) or permanent complications. Because of bacteriolytic (Herxheimer) reactions, chloramphenicol should be started carefully and increased gradually over 3 days. These reactions appear to be unimportant with co-trimoxazole.

Co-trimoxazole should be given in high dosage of 2.4 g of sulphamethoxazole + 0.48 g of trimethoprim a day (3 tablets twice a day). The blood count should be regularly checked. Since co-trimoxazole is generally well tolerated, treatment should be continued until the 10th day after defervescence.

Chloramphenicol can be used for patients with sulphonamide allergy or when co-trimoxazole has failed. Chloramphenicol is preferably given by mouth but can be given parenterally in unconsciousness or vomiting. Resistance to chloramphenicol can occur and sensitivity testing is advisable.

A suitable regimen for oral or parenteral chloramphenicol in 3 divided doses is
day 1: 1 g for adults, 10–20 mg/kg for children,
day 2: 2 g for adults, 30–40 mg/kg for children,
day 3: 3 g for adults, 40–60 mg/kg for children.

The chloramphenicol dose of 3 g (or 40–60 mg/kg) is given until defervescence, and followed by 1.5–2 g or 30 mg/kg a day for a further 10–14 days. When the critical total amount of chloramphenicol of 25–30 g or 700 mg/kg (for children) has been given, treatment should preferably be continued with co-trimoxazole or amoxycillin in order to avoid haematotoxicity.

Prednisone (20–60 mg/day for 2–3 days) may be given for shock usually at the start of treatment or for particularly severe disease. Because of the risk of intestinal perforation, prednisone is contraindicated after the 3rd week of illness or in the presence of intestinal complications such as haemorrhage or peritonitis. The combination of chloramphenicol, clindamycin and gentamicin is useful for intestinal perforation when a mixed aerobic and anaerobic peritonitis can arise. Salicyclates should not be used as antipyretic agents because hypersensitivity can give rise to hypothermia.

Ampicillin only achieves a slow resolution of fever and a delayed improvement in clinical symptoms. It is therefore inferior to both co-trimoxazole and chloramphenicol. When *in vitro* activity is established, however, ampicillin can be used in the late treatment of metastatic foci of infection and relapses, and for the clearance of chronic carriage. Adults should receive 4–8 g a day and children 100–200 mg/kg parenterally in 4 divided doses. *Amoxycillin* is apparently superior to ampicillin for the treatment of typhoid; it can also be used for the clearance of chronic carriers.

Despite good *in vitro* activity and high biliary concentrations, *tetracycline* fails in typhoid and paratyphoid fevers. The older cephalosporins and aminoglycosides are clinically ineffective and, despite strong *in vitro* activity, the β-lactamase-stable cephalosporins are also of little value in abdominal typhoid, although they may be used for local suppuration due to S. typhi.

Since bacterial resistance is not generally expected, relapses can be treated with a further course of co-trimoxazole, chloramphenicol or amoxycillin. *Metastatic infective foci* in other organs (osteomyelitis, spondylitis, cholecystitis, gall bladder empyema, meningitis, orchitis) should be treated with chloramphenicol initially as above, followed by amoxycillin, with additional gentamicin in severe cases, until complete resolution has occurred.

b) Salmonella Enteritis

The *causative organisms* are food-poisoning strains of salmonella (many serotypes), which cannot generally be isolated from either blood or urine, but can be cultured from the stool from the onset of the illness. The infection is generally acquired from contaminated food (see p. 360) and gives rise to a febrile enteritis which can be severe or even life-threatening in patients with impaired resistance or severe dehydration.

Severe enteritis with bacteraemia (high fever and signs of septicaemia) is best *treated* with co-trimoxazole in standard dosage (2 tablets twice a day in adults), or with high doses of ampicillin (when proven sensitive) in combination with gentamicin. Salmonella meningitis can be treated with cefotaxime or chloramphenicol.

c) Salmonella Carriers

Carriers of salmonellae fall into two distinct categories, namely:
1. *Excretors of S. typhi and S. paratyphi,* who have a reservoir of organisms in the gall bladder, urinary tract or intestine which is unlikely to clear spontaneously.
2. *Excretors of food-poisoning strains of salmonella* who pass the organisms in the faeces after an attack of enteritis for a variable period, sometimes 1–12 months, followed by spontaneous clearance.

α) Chronic Carriage of Salmonella Typhi and S. Paratyphi

Chronic carriers continue to excrete Salmonella typhi or S. paratyphi A or B in the urine or faeces for months or years after completion of treatment and resolution of the acute illness. They often have chronic cholecystitis or gallstones. Duodenal fluid should be examined bacteriologically and a cholecystogram performed before attempting to cure a chronic typhoid carrier. If chronic gall bladder disease is present, removal of the carrier state will only be achieved by cholecystectomy under antibiotic cover (see below). The risk of operation must be balanced against the dangers of carriage in each case. If the gall bladder is normal and free of stones, cholecystectomy is not usually necessary and large doses of ampicillin should first be tried.

Treatment of chronic carriers: Ampicillin, 5–10 g a day in several short infusions, possibly in combination with probenecid, 0.5 g 4 times a day, to increase blood concentrations, for 14 days or more. The sensitivities of the salmonella should first be tested *in vitro*. This regimen may be followed by 4 g of ampicillin a day by mouth for 2 months or 2–3 g of amoxycillin by mouth.

Good results have also been achieved with co-trimoxazole, 2 tablets twice a day for 2–4 months, which may become accepted as the best method of salmonella clearance in the future because of its good tolerance.

Chloramphenicol should not be used in chronic typhoid and paratyphoid carriage because of its toxicity and clinical ineffectiveness.

β) Excretion of Food Poisoning Salmonellae

The reservoir of organisms in chronic carriers of food-poisoning salmonellae, e. g. Salmonella typhi-murium, is usually the intestine, and only rarely the gall bladder. The faeces almost always becomes free of pathogens in a few weeks or months without further treatment. Indeed, antibiotics may even prolong the excretion of salmonellae. If treatment is attempted nevertheless because the patient is a food-handler, oral polymyxin or co-trimoxazole should be used (see p. 152, 200 for dosage). Person-to-person spread is uncommon, but has been described in hospitals, particularly in children's wards and institutions for the mentally subnormal.

References

AFIFI, A. M.: Amoxycillin in the treatment of typhoid fever. Brit. med. J. *II:* 1033 (1976).
BUTLER, T., N. N. LINH, K. ARNOLD, M. D. ADRICKMAN, D. M. CHAU, M. M. MUOI: Therapy of antimicrobial-resistant typhoid fever. Antimicrob. Ag. Chemother. *11:* 645 (1977).

CLEMENTI, K. J.: Treatment of Salmonella carriers with trimethoprim-sulfamethoxazole. Canad. med. Assoc. J. *112:* 28 (1975).

GEDDES, A. M., R. N. H. PUGH, F. J. NYE: Treatment and follow-up studies with co-trimoxazole in enteric fever and in typhoid carriers. J. Antimicrob. Chemother. *1:* 51 (1975).

GILMAN, R. H.: Comparison of trimethoprim-sulfamethoxazole and amoxycillin in therapy of chloramphenicol-resistant and chloramphenicol-sensitive typhoid fever. J. infect. Dis. *132:* 630 (1975).

KAZEMI, M., T. G. GUMPERT, M. I. MARKS: A controlled trial comparing sulfamethoxazole-trimethoprim, ampicillin, and no therapy in the treatment of Salmonella gastro-enteritis in children. J. Pediat. *83:* 646 (1973).

LAWRENCE, R. M., E. GOLDSTEIN, P. D. HOEPRICH: Typhoid fever caused by chloramphenicol-resistant organisms. JAMA. *224:* 861 (1973).

NOLAN, C. M., P. C. WHITE Jr.: Treatment of typhoid carriers with amoxicillin. JAMA *239:* 2352 (1978).

OVERTURF, G., K. I. MARTON, A. W. MATHIES, Jr.: Antibotic resistance in typhoid fever. New Engl. J. Med. *289:* 463 (1973).

PICHLER, H., K. H. SPITZY: Sanierungsergebnisse an Typhus- und Paratyphus-B-Dauerausscheidern mit Trimethoprim-Sulfamethoxazol. Dtsch. med. Wschr. *97:* 1401 (1972).

PILLAY, N., E. B. ADAMS, D. NORTH-COOMBES: Comparative trial of amoxycillin and chloramphenicol in treatment of typhoid fever in adults. Lancet *II:* 333 (1975).

SCRAGG, J. N.: Further experience of typhoid fever with amoxycillin in children. Brit. med. J. *II:* 1031 (1976).

SNYDER, M. J., J. PERRONI, O. GONZALEZ: Comparative efficacy of chloramphenicol, ampicillin, and co-trimoxazole in the treatment of typhoid fever. Lancet *2:* 1155 (1976).

24. Brucellosis

Causative organisms: Brucella abortus, Brucella melitensis, Brucella suis. The infection is transmitted to man by cattle (B. abortus), sheep and goats (B. melitensis) and pigs (B. suis) and causes septicaemia with an acute, subacute or chronic course.

Complications include osteomyelitis, spondylitis, endocarditis, meningoencephalitis, granulomatous hepatitis, pneumonia, abortion etc. Epithelioid cells are seen histologically in the granulomas. The peripheral white cell count is normal or low. The organisms can be cultured from the blood by using special media with CO_2 enrichment. Agglutinating and complement-fixing antibodies may be found in the patient's serum although the serological response does not always reflect the clinical picture.

Treatment is difficult, particularly of the subacute and chronic disease. Relapses are frequent despite chemotherapy with tetracycline and streptomycin. Patients become weak and easily fatigued, so general supportive measures are necessary. Tetracycline 2 g a day by mouth (50 mg/kg in children) or doxycycline 200 mg a day for 3–4 weeks used to be the drug of choice, combined in severe cases with streptomycin i. m. for 2 weeks in a dose of 500–750 mg a day (25 mg/kg in children). Because of the risk of ototoxicity, gentamicin is now preferred. Co-trimoxazole (1.92 g a day for 6 weeks) is also effective in the acute illness, as is rifampicin (300 mg twice a day).

A Herxheimer reaction should be treated with 50–80 mg a day of prednisone for 1–3 days.

Tetracycline is usually effective in *relapses* and resistance has not been observed.

Chronic brucellosis with, for example, endocarditis or osteomyelitis should be treated with tetracyclines in maximal dosage for 6 weeks in combination with gentamicin i. m. for 3–4 weeks.

References

Center for Disease Control: Brucellosis Surveillance: Annual Summary 1976. October 1977.
HASSAN, A., M. M. ERIAN, Z. FARID, S. D. HATHOUT, K. SORENSEN: Trimethoprim-sulphamethoxazole in acute brucellosis. Brit. med. J. *3:* 159 (1971).
LAL, S., K. K. MODAWAL, A. S. E. FOWLE, P. PEACH, R. D. POPHAM: Acute brucellosis treated with trimethoprim and sulphamethoxazole. Brit. med. J. *3:* 256 (1970).
LÜBECKE, P., V. FREITAG: Therapeutische Aspekte der menschlichen Brucellose. Dtsch. med. Wschr. *100:* 431 (1975).
SAMRA, Y., Y. SHAKED, M. HERTZ, G. ALTMAN: Brucellosis: difficulties in diagnosis and a report on 38 cases. Infection *11:* 310 (1983).
STREET, L. JR., W. W. GRANT, J. D. ALVA: Brucellosis in childhood. Pediatrics *55:* 416 (1975).

25. Tularaemia

Causative organism: Francisella tularensis. Transmitted by rodents, infected meat, droplets, animal bites and insect vectors. The primary focus is a sharply defined ulcer in the skin with marked swelling and even suppuration of the regional lymph nodes. Pneumonia, conjunctivitis and septicaemia can also occur. Agglutinins may be demonstrated in the serum, a titre greater than 1:160 being considered significant. Animal inoculation is also used, and the organism may be cultured on special media.

Treatment: Because of its good bactericidal activity, streptomycin has up to now been the most effective agent, though resistance develops rapidly. Good results have also been obtained with a tetracycline when given early; a combina-

tion of streptomycin and a tetracycline is likely to be effective. Oral tetracyclines
are the best agents to prevent relapse.

Dosage: Streptomycin, 1 g a day i.m., or in combination with doxycycline,
200 mg a day by mouth for 10–14 days for pneumonia or septicaemia until at least
5 days after defervescence. Gentamicin is apparently also effective.

References

ALFORD, R. H., J. T. JOHN, R. E. BRYANT: Tularemia treated successfully with gentamicin.
Amer. Rev. resp. Dis. *106:* 265 (1972).
BLOOM, M. E., W. T. SHEARER, L. L. BARTON: Oculoglandular tularemia. Pediatrics *61:* 660
(1978).
BUTLER, T.: Plague and tularemia. Pediat. Clin. North Amer. *26:* 355 (1979).
HALSTED, C. C., H. P. KULASINGHE: Tularemia pneumonia in urban children. Pediatrics *61:*
660 (1978).
HORNICK, R. B.: Tularemia. In: HOEPRICH, P. D. (ed.): Infectious Diseases, ed. 2,
pp. 1043–1049. Harper & Row, Hagerstown 1977.

26. Pertussis

Pertussis can occur in infants during the first year of life who have not acquired
maternal antibody. The disease most commonly occurs in young children, though
a mild form is also found in adults. The cough in the catarrhal phase is not
characteristic of pertussis, but typical paroxysms occur later. There is a peripheral
lymphocytosis, and Bordetella pertussis can be cultured on Borget-Gengou and
other selective media prior to antibiotic treatment.

A pernasal swab should be inoculated as soon as possible on to the culture
media; this is valuable for early diagnosis, in unclear cases and for the
differentiation of potentially pathogenic bacteria. Bordetella parapertussis is
sometimes also found in whooping-cough.

There is now a rapid immunofluorescent method for the demonstration of
bordetellas in a pernasal swab soon after collection; false positive and false
negative results are found. Best results are obtained when the patient attends the
laboratory. Pertussis-like symptoms can occur in children with Haemophilus
influenzae, Branhamella catarrhalis, Mycoplasma pneumoniae, Chlamydia
trachomatis (in the first year of life) and adenovirus infections. Foreign body
aspiration should also be considered.

Antibiotics for whooping-cough are used not only to eliminate the bordetellas
but also to prevent and treat complications. Early treatment in the catarrhal phase
and at the beginning of the convulsive stage is generally only indicated in infants

and young children who are at particular risk of pneumonia and encephalopathy. Antibiotics are not necessary for children of school age unless they have impaired immunity (e.g. leukaemia) or have had brain injury.

Treatment: Erythromycin, 50 mg/kg a day by mouth, or parenteral ampicillin, 100 mg/kg/day for 2 weeks or longer in patients who are vomiting; the bacteria disappear quickly but the paroxysmal phase is not shortened. The patient who has received erythromycin for 2 weeks may thus be assumed to be non-infectious.

Alternative treatments are amoxycillin, 50 mg/kg a day, azidocillin (60 mg/kg/day), or a tetracycline, e.g. doxycycline syrup (4 mg/kg once a day, from the 7th year on). Pertussis hyperimmune globulin is useless, and active immunisation should not be given once symptoms have developed.

Additional treatment: Fresh air, sedation (e.g. diazepam), broncholytics, frequent small meals, hospital care, careful aspiration of mucus or vomit, humidification of respired air, with an oxygen tent, if necessary. Codeine should not be given because of the increased risk of atelectasis and secondary pneumonia. Supportive measures are prednisone for encephalopathy, possibly also an anticonvulsant and lumbar puncture to relieve the cerebrospinal pressure; bronchoscopy and aspiration of secretion in persistent major pulmonary atelectasis.

Pertussis pneumonia is often accompanied by secondary infection with staphylococci, Haemophilus influenzae, pneumococci or other organisms; additional treatment with cefuroxime i.v. (60 mg/kg a day), or cefaclor by mouth (50–100 mg/kg daily) is therefore advisable.

Chemoprophylaxis after exposure of infants or young children at particular risk, e.g. with heart defects, cystic fibrosis etc.: amoxycillin syrup, 50 mg/kg a day, or erythromycin (30 mg/kg a day) for 10 days or longer if contact is prolonged.

References

ALTEMEIER, W. A., E. M. AYOUB: Erythromycin prophylaxis for pertussis. Pediatrics *59:* 623 (1977).
BAROFF, L. J., J. WILKINS, P. F. WEHRLE: The role of antibiotics, immunizations and adenoviruses in pertussis. Pediatrics *61:* 224 (1978).
HALSEY, N. A., M. A. WELLING, R. M. LEHMAN: Nosocomial pertussis: A failure of erythromycin treatment and prophylaxis. Amer. J. Dis. Child. *134:* 520 (1980).
LAUTROP, H.: Epidemics of parapertussis. Lancet *1:* 1195 (1971).
OLSON, L.: Pertussis. Medicine *54:* 427 (1975).

27. Leptospirosis

Causative organisms: Various subspecies of Leptospira interrogans infect man, the commonest in Europe being Leptospira icterohaemorrhagiae (Weil's disease), L. grippotyphosa (swamp fever), L. canicola and L. pomona (lymphocytic meningitis), and L. hardjo (associated with cattle).

Diagnosis: Agglutinins and complement-fixing antibodies may be shown in the patient's blood from the third week onwards; IgG antibodies can be detected by ELISA. Leptospires can be cultured from blood and CSF in the first week, and from alkaline urine from the second week onwards.

Treatment: The prognosis depends largely on the virulence of the organisms and the patient's age and is less favourable in the elderly. Antibiotic treatment is usually only successful if started early on the first or second day of illness. This will reduce the likelihood of meningitis or shorten the disease. After the fourth day of illness, antibiotics are unlikely to be of value. Even early antibiotic treatment has little chance of success in Weil's disease. Tetracycline used to be recommended, giving doxycycline i.v., 200 mg once a day, even in renal failure, and continuing by mouth when the first signs of improvement appear.

Large doses of benzyl penicillin (10–20 megaunits a day for 7 days) or of ampicillin i.v. are considered to be more effective. Herxheimer reaction may occur at the start of therapy.

References

CLEIN, L.: Penicillin in leptospirosis. Brit. med. J. *3:* 354 (1973).
LAWSON, H. J.: Letter: Penicillin in leptospirosis. Brit. med. J. *4:* 109 (1973).
TURNER, L. H.: Leptospirosis. Brit. med. J. *1:* 537 (1973).
WONG, M. L., S. KAPLAN, L. M. DUNKLE, B. STECHENBERG, R. D. FEIGIN: Leptospirosis: A childhood disease. J. Pediat. *90:* 532 (1977).

28. Rickettsial Infections

Types: Apart from a few late relapses, recrudescent epidemic louse-born typhus (Brill-Zinsser disease) due to Rickettsia prowazeki and other rickettsial infections have become very uncommon in Northern and Central Europe. Q-fever, which is due to Coxiella burneti and often causes an interstitial pneumonia, is rare. Exotic forms of typhus are occasionally imported. Cases of "fièvre boutonneuse" due to Rickettsia conorii sometimes occur after travel to the Mediterranean and Africa.

The clinical diagnosis can be confirmed by the demonstration of a rise in antibody titre, or a single high convalescent titre in the patient's blood by agglutination, ELISA or immunofluorescence.

Treatment of the various types of *typhus* and *Brill-Zinsser disease:*
Doxycycline, 200 mg once a day, initially i. v., then orally, up to 6 days after defervescence. Single dose treatment and prophylaxis was studied successfully in Africa. Chloramphenicol has also been used in daily doses of 3 g by mouth initially, then 2 g a day after defervescence. 25–50 mg of prednisone may also be given for a few days in severe cases.

Treatment of Q-fever:
Doxycycline i. v. or by mouth, 200 mg on the first day, then 100 mg every 24 h. Children should receive 4 mg/kg on day 1, then 2 mg/kg/day. Q-fever endocarditis: see p. 316.

References

BERMAN, S. J., W. D. KUNDIN: Scrub typhus in South Vietnam. Ann. intern. Med. *79:* 26 (1973).
BURGDORFER, W.: Rickettsiae and Rickettsial Diseases. Academic Press, New York 1981.
KELSEY, D. S., R. L. ANACKER: Rocky Mountain spotted fever. Pediat. Clin. North Amer. *26:* 367 (1979).
MURRAY, E. S.: The rickettsial diseases. In: CONN, H. F. (ed.): Current Diagnosis. Saunders, Philadelphia 1977.
SALIH, S. Y., D. MUSTAFA: Louse-borne relapsing fever: II. Combined penicillin and tetracycline therapy of 160 Sudanese patients. Trans. roy. Soc. trop. Med. Hyg. *71:* 49 (1977).

29. Influenza

Antibacterial chemotherapy is not generally required for true influenza due to influenza virus A or B, which should not be confused with other influenza-like viral infections of the upper respiratory tract or with acute bronchitis due to Haemophilus influenzae. Uncomplicated cases of influenza are treated symptomatically with drugs such as codeine and salicylates. Superinfection with virulent bacteria can have serious consequences. Hospital admission, and hence exposure to the hospital bacterial flora, should be avoided if possible. Since influenza predisposes to pneumonia with Staphylococcus aureus, pneumococci and Haemophilus influenzae, appropriate *antibiotics* should be given early to patients at particular risk such as the elderly, diabetics, pregnant women in the last trimester, and patients with cardiac failure, mitral valve defects, hepatic cirrhosis and bone-marrow insufficiency; such early treatment probably reduces the incidence of secondary bacterial pneumonia. Broad-spectrum combinations such as ampicillin plus cloxacillin or flucloxacillin, 5 g a day, or cefaclor, 3 g a day are active against pneumococci, staphylococci and Haemophilus influenzae. Co-trimoxazole and erythromycin are also useful. Prompt active immunisation with a vaccine containing the epidemic strain gives effective protection, which is particularly important for the chronically ill and elderly. Daily amantadine is not practicable as prophylaxis.

Influenzal pneumonia occurs in two forms. A *primary haemorrhagic viral* pneumonia can occasionally develop early in the infection, whereas a *secondary bacterial bronchopneumonia* is a common complication of influenza. Since superinfection with staphylococci or other organisms also occurs after primary viral pneumonia, the patient should be treated initially with high doses of amoxycillin plus flucloxacillin, or a cephalosporin such as cefazolin, intravenously. *Bacterial bronchopneumonia in* the elderly or in patients with impaired resistance is usually due to pneumococci, staphylococci or Haemophilus influenzae and accompanied by a high peripheral white blood cell count. A broad-spectrum combination such as ampicillin 4 g a day i. v. plus cloxacillin 4 g a day i. v., or a cephalosporin such as cefuroxime, cefamandole or cefazolin, 4–6 g a day i. v., is likely to be effective against most expected bacterial pathogens. Most strains of staphylococci are resistant to tetracycline.

Other complications include otitis media and sinusitis, which are sometimes caused by bacteria, laryngo-tracheitis (influenzal croup) and toxic myocarditis.

References

DAVENPORT, F. M.: Influenza viruses. In: EVANS, A. S. (ed.): Viral Infections of Humans, p. 273. Plenum Press, New York 1976.

FOY, H. M., M. K. COONEY, J. ALLAN: Rates of pneumonia during influenza epidemics in Seattle 1964–1975. JAMA *241:* 253 (1979).

GERBER, G. J., W. C. FARMER, L. L. FULKERSON: β-Hemolytic streptococcal pneumonia following influenza. JAMA *240:* 242 (1978).

PAISLEY, J. W., F. W. BRUKER, B. A. LANER: Type A_2 influenza viral infections in children. Amer. J. Dis. Child. *132:* 34 (1978).

30. Actinomycosis

Causative organism: Actinomyces israeli, which is not a true fungus, but an anaerobic, branching filamentous bacterium. Clinically, actinomycosis gives rise to chronic inflammation with a tendency to form abscesses and fistulae. Cervicofacial actinomycosis is the commonest form, and thoracic (sometimes with empyema) and abdominal actinomycosis account for only about 20% of cases. Metastatic spread to the skin, bones, liver, kidneys, testes, cardiac valves or brain (causing cerebral abscess) are rare. The organisms can be seen microscopically in microcolonies (»sulphur granules«) in pus as branching, filamentous gram-positive bacilli. For this reason, pus should always be sent to the laboratory in preference to a swab. Culture is on special media for at least 10 days under anaerobic conditions. The diagnosis may also be made histologically.

Treatment: A. israeli is very sensitive to benzyl penicillin and has a minimal inhibitory concentration of 0.1 units/ml. As with other chronic infections, long courses at high dosage have to be given because of poor antibiotic penetration into the granulation tissue.

Dosage: Thoracic and abdominal actinomycosis should be treated with 10 megaunits of benzyl penicillin twice a day in short i. v. infusions for 4–6 weeks, followed by 2–5 megaunits a day of a depot or oral penicillin for 2–6 (−12) months. Patients with penicillin allergy or in whom penicillin has failed may be given tetracycline, 2 g a day. Fusidic acid or clindamycin i. v. are also effective. Lower doses of penicillin (3 megaunits a day for 6 weeks) may suffice in cervical actinomycosis.

Mixed infections with penicillin-resistant staphylococci or anaerobes (Actinobacillus actinomycetem concomitans, Haemophilus aphrophilus, Bacteroides, streptococci etc.) should be treated additionally with flucloxacillin (for staphylococci) or metronidazole (for anaerobes). Combinations of sulphonamides with penicillin as formerly recommended do not improve the results. Surgical treatment such as resection, incision or drainage is also necessary in some cases. If antibiotic treatment fails, the rare but clinically and microscopically similar nocardiosis should be considered; this infection usually responds to large doses of sulphonamides or rifampicin.

References

DRAKE, D. D., R. J. HOLT: Childhood actinomycosis. Arch. Dis. Child. *51:* 979 (1976).
FEIFEL, G., B. WIEBECKE, J. BEYER: Chirurgische Aspekte zur Diagnostik und Therapie der Aktinomykose. Dtsch. med. Wschr. *99:* 1016 (1974).
LERNER, P. J.: Susceptibility of pathogenic actinomycetes to antimicrobial compounds. Antimicrob. Ag. Chemother. *5:* 302 (1974).
MOHR, J. A., E. R. RHOADES, H. G. MUCHMORE: Actinomycosis treated with lincomycin. JAMA *212:* 2260 (1970).
ROSE, H. D., M. W. RYTEL: Actinomycosis treated with clindamycin. J. Amer. med. Ass. *22:* 1052 (1972).
WEISSE, W. C., J. SMITH: A study of 57 cases of actinomycosis over a 36-year-period. Arch. intern. Med. *135:* 1562 (1975).

31. Tuberculosis

Since the introduction of antituberculous drugs, the mortality of tuberculosis has been dramatically reduced and the prognosis greatly improved. New infections still occur in young adults, the elderly, immigrants and patients with severe underlying disease. Since chemotherapy has to be given for a long period and carries the risk of side effects, the diagnosis must be confirmed by bacteriological and other means.

The following **diagnostic procedures** should be performed before starting treatment:

1. *Microscopical examination* of sputum, gastric juice etc. The presence of acid and alcohol fast bacteria stained by the Ziehl-Neelsen method is suspicious but not in itself diagnostic of tuberculosis, since saprophytic and »atypical« mycobacteria also stain in this way. The numbers of acid-fast bacilli in the sputum may be estimated from the Gaffky scale.

2. *Culture* is essential for confirmation of the diagnosis and for sensitivity determination. Where appropriate, sputum, a laryngeal swab, fasting gastric washings in children, pus, urine, CSF, needle biopsy material and possibly bronchial secretion taken at bronchoscopy should be sent to a laboratory for culture. Excised tissue should always be cultured in addition to histological examination.

3. *Animal inoculation* for primary isolation of Mycobacterium tuberculosis is no longer necessary because of improvements in culture in vitro; it is still useful occasionally for differentiation of the mycobacteria grown. A negative result does not rule out the presence of tubercle bacilli in the specimen because isoniazid-resistant strains of M. tuberculosis can have reduced virulence in the guinea pig.

4. The *tuberculin test* is still of great practical value in children. In developed countries where BCG vaccination is not routinely given to schoolchildren in their early teens, up to 60–80% of healthy young adults may be tuberculin-negative and a strongly positive test would be of diagnostic significance in these cases. Patients with active tuberculosis generally have a positive skin test at low tuberculin concentrations (1/100, 1/10 or 1 unit). Reactions which are negative at 1, 10 and 100 tuberculin units normally exclude active tuberculosis; false negatives occur in less than 1% of patients and are due to very early infection (preallergic phase), negative anergy, steroid or cytotoxic therapy, measles, AIDS etc. A positive tuberculin test is not proof of human or bovine tuberculosis, but is merely evidence of past or present infection with acid-fast

bacteria which can include other species such as Mycobacterium fortuitum, M. kansasii, M. avium-intracellulare etc. A positive tuberculin test is found for 5—10 years after BCG vaccination.

5. The mycobacteria isolated should be tested for *sensitivity to a full range of antituberculous drugs*, both initially and later if the sputum does not convert to negative, in case the infecting organisms have developed resistance during therapy. In vitro testing is not always reliable and may need to be repeated. Complete or partial resistance to a number of drugs early in the disease is suspicious of atypical mycobacteria or saprophytes, which should be identified. Cross-resistance is found between ethionamide and prothionamide and also between some antibiotics of the streptomycin group (streptomycin, kanamycin, capreomycin).

6. *Histopathology:* Tissue granulomas with epitheloid and giant cells in biopsies or excised material are not pathognomic of tuberculosis; they are also found in other mycobacterial infections, fungal infections, brucellosis etc. The differentiation between non-caseous tuberculosis and sarcoidosis can be difficult.

Differentiation of pulmonary tuberculosis in uncomplicated and complicated cases:

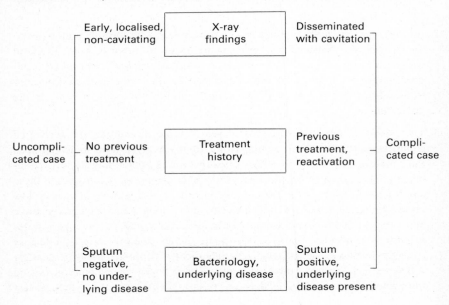

a) Principles of Antituberculous Chemotherapy

1. In developed countries, every measure necessary to produce a definitive cure should be taken. New cases should be admitted to a special ward in a hospital with a full range of diagnostic facilities and should be followed up after discharge by a chest specialist.

The distinction between complicated and uncomplicated cases (see table) is of practical importance because there are some differences in the principles of treatment of the two groups of patients. The combination of more than one antituberculous agent in full dosage for a long period is common to both groups, however. Triple therapy with isoniazid, streptomycin and PAS was the standard regimen for many years. PAS, which is poorly tolerated, was then replaced by ethambutol. When rifampicin, which is bactericidal, was introduced, the duration of treatment could be reduced from 2 years to 6–12 months.

The **treatment of the uncomplicated case** can differ considerably from that needed in complicated cases, and is based on six standard drugs, namely rifampicin, isoniazid, ethambutol, pyrazinamide, streptomycin and prothionamide. An initial intensive course of 2–3 months is followed by 4–7 months of consolidation therapy (Table 52). The treatment during this second phase may be given intermittently as a single dose twice a week. The following regime which lasts for only 6 months altogether has proved effective and has a recurrence rate of less than 1%.

First 2 months	*Subsequent 4 months*
Rifampicin	Rifampicin + Isoniazid
Isoniazid	
Pyrazinamide	
Streptomycin	

A combination of agents must always be used because it increases antibacterial activity and prevents the emergence of resistance. Single drug therapy of tuberculosis constitutes malpractice because the agent rapidly becomes ineffective as resistance develops.

The **chemotherapy of the complicated case** is not easily schematized. Non-pulmonary tuberculosis always comes into this category because of the likelihood of relapse, the emergence of resistant strains and the presence of underlying disease such as diabetes, alcoholism, neoplasia or corticosteroid therapy which impairs the resistance of the host. If the disease progresses or is reactivated despite treatment, the use of untested antituberculous agents should

Table 52. Dosage of antituberculous agents when given daily or intermittently.

Drug	Daily dose (mg/kg)	Usual total dose (g/day)	Intermittent dose
Rifampicin	10	0.45–0.6 (maximum 0.75)	10 mg/kg (maximum 0,75 g)
Isoniazid	5	0.3	15 mg/kg
Ethambutol	15–25	1.0–1.6	40–50 mg/kg
Pyrazinamide	30–35	1.5–2.0	60 mg/kg (3–4 g)
Streptomycin	15	0.75–1.0	0.75–1 g
Prothionamide	8–10	0.5–1.0	0.5–1 g

be avoided. Further treatment should always receive a full course of treatment, and is best managed by a tuberculosis specialist.

Length of treatment: Treatment with an effective triple combination should be given to *open cases* of pulmonary tuberculosis at least until sputum conversion (the absence of microscopically evident acid-fast bacilli in the sputum) which usually occurs within 2–3 months, and should be followed with an effective combination of two drugs, one of which should if possible be rifampicin for 6–9 months. *Closed cases* (primary tuberculous pleurisy or culture-negative pulmonary tuberculosis with minimal changes) may be treated with a combination of two drugs such as isoniazid + ethambutol or isoniazid + rifampicin for 6–9 months from the outset. The treatment of tuberculosis requires a great deal of understanding and cooperation from the patient; failure by the physician to obtain this compliance is nowadays the main reason for failure.

Patients who are unlikely to take their medication reliably should be treated parenterally at first. Isoniazid, rifampicin, ethambutol, streptomycin and prothionamide may all be given by this route.

Active tuberculosis in **pregnancy** can be treated with isoniazid, ethambutol and PAS without serious risk to the fetus. Rifampicin may be used in the second half of pregnancy if necessary. Streptomycin, capreomycin and kanamycin should be avoided, as should ethionamide, prothionamide and rifampicin in early pregnancy.

In patients with **pre-existing liver damage,** streptomycin and ethambutol carry the lowest risk of side effects. Isoniazid can be continued if the liver function does not deteriorate.

In **renal impairment,** isoniazid and rifampicin may be given in normal dosage since they are largely metabolized by the liver. The dose of ethambutol (see p. 234), pyrazinamide, streptomycin and capreomycin should be reduced and the two aminoglycosides should be avoided in severe renal failure. Cycloserine, ethionamide and prothionamide, PAS and kanamycin should be avoided if possible.

Children should be treated according to the same principles as adults.

Congenital tuberculosis is very rare; if treatment is required during the first month of life, potentially ototoxic antibiotics such as streptomycin, capreomycin etc. should only be given in reduced doses because of the immature renal function and risk of accumulation.

2. **Bacterial resistance** is rare in new cases of tuberculosis in Europe and occurs only in 1–5% with isoniazid, streptomycin, PAS and ethambutol; it is more frequent in recurrent infections and has to be considered for therapy. Primary resistance to rifampicin and pyrazinamide is much less common. Treatment of relapse or failure of therapy is started with a combination of three drugs, two of which must not have been used before (e.g. ethambutol + prothionamide + capreomycin). Subsequent treatment is based on the results of sensitivity testing, which is usually available after about 6 weeks. If one of the antituberculous drugs is found during treatment to be ineffective, a number of alternatives should be considered; ethionamide or prothionamide in combination with another drug has been proved effective. Capreomycin or kanamycin should be used in streptomycin resistance only when their sensitivity has been demonstrated in the laboratory, since cross-resistance sometimes occurs. Neither should be used in the presence of inner ear damage due to streptomycin because their ototoxicity is additive. The antituberculous activity of PAS is poor and the drug often causes side effects; its main value is the prevention of development of resistance in combined treatment. Thioacetone and cyloserine also give rise frequently to side effects when given in full dosage.

3. **Supplementary measures** include, in relation to the severity of the disease, physiotherapy, breathing exercises and psychotherapy; surgical excision is still occasionally necessary. The patient should remain in hospital until he ceases to be infectious and his condition has improved sufficiently for discharge. He should then attend regularly as an outpatient, provided that he can be effectively managed in other ways at home.

4. **Corticosteroids** with antituberculous cover are primarily used in tuberculous meningitis, miliary tuberculosis, tuberculous pericarditis and empyema. They are of little value in other forms of tuberculosis. The general contraindications

Table 53. Possible side effects of the main antituberculous agents at normal dosage.

Side effects	Isoniazid	Rifampicin	Ethambutol	Streptomycin	Prothion-amide	Pyrazin-amide
Normal daily dose for adults	0.3–0.5 g (6 mg/kg)	0.45–0.75 g (10 mg/kg)	1–2 g (15–25 mg/kg)	0.75–1 g (15 mg/kg)	0.5–1 g (8–15 mg/kg)	1.5–2.5 g (35 mg/kg)
Stomach and intestine	+	(+)			+	(+)
Liver	+	+			+	+
Kidneys		(+)		(+)		
Central nervous system	(+)		+	++	(+)	
Peripheral nervous system	+		(Optic nerve)	(Vestibular nerve)		
Bone marrow	(+)	(+)			(+)	
Skin	(+) (Pellagroid)				(+) (Pellagroid)	(+) (Photodermatosis)
Joints						+(gout)
Precautions and contraindications	Consumption of alcohol, epilepsy, psychiatric illness	Liver damage, early pregnancy	Eye damage, consumption of alcohol	Renal failure, hearing loss, pregnancy	Liver damage, psychosis, epilepsy, alcohol abuse, early pregnancy, diabetes	Renal failure, liver damage, gout

of corticosteroids must always be considered, and particular care taken when using them in the presence of severe underlying disease such as leukaemia, where they may impair the activity of the antituberculous drugs and thus actively encourage dissemination of the disease. In such cases, steroid treatment should be withheld until an effective combination of antituberculous drugs has been given in full dosage.

Dosage of prednisone: 30–50 mg a day initially for adults, or 0.5–1 mg/kg by mouth for children, which should then be progressively reduced. Prednisone is given until exudative features regress and the patient's general condition has improved, usually after 4–6 weeks.

5. The risk of irreversible drug toxicity is small, provided the patient is continuously monitored for **side effects** and the appropriate agent stopped at the first signs of intolerance (Table 53). Isoniazid can interfere with pyridoxine metabolism, so 25–50 mg of pyridoxine (Vitamin B_6), i.e. 10 mg for every 100 mg of isoniazid, should be given daily during isoniazid therapy. Because of its *ototoxicity,* regular audiograms and vestibular tests are necessary with streptomycin and an alternative, non-aminoglycoside drug must be given at the first signs of ototoxicity, which may appear after a total dose of only 30–80 g of streptomycin. *Hepatotoxicity* may be enhanced with combinations which contain rifampicin and the plasma transaminases and bilirubin should be monitored regularly.

Aminoglycosides (streptomycin, capreomycin, kanamycin and gentamicin) must never be combined with one other. When an aminoglycoside has been given over a period, a different aminoglycoside should only be substituted if the audiogram is normal and cochlear and vestibular function are regularly checked. The fixed combination of dapsone, isoniazid and prothionamide, which is used for the treatment of leprosy, is not suitable for treatment of tuberculosis in Europe.

If *allergic symptoms* develop during combined therapy, the most likely cause (streptomycin) should be stopped and replaced with an alternative antituberculous agent.

Women receiving antituberculous therapy should take adequate contraceptive precautions because of the risk of teratogenicity. Rifampicin interferes with the oral contraceptives.

6. The **criteria for successful treatment** are a decrease in acid fast bacilli (which may be estimated using the Gaffky scale) or their disappearance (sputum conversion), the involution of a cavity or infiltrate, reduction in ESR and defervescence.

Failure of chemotherapy may be due to:
1. too short or irregular a course,
2. use of a single agent only,
3. primary or secondary bacterial resistance,
4. underlying diseases (silicosis, leukaemia, Hodgkin's disease etc.),
5. inadequate initial treatment (underdosage, omission of a highly active drug in the initial combination),
6. infection with atypical myobacteria.

Clinical improvement in pulmonary tuberculosis usually begins after 2–4 weeks and is followed by progressive improvement in the radiological changes. The sputum usually converts after 4–8 weeks. If acid-fast bacilli are still present after 6 months of combined chemotherapy, they are almost always resistant to one or more of the drugs given.

7. **Chemoprophylaxis** may be given to *children* and older family contacts even when symptoms are absent and the tuberculin test is negative. 6–10 mg/kg/day of isoniazid should be given for at least 3 months. If, after this period, the child is still tuberculin-negative (up to 100 units intradermally), BCG vaccination is recommended. The child should then be kept away from any possible source of infection for at least 6 weeks. During chemoprophylaxis, regular tests for the possible emergence of tuberculin allergy or of lung infection should be carried out. Immediate contacts of the patient should be tuberculin tested and have serial chest x-rays where necessary.

The *newborn infant* of a mother who has been adequately treated during pregnancy or earlier and has no active tuberculosis does not need to be separated from the mother after delivery. The baby does not require isoniazid and may be given BCG. When the mother shows signs of active tuberculosis and is infectious, the safest course is to separate mother and baby immediately after birth, give chemoprophylaxis with isoniazid for 3 months followed by BCG (if the baby remains tuberculin-negative), and maintain the separation until the baby becomes tuberculin-positive (usually 6–12 weeks after BCG). Congenital tuberculosis should always be excluded. If the temporary separation of mother and child is impractical, the baby should receive prophylactic isoniazid for 1 year, under continuous medical supervision, and should then be given BCG if still tuberculin-negative.

8. **Preventive chemotherapy** with isoniazid, possibly in combination with a second drug such as rifampicin, is recommended in the following situations:
   a) When tuberculin conversion occurs during childhood, either before the age of 6 or during puberty, particularly when the source of infection is known or is found from screening of family and other contacts. *Dosage:* isoniazid

6–10 mg/kg/day up to a maximal daily dose of 300 mg, for 6 months to 1 year.

b) When there is a risk of reactivation of old tuberculosis by measles, whooping cough, leukaemia, corticosteroid or immunosuppressive therapy. The dosage of isoniazid for adults is 300 mg a day, and for children 10 mg/kg/day for the period of exposure. Isoniazid is hepatotoxic and should be used with caution in the elderly and patients with liver disease. If radiological changes are detected by regular chest x-rays, combined chemotherapy should be given as in the acute case.

b) Clinical Forms of Tuberculosis and Their Chemotherapy

Pulmonary tuberculosis: Initial treatment is with a bactericidal combination, preferably isoniazid, rifampicin and ethambutol. The addition of pyrazinamide accelerates the elimination of the bacilli. The following regimens may be used for uncomplicated pulmonary tuberculosis:

Initial treatment			Consolidation phase	
I. Rifampicin Isoniazid Ethambutol	10 mg/kg 5 mg/kg 20–25 mg/kg	} 2–3 months	Rifampicin Isoniazid	} further 6–9 months
II. Rifampicin Isoniazid Streptomycin	10 mg/kg 5 mg/kg 15 mg/kg	} 2–3 months	Rifampicin Isoniazid	} further 6–9 months
III. Rifampicin Isoniazid Streptomycin Pyrazinamide	10 mg/kg 5 mg/kg 15 mg/kg 30–35 mg/kg	} 2 months	Rifampicin Isoniazid	} further 4–7 months

The *consolidation phase of treatment* is generally given as an outpatient. The regular intake of drugs must be ensured and unreliable patients may need readmission. Close medical supervision including x-rays, blood count, ESR, and bacteriological sputum examinations are essential. Serum transaminases should be monitored in treatment with rifampicin, isoniazid, prothionamide and pyrazinamide. Regular tests of vision, visual fields, colour vision and fundoscopy must be carried out during treatment with ethambutol. Blood counts are important in treatment with isoniazid and rifampicin.

In *absorption atelectasis* secondary to bronchial obstruction by caseous material, a bronchoscopy may be necessary to drain bronchial secretions and avoid persistent pulmonary induration.

Segmental resection or lobectomy are nowadays rarely needed, if at all for a localised lesion, such as a unilateral cavity, which will not resolve with chemotherapy.

Exudative pleurisy: Treat for several months with isoniazid + ethambutol + rifampicin (or streptomycin) as for pulmonary tuberculosis. Give a steroid initially to accelerate absorption of the effusion and avoid extensive scarring.

Dosage: 30–50 mg of prednisone initially, reducing to 10–20 mg for about 4 weeks. Streptomycin, PAS or kanamycin were formerly instilled intrapleurally, though this is not usually necessary today.

Empyema: Systemic treatment is as for pulmonary tuberculosis, and instillation into the pleural cavity is advisable. Surgery may be necessary. Secondary staphylococcal infection frequently occurs and should be treated with flucloxacillin.

Tuberculosis of the cervical lymph nodes with human or bovine strains should be treated for several months with isoniazid, ethambutol and/or rifampicin, particularly when complete operative removal is not possible and there is a risk of recurrence. Surgical removal of the lymph nodes shortens the course of the disease and reduces the likelihood of complications.

The *treatment* of cervical lymphadenitis due to atypical myobacteria depends on the species and the outcome of sensitivity testing.

The following agents are recommended for

Mycobacterium scrofulaceum: cycloserine, ethambutol, prothionamide, ethionamide;

Mycobacterium kansasii: isoniazid in large doses, rifampicin, and possibly also cycloserine, prothionamide or ethionamide;

Mycobacterium avium-intracellulare: ethambutol, cycloserine, rifampicin, prothionamide, ethionamide.

When the primary focus is in the tonsils or adenoids, tonsillectomy or adenoidectomy may be useful.

Tuberculosis of the mesenteric lymph nodes is nowadays usually due to haematogenous spread in patients with open pulmonary tuberculosis. Combined chemotherapy should be given as for pulmonary tuberculosis, and isoniazid should never be given alone.

Miliary tuberculosis: Triple therapy with isoniazid, streptomycin and ethambutol or rifampicin. A corticosteroid may be given in addition for a short period in patients with severe dyspnoea or toxicity. A lumbar puncture should be performed to exclude meningitis. A long course of treatment is essential, even if there is rapid improvement.

Tuberculous meningitis: Treatment should begin immediately with four drugs *in maximum dosage,* once a specimen of CSF has been examined. These are:

Isoniazid, 10 mg/kg initially, then 5–7 mg/kg after 3–4 weeks in adults; 15–20 mg/kg initially, then 10 mg/kg after 3–4 weeks in children. The maximum daily dose for adults is 1 g and for children 500 mg.

Rifampicin, 10 mg/kg/day, up to a maximum adult daily dose of 750 mg.

Streptomycin, 30 mg/kg i. m., with a maximum daily dose of 1–1.5 g in adults, for 1 month, reducing to twice a week from the second month onwards.

Ethambutol, 25 mg/kg for the first 2 months, then 15 mg/kg.

If the infecting tubercle bacilli become resistant to one of these agents, treatment is continued with ethionamide, prothionamide or pyrazinamide (Table 52, p. 464), all of which pass into the CSF. Pyrazinamide may be used initially in place of ethambutol in a daily dose of 35 mg/kg (maximum 2 g). After 2–3 months, treatment may be changed to a combination of isoniazid and rifampicin for a further ten months, if the clinical condition permits.

Prednisone may be given in severe cases in a dose of 50–100 mg for adults and 1–2 mg/kg for children, reducing to a maintenance dose when improvement is established.

Isoniazid need not be given intrathecally because the drug passes into the CSF well. Intrathecal streptomycin sulphate is harmful and unnecessary.

Peritoneal tuberculosis: Treat as miliary tuberculosis.

Urogenital tuberculosis: Treat with a combination of agents, as other severe organ tuberculosis, preferably with isoniazid, ethambutol and rifampicin. Of these three agents, only the dose of ethambutol has to be reduced in impaired renal function. A long course of treatment is necessary to prevent relapse. Surgery is seldom necessary nowadays. The prognosis is worse if secondary infections develop, and procedures such as catheterisation and cystoscopy should be avoided unless absolutely necessary.

Tuberculosis of bones and joints: Long course of combined chemotherapy as for other forms of organ tuberculosis, with surgical removal of foci if necessary, and orthopaedic measures.

Skin tuberculosis: Isoniazid, streptomycin and other antituberculous measures, and surgical treatment if necessary.

References

COMSTOCK, G. W., C. BAUM, D. E. SNIDER: Isoniazid prophylaxis among Alaskan Eskimos. Amer. Rev. resp. Dis. *119:* 827 (1979).

DELAGE, G., M. DUSSEAULT: Tuberculous meningitis in children: A retrospective study of 79 patients with an analysis of prognostic factors. Canad. med. Assoc. J. *120:* 305 (1979).

Deutsches Zentralkomitee zur Bekämpfung der Tuberkulose: Expertisen – Die Chemotherapie der Tuberkulose. Hamburg 1980.

FOX, W., D. A. MITCHISON: Short-course chemotherapy for pulmonary tuberculosis. Amer. Rev. resp. Dis. *111:* 325, 845 (1975).

GLASSROTH, J., A. G. ROBINS, D. E. SNIDER: Tuberculosis in the 1980's. New Engl. J. Med. *302:* 1441 (1980).

Joint American Thoracic Society: Guidelines for short-course tuberculosis chemotherapy. Amer. Rev. resp. Dis. *121:* 611 (1980).

LOOS, U., E. MUSCH, K. G. MACKES: Intravenöse Rifampicin-Therapie offener Lungentuberkulosen. Med. Welt *34:* 701 (1983).

MARGILETH, A. M.: Tuberculosis. In: SHIRKEY, H. C. (ed.): Pediatric Therapy. p. 440, 6th Ed. Mosby Co., St. Louis 1980.

OVERRATH, H.: Chemotherapie der Lungentuberkulose bei Leberschäden. Prax. Pneumol. *27:* 182 (1973).

RAHAJOE, N. N., N. RAHAJOE, I. BOEDIMAN: The treatment of tuberculous meningitis in children with a combination of isoniazid, rifampin and streptomycin: Preliminary report. Tubercule *60:* 245 (1979).

SCHUITT, K.: Mycobacterial lymphadenitis in childhood. Amer. J. Dis. Child. *132:* 675 (1978).

SIFONTES, J. E.: Rifampin in tuberculous meningitis. J. Pediat. *87:* 1015 (1975).

STEINER, M., P. STEINER, M. RAO, R. PADRE, R. GOLDBERG: Primary drug-resistant tuberculosis in children, 1961 to 1971. Amer. Rev. resp. Dis. *108:* 321 (1973).

TAUCHNITZ, Ch., W. STORCH, M. ELLORHAOUI: Chronische Meningitis tuberculosa bei bekannter Infektion mit Mycobacterium kansasii. Z. inn. Med. *29:* 493 (1974).

WOLINSKY, E.: New anti-tuberculosis drugs and concepts of prophylaxis. Med. Clin. North Amer. *58:* 697 (1974).

WOLINSKY, E.: Non-tuberculous mycobacteria and associated diseases. Amer. Rev. resp. Dis. *119:* 107 (1979).

YOUMANS, E. P.: Tuberculosis. Saunders, Philadelphia 1979.

32. Fungal Infections

Diagnosis: The fungi pathogenic to man make up a large group of very different organisms. For practical purposes, they may be grouped as follows:

1. *Dermatophytes* (Trichophyton, Microsporum, Epidermophyton etc.).
2. *Facultative pathogenic yeasts* (Candida, Torulopsis etc.).
3. *Facultative pathogenic moulds* (Aspergillus, Mucor etc.).
4. *Dimorphous fungi* (causes of systemic mycoses such as Histoplasma, coccidioides etc.).

Filamentous bacteria such as actinomycetes and nocardia were at one time classified with the fungi; their similarities are morphological only, however, since they are, like bacteria, inhibited by antibacterial agents.

Fungi are easily identified microscopically and in culture. Since they can be part of the normal body flora or present in the environment, however, the interpretation of the significance of positive isolates can be difficult. The presence of fungi on the skin can be shown by a squash preparation on a microscope slide in 10% potassium hydroxide. The best material is scraped from the edge of the lesion or, with vesicles, from the vesicle wall (not the base or the fluid). Hair should be removed intact with forceps. Nail clippings should be full thickness and taken as near to the base of the nail as possible. Identification is important with yeasts and moulds since certain species, such as Candida albicans and Aspergillus fumigatus are more important clinically than other species. Correlation with the clinical picture is also important, and an isolate in the absence of supportive clinical features does not normally justify antifungal therapy.

The diagnostic procedures in fungal septicaemia and organ mycoses are described elsewhere. The failure of "blind" antibiotic therapy is often attributed to systemic fungal infection, although this only occurs in practice in patients with bone marrow suppression. There are usually other reasons in patients with normal immunity.

Dermatophyte infections: Various species of Trichophyton and Epidermophyton may be pathogenic and are usually transmitted by direct contact (e.g. from animals). Their culture and identification requires special mycological techniques, though these are not essential when the clinical picture is unequivocal. The distinction between a candida and a dermatophyte infection by culture is, however, important in inflammatory intertrigo, since griseofulvin and tolnaftate are not effective against Candida. Many sites may be affected (tinea) but invasion of deep tissues or mucous membranes is unknown. Occasionally an allergy to the infection can arise, with blisters on non-infected areas of skin as well.

Treatment of severe infections: The systemic treatment of choice is griseofulvin, in a single daily dose of 500 (−750) mg or 10 mg/kg with a fatty meal, and taken for 3–6 weeks or longer if necessary. Contraindications are pregnancy and liver damage. Infections of the scalp and hair should always be treated systemically. An alternative to griseofulvin is ketoconazole (200 mg a day). Acute inflammatory features should be treated symptomatically at the same time.

Mild infections respond well to local preparations. Apart from a number of old benzoic acid derivatives, tolnaftate is the drug of choice for local therapy. Newer preparations such as the imidazoles (clotrimazole, miconazole, tinidazole, econazole) or ciclopiroxolamine have the additional advantage of activity against Candida albicans. A longer course of local therapy is recommended.

Fungal infections of the nails: The most frequent causes are dermatophytes, although Candida species and moulds (Scopulariopsis, Hendersonula, Aspergillus etc.) can give rise to clinically similar infections of the nails. Mixed infections, e. g. with candida and a dermatophyte, are not uncommon, and more commonly affect toe nails, either alone or in the presence of tinea pedis or tinea at other sites. Oral griseofulvin has proved effective and should be continued for long enough for the inhibited, but not dead, fungi to grow out of the nail. Dermatophyte infections of the finger nails normally require 4–8 months of treatment. A new alternative is oral ketoconazole. Systemic treatment should be supplemented by local antifungal agents (clotrimazole, miconazole, ciclopiroxolamine, tolnaftate) and mechanical measures (nail filing). Infections of the toe-nails are more difficult to treat and the nails may have to be removed operatively.

Microsporum infections affect the scalp, involve anthropophilic strains (Microsporum audouinii) and are very contagious, particularly among school children. The scalp hair is fluorescent under Wood's light. The differential diagnosis in tinea capitis is trichophytosis.

The *treatment of choice* is griseofulvin by mouth.

Pityriasis versicolor: Is caused by Pityrosporum (Malassezia) furfur. Its occurrence is very dependent on host and environmental factors, such as heat, sweating or corticosteroids. Many local agents are effective. The *drug of choice* is selenium sulphide, 2.5%. The skin foci should be thoroughly painted overnight on two occasions 8 days apart. Clotrimazole and miconazole are also effective locally.

Candida infections: The commonest pathogen is Candida albicans. Other species of Candida are less common (C. tropicalis, C. pseudotropicalis etc.), as well as Torulopsis species. C. albicans is a common component of the normal body flora (mouth, gut) and can be selected by antibiotics, oral contraceptives, pregnancy, diabetes, iron deficiency and impaired host defences. In many patients, the reason for the candida infection is unknown.

Genital thrush occurs in women as vulvitis and vaginitis with redness, itching, whitish patches and a creamy discharge. Men have balanitis and both sexual partners may be infected. *Local treatment:* Imidazoles such as clotrimazole, miconazole, econazole, but also ciclopiroxolamine and nystatin. Povidone iodine or amphotericin B may also be applied locally. Length of treatment: (3–)6–14 days. The partner should also be treated if possible. There is a high tendency to relapse but resistance almost never develops.

Oral thrush is common in the newborn and in infants with impaired resistance, in patients with lowered resistance receiving antibiotic therapy and in the elderly with severe illnesses. The *treatment of choice* is oral nystatin given as a suspension (1 ml containing 100,000 units/ml) instilled around the mouth every 3–6 hours. The suspension should then be swallowed since the oesophagus is also often affected. Lozenges containing pimaricin and amphotericin B are also available.

Candida oesophagitis is a relatively common and serious complication in patients with bone marrow suppression, in whom it is associated with oral thrush. It is rare in other patients. The diagnosis is difficult, requiring a barium swallow or oesophagoscopy. Since candida oesophagitis can be the focus for a fungaemia, treatment is justified on suspicion. The *treatment of choice* is an oral suspension of nystatin or amphotericin B. Severe cases or where there is marked impairment of resistance should receive systemic amphotericin B, flucytosine, miconazole or ketoconazole.

Candida enteritis is rare. Yeasts found in faeces are normally of no clinical importance. Candida albicans only causes inflammatory changes in the gut in oncological patients with severely impaired resistance. The intestinal tract can, however, serve as a reservoir for further infection in recurrent genital candidiasis; in such cases, nystatin should be given orally.

Candida pneumonia is rare and only affects patients with markedly lowered resistance. It usually results from haematogeneous spread from candida septicaemia but sometimes arises through aspiration. Yeasts found in expectorated sputum are usually oral contaminants and do not support the diagnosis of candida pneumonia, for which Candida should also be found in large amounts in a transtracheal aspirate. Yeasts are commonly found in tracheal secretions in patients who have been intubated or ventilated for long periods, even in the absence of pneumonia.

Established cases of candida pneumonia should be *treated systemically* with amphotericin B + flucytosine; milder infections may be treated with i.v. miconazole or oral ketoconazole. Nystatin inhalations are not useful on account of the large particle size.

Candida infections of the urine: The presence of yeasts in normal urine is rare and very small numbers are then found. Torulopsis glabrata and Candida tropicalis may be isolated but they are usually of little clinical importance. Yeasts often do not originate in the bladder but are vaginal contaminants. A suprapubic aspirate is therefore always advisable before starting antifungal chemotherapy, which always carries some risk. A symptomless funguria with high fungal counts can disappear spontaneously in a very short time. Diabetes mellitus, indwelling catheters and renal transplantation are all predisposing factors for urinary infections with yeasts. Candida albicans is often isolated in small amounts in the urine in patients with candida septicaemia with multiple foci in the kidneys and sometimes mucous membranes of the bladder. Flucytosine is the best agent where the organism is sensitive, since high urinary concentrations are attainable.

The *treatment* should be monitored by fungal culture because resistance to flucytosine can develop. Intravenous amphotericin B is only justifiable in cases of proven candida septicaemia, and renal function must be closely monitored when it is used. Imidazole derivatives such as miconazole or ketoconazole give only low urinary concentrations and are not therefore useful in this situation.

Candida septicaemia: The most common portals of entry are long intravenous lines. A rare but very dangerous condition is postoperative endocarditis after the implantation of an artificial heart valve. Candida albicans sometimes enters the blood-stream in immunosuppressed patients, but candida septicaemia is otherwise very rare. The most important symptom is fever; metastatic colonies are fairly commonly found in the retina, brain and kidney.

The *treatment of choice* is a combination of amphotericin B + flucytosine. An infected foreign body should be removed wherever possible. The symptoms usually regress after the removal of an infected venous catheter. Patients with candida endocarditis usually require replacement of the infected valve. For less severe cases with a transient fungaemia, i. v. miconazole or oral ketoconazole may be adequate.

Candida infections of the skin are a fairly common inconvenience though they are not dangerous. Intertrigo, perianal eczema, napkin dermatitis, balanitis, chronic paronychia, perlèche and otitis externa are all caused predominantly by Candida albicans. Local maceration of the skin with bacterial superinfection can play a part in the pathogenesis. Congenital cutaneous candidiasis is described on p. 500. Redness, considerable itching and peeling (hyperkeratosis) are all suggestive of cutaneous candidiasis. Small children can also develop Candida granulomas, particularly on the face and scalp. The demonstration of the fungus is very straightforward.

Treatment consists of local antifungal agents. Polyenes (nystatin, amphotericin B) or imidazole derivatives (clotrimazole, miconazole) are generally used as ointments, creams or solutions. Alternatives are ciclopiroxolamine, haloprongin, pimaricin, and povidone iodine.

Griseofulvin and tolnaftate have no effect on yeast infections. Flucytosine should be avoided because of the danger of resistance. Ketoconazole is indicated in severe infections. Severe itching may be a sign of an allergy associated with the infection. If such is the case, a short course of a topical corticosteroid is sometimes effective. Predisposing factors such as macerated skin should be removed where possible.

Chronic mucocutaneous candidiasis (candidiasis granulomatosa) is mainly found in children. The cause is always a primary or an acquired immune defect, either an isolated or a combined immune deficiency (with T-cell deficiency) which can often only be characterised by complex immunological techniques.

The *treatment* of chronic mucocutaneous candidiasis is difficult. Improvement or cure in primary immune defects is usually not possible. Long-term topical therapy is often ineffective. Oral ketoconazole over a long period seems at present to be the best alternative. Relapses are to be expected. The combination of amphotericin B + flucytosine should be considered when the infecting organisms are resistant to other forms of treatment.

Aspergillus infections: Aspergillus fumigatus is the commonest cause. Other species of aspergillus are only occasionally involved (A. nidulans, A. glaucus). A flavus is medically important through the production of aflatoxins in food, but does not cause infection. A. fumigatus is widespread in the inanimate environment (earth, damp areas, flower pots, dust) and the spores are generally inhaled and expectorated with no ill effect. An isolated finding of A. fumigatus in sputum is not indicative of disease; the organisms must be present repeatedly or in large amounts and with associated clinical evidence since A. fumigatus is not part of the normal body flora. Aspergilli are best cultured on a fungal medium incubated at 40–45° C. The antigen of Aspergillus fumigatus can be detected in serum, e. g. by ELISA. A. fumigatus can cause several types of disease, namely:

1. **Bronchopulmonary aspergillosis:** In addition to the purely allergic form which arises through the inhalation of spores, there is an invasive disease in which the bronchi are attacked and the bronchial wall destroyed. Chemotherapy is only justifiable when the pathogen has been cultured and identified. Purely allergic forms should be treated with corticosteroids.

2. **Aspergilloma** is a non-invasive infection of pre-formed cavities (pulmonary cysts or bullae, old tuberculous cavities). The chest x-ray is typical and shows a fungal mass containing crescents of air. Haemoptysis often occurs. Aspergilloma does not respond to systemic or local chemotherapy and must be removed surgically.

3. **Invasive pulmonary aspergillosis** presents as a pneumonia which is resistant to other forms of therapy in patients with severe immunosuppression (e. g. leukaemia); cavitation and haemoptysis sometimes occur.

4. **Aspergillus septicaemia:** Occurs in immunocompromised patients. The portal of entry is sometimes an infected venous catheter, but is often unknown.

Haematogenous spread leads to infected infarcts and metastatic abscesses, usually in the brain, kidneys or myocardium. Blood culture is usually negative.

5. **Eye infections, otitis externa, sinusitis** and colonisation of chronic **skin ulcers** or burns are rare.

The *treatment* of aspergillus infections is difficult and the relatively toxic combination of amphotericin B and flucytosine at full dosage as a long course (p. 175, 182) is still recommended. Imidazole derivatives (miconazole i. v., ketoconazole orally) are less promising. Local treatment such as inhalations of amphotericin B in bronchopulmonary aspergillosis is seldom effective. The *prognosis* of invasive aspergillus infections in leukaemia is bad, even with the best treatment available.

Phycomycoses are caused by various phycomycetes such as Rhizopus and Mucor. The portals of entry are the skin, mucous membranes, and infected venous catheters. In immunosuppressed patients, but also in ketoacidotic diabetics the fungi can penetrate arterial walls and cause thrombosis and infarcts in the brain and other organs. Superficial infections of the skin, external ear and oesophageal and gastric mucosa can give rise to purulent necrosis which is more readily diagnosed than pulmonary infection (infarcts), infections which spread to the brain (e. g. from the orbits) and disseminated disease. Amphotericin B is sometimes effective.

Histoplasmosis: See p. 350.

Cryptococcosis: See p. 331.

The **coccidioidomycoses** are caused by Coccidioides immitis and occur in North, Central and South America. They occur in 3 forms, namely a primary pulmonary form, a primary extrapulmonary form and a disseminated form. The diagnosis is made microscopically, culturally, serologically and sometimes through a skin test. Amphotericin B and miconazole are effective though not very reliable.

References

LEVINE, H. (ed.): Ketoconazole in the Management of Fungal Diseases. Adis, Balgowlah 1982.
SPELLER, D. C. E.: Antifungal Chemotherapy. Wiley, Chichester 1980.
UTZ, J. P.: Antifungal agents. In: B. KAGAN: Antimicrobial Therapy. Saunders, Philadelphia 1980.

33. Toxoplasmosis

The **diagnosis** of toxoplasmosis should be adequately confirmed if a combination of pyrimethamine and a sulphonamide is to be used, since this regime carries the risk of damage to the bone marrow.

Low antibody titres are not in themselves evidence of toxoplasmosis since 20–80% of the population have latent infection and positive serological reactions are therefore quite common.

The *following criteria* are regarded as diagnostic of toxoplasmosis:

1. In congenital toxoplasmosis and during the first few months of life, toxoplasma can be demonstrated microscopically in a stained CSF deposit. The CSF has a high protein content and low cell count with erythrocytes and occasional eosinophils. A marked eosinophilia is sometimes found in the peripheral blood.

2. A significant (four-fold) rise in serum antibody titre in the Sabin-Feldman dye test, complement fixation test, indirect toxoplasma immunofluorescence, or ELISA, in the presence of clinical symptoms. A single high titre is suspicious but not diagnostic. On the other hand, the presence of toxoplasma-specific IgM in a child and its subsequent disappearance is sufficient proof. To exclude experimental error, the patient's pair of sera should whenever possible be examined in parallel on the same occasion. Any serological results should be interpreted critically in view of the relative rareness of florid infection. Toxoplasma antibodies (other than complement-fixing ones) persist for life in silent infections as well.

   The newborn can have maternal IgG antibodies which have crossed the placenta and fall gradually during the first few months of life. An increased total IgM content in the presence of a positive Sabin-Feldman dye test is suggestive of active infection in the child. The demonstration of toxoplasma IgM antibodies by immunofluorescence in the newborn is proof of infection. Toxoplasma-specific IgM during pregnancy indicates that the mother has recently contracted the infection since these antibodies disappear after a few weeks, while IgG antibodies persist for a long time. In fact, quite a high percentage of neonates with congenital toxoplasmosis have still not formed toxoplasma-specific IgM in the first weeks of life. Specific IgM can still sometimes be detected in the mother, however.

   In immunosuppressed patients with active toxoplasmosis, serological tests are often unreliable and titres may be strikingly low in isolated toxoplasma chorioretinitis or brain abscess.

3. Histological demonstration of toxoplasma or a typical histological picture in lymph nodes in the lymphoglandular form of the disease or in the septicaemic form with lymphadenitis confirm the diagnosis.

4. Demonstration of the organisms in CSF, blood, freshly removed organs or placenta, by inoculation into mice, guinea pigs or hamsters, are confirmatory. Naturally acquired infection in the test animals must be excluded beforehand.

Clinical symptoms are very varied and none are specific for toxoplasmosis. The organ changes in the congenital disease, such as encephalitis, intracerebral calcifications, chorioretinitis, hydrocephalus, microcephaly, hepatosplenomegaly and jaundice are also found in congenital cytomegalovirus infection. Acquired toxoplasmosis is equally difficult to recognise clinically, since other infective agents can cause similar symptoms (septicaemia, encephalitis and lymphadenopathy). Patients with lymphoma or AIDS and those receiving immunosuppressive therapy occasionally develop a disseminated toxoplasmosis with encephalitis, pneumonia, myocarditis etc., which can be fatal. This is probably reactivation of an infection acquired earlier.

Treatment: Both pyrimethamine and sulphonamides inhibit folic acid synthesis in the parasites, but have different, sequential points of attack in the pathway. They act synergistically on extracellular, actively multiplying but not on intracellular parasites or pseudocysts. This treatment can only succeed in the active phase of the infection. At best, active infection is converted into an inactive form in which spontaneous healing is encouraged. Antibody titres remain high despite effective treatment.

There are a number of therapeutic regimen and dosage recommendations. If the dosage is too low, the treatment may be ineffective; if too high, the risk of blood dyscrasias is increased. A suitable regimen is as follows:

In the first three days, adults receive 50 mg of pyrimethamine a day and children 1 mg/kg up to a maximum of 25 mg/day, then half this dose for up to 4 weeks. A sulphonamide such as sulphadiazine in a daily dose of 2–4 g in adults or 100 mg/kg in children should be given at the same time. 2–3 single doses of pyrimethamine a week may be sufficient, e. g. 12.5 mg twice a week for infants, 12.5 mg three times a week for small children or 12.5 mg on alternate days for older children. Sulphadiazine is given in standard dosage (see above). Prednisone is recommended in a dose of 1–2 mg/kg/day up for to a maximum of 75 mg until improvement is established, when it should be tailed off. Folinic acid 1–10 mg orally or i. v. should be given 2–3 times a week during this therapy to reduce the risk of bone marrow suppression (see below). If necessary, a further course may be given after an interval of several weeks. The addition of steroids is always recommended for chorioretinitis.

If this treatment cannot be tolerated, a long-acting sulphonamide can be used. An alternative to pyrimethamine is clindamycin orally or i. v. (300 mg 4 times a day) in combination with sulphadiazine, although this regime has only so far been shown to be effective in animals. Co-trimoxazole is less effective in animals than pyrimethamine plus sulphadiazine. The activity of spiramycin on toxoplasma is unreliable.

The common **side effects** of pyrimethamine are leucopenia, thrombocytopenia and anaemia. Central nervous effects such as convulsions may occur in patients with underlying CNS disease, and a slow increase in dose is advisable in such patients. The side effects of sulphonamides include leucopenia, haematuria, fever and transient rashes. A white cell and platelet count should be done every 2–3 days and the dose reduced at the first signs of bone marrow toxicity; folinic acid 6 mg a day i. m. for 3 days in adults is given as an antidote. The blood count usually returns to normal and treatment with pyrimethamine and sulphonamide can be resumed at lower dosage. Otherwise, the treatment must be discontinued and resumed later with clindamycin in combination with a sulphonamide.

Because of the risks of teratogenesis, pyrimethamine should be avoided during the first four months of pregnancy. If treatment is necessary during this period, sulphonamides, possibly in combination with clindamycin, can be given in normal dosage. Treatment with pyrimethamine and sulphadiazine during the second half of pregnancy is only indicated if there are good reasons for suspecting a fresh infection. A previous child with congenital toxoplasmosis is not an indication for treatment during subsequent pregnancies because congenital toxoplasmosis does not generally affect later siblings.

References

DESMONS, G., J. COUVREUR: Congenital toxoplasmosis. A prospective study of 378 pregnancies. New Engl. J. Med. *290:* 1110 (1974).

KOCHER, R., G. HAENSCH: Neuere Gesichtspunkte zur Behandlung der Toxoplasmose. Dtsch. med. Wschr. *98:* 1920 (1973).

NICHOLSON, D. H., E. B. WOLCHOK: Ocular toxoplasmosis in an adult receiving long-term corticosteroid therapy. Arch. Ophthalmol. *94:* 248 (1976).

RUSKIN, J., J. S. REMINGTON: Toxoplasmosis in the compromised host. Amer. intern. Med. *84:* 193 (1976).

SCHLAEGEL, T. F., Jr.: Ocular Toxoplasmosis and Pars Planitus. Grune and Stratton, New York 1978.

WEITBERG, A. L., J. C. ALPER, I. DIAMOND, A. FLIGIEL: Acute granulomatous hepatitis in the course of acquired toxoplasmosis. New Engl. J. Med. *300:* 1093 (1979).

34. Malaria

Many cases of malaria are imported every year into Europe in travellers returning from the tropics, usually in persons who took insufficient antimalarial prophylaxis. As in the endemic regions themselves, several species of the malaria parasite and forms of malaria are seen, namely:

1. *Tertian malaria* (Plasmodium vivax or rarely P. ovale) with attacks of fever every 48 hours.
2. *Quartan malaria* (P. malariae) with bouts of fever every 72 hours.
3. *Falciparum malaria* (P. falciparum) with irregular attacks. This is the most severe form and has the greatest variability of symptoms.
4. *Double infections.*

Malaria can develop in the patient at a variable time after the patient has left the malarious area and can in the case of falciparum malaria be severe and often fatal. The diagnosis must be made rapidly and treatment started as soon as possible. The laboratory diagnosis is best made from a thick and thin blood film, stained by the Giemsa method, which can also be taken between attacks of fever. Specific serum antibodies can be demonstrated by indirect immunofluorescence, which is useful when the blood film is temporarily negative, as sometimes occurs in falciparum malaria. Daily blood films are advisable to monitor treatment.

Choice of drugs: *Chloroquine,* a 4-aminoquinoline, acts on the schizonts and trophozoites (ring forms) which are found in the erythrocytes, and can achieve a clinical cure of falciparum malaria, in which exoerythrocytic tissue forms are not found. The gametes and exoerythrocytic forms, but not the schizonts, of tertian and quartan malaria are only eliminated by *primaquine,* an 8-aminoquinoline, which should be given for two weeks in conjunction with chloroquine if these forms are to be eradicated. In falciparum malaria too, only primaquine eliminates the gametes to give a radical cure, so that these patients are also first treated with chloroquine and then with primaquine. *Pyrimethamine,* a diaminopyrimidine, acts primarily on exoerythrocytic forms. It is used in combination with a sulphonamide (sulfadoxine) as Fansidar to treat chloroquine-resistant falciparum malaria. *True prophylaxis* of malaria, that is, the prevention of infection, is not yet possible because no drug has so far been developed which kills the sporozoites at the time of transmission by the mosquito. The regular intake of chloroquine and other drugs as prophylaxis (Table 54) is therefore more correctly a means of suppression which inhibits the development of blood schizonts and thus prevents the clinical disease.

Treatment of the malarial attack: Non-immune persons (Europeans) receive 600 mg of chloroquine base, which corresponds to 1 g of chloroquine diphosphate, initially, followed by 300 mg of chloroquine base after 6 h, 24 h, and 48 h. Infants, pre-school children and school children are given 100, 200 or 300 mg respectively at first, followed by 50, 100 or 150 mg respectively after 6 h, 24 h, and 48 h. Adults then receive 15 mg a day of primaquine base corresponding to 26 mg of diphosphate for 2 weeks to eliminate the gametes and tissue forms. The daily dose in children is 0.25 mg/kg, and never more than 15 mg. Patients with glucose-6-phosphate dehydrogenase deficiency may undergo haemolysis if they receive primaquine, and patients at risk should be screened beforehand for this defect; if present, regular erythrocyte counts should be performed during treatment. Chloroquine and primaquine should always be taken after meals to avoid gastric irritation. Every patient with suspected falciparum malaria in Europe should be managed in a hospital with suitable intensive care facilities, because of the serious,

Table 54. Chemoprophylaxis of malaria (treatment until 6 weeks after leaving the endemic area).

Name	Proprietary names	Dosage	
		Adults	Children
Chloroquine	Aralen, Avloclor, Malarivon, Resochin, Nivaquine	300 mg of base a week or 75 mg a day	<1 y. 50 mg of base 1–3 y. 75 mg of base 4–6 y. 100 mg of base 7–10 y. 150 mg of base 11–16 y. 200–300 mg of base (all once a week)
Pyrimethamine	Daraprim	25 mg a week	1–2 y. 6.25 mg a week 3–10 y. 12.5 mg a week >10 y. 25 mg a week
Proguanil	Paludrin	100(–200) mg a day	2 y. 25–50 mg a day 3–6 y. 50–75 mg a day 7–10 y. 100 mg a day
Pyrimethamine-sulphadoxine:	Fansidar	25 mg of pyrimethamine + 500 mg of sulfadoxine a week (= 1 tab.)	Pyrimethamine: see above Sulfadoxine: ½–1 y. 125 mg 1–3 y. 250 mg 4–8 y. 500 mg 9–14 y. 750 mg
Pyrimethamine-dapsone	Maloprim	12.5 mg of pyrimethamine + 100 mg of dapsone (= 1 tab.) once a week	For children aged less than 4 years only: 0.2 mg/kg of pyrimethamine + 1.6 mg/kg of dapsone (once a week)

and sometimes fatal nature of the disease. Severe falciparum malaria with hyperpyrexia, vomiting, circulatory collapse, pulmonary oedema, coma or cerebral malaria should be treated with intramuscular chloroquine, 200–400 mg initially, followed by 200 mg after 4 h, 24 h and 48 h, changing to the oral route as soon as possible. Because of the risk of circulatory collapse, chloroquine should not be given parenterally to infants and young children.

The first signs of renal failure or blackwater fever, which results from massive intravascular haemolysis, should be carefully watched for. Smaller doses of chloroquine may be sufficient to treat malaria in patients with partial immunity such as adult inhabitants of endemic regions who do not take regular drug prophylaxis.

Chloroquine-resistance: Chloroquine-resistant falciparum malaria is found in South America, Kenya and Tanzania, and Southeast Asia. It is recognised by the persistence of trophozoites (ring forms) in the blood and the absence of defervescence after 2 days of treatment with chloroquine, in mild forms only during relapses. Since the sensitivity of causative strains varies considerably, there are several recommendations for treatment. A combination of the following drugs is generally used in the U.S.A.: quinine, 650 mg every 8 h for 10 days plus pyrimethamine, 25 mg every 12 h for 3 days, plus sulphadiazine, 25 mg/kg 4 times a day for 10 days or sulphisoxazole, 500 mg every 8 h for 10 days. If one of these drugs is ineffective, dapsone can be substituted in a dose of 25 mg a day for 4 weeks. Mefloquine is a promising new agent for chloroquine-resistent malaria.

Malaria prophylaxis (suppression): Chloroquine base, 300 mg corresponding to 500 mg of diphosphate, or 2 tablets, once a week; 50 mg for children in their first year, 50–100 mg for children aged 1–4 years, 100–150 mg for children aged 5–8 years and 150–300 mg for children aged 9–15 years, starting one week before entering the endemic region until 6 weeks after leaving. When the risk is increased or the disease is suspected, a course of primaquine, 15 mg a day for 2 weeks, should be added in order to avoid later disease with exoerythrocytic forms of Plasmodium vivax or ovale. Larger doses of chloroquine are recommended in hyperendemic regions, e.g. 300 mg of base twice a week. If chloroquine phosphate is not tolerated, chloroquine sulphate may be used. Alternatives to chloroquine (see Table 55) are pyrimethamine, 25 mg once a week and proguanil, 100 mg a day. Another alternative is to take 300 mg of chloroquine base and 45 mg of primaquine base simultaneously once a week as a combined tablet until 8 weeks after leaving the endemic region. The combination of pyrimethamine and sulfadoxine (Fansidar) has been successful for prophylaxis in regions with chloroquine-resistant falciparum malaria. This combination is not reliable in Africa on account of the frequent resistance there to pyrimethamine.

References

BENSON, L. E., A. J. SIEGEL, R. E. LYMCH, E. J. COLWELL, J. P. CANBY: Drug resistance in malaria. Lancet *1:* 743 (1972).
Center for Disease Control: Chemoprophylaxis of malaria. Morbidity and Mortality Weekly Report *27:* 81 (1978).
HALL, A. P.: The treatment of malaria. Brit. med. J. *1:* 323 (1976).
HALL, A. P.: The treatment of severe falciparum malaria. Trans. roy. Soc. trop. Med. Hyg. *71:* 367 (1977).
WERNSDORFER, G., W. WERNSDORFER: Maßnahmen zur Malariaprophylaxe. Dtsch. Ärztebl. *76:* 557 (1979).
WHO: Informations on malaria risk for international travellers. WHO Wkly. Epidem. Rec. *25:* 181 (1978).
World Health Organization: Chemotherapy of Malaria and Resistance to Antimalarials. WHO Tech. Rep. Series No 529 (1973).

35. Antiparasitic Chemotherapy

The main helminthic infestations in Europe are with *roundworms* (nematodes) such as ascariasis, oxyuriasis, trichuriasis and trichinosis, and *tapeworms* (cestodes) such as taeniasis, cysticercosis, fish tapeworm infestation and echinococcosis. Travellers outside Europe may encounter other species such as trematodes (schistosomiasis and distosomiasis).

Table 55. Spectra of activity of antihelminthic agents.

Parasites	Thiaben-dazole	Pyran-tel	Mebenda-zole	Pipera-zine	Pyrvi-nium	Bephe-nium
Ascaris	+++	+++	+++	+++	++	+++
Enterobius	+++	+++	+++	++	+++	++
Trichuris	+++	++	++	0	0	0
Hookworm	+++	+++	+++	0	0	+++
Strongy-loides	+++	+++	+++	0	0	+
Trichinella	+++	++(?)	++(?)	0	0	0
Cutaneous larva migrans	+++	?	++(?)	0	0	0

Effect: +++ = good, ++ = moderate, + = slight, 0 = nil.

Table 56. Treatment of worm infestations.

Disease	Drug of choice and dosage	Remarks	Other treatment
Ascariasis	Pyrantel, 11 mg/kg in a single dose (maximum of 1 g of base)	Side effects: diarrhoea, nausea, vomiting. Do not give in pregnancy	Thiabendazole, piperazine, mebendazole
Enterobiasis (Oxyuriasis)	Pyrantel in a single dose of 11 mg/kg up to a maximum of 1 g of base. Repeat after 1 week	Treat the whole family (reinfection frequent)	Mebendazole, pyrvinium, piperazine
Trichuriasis (Whip worm)	Mebendazole, 100 mg twice a day for 3 days for adults and children	Side effects: diarrhoea, abdominal pain. Do not give during pregnancy	Thiabendazole
Trichinosis	Thiabendazole, 25 mg/kg twice a day for 3 days (only effective in the intestine). Maximum daily dose for adults: 3 g	Central nervous disorders, so give only on rest days. Avoid in patients with liver disease	
Strongyloidiasis	Thiabendazole, 25 mg/kg twice a day for 3 days. Repeated after 1 week. Maximum daily dose: 3 g (for adults)	Treat asymptomatic cases as well because of the risk of generalisation	Mebendazole
Filariasis	Diethylcarbamazine, 2 mg/kg 3 times a day for 2–3 weeks	Allergy due to lysis of parasites (fever, urticaria), possibly needing steroids	Mebendazole?
Dracunculosis	Niridazole, 25 mg/kg in 3 single doses for 10 days. Maximum daily dose: 1.5 g	Remove worms where possible	Diethylcarbamazine to prevent reinfection
Hookworm infection (Ancylostoma duodenale)	Pyrantel, 11 mg/kg/ day for 3 days. Maximum dose: 1 g of base	Side effects: gastrointestinal upset, fever, rashes. Do not use with impaired liver function	Mebendazole

Table 56. (Continued)

Disease	Drug of choice and dosage	Remarks	Other drugs
Cutaneous larva migrans	Thiabendazole, 25 mg/kg twice a day for 3 days. Repeated after 1 week. Maximum daily dose: 3 g (for adults)	Failure in forms not caused by hookworm larvae (e. g. sparganosis, myiasis)	Freezing with chlorethyl spray
Schistosomiasis (Bilharziasis)	Praziquantel, 40 mg/kg (single dose)	Side effects (of short duration): abdominal pain, headache, urticaria	Niridazole, oxamniquine, albendazole
Paragonimiasis (Lung fluke)	Praziquantel, 3 doses of 25 mg/kg in one day	Experience with praziquantel is still small	Bithionol
Clonorchiasis (Chinese liver fluke)	Praziquantel, 3 doses of 25 mg/kg in one day	Experience with praziquantel is still small	Chloroquine
Fasciola hepatica infection (Liver fluke)	Praziquantel	Experience with praziquantel is still small	Bithionol, emetine
Taeniasis (Taenia saginata, Taenia solium)	Niclosamide, a single dose of 2 g in adults, 1 g in children aged 2–8 and 500 mg in children under 2 years	Well tolerated, no laxative effect, elimination of scolex is necessary	Praziquantel (against cysticercosis
Fish tapeworm infestation (Diphyllobothrium latum)	Niclosamide as above, plus Vit. B_{12}	See taeniasis	See taeniasis
Echinococcosis (Dog tapeworm)	Initial treatment with mebendazole in large doses, possibly long-term	Parasitolysis may occur with rupture of cysts. Cysts may not be completely eliminated	Surgery, praziquantel
Infestation with Hymenolepis nana	Niclosamide as above, repeated after 10 and 20 days	See taeniasis	See taeniasis

Diagnosis is based on the clinical picture and the demonstration of the worm at some stage of its life cycle. Worm eggs may be found in a single faecal suspension, or after enrichment with common salt or some other concentration procedure. The salt method is unsuitable for trematodes and fish tapeworms. A loopful of faeces (avoiding large particles) is mixed with 1 drop of water on a slide and covered with a cover-slip. The eggs are concentrated by mixing 1 part of faeces with 20 parts of saturated NaCl solution. After standing for 20 min, a loop of ½ cm diameter and bent at a right angle is applied horizontally to the surface of the liquid, and three drops so obtained put on to a slide which is examined microscopically without a cover-slip by focusing on to the surface of the suspension. Eggs of Enterobius and Taenia saginata are best obtained either with a sellotape slide, in which the sticky side is applied to the anal skin, or from a moist cotton-wool swab applied to the anal margin; they are then examined unstained on a microscope slide.

Treatment: The main antihelminthic agents are summarised in Tables 55 and 56.

The treatment of choice of *tapeworm infections* is niclosamide, as a single dose of 2 g (4 tablets) in adults.

Constipated patients should empty their bowels before treatment. The cure-rate is greater than 95%. The course can be repeated if further proglottides are passed. Hymenolepis nana is more resistant and requires an initial dose of 2 g, then 1 g a day for 6 days.

The treatment of *roundworm infections* is more difficult, but the results have improved with the new drugs pyrantel, mebendazole and thiabendazole, whose particular advantage is their broad range of activity, since patients from developing countries are often multiply infested, e. g. with ascaris, hookworm and trichuris. A single dose is sufficient for pyrantel and pyrvinium.

Pyrantel, mebendazole and thiabendazole are also well tolerated.

Praziquantel is almost always effective in *schistosomiasis* and infections with *flukes* and *cestodes* and is effective as a single-dose treatment in Schistosoma mansoni infections.

References

ADAMS, E. B., I. N. MACLEOD: Invasive amebiasis: II. Amebic liver abscess and its complications. Medicine *56:* 325 (1977).

BEARD, T. C., M. D. RICKARD, H. T. GOODMAN: Medical treatment for hydatids. Med. J. Aust. *1:* 633 (1978).

BEKHTI, A., J. P. SCHAAPS, M. CAPRON, J. P. DESSAINT, F. SANTORO, A. CAPRON: Treatment of hepatic hydatid disease with mebendazole: Preliminary results in four cases. Brit. med. J. *2:* 1047 (1977).

BURKE, J. A.: Strongyloidiasis in childhood. Amer. J. Dis. Child. *132:* 1130 (1978).
HARDMAN, E. W., R. L. H. JONES, A. H. DAVIES: Fascioliasis: A large outbreak. Brit. med. J. *3:* 502 (1970).
JONES, W. E., P. M. SCHANTZ, K. FOREMAN, W. K. SMITH, E. J. WITTE, D. E. SCHOOLEY, D. D. JURANEK: Human toxocariasis in a rural community. Amer. J. Dis. Child. *134:* 967 (1980).
MAHMOUD, A. F.: Schistosomiasis. New Engl. J. Med. *297:* 1329 (1977).
MERRILL, J. R., J. OTIS, W. D. LOGAN, M. B. DAVIS: The dog heartworm (Dirofilaria immitis) in man. JAMA *243:* 1066 (1980).
RODE, H., M. R. Q. DAVIES, S. CYWES: Amoebic liver abscesses in infancy and childhood. S. Afr. J. Surg. *16:* 131 (1978).
SCHANTZ, P. M., L. T. GLICKMAN: Toxocaral visceral larva migrans. New Engl. J. Med. *298:* 436 (1978).
ZINKHAM, W. H.: Visceral larva migrans: A review and reassessment indicating two forms of clinical expression: Visceral and ocular. Amer. J. Dis. Child. *132:* 627 (1978).

E. Special Therapeutic Problems

1. Treatment of Pyrexia of Unknown Origin

Pyrexia of unknown origin (PUO) in patients outside hospital is often due to viral infection. Patients with prolonged fever usually require investigation in hospital. The differential diagnosis of PUO is one of the most difficult subjects in medicine. Only one-third of cases are caused by infection; a further third are due to allergy, tumours, deep venous thrombosis etc., and the remainder are due to other causes. Bacterial endocarditis, typhoid fever, malaria, amoebic abscess and miliary tuberculosis are the most serious infectious causes and should be excluded first.

The following **factors** should be systematically considered:

1. *Epidemiological history* (known contact with an infectious disease, occupation, travel, contact with animals, hobbies, past medical history including tuberculosis, injuries).
2. *Clinical findings* (type of fever, lymphadenopathy, splenic enlargement, palpable liver, pulmonary consolidation, peripheral blood count, ESR or plasma viscosity, protein electrophoresis, urine examination, serum transaminases, cerebrospinal fluid examination at the slightest sign of meningitis, fundoscopy, examination of the sinuses and genitalia), tuberculin testing and chest x-ray for suspected tuberculosis, and ultra-sound (liver, abdomen, echocardiography).
3. *Bacteriological examination* of blood, urine, faeces, sputum, nose and throat swabs, and pus from wounds, where applicable.
4. *Serological examination* for typhoid, paratyphoid, brucellosis, ornithosis, Q-fever, leptospirosis, toxoplasmosis, infectious mononucleosis, syphilis, rheumatic disease and streptococcal and staphylococcal antibodies. Where clinically indicated, viral culture should be performed, and acute and convalescent sera tested in parallel for a rise in specific viral antibody titres. Tropical diseases (e. g. malaria) should be considered in patients who have been exposed to them.

In the absence of characteristic symptoms, the following should be considered initially: bacterial endocarditis, septicaemia, typhoid fever, tuberculosis, osteomyelitis, abscesses of internal organs, intra-abdominal inflammation (diverticulitis, appendicitis, mesenteric lymphadenitis), adnexitis, collagen diseases (rheumatic fever etc.) and allergies. Further relevant investigations should be carried out.

Non-infectious diseases associated with fever, such as lymphogranulomatosis, polyarteritis nodosa, lupus erythematosus, malignant tumours, drug fever, habitual hyperthermia, thyrotoxicosis, Addison's disease and factitious fever should be excluded. When the cause of the fever is not found soon after hospital admission and the symptoms are mild, antibiotics may be withheld pending further observation and investigations. Antipyretics should be avoided in such cases, since the pattern of fever can provide important clues to the nature of the disease.

If the patient is very ill, antibiotics may have to be given before a diagnosis can be made. Since the response to a given treatment may help to reach a diagnosis, it is better not to start with a very broad spectrum combination. Benzyl penicillin may be given initially and, if the temperature does not fall within 3 to 5 days, alternatives should be considered. Possible chlamydial, rickettsial or mycoplasma infections may be treated with doxycycline. Anaerobic and staphylococcal infections should respond to clindamycin. Metronidazole would also be effective in anaerobic infections and in amoebic liver abscess. If antituberculous agents are tried, a combination which is inactive against other organisms, such as isoniazid + ethambutol is preferable. Rifampicin is less useful because of its additional activity against staphylococci, chlamydiae and Legionella. Tuberculosis is still the main cause of PUO in young immigrants, though other causes must be considered in the light of the individual clinical circumstances. Steroids are not recommended in PUO because they may impair the immune response in the early stages of a bacterial infection. Some infections improve in the short term with corticosteroids but the clinical picture can become confused. The steroid treatment which is essential in cases of collagen disease must, therefore, be carefully considered. The use of immunoglobulins without a clear indication (e. g. immunodeficiency) in PUO is not recommended and can be dangerous in systemic lupus erythematosus.

2. Antibiotics in Pregnancy

Tolerance: Chemotherapeutic agents should only be given during pregnancy when there is no possibility of injury to the patient or to the developing embryo or fetus. Tetracyclines are hepatotoxic in pregnancy, particularly when given in high parenteral dosage and in the presence of renal disease. Other antibiotics which can cause liver damage (e. g. rifampicin) should only be used for firm indications if liver function is continually monitored. When there is pre-existing renal damage (e. g. pyelonephritis of pregnancy) potentially nephrotoxic antibiotics should only be used with great care.

The *teratogenicity* of antibiotics in man is poorly understood but has been little studied to date. Chemotherapeutic agents with a potential cytotoxic effect (e. g.

Table 57. Use of important antimicrobials in pregnancy.

Period	Generally safe	Safety not demonstrated	Potentially teratogenic or cytotoxic	Toxic
First trimester	Benzyl penicillin, phenoxymethyl penicillin, ampicillin, amoxycillin, cefazolin, cefuroxime, cefoxitin, erythromycin, sulphonamides	New penicillins, new cephalosporins (risk obviously very slight), other new substances, clindamycin	Trimethoprim, tetroxoprim, pyrimethamine, rifampicin, ethionamide, chloramphenicol, flucytosine, nitrofurantoin, nitroimidazoles, griseofulvin	Tetracyclines, aminoglycosides, nalidixic acid (and other quinolones), amphotericin B, flucytosine
Second and third trimester	As first trimester	–	–	As first trimester
Last week before delivery	As first trimester (except for sulphonamides)	–	–	As first trimester plus sulphonamides, co-trimoxazole, nitrofurantoin

griseofulvin, nitrofurantoin, co-trimoxazole, pyrimethamine, flucytosine, amphotericin B, rifampicin, chloramphenicol etc.) should not, therefore, be given during the *first trimester* of pregnancy (Table 57).

Substances not mentioned in Table 57 should generally be considered unsuitable for use during pregnancy.

Tetracyclines, which impair skeletal growth and stain teeth, should only be given during the *second and third trimesters* after other antibiotics have failed. Ototoxic antibiotics (aminoglycosides) have caused damage to the child's inner ear during pregnancy. Aminoglycosides should, therefore, be avoided whenever possible, as should vancomycin and spectinomycin, for which less toxic alternatives are readily available. Flucytosine can damage the fetal blood cells and is contraindicated throughout pregnancy, as is amphotericin B. New antibiotics should in general be given with great care to pregnant women.

Sulphonamides and co-trimoxazole should be avoided in the *last week* before the estimated date of delivery since they can cause neonatal jaundice by displacement of bilirubin from its binding sites on plasma proteins, leading to bilirubin encephalopathy (kernicterus). Nitrofurantoin shortly before birth can give rise to haemolytic anaemia in the newborn as a result of immaturity of enzyme systems.

Penicillins, cephalosporins, erythromycin and fusidic acid are *well tolerated in pregnancy* and should always be considered first. The new penicillins and cephalosporins, particularly cefotaxime, cefoxitin and ceftazidime have greatly increased the spectrum of activity of the β-lactam antibiotics so that aminoglycosides and other potentially toxic antibiotics can now generally be avoided, even in severe infections.

Suggestions for treatment: *Respiratory and urinary infections* are best treated in pregnancy with agents shown in Table 57. Prompt antibiotic treatment following bacteriological examination is important, since unnecessary prolongation of an infection can put the pregnancy at risk. The risks from the infection should always be weighed against the risks of antibiotic side effects. If treatment is considered necessary, it should not be withheld for fear of teratogenicity or toxicity since infection itself can also damage the fetus. Potentially toxic agents are occasionally unavoidable; for example, ornithosis occurring in pregnancy should be treated with doxycycline, even though tetracyclines should normally be avoided.

Chorioamnionitis (amniotic infection syndrome) is particularly difficult to treat. The causative organism is not generally known and the infection is almost always mixed, with streptococci, enterobacteria and anaerobes. Listeria, chlamydiae and clostridia can also be involved. Many antibiotics do not cross the placenta.

Placental passage: Penicillins and cephalosporins appear to different extents in the fetal circulation. The concentrations of benzyl penicillin, the acylamino penicillins and cephalosporins in the umbilical cord blood are known to be about 50% of those in the mother's serum. Aminoglycosides, erythromycin and clindamycin cross the placenta poorly and the polymyxins not at all. Chloramphenicol, which crosses the placenta best, should not be given because of its haematotoxicity. Penicillins and cephalosporins, which are predominantly excreted by the kidneys, are concentrated in the amniotic fluid as a result of fetal renal excretion. They are then swallowed and so are partially reabsorbed in the fetal gut. When given continuously in sufficient dosage, therefore, these antibiotics can be present at much higher serum concentrations in the fetus than in the mother, and therapeutically effective concentrations of such antibiotics are readily achieved in the fetus.

The *causative organisms* of intra-amniotic infections are difficult to show. One approach is to culture cervical and vaginal secretions before delivery (Table 58) and use the results later, should chorioamnionitis develop. This information can be misleading, however, and these infections are usually mixed. Clinical signs such as fever, premature rupture of the membranes or foul, offensive amniotic fluid are

Table 58. Facultative pathogens in the vagina and methods for their detection.

Species	Detection
Neisseria gonorrhoeae	Immediate inoculation into Thayer-Martin medium
Chlamydia trachomatis	Special transport medium and culture in McCoy cells. Microscopic examination of a smear stained by Giemsa, or by specific immunofluorescence
Candida	Microscopic examination of a wet preparation, culture on Sabouraud's or malt agar
Mycoplasma	Send swab in special liquid medium
Herpes simplex virus	Microscopic examination of a smear by immuno-fluorescence, or with Papanicolaou stain. Swab in special transport medium for viral culture.
Group B streptococcus	Culture on selective medium
Gardnerella vaginalis	Blood agar, microscopy

initially more useful than bacteriological results and antibiotics are generally given without knowledge of the pathogen.

The frequency of mixed aerobic and anaerobic infections makes rapid delivery safer than conservative management after premature rupture of the membranes with signs of infection.

Cefoxitin, cefotaxime, mezlocillin and piperacillin have suitable spectra of activity and pharmacokinetics for the treatment of intra-amniotic infections. When intrauterine sepsis or pneumonia are suspected, several blood cultures and platelet counts should be collected from the baby, starting immediately after birth. If signs of amniotic infection are present, the baby should be treated with antibiotics such as cefuroxime or cefotaxime plus piperacillin.

References

HIRSCH, H. A.: The use of cephalosporin antibiotics in pregnant women. Postgrad. med. J. (Suppl.) *47:* 90 (1971).

HIRSCH, H. A.: Infektionsgefahren bei vorzeitigem Blasensprung. In: SIMON, C., V. v. LOEWENICH (eds.): Neugeboreneninfektionen. Enke, Stuttgart 1978.

SABATH, L. B.: Use of antibiotics in obstetrics. In: D. CHARLES, M. FINLAND (ed.): Obstetric and Perinatal Infections, p. 563. Lea and Febiger, Philadelphia 1973.

SALING, E.: Ein neuer Weg zur Senkung der subpartualen Infektionsgefährdung. In: SIMON, C., V. v. LOEWENICH (eds.): Neugeboreneninfektionen. Enke, Stuttgart 1978.

3. Antibiotic Therapy in the Neonatal Period

Range of organisms: Neonatal infection can be caused by bacteria (Table 59), viruses or fungi and can become established before, during or after birth. Common causes are amniotic infection after premature rupture of the membranes, aspiration, mechanical ventilation, intravascular lines, superficial injuries during birth and immunodeficiency.

Gram-negative bacilli (Escherichia coli, Klebsiella, Enterobacter, Pseudomonas and Bacteroides sp.) cause pneumonia and septicaemia mainly as a result of amniotic infection, aspiration and mechanical ventilation. Such infections are often mixed. Enterotoxigenic Escherichia coli gives rise to severe enterocolitis, which can develop rapidly into intestinal perforation and paralytic ileus. Gram-negative bacilli vary considerably in their antibiotic sensitivity patterns, but are still generally susceptible to cefoxitin (β-lactamase-stable), cefotaxime and amikacin or another aminoglycoside. Campylobacter septicaemia with meningitis responds best to gentamicin + chloramphenicol. Azlocillin and piperacillin are anti-pseudomonal penicillins. In neonatal peritonitis, Bacteroides species are frequent components of mixed infections and are generally sensitive to clindamycin, cefoxitin and metronidazole.

Of the *gram-positive organisms*, the newborn baby seems particularly predisposed to infection with Staphylococcus aureus. Group B streptococcal infections have increased considerably in recent years. The early onset form usually presents as a fulminating septicaemia which originates in utero, and the late onset form as purulent meningitis. Neonatal listeriosis can arise both before and during birth (from bacteria in the mother's vagina) and give rise to pneumonia, enteritis, septicaemia or meningitis. Clostridium tetani only causes neonatal tetanus (mainly of umbilical origin) when the mother has no tetanus antitoxin so the child lacks passive protection.

Neisseria gonorrhoeae may be carried asymptomatically in the vagina and can cause purulent conjunctivitis, rhinitis and occasionally even septicaemia if amnionitis arises after premature rupture of the membranes.

Chlamydia from the mother's vagina can infect the conjunctiva of the baby and lead to inclusion blenorrhoea in the second week of life. This normally heals rapidly with sulphonamide or tetracycline eye drops. Chlamydial pneumonitis is found in the first 6 months and requires systemic erythromycin. Any infant in the first few months of life with pneumonia following unexplained conjunctivitis or eosinophilia should be treated with erythromycin.

Candida albicans occurs in the maternal vagina (perinatal infection) or in the environment (postnatal infection). Stomatitis and dermatitis of the nappy (diaper)

Table 59. Bacterial infections in the neonatal period.

Organism	Occurrence	Infection	Antibiotic therapy
Staphylococcus aureus	Umbilical wound, skin, nose	Septicaemia, meningitis, pneumonia, omphalitis, conjunctivitis, osteomyelitis, scalded skin syndrome, abscesses (skin, breast glands, parotid gland)	Penicillinase-stable penicillins (e. g. flucloxacillin), cefazolin, occasionally benzyl penicillin
Streptococci (group A or B)	Birth canal, wounds	Septicaemia, meningitis, pyoderma, erysipelas	Benzyl penicillin
Clostridium tetani	Wounds, faeces, umbilicus	Tetanus	Benzyl penicillin
Listeria monocytogenes	Birth canal, intrauterine infection	Septicaemia, meningitis, enteritis	Ampicillin, piperacillin
Neisseria gonorrhoeae	Birth canal	Gonoblennorrhoea, rhinitis, septicaemia (if amnionitis)	Benzyl penicillin, or if resistent, cefuroxime
Campylobacter	Birth canal, intestine	Septicaemia, serous meningitis	Gentamicin + chloramphenicol
Escherichia coli	Umbilical wound, intestine, infected amniotic fluid	Septicaemia, meningitis, pneumonia, omphalitis, enteritis, pyelonephritis	Mezlocillin, cefuroxime, cefotaxime
Proteus, Enterobacter, Klebsiella	Umbilical wound, intestine, infected amniotic fluid	Septicaemia, meningitis, pyelonephritis	Cefotaxime, cefoxitin, cefuroxime, possibly with an aminoglycoside
Pseudomonas aeruginosa	Umbilical wound, skin, ventilating apparatus	Septicaemia, meningitis, pneumonia, omphalitis, conjunctivitis	Azlocillin, piperacillin, tobramycin, amikacin, cefsulodin, ceftazidime
Non-sporing anaerobes (Bacteroides, peptostreptococci, peptococci etc.)	Birth canal, intestine, infected amniotic fluid	Pneumonia, septicaemia, peritonitis (often mixed infection)	Cefoxitin, clindamycin, possibly benzyl penicillin
Chlamydia trachomatis	Birth canal	Conjunctivitis, pneumonia	Erythromycin

area are relatively common. Fungal sepsis is rare and probably implies a special reduction in resistance (serious illness, corticosteroid therapy, prematurity).

Amnionitis following premature rupture of the membranes can result in a congenital generalised cutaneous candidiasis, usually without involvement of the oral mucosa or internal organs.

Virus infections of the newborn (e. g. cytomegalovirus infection) are very difficult to influence therapeutically (see p. 532). Cases of disseminated Herpes simplex infection or varicella should be treated with acyclovir (see p. 536). When a mother is positive for HB_sAg during pregnancy and has no anti-HB_s, the baby should be given active immunisation together with hepatitis-specific immuno-globulin immediately after birth.

Table 60. Causes of neonatal pneumonia.

Antenatal	Perinatal and postnatal
Treponema pallidum	Gram-negative bacilli (Klebsiella, Serratia,
Listeria	Pseudomonas, Proteus etc.)
Toxoplasma	Anaerobes (Bacteroides, Peptostreptococcus,
Cytomegalovirus	Peptococcus)
Rubella virus	Streptococci (groups A and B)
Herpes simplex virus	Chlamydia trachomatis
Enteroviruses	Staphylococcus aureus
Gram-negative bacilli	
Anaerobes	
Group B streptococci	

Table 61. Causes of non-pyogenic meningitis in the newborn, and their demonstration.

Causative organism	Method of detection
Coxsackie virus	Tissue culture, CFT
Herpes simplex virus	Microscopy (immunofluorescence), tissue culture
Cytomegalovirus	Tissue culture, microscopy; giant cells (urine), specific IgM (serum)
Treponema pallidum	Specific serological tests
Campylobacter	Culture on special media
Anaerobes	Strictly anaerobic transport and culture
Listeria	Microscopy, culture
Candida	Microscopy, culture

Table 62. Causes of inflammatory skin blisters in the newborn, and their detection.

Causative organism	Method of detection
Staphylococci, streptococci, Candida	Culture, microscopy
Treponema pallidum	Dark field microscopy, serological tests
Herpes simplex virus Varicella-zoster virus	Microscopy (immunofluorescence), culture, specific IgM (serum)
Coxsackie A virus (hand, foot and mouth disease)	Culture

Microbiological diagnosis: In the premature and full-term neonate, it may be difficult to establish the presence and site of an infection because of the nonspecific nature of the clinical symptoms. Whenever infection is suspected, appropriate investigations (blood cultures, CSF, x-rays, blood counts) should be started. Isolation of the causative organism is more difficult, e.g. in neonatal pneumonia (Table 60) and serous meningitis (Table 61) since a large range of organisms must be considered. Inflammatory skin blisters whose cause is unclear (Table 62) may be due to a number of agents, and a direct or indirect attempt to identify the cause of such infections in the newborn should always be made so that antibiotic therapy can be based on tested sensitivities. New transport media should be used, particularly for anaerobes, chlamydiae, campylobacters, gonococci etc. Blood cultures should be taken as soon as possible. Certain agents such as treponemes, gonococci, Candida and Chlamydia are readily demonstrated by direct microscopy. Some viruses can be shown by immunofluorescence techniques. Modern serological methods (e.g. immunofluorescence for the detection of specific IgM) provide important diagnostic information.

Tolerance to antibiotics: The newborn baby, particularly when premature, does not metabolise or detoxify certain antimicrobials in the usual way because of hepatic immaturity. Chloramphenicol in the otherwise normal dose of 80 mg/kg causes the grey baby syndrome in the newborn (see p. 127) so that only 25 mg/kg may be given in the 1st – 2nd weeks of life and 50 mg/kg in the 3rd–4th weeks. Sulphonamides, nitrofurantoin and tetracyclines are unsuitable for the reasons given in the previous chapter.

Penicillins given in high doses to the newborn, particularly when premature, can accumulate because of renal immaturity and cause convulsions which cease when the drug is stopped. For certain antibiotics, e.g. the nitroimidazoles, which are excellent in anaerobic infection, experience in the newborn is limited.

Antibiotics are not generally licensed for use in the newborn until experience has accumulated in adults.

Antibiotics in breast milk. Certain antimicrobials given to the mother when breast feeding, particularly sulphonamides, tetracyclines, chloramphenicol and isoniazid, pass into the breast milk. Any drugs contra-indicated in the newborn should not therefore be given to the mother at this time. Penicillins, aminoglycosides and cephalosporins are generally harmless unless the child is already allergic to the drug, since they only pass in small quantities into the milk.

Pharmacokinetics: The pharmacokinetics of antibiotics in the newborn differ markedly from those of adults as a result of:
1. renal immaturity,
2. liver immaturity,
3. reduced plasma protein binding,
4. increased vascular permeability and
5. a larger extracellular space.
The absorption of some antibiotics by the oral route is less than in older children. All these factors affect antibiotic therapy.

Renal immaturity: The mean half-life of almost all antibiotics varies in the newborn according to the week of life (Table 63); for carbenicillin, for example, it is 5 h in the 1st week, 3 h in the 2nd week and 2.5 h in the 3rd and 4th weeks, after which it converges on the adult value of about 1 h. Erythromycin, which is incompletely absorbed, almost completely metabolised, and mainly eliminated in the bile, is the only antibiotic with a constant half-life in this age-group. The differences in half-lives according to the week of life for the penicillins and cephalosporins, which are well tolerated, are not so important. Unexplained convulsions in a newborn baby receiving penicillin in high dosage, especially in the first few days of life, should be considered as possible side effect of the antibiotic, however.

There are considerable differences in half-life between the immature and the full-term neonate, as far as has been investigated, but these are not usually taken into account when calculating the dosage. Aminoglycoside dosage in very early premature babies should be monitored with particular care.

After the 1st month of life, the antibiotic half-life begins to approach the adult value. Thus the half-life of phenoxymethyl penicillin is 3–6 times the adult value in the newborn after an oral dose and twice the adult value in children aged ½–1½ years. The adult half-life is about 30 min.

Renal function is known to mature after 1–2 years and glomerular filtration matures faster than tubular secretion. For this reason, antibiotics in infants after

Table 63. Antibiotic half-lifes in the premature and full-term neonate and in adults.

| Drug | Half-life (h) in | | | | |
| | Premature neonates (0–6d) | Full-term neonates aged | | | Adults |
		0–6d	7–13d	14–18d	
Benzyl penicillin	–	3.2	1.7	1.4	0.5
Phenoxymethyl penicillin	–	3	1.7	1.4	0.5
Ampicillin	4.7	4.0	2.8	1.7	1
Amoxycillin	–	–	3	3	1.5
Oxacillin	1.6	1.2	0.8	0.6	0.5
Azlocillin	2.6	2.6	2.6	2.6	1.2
Mezlocillin	2.1	1.8	1.8	1.8	0.9
Piperacillin	–	2.1	2.1	2.1	1.0
Cefazolin	–	4	4	3	1.5
Cefoxitin	6	4	3	2	0.7
Cefuroxime	–	5	4	2	1.2
Cefotaxime	2.4	1.5	1.5	–	1
Ceftazidime	–	3	–	–	2
Cephalexin	–	4	3	2	1
Gentamicin, Tobramycin	11	5	3	3	2
Amikacin	8	6	6	6	2.5
Chloramphenicol	24	15	–	–	3
Erythromycin	–	2	2	2	2

the first month of life are dosed in the same way as in young children, that is, based on body weight, since the blood concentrations are not significantly higher because the extracellular space is relatively larger.

Liver immaturity: Immature hepatic function not only increases the half-life of a drug such as chloramphenicol; nafcillin, a penicillin used in the USA for staphylococcal infections in the newborn, is also affected. Only 15–30% of a parenteral dose of nafcillin is eliminated in active form in the urine. In spite of this, the half-life in premature babies is increased 10-fold and in mature neonates 4-fold because of a small degree of liver metabolism. The drug is very well tolerated and so a reduction in dosage is not necessary, but a relatively low dose of 50 mg/kg is sufficient in the newborn, compared with 100 mg/kg in infants.

Plasma protein binding: The plasma protein binding of antibiotics in the newborn has been studied *in vitro* in cord blood. The concentrations which could be achieved therapeutically differed significantly between the newborn and adults for certain antibiotics, e. g. cefazolin (for 26%) but for others (cephradine and clindamycin) was not statistically significant (for 4% and 3% respectively). The lesser protein binding with cefazolin is due not to the low-grade hypoalbuminaemia sometimes found in the newborn, but rather to the low binding affinity of neonatal albumin. Similar results have been observed with other antibiotics, diphenylhydantoin and barbiturates. The effect of reduced plasma protein binding on the tolerance and tissue distribution of these drugs is not yet clear.

Further studies are necessary to establish the reason for the reduced plasma protein binding and to decide whether the dose of certain drugs should be modified for this reason.

Absorption: The absorption of chloramphenicol after oral dosage as an ester has been shown in infants to be reduced. Pivampicillin, an ester of ampicillin, is also less well absorbed in the first year of life than in small children. Pivampicillin is de-esterified by an esterase in the intestinal wall to pivalic acid and ampicillin hydroxymethyl ester; infants are apparently less well able to do this. All absorption esters (carindacillin, carfecillin, bacampicillin, talampicillin, pivmecillinam) should therefore be examined for bioavailability in the infant.

Dosage: The daily dose specified for the newborn is generally similar to that recommended for infants, and based on body weight. These doses are calculated from empirical data such as the sensitivity of the causative organism, the tolerance and pharmacokinetics of the antibiotic and the site of the infection. The doses of penicillins and cephalosporins may be increased several times without harm. An average daily dose is recommended for infections with organisms of normal sensitivity and a higher dose for those with moderate or only slight sensitivity. The normal dose interval in the newborn may be doubled to take account of the renal immaturity.

Published reports often suggest a higher dosage (5–6 mg/kg) of gentamicin than that given in Table 30, p. 263, since the blood concentrations in the newborn given adequate dosage are less than those found in adults. The reason for this is not clear, but could be that gentamicin is deposited to a greater extent in the kidney of the neonate than in adults. The accumulation of gentamicin in the kidney explains the prolonged urinary excretion of the antibiotic after cessation of therapy.

References

AMON, I., K. AMON: Zum Übertritt von Arzneimitteln in das Fruchtwasser. Zbl. Gynäk. *98:* 961 (1976).

EHRNEBO, M., S. AGURELL, B. JALLING, L. O. BOREUS: Age differences in drug binding by plasma proteins: studies on human foetuses, neonates and adults. Europ. J. Clin. Pharmacol. *3:* 189 (1971).

FINITZO-HIEBER, T., G. H. McCRACKEN Jr., R. J. ROESSER: Ototoxicity in neonates treated with gentamicin and kanamycin. Results of a four-year controlled follow-up study. Pediatrics *63:* 443 (1979).

KAPLAN, J. M., G. H. McCRACKEN, M. L. THOMAS: Clinical pharmacology of tobramycin in newborns. Amer. J. Dis. Child. *125:* 656 (1973).

KAPLAN, J. M., G. H. McCRACKEN Jr., L. J. HORTON, M. L. THOMAS, N. DAVIS: Pharmacologic studies in neonates given large dosages of ampicillin. J. Pediatrics *84:* 571 (1974).

KIOSZ, D.: Therapie der Neugeborenen-Sepsis. Fortschr. antimikrob. Chemother. (FAC) *3-1:* 65 (1984).

KIOSZ, D., C. SIMON: In-vitro-Untersuchungen zur Therapie gefährlicher bakterieller Neugeborenen-Infektionen. Fortschr. antimikrob. Chemother. (FAC) *3-1:* 15 (1984).

KIOSZ, D., C. SIMON, V. MALERCZYK: Die Plasmaeiweißbindung von Clindamycin, Cephazolin und Cephradin bei Neugeborenen und Erwachsenen. Klin. Pädiatrie *187:* 71 (1975).

KLEIN, J. O., M. MARCY: Bacterial infections. In: REMINGTON, J. S., J. O. KLEIN (eds.): Infectious Diseases of the Fetus and Newborn Infant, p. 1020. Saunders, Philadelphia 1983.

MARKS, M. I.: Common bacterial infections in infancy and childhood. MTP Press, Lancaster 1979.

MARGET, W., B. H. BELOHRADSKY, R. ROOS: Guidelines for adequate chemotherapeutic dosage in newborns and infants with septicaemia and meningitis. Infection *8, Suppl. 1:* 582 (1980).

McCRACKEN, G. H., jr., J. D. NELSON: Antimicrobial Therapy for Newborns. Grune and Stratton, New York 1977.

McCRACKEN, G. H., jr.: Group B streptococci: The new challenge in neonatal infections. J. Pediat. *82:* 703 (1978).

PHILIPSON, A., L. D. SABATH, D. CHARLES: Transplacental passage of erythromycin and clindamycin. New Engl. J. Med. *288:* 1219 (1973).

SIMON, C.: Infektionen des Neugeborenen. In: W. STILLE (ed.): Unspezifische Infektionen, p. 148. Thieme, Stuttgart 1982.

SIMON, C., A. MOHÁCSI: Cefazolin in der Neugeborenenperiode. Med. Welt (N. F.) *28:* 1918 (1977).

SIMON, C., C. D. KIOSZ: Zur Pneumonie bei Langzeitbeatmung im ersten Lebensmonat. Fortschr. antimikrob. Chemother. (FAC) *2-1:* 65 (1983).

WASZ-HÖCKERT, O., S. NUMMI, S. VUOPALA, P. A. JÄRVINEN: Transplacental passage of azidocillin and penicillin G during early and late pregnancy. Scand. J. infect. Dis. *2:* 125 (1970).

WEINSTEIN, A. J., R. S. GIBBS, M. GALLAGHER: Placental transfer of clindamycin and gentamicin in term pregnancy. Amer. J. Obstet. Gynec. *124:* 688 (1976).

YOSHIOKA, H., T. MONMA, S. MATSUDA: Placental transfer of gentamicin. J. Pediatrics *80:* 121 (1972).

4. Antibiotic Therapy in Abnormal Liver Function

Metabolism in the liver: The liver plays an important role in the metabolism and detoxification of drugs. Antibiotics which cannot be detoxified because of hepatic insufficiency can produce serious side effects. Chloramphenicol, nalidixic acid, norfloxacin and sulphonamides are bound to glucuronic acid in the liver and eliminated in this form in the urine. They are therefore contra-indicated in severe liver disease and particularly in hepatorenal failure since the blood concentrations of the free antibiotics are then markedly raised. Clindamycin is also metabolised in the liver and accumulates when liver function is impaired.

Excretion through the liver: Antibiotics which are excreted through the liver into the intestine (e.g. erythromycin, fusidic acid, nafcillin, mezlocillin, cefoperazone, ceftriaxone) should only be given with caution to patients with *hepatitis* and *cirrhosis*. Serious side effects have not, however, been reported with these substances in patients with liver disease. Antibiotics which are mainly eliminated unchanged through the kidney (benzyl penicillin, cephalexin, cefoxitin, cefuroxime, gentamicin) may be safely used in cases of severe liver damage.

Because serious liver disease is often accompanied by coagulopathies, antibiotics which themselves give rise to a bleeding tendency (carbenicillin, latamoxef, cefoperazone) are best avoided.

Direct hepatotoxicity is unlikely to be caused by commercially available antibiotics, especially when given in normal dosage to patients with normal renal function. Certain antibiotics (see below) can, however, exacerbate pre-existing liver damage, particularly when overdosed. Two principal patterns of drug-induced hepatotoxicity are described (Table 64).

The *tetracyclines* can lead to potentially fatal toxic liver damage (hepatic dystrophy and fatty degeneration) when given parenterally in large doses (2–4 g i.v. a day). The not uncommon incidence of such toxicity in pregnancy suggests that tetracyclines can cause hepatopathy of pregnancy; the extent to which pre-existing renal insufficiency or liver damage is responsible remains unclear.

In patients with normal liver function given the correct dosage (1–2 g by mouth or 0.5–0.75 g parenterally) the tetracyclines would not be expected to cause liver damage. Tetracyclines should be avoided, however, in cases of hepatitis, cirrhosis and hepatic coma.

Rifampicin often induces liver enzymes and gives rise to raised transaminases and other liver disorders (sometimes accompanied by jaundice) which have, in a few cases, been fatal. Active liver disease particularly acute hepatitis, is a contra-indication for rifampicin.

Table 64. Potential hepatotoxicity of antimicrobial agents.

Direct liver cell damage (Raised transaminases as in mild hepatitis, sometimes associated with fatty change and possibly enzymatic induction)	Intrahepatic cholestasis (Features of obstructive jaundice, with increased alkaline phosphatase, and also eosinophilia and fever, apparently of allergic origin)
Tetracyclines Ketoconazole Griseofulvin Rifampicin Sulphonamides Isoniazid Ethionamide Pyrazinamide PAS	Erythromycin estolate = erythromycin lauryl sulphate Triacetyl oleandomycin Sulphonamides Lincomycin Clindamycin Nitrofurantoin PAS

Griseofulvin can be hepatotoxic in patients with pre-existing liver damage, and should never be used for the long-term treatment of fungal infections in patients with liver disease.

Potentially toxic antimicrobials should not be given to patients with viral hepatitis; urinary tract infections in such patients should not, therefore, be treated with *co-trimoxazole*.

Intrahepatic cholestasis may be caused by several drugs.

Erythromycin estolate (erythromycin lauryl sulphate) and *triacetyl oleandomycin* can give rise to an allergic cholestatic hepatosis when given for periods of more than 10 days or in repeated courses. Features of obstructive jaundice with an increase in alkaline phosphatase, fever and eosinophilia appear. These changes are temporary and rapidly disappear after treatment has stopped but are the reason for which erythromycin ethyl succinate and stearate are given instead.

Lincomycin and *clindamycin* have a prolonged half-life in hepatic insufficiency and should therefore be carefully dosed. Jaundice and abnormal liver function tests are occasionally seen during clindamycin therapy. The other antimicrobial agents listed in Table 64 should also be used with caution in hepatic insufficiency and stopped at once if marked changes in liver function are seen.

In **hepatic coma**, an oral aminoglycoside (e.g. neomycin) may be given to reduce the intestinal production of ammonia. This has led to an improvement in many patients, the basis for which is not entirely clear. Oral aminoglycosides cannot sterilise the intestine although they can reduce the enteric bacterial counts considerably. Prolonged oral treatment with aminoglycosides may lead to small-intestinal villous atrophy and is not therefore recommended.

5. Antibiotic Therapy in Renal Insufficiency

Mode of excretion: Whereas benzyl penicillin, cefazolin, gentamicin and vancomycin, are almost entirely eliminated in the urine, most other antibiotics are only partially eliminated by the kidneys, either in unchanged active form or as inactive metabolites, with the remainder eliminated through the bile and gut.

The *urinary recovery* is an important basic parameter in chemotherapy. Minocycline, erythromycin, fusidic acid, oxacillin and cefoperazone mainly appear in the faeces. Accumulation and prolongation of the elimination half-life (Table 65, p. 509) is seen in renal insufficiency and depends on the mode of excretion and rate of metabolism of the antibiotic given. The degree of renal failure is best shown by the reduction in creatinine clearance (and less well by serum urea and creatinine values).

A *creatinine clearance* of 40 ml/min usually corresponds to a serum creatinine of 2 mg/dl, a creatinine clearance of 20–40 ml/min to a serum creatinine of 2–4 mg/dl and a creatinine clearance of 10–20 ml/min to a serum creatinine value of 4–8 mg/dl. The risk of side effects depends not only on the degree of accumulation but also on the potential toxicity of the antibiotic. From this, certain rules can be drawn up for the dosage of antibiotics in renal failure (Table 65).

Potentially nephrotoxic antibiotics include *amphotericin B* (used for the treatment of generalised fungal infections and contra-indicated in severe renal insufficiency), *bacitracin, neomycin and paromomycin* which are only used topically as local agents.

Cephaloridine, which is now obsolete, can cause tubular necrosis at high dosage (>4–6 g/day). *Cephalothin* and *cephradine* are also nephrotoxic at very high dosage. The nephrotoxicity of the *newer cephalosporins*, however, is very low.

Polymyxins can accumulate in renal insufficiency and cause a number of symptoms of neurotoxicity; they should, therefore, no longer be used systemically.

Streptomycin, kanamycin, amikacin, gentamicin, sisomicin, tobramycin, netilmicin, capreomycin and *vancomycin* are also potentially nephrotoxic; to a lesser extent they are also neurotoxic on accumulation and should be given to patients with renal insufficiency only for severe infections, at reduced dosage and with blood level monitoring. Test kits are now commercially available for the determination of blood concentrations of gentamicin, tobramycin, netilmicin and

Table 65. Half-lifes of antibiotics which require the interval between normal individual doses to be modified in renal failure.

Antibiotic	Half-life (h)		Dose-interval (h) at a creatinine clearance (ml/min) of				% Urinary recovery (parenteral dose, normal renal function)
	Normal	Severe renal failure	>80	50–80	10–50	<10	
Benzyl penicillin	0.65	7–10	6	8	8	12	90
Oxacillin	0.4	2	4–6	6	6	8	25
Flucloxacillin	0.75	8	6	8	8	12	35
Ampicillin	1.0	8.5	6	8	12	12–24	60
Ticarcillin	1.1	16	6	8	12	12–24	95
Azlocillin	1.25	8–10	6	8	8	12–24	60
Mezlocillin	0.8	6–14	6	8	8	12–24	60
Piperacillin	1.0	6–10	6	8	8	12–24	60
Cefalothin	0.65	3–18	4–6	6	6	8	65
Cefazolin	1.5	5–20	6	8	12	24–48	90
Cefuroxime	1.2	5–20	6	8	12	24–48	90
Cefoxitin	0.75	5–10	6	8	12	24	90
Cefotaxime	1.0	14	8	8	8	12	50
Cefoperazone	2.0	5–10	8	8	8	12	20
Latamoxef	2.0	5–20	8	8	12	24	75
Cephalexin	1.0	30	6	6	8	24–48	90
Cefaclor	1.0	6–10	6	8	8	12	60
Gentamicin	2	60	8	12	18–24	48	90
Amikacin	2.3	72–96	8	24	24–72	72–96	90
Vancomycin	6	216	12	72	240	240	85
Tetracycline	8–9	30–128	6	12	48	72–96	60
Lincomycin	5	10–13	8	8	12	12	40
Clindamycin	3	3–5	6	6	8	12	40
Co-trimoxazole	10 and 12	12–24	12	12	24	–	60 and 80
Flucytosine	3–4	6–12	6	8	12–24	24–48	90
Metronidazole	7	8–12	8	8	12	24	30

amikacin. Except for vancomycin the ototoxicity of aminoglycosides is increased by the simultaneous administration of certain diuretics, e.g. frusemide (see p. 136). The blood concentration immediately before a dose (trough level) is particularly useful and, if the dose interval is correct, need not be significantly greater than the concentration with a healthy kidney and normal dose interval.

Renal damage has been reported with *methicillin* so that this antibiotic, which can be readily replaced by flucloxacillin and dicloxacillin, is not suitable in renal insufficiency. *Nalidixic acid* and other quinolones (gyrase inhibitors) are not usually effective in severe renal failure because of the low urinary concentrations; for this reason, and the increased risk of side effects, they should be avoided.

Antibiotics whose dose must be reduced in renal failure: The *tetracyclines* are 10–25% excreted by the kidneys when given orally and 50–70% when given i. v. They can accumulate in patients with renal insufficiency and cause toxic kidney damage. Because of the catabolic effect of the tetracyclines, the serum concentrations of substances normally eliminated in the urine are increased during tetracycline therapy. *Demeclocycline* can cause a nephrogenic diabetes insipidus and should not be used in patients with pre-existing renal damage. *Doxycycline* and *minocycline,* however, do not accumulate in renal failure.

All *β-lactam antibiotics* should be carefully dosed during renal insufficiency and very high doses avoided. A combination with gentamicin or other potentially nephrotoxic antibiotics (see above) should be avoided in impending acute renal failure.

Lincomycin and *clindamycin* are given at ¼ to ⅓ the normal dose in severe renal insufficiency. The dose of *flucytosine* (Table 65 and p. 182) and of *metronidazole* (Table 65 and p. 221) must also be reduced.

Most *short* and *long-acting sulphonamides* are now more water-soluble and less acetylated than the early components. They do not, therefore, cause renal damage under normal conditions but should be given in reduced dosage in renal insufficiency (see below). This is especially true for sulphadiazine which should not be given to patients with severe dehydration, uraemia, or pre-existing renal damage.

The elimination of *sulphamethoxydiazine* and other *long-acting sulphonamides* is retarded at creatinine clearance values below 30 ml/min so that the daily dose should be halved. Sulphonamides should not be given to patients whose creatinine clearance is less than 20 ml/min. *Co-trimoxazole* should not be used when the creatinine clearance is less than 15 ml/min and at values of 15–30 ml/min, the daily dose should be halved.

Nitrofurantoin leads to severe neurotoxic effects (polyneuritis etc.) in renal insufficiency due to marked accumulation. It should be avoided wherever possible even in low grade renal insufficiency.

Fixed combinations may lead to different accumulation of the consisting components. This will play a role with imipenem in combination with cilastatin where cilastatin particularly increases in renal insufficiency.

Antibiotics which require no dose reduction in renal insufficiency: *Benzyl penicillin* is so non-toxic that it can be given in the normal daily dose even though considerable accumulation occurs in renal insufficiency. The interval may, however, be prolonged in severe renal impairment. Doses of benzyl penicillin exceeding 10 megaunits a day can produce convulsions in patients with uraemia; this limit should not, therefore, be exceeded. *Ampicillin, azlocillin, mezlocillin, piperacillin, oxacillin, flucloxacillin* and *dicloxacillin* may be administered in moderate doses in renal insufficiency.

In uraemia, the electrolyte content of the antibiotic must be taken into account, especially of the disodium salts *ticarcillin, fosfomycin* and *ceftriaxone* and *benzyl penicillin potassium. Cefotaxime, cefoperazone, ceftriaxone, cephalothin, cefacetrile* and *cefapirin* are about one-third metabolised in the body and therefore accumulate less than other cephalosporins. In patients with severe renal insufficiency, therefore, the dose interval has to be increased accordingly, but the normal dose of all cephalosporins may still be given. *β-lactam antibiotics* with significant biliary elimination (cefoperazone, mezlocillin) accumulate less than those derivatives with a predominantly renal elimination. Cephalosporins should not be combined with potentially nephrotoxic antibiotics in patients with pre-existing renal damage since cephalosporins have been shown to produce renal damage at high dosage in animal experiments.

Erythromycin, fusidic acid and *rifampicin* are well tolerated in renal insufficiency if the liver function is normal. *Doxycycline* and *minocycline* can also be used without restriction in renal failure. The daily dose of *chloramphenicol,* which is predominantly excreted in the urine, does not have to be reduced in patients with reduced renal function and accumulation of the antibacterially inactive metabolites does not apparently give rise to side effects. When liver function is also impaired, however, and glucuronidation is reduced, chloramphenicol should not be given. *Miconazole* and *ketoconazole* may also be given at normal dosage in renal failure.

Antibiotic therapy in anuria: In acute anuria, antibiotics which require no dose reduction in renal impairment may be given at full dosage. These are the penicillins (except carbenicillin and ticarcillin), doxycycline, chloramphenicol, erythromycin, fusidic acid and rifampicin. In patients on intermittent haemodialysis or peritoneal dialysis, antibiotics are often necessary for intercurrent infection, e. g. of an arteriovenous shunt. If substances which do not accumulate are not appropriate for the infection present, other antibiotics which have to be given at greater intervals should be considered. The dose depends on the residual diuresis, the possibility of extra-renal elimination, the frequency of dialysis and whether the antibiotic can be dialysed. Plasma urea and creatinine values are unsuitable criteria for deciding the antibiotic dose in dialysis patients. Certain toxic antibiotics such as amphotericin B and vancomycin should generally only be given once to dialysis patients. Since they are not dialysable and have virtually no extra-renal pathway of elimination, they persist for weeks in sufficient quantities in the blood. A further dose should be given after a long interval and after an assay has been performed. Antibiotics are generally given parenterally to uraemic patients since the absorption and tolerance of oral doses can be affected by uraemic gastritis. The normal dose should be given at the end of each dialysis session since most antibiotics are dialysable (with the exception of colistin, polymyxin B, lincomycin, clindamycin, fusidic acid, vancomycin and probably also rifampicin). Benzyl penicillin and the penicillinase-stable penicillins such as flucloxacillin are only partially removed by dialysis. Published data about the half-lifes of antibiotics during dialysis are very variable, probably because of differences in the properties of the membranes used in various dialysis systems, and variation in the period of dialysis. The possible addition of antibiotics to the dialysis fluid should be considered as part of the dosage since most antibiotics diffuse into the blood.

Peritoneal dialysis is less effective and certain antibiotics, e. g. benzyl penicillin and cefazolin, which can be removed by haemodialysis, are not, or incompletely removed. Most antibiotics behave similarly in peritoneal and haemodialysis. If an antibiotic is added to the fluid during peritoneal dialysis, it can diffuse into the blood and cause side effects. Ampicillin, oxacillin, cloxacillin, cefotaxime and cephalothin may be added relatively safely to the dialysis fluid in peritonitis at 50 mg/l, causing an initial increase in the serum concentration; this decreases afterwards through metabolism and extra-renal excretion. Aminoglycosides should not be given intraperitoneally because of the danger of neuromuscular blockade. Fungal peritonitis following peritoneal dialysis can be treated by instillation of amphotericin B or miconazole.

The risk of side effects in renal insufficiency should not deter the physician from carrying out life-saving treatment, e. g. during an acute exacerbation of chronic pyelonephritis.

References

ALESTIG, K.: Studies on doxycycline during intravenous and oral treatment with reference to renal function. Scand. J. infect. Dis. *5:* 193 (1973).
BENNETT, W. M., I. SINGER, T. GOLPER, P. FEIG: Guidelines for drug therapy in renal failure. Ann. intern. Med. *86:* 754 (1977).
CHAN, R. A., E. J. BENNER, P. D. HOEPRICH: Gentamicin therapy in renal failure: A nomogram for dosage. Ann. intern. med. *76:* 773 (1972).
CUTLER, R. E., A. GYSELYNCK, W. P. FLEET, A. W. FORREY: Correlation of serum creatinin concentration and gentamicin half-life. JAMA *219:* 1037 (1972).

GIBSON, T. P., H. A. NELSON: Drug kinetics and artificial kidneys. Clin. Pharmacokinetics *2:* 403 (1977).

LÜTHY, R., W. SIEGENTHALER: Die Dosierung von Antibiotika bei Niereninsuffizienz. Schweiz. med. Wschr. *103:* 740 (1973).

McHENRY, M. C., T. L. GAVAN, D. G. VIDT, S. JAMESON, J. G. WAGNER: Minocycline in renal failure. Clin. Pharmacol. Ther. *13:* 146 (1972).

6. Antibiotic Therapy in Bone-Marrow Suppression and Immune Defects

a) Bone-Marrow Suppression

In bone marrow suppression, particularly in the advanced stages of leukaemia, agranulocytosis or pancytopenia (a fall in the peripheral white cell count to less than 700/µl), the body's resistance is lowered to such an extent that the further course of the disease is dominated by severe infections of the skin, mucous membranes or internal organs. Resistance to infection is also markedly reduced by the immunosuppressive properties of most cytotoxic agents.

Table 66. Common pathogens of fever in patients with myeloid insufficiency.

Common site	Infected venous catheters (with thrombophlebitis) Pneumonia Enteritis Oesophagitis Skin infections (abscesses, ecthyma etc.) Septicaemia or bacteraemia Underlying lesions (necrosis etc.) Blood transfusion Drug fever
Common pathogens	Bacterial infection (including enterobacteria, Pseudomonas, Legionella, staphylococci, anaerobes, Listeria, mycobacteria) Virus infections (hepatitis, parotitis, cytomegalovirus, herpes simplex, herpes zoster, varicella, papova viruses etc.) Fungal infections (Candida, Aspergillus, Mucor, Cryptococcus, Torulopsis etc.) Parasitic infections (Pneumocystis carinii, Toxoplasma gondii, Giardia lamblia etc.)

Pathogens: The most important pathogens (Table 66) are Pseudomonas, Bacteroides, Klebsiella, Escherichia coli and staphylococci. The whole range of facultative pathogens must be considered, however. The main reservoir is the normal colonic and oral flora. Exogenous infections can spread rapidly under suitable conditions, so that meningococci, Listeria, Legionella, salmonellae and Clostridium welchii are often found. Tuberculosis is also not uncommon in this situation, usually as an exacerbation of an earlier infection. Fungal infections (Candida, Cryptococcus, Aspergillus etc.) or protozoal infections (pneumocystis, toxoplasma) often appear. Virus infections (cytomegalovirus, varicella, herpes) are usually severe.

Treatment: There are many possible causes of fever in bone marrow insufficiency, and antibiotic therapy often cannot be directed against a particular pathogen. Even when an organism has been isolated, the entire range of facultative pathogens should be covered by the antibiotic combination. Narrow-spectrum chemotherapy often causes the infecting organism to change. Any previous antibiotic treatment should be taken into account when choosing the best antibiotic regimen and, wherever possible, a combination should be used which has not been given in the recent past. Combinations which have wide activity are cefoxitin + azlocillin or cefotaxime + azlocillin. Such combinations should include an aminoglycoside such as gentamicin to potentiate the bactericidal effect. Overt infections in patients with bone marrow insufficiency have a poor prognosis. Septicaemia often develops with shock, or large areas of necrosis appear with no cellular reaction. The lack of functional granulocytes cannot be completely compensated for by the antibiotic therapy. A granulocyte transfusion may be performed, especially when the marrow suppression is reversible.

A prompt start to antibiotic therapy is very important in the neutropenic patient. Once specimens have been collected for culture, a bactericidal combination should be started without delay. The most important index of effective therapy is defervescence. The response to antibiotic therapy is, however, often difficult to assess. Persistence of the fever over long periods suggests the presence of resistant pathogens. Non-bacterial infections may be present, such as pneumocystis, Aspergillus fumigatus or cytomegalovirus. Treatment must sometimes be based only on the clinical picture because these opportunistic organisms are frequently not demonstrated in life; the diagnosis usually requires a tissue biopsy, a procedure which is generally too dangerous for leukaemic patients. Nevertheless, every effort should be made to isolate the causative organism of a pneumonia (Table 67) or gastroenteritis (Table 68). Treatment is almost always given without knowledge of the pathogen. If an antibacterial agent fails, a trial of antifungal therapy, e. g. miconazole + flucytosine, may be worthwhile.

Table 67. Pathogens of pneumonia in patients with myeloid insufficiency.

Causes of pneumonia	Demonstration
Pneumococci Haemophilus	Culture, microscopy (sputum), latex agglutination test (serum, urine)
Staphylococci	Culture (sputum), possibly blood culture
Mycobacterium tuberculosis	Culture, microscopy (sputum, tracheal secretion)
Enterobacteria Pseudomonas Anaerobes	Culture (tracheal secretion)
Cytomegalovirus, measles virus, varicella virus	Tissue culture, microscopy (immunofluorescence), possibly serology
Candida albicans Cryptococcus neoformans	Culture (tracheal secretion), latex agglutination test (serum)
Pneumocystis carinii Toxoplasma gondii	Microscopy (biopsy, possibly tracheal secretion), possibly serological (fluorescent antibodies)

Superficial candida infections, which are encouraged both by the underlying disease and its steroid or cytotoxic treatment, require intensive treatment of the skin and mucous membranes with nystatin. If there is reasonable suspicion of a *generalised candida infection* or localised involvement (e. g. of the lungs or oesophagus), flucytosine (6–10 g a day by mouth) may be given in combination with amphotericin B. Oral ketoconazole is not sufficiently reliable but may be worth trying. *Aspergillus infection* is often only detectable as a fever, and occasionally as a resistant pneumonia; the fungus is difficult to demonstrate and is

Table 68. Pathogens of enteritis in patients with myeloid insufficiency.

Causes of enteritis	Demonstration
Salmonellae Shigellae Yersinia Pseudomonas	Culture
Campylobacter jejuni Clostridium difficile	Culture, microscopy
Rotaviruses	ELISA technique
Candida	Microscopy, culture
Cryptosporidium	Microscopy
Giardia lamblia	Microscopy, ELISA technique

often only found post-mortem. Treatment may, therefore, have to be started on clinical suspicion. Other fungal species such as Cryptococcus neoformans and Mucor are also found (see p. 349). Acyclovir is effective in *herpes simplex* and *varicella zoster* infections. High doses of co-trimoxazole are indicated if there is radiological evidence of *pneumocystis pneumonia*. The standard treatment of *toxoplasmosis* is still pyrimethamine + sulphadiazine but, because of the relative safety of trimethoprim in comparison with pyrimethamine, co-trimoxazole may also be considered. Intestinal *giardiasis* should be treated with metronidazole (see p. 365). The treatment of *Cryptosporidium* enteritis is not yet established.

The poor prognosis of established infection in granulocytopenics is the reason for **prophylaxis.** The most sophisticated technique is protective isolation in an isolator with decontamination. Several isolators are available (incubators, "Life Island", a sterile ward, the Trexler isolator, laminar air flow systems etc.). The function of these systems is to prevent contact with exogenous pathogens. All systems are expensive and personnel-intensive; they are not, therefore, available for all patients. They can also cause psychological problems for the patients. It is, moreover, still not clear whether exogenous or endogenous infections are more frequent. There is no doubt that endogenous infections play an important role. Isolation units per se are of no value unless used in conjunction with decontamination of the patient, i. e. a marked reduction and, if possible, elimination of the body's own bacterial flora. Decontamination consists essentially of a reduction in the intestinal and mouth flora and the almost complete elimination of the skin flora. There is no best way of achieving intestinal decontamination (sometimes mis-named sterilisation). A combination of neomycin (2–4 g/day), polymyxin B (0.4–0.6 g/day) and nystatin (1.5–3 million units/day) is often given by mouth. Bacteroides sp. are unaffected by this combination. The large number of tablets required (ca. 20/day) is also a problem and the antibiotics may be given as a powder. Oral gentamicin, vancomycin and other antibiotics are used in the USA. The mouth flora may be reduced by various local antibiotics and disinfectants, but complete suppression of the bacterial flora is seldom achieved. Well tolerated antibacterial disinfectants should be used for skin decontamination, paying special attention to skin creases (the axillae, anal cleft etc.). Even decontamination carries the risk of selection of resistant organisms, and regular bacteriological surveillance is advisable.

The ideal procedure would be *selective decontamination* in which facultative pathogens are eliminated but non-pathogenic flora (e. g. lactobacilli) remain unaffected. Co-trimoxazole, nalidixic acid and the polymyxins are suitable agents for this purpose.

Agranulocytopenic patients for whom no isolation system is available should be given antibiotic prophylaxis; without this, they often die in the early stages of their illness from fulminant infections with streptococci, pneumococci, Escherichia coli, Klebsiella etc. Many studies have shown the effectiveness of prophylactic intestinal decontamination with or without systemic antibiotics in reducing the frequency of bacterial superinfection in neutropenic patients. A practical regimen is cefotaxime, 2 g twice a day, gentamicin, 80 mg twice a day, and daily oral doses for intestinal decontamination of neomycin 3 g, polymyxin B 0.5 g and nystatin 2 million units. Gammaglobulins are only justified where immunoglobulin deficiency has been demonstrated. Cytomegalovirus immunoglobulin is available to protect against CMV infection in, for example, bone marrow transplantation. Prophylactic co-trimoxazole (p. 200) may be used against pneumocystis pneumonia.

b) Immune Deficiencies

Opportunistic infections with bacteria, viruses, fungi and protozoa can affect patients with congenital and acquired immune deficiencies. A variety of bacterial infections may be expected in patients with isolated B-cell deficiencies whereas viral, fungal and parasitic infections are more common in patients with isolated T-cell deficiencies.

The **acquired immune deficiency syndrome (AIDS),** which is now more common than congenital immunological defects (4000 cases in the USA 1981–84) is of particular current interest. The disease has a very high mortality and treatment is often ineffective. The cause is apparently a virus, transmitted by blood products or sexual contact, particularly between homosexuals. The incubation period is 2 months to 5 years. The disease is expressed as a viral-induced suppression of immunity which leads in previously healthy young adults to severe infections and malignancies (Table 69). The population affected in the USA has been homosexuals (71%), heroin addicts (17%), Haitians (5%), haemophiliacs (1%), recipients of blood transfusions, heterosexual partners of patients and the babies of mothers with the disease. The diagnosis is supported by the following laboratory investigations: a lymphocytopenia (in particular a T-cell deficiency) with a relative reduction in helper-cells and a relative increase in suppressor cells, a reduced response of the lymphocytes to mitogens (e. g. phytohaemagglutinin) and the absence of killer activity. Immunoglobulins are usually increased. Previously positive tuberculin skin tests are negative (anergy).

Prophylaxis and treatment: The commonest infection is pneumocystis pneumonia which may be treated with co-trimoxazole (see p. 351). Patients with haemophilia A, who almost always suffer from pneumocystis pneumonia if they develop AIDS, should be given co-trimoxazole as soon as fever and the blood

Table 69. Opportunistic infections and tumours (in order of frequency) in the Acquired Immune Deficiency Syndrome (AIDS).

Opportunistic infections by	Tumours
Pneumocystis carinii	Kaposi's varicelliform sarcoma (visceral,
Cytomegalovirus	atypically on the skin)
Herpes simplex virus	Burkitt-like lymphomas
Candida species	Non-Hodgkin lymphomas
Mycobacterium avium-intracellulare	CNS lymphomas
Mycobacterium tuberculosis	Angioblastic lymphadenopathy
Cryptococcus neoformans	Lymphoblastic pre-leukaemia
Toxoplasma gondii	
Salmonellae	
Cryptosporidium	
Isospora belli	
Papovaviruses (progressive multi-focal	
leucoencephalopathy)	
Nocardia asteroides	
Histoplasma capsulatum	

changes described (lymphocytopenia etc.) occur. Toxoplasmosis (usually encephalitis) is treated with pyrimethamine + sulfadiazine. Acyclovir (see p. 536) is now available for herpes zoster and for herpes simplex infections, which are common in the anal region. No treatment, however, is available for cytomegalovirus infections which may present as pneumonia, hepatitis and retinitis. Locally invasive or disseminated infections with Candida respond to amphotericin B and flucytosine, as do cryptococcal infections of the lung and central nervous system and histoplasmosis.

Mycobacterial infections (p. 470) and salmonellosis (p. 449) may be treated with antibiotics as may nocardiosis (see p. 460). No treatment is currently available for certain protozoal infections such as Cryptosporidium or Isospora enteritis or for Papova (warts) virus infections which can lead to progressive multi-focal encephalopathy (PML). Malignant conditions may be treated in the usual way.

Prophylaxis against exposure is not practical for these generally endogenous infections. The viral cause of AIDS apparently occurs in blood and probably in seminal fluid. Patients at risk should be warned against promiscuity in sexual contact and encouraged to avoid exposure. Haemophiliacs may be protected by treatment predominantly with cryoprecipitate and homosexuals should not be accepted as blood donors. The indications for blood transfusion should be more strictly enforced than hitherto.

References

ALLEN, J. (ed.): Infection and the Compromised Host. Williams and Wilkins, New York 1981.

BARRE-SINOUSSI, F., J. C. CHERMAN, F. REY: Isolation of a T-lymphotropic retrovirus from a patient at risk for acquired immune deficiency syndrome. Science *220:* 868 (1983).

BELOHRADSKY, B. H., W. THEIL, S. DÄUMLING: Gnotobiotische Ergebnisse bei der Knochenmarktransplantation von Kindern mit akuter lymphoblastischer Leukämie. Z. antimikrob. Chemother. *1:* 5 (1983).

BODEY, G., V. RODRIGUEZ: Hospital Associated Infections in the Compromised Host. Dekker, New York 1979.

BRUNET, J. B., E. BRUVET, J. CHAPERON: Acquired immunodeficiency in France. Lancet *1:* 700 (1983).

EBBESEN, P., R. J. BRIGGAR, M. MELBYE: AIDS in Europe. Brit. med. J. *287:* 1324 (1983).

EORTC International Antimicrobial Therapy Project Group: Three antibiotic regimens in the treatment of infection in febrile granulocytopenic patients with cancer. J. infect. Dis. *137:* 14 (1978).

GAYA, H., J. KLASTERSKY, S. C. SCHIMPFF, D. FIÈRE, S. WIDMAIER, G. NAGEL: Prospective randomly controlled trial of three antibiotic combinations for empirical therapy of suspected sepsis in neutropenic cancer patients. Europ. J. Cancer *11:* 5 (1975).

HARTLAPP, J. H.: Empirische Antibiotikatherapie bei leukopenischen Patienten. Fortschr. antimikrob. Chemother. *3–1:* 39 (1984).

JONES, P.: Acquired immunodeficiency syndrome, hepatitis and haemophilia. Brit. med. J. *287:* 1737 (1983).

KLASTERSKY, J.: Therapy with antibiotics in leukemic patients. Infection *11:* 97 (1983).

KLASTERSKY, J. (ed.): Infections in Cancer Chemotherapy. Pergamon Press, Oxford 1976.

LEVINE, A. S., R. A. ROBINSON, J. M. HAUSER: Analysis of studies on protected environments and prophylactic antibiotics in adult leukemia. Europ. J. Cancer *11:* 57 (1975).

MEURET, G., A. ROUX, M. E. HEIM: Zur Behandlung der schweren febrilen Neutropenie. Dtsch. med. Wschr. *105:* 1776 (1980).

MUTTON, K., J. GUST: Acquired immune deficiency syndrome. Med. J. Austr. *1:* 540 (1983).

PINCHING, A. J.: Studies of cellular immunity in male homosexuals in London. Lancet *2:* 126 (1983).

STORRING, R. A., T. J. McELWAIN, B. JAMESON, E. WILTSHAW: Oral non-absorbed antibiotics prevent infection in acute non-lymphoblastic leukaemia. Lancet *2:* 837 (1977).

TILLMANN, W., G. PRINDULL, R. KÖNIG, A. BORNSCHEUER, W. WEIGEL: Sepsisverdacht bei leukämischen Kindern: Erfahrungen mit einer Kombination aus Cefotaxim und Gentamicin. Fortschr. antimikrob. Chemother. *2–1:* 117 (1983).

7. Chemoprophylaxis

In practice, the distinction between prophylaxis and early treatment is often blurred. Indiscriminate antibiotic prophylaxis is clearly as misguided as its total avoidance. The rules for antibiotic prophylaxis differ in operative and non-operative medicine. There are a number of well-founded rules which are now generally agreed. The following should be distinguished:

1. Chemoprophylaxis during the incubation period of an infection, e.g. with scarlet fever (after exposure) or malaria.
2. Prophylaxis of relapse after certain diseases (e.g. rheumatic fever).
3. Prophylaxis of otherwise unavoidable infectious complications (e.g. after major open-heart operation, or a contaminated wound).

1. **Chemoprophylaxis during the incubation period of an infection** is only used in certain situations because if applied indiscriminately, there would be a high failure rate and overgrowth of resistant bacteria and fungi would be promoted. The value of chemoprophylaxis in *malaria* is universally accepted, for example by taking chloroquine once or twice a week (300 mg base = 500 mg diphosphate or 2 tablets) up to 6 weeks after leaving the malarious area (p. 484).

Specific, properly dosed and continued antimicrobial suppression during the incubation period of a bacterial disease can prevent, attenuate or delay the infection:

Infants and children with a severe underlying disease (leukaemia, nephrosis etc.) should be treated after exposure to *whooping cough* with erythromycin or amoxycillin in normal dosage for 1–2 weeks and longer in persistent cases.

Tuberculin conversion in non-vaccinated children with no clinical signs of tuberculosis is an indication for isoniazid treatment for at least six months. Antituberculous chemoprophylaxis is also justified in infants with close family contacts with open tuberculosis.

Exposure to *syphilis* is justification for prophylactic benzyl penicillin, e.g. 2.4 megaunits of benzathine penicillin. If the dose of penicillin is too low, syphilis can be masked.

For post-exposure prophylaxis of *scarlet fever* phenoxymethyl penicillin should be given for 5–10 days in a daily dose of 250 mg (infants), 500 mg (school-children) and 1 g (adults).

Close contacts in an epidemic of *meningococcal disease,* and household contacts of a single case should be given prophylaxis. If the isolate is sensitive to sulphonamides, sulphadiazine should be given in a twice daily dose for 2 days of 250 mg (infants), 500 mg (children aged 1–12 years) and 1 g (older children and adults). If sulphonamide-resistant, rifampicin should be given in a twice daily dose for 2 days of 5 mg/kg (infants <1 year), 10 mg/kg (children aged 1–12 years) and 600 mg (patients over 12 years). Minocycline is an alternative.

2. **Prophylaxis of relapse:** The risk of relapse of *rheumatic fever* through a new streptococcal infection can be greatly reduced by the regular administration of phenoxymethyl penicillin. If the patient can be relied on, an oral dose of 250–500 mg a day is sufficient. A more certain method is to give 1.2 megaunits of benzathine penicillin i.m. once a month. This cannot, however, be used when penicillin allergy is suspected; in such cases, erythromycin, a sulphonamide or cephalexin should be given.

Prophylaxis of *endocarditis* is important in patients with abnormal or damaged heart valves, after an earlier attack of bacterial endocarditis in congenital heart disease, or after heart operations, or whenever the patient requires a surgical procedure which may give rise to transient bacteraemia (e.g. dental extraction, urological or gynaecological operation). As penicillin, erythromycin or vancomycin are used and detailed regimens are described in Part D, Chapter 3, p. 317.

Prevention of *recurrent ascending urinary infection:* Young women not infrequently suffer from recurrent cystitis, often related to sexual activity (e.g. honeymoon cystitis), but sometimes due to anatomical or physiological anomalies such as a short urethra or micturition which is too infrequent. The frequency of recurrence can be reduced by taking a small dose of an antimicrobial post-coitally or regularly every evening. This could be 50 mg of nitrofurantoin, 240 mg of cotrimoxazole or 250 mg of cephalexin. Such prophylaxis should continue over a long period and should not be confused with suppressive therapy at full dosage, e.g. in infected renal calculus.

Patients with *recurrent erysipelas* may be protected by long-term phenoxymethyl penicillin or a monthly i.m. injection of benzathine penicillin.

3. **Prophylaxis of infectious complications** resulting from mucosal ulceration, contaminated skin wounds, or certain operations such as colonic surgery, is often effective. Since the bacterial load can only be reduced temporarily by this means, this type of prophylaxis carries risks of superinfection or of changes of infecting agent. The effect is only temporary.

Patients who have *aspirated* material (unconsciousness, drowning, poisoning etc.) require antibiotic treatment of incipient pneumonia. Since non-sporing anaerobes are an important cause of aspiration pneumonia, an antibiotic active also against Bacteroides sp. should be used.

Patients undergoing high dose *corticosteroid therapy* are at risk of fulminant streptococcal, pneumococcal or meningococcal infections; this risk can be reduced by standard doses of a penicillin by mouth.

Patients with a history of tuberculosis who require high dose prednisone therapy should be given prophylactic isoniazid (5 mg/kg/day) because of the danger of reactivation of old tuberculosis. The threshold dose of prednisone above which an infection may be reactivated is 20 mg a day.

Patients with *bone marrow suppression* should be given parenteral antibiotics when severely granulocytopenic. The full range of possible infecting organisms should be covered. The prophylaxis can be extended by intestinal decontamination, with, for example, neomycin, polymyxin B and nystatin. Even so, some gaps in antibiotic activity will remain and infection with resistant organisms can still occur.

Prophylaxis in *patients on mechanical ventilators* is difficult, since systemic antibiotics are only likely to suppress some lung infections. The instillation of gentamicin locally into the trachea may reduce upper respiratory colonisation with gram-negative bacilli and the consequent pneumonia which sometimes occurs with these organisms. The patients are given 1–2 ml of a dilute gentamicin solution (2–10 mg/ml) every time the trachea is aspirated. Little gentamicin is likely to be absorbed by this route. Because the colonising flora may change, regular bacteriological cultures should be carried out.

The most important *indications for prophylaxis in surgery* are:
operations in infected areas (particularly the colon and uterus),
sternotomy,
neurosurgical operations,
implantation of intravascular devices,
bites, penetrating and crush injuries, including stab and bullet wounds,
trauma involving the paranasal sinuses or joints,
fracture of the base of the skull,
limb amputation for ischaemia,
gas-gangrene prophylaxis.

Various antibiotics may be given parenterally for these indications (p. 386). Benzyl penicillin, an acylamino penicillin, an antistaphylococcal penicillin (e.g. flucloxacillin), a cephalosporin or an aminoglycoside may be used. Metronidazole and clindamycin are particularly effective against anaerobes.

To prevent *gas gangrene* after contaminated wounds or lower limb amputation for ischaemia, moderate doses of benzyl penicillin are sufficient.

Staphylococci are important causes of infection after sternotomy, intravascular implantation of foreign bodies and in neurosurgery and prophylaxis must be active against penicillin-resistant strains. *Anaerobes* are important in abdominal and gynaecological operations and prophylaxis for these should cover Bacteroides fragilis.

Antibiotic prophylaxis in surgery was often started too late and continued too long. Antibiotics should start shortly before or during the operation; if an unexpected situation arises which needs antibiotic cover (e.g. the opening of a viscus), they should be given without delay by the anasthesist. Controlled studies have shown that prophylaxis given for too long is of no value and may even be harmful by encouraging colonisation by resistant flora. Views on the optimal duration of perioperative prophylaxis vary from one dose to 3 days, but *correct timing is very important,* and a start just before the operation is the best. The distinction between prophylaxis and early treatment is often blurred, but an established infection should be properly treated for as long as necessary.

References

CHODAK, G. W., M. E. PLAUT: Use of systemic antibiotics for prophylaxis in surgery: A critical review. Arch. Surg. *112:* 326 (1977).

CLARKE, J. S., R. E. CONDON, J. G. BARTLETT, S. L. GORBACH, R. L. NICHOLS, S. OCHI: Preoperative oral antibiotics reduce septic complications of colon operations: Results of prospective randomized double-blind clinical study. Ann. Surg. *186:* 251 (1977).

GARROD, L. P.: Chemoprophylaxis. Brit. med. J. *4:* 561 (1975).

MYEROWITZ, P. D., K. CASWELL, W. G. LINDSAY, D. M. NICOLOFF: Antibiotic prophylaxis for open-heart surgery. J. thorac. cardiovasc. Surg. *73:* 625 (1977).

WARREN, J. W., R. PLATT, R. J. THOMAS: Antibiotic irrigation and catheter-associated urinary tract infection. New Engl. J. Med. *299:* 570 (1978).

8. Hospital Infections

Range of organisms: The commonest causes of hospital (nosocomial) infections are resistant strains of Staphylococcus, Klebsiella and Pseudomonas aeruginosa. Other gram-negative bacilli such as Serratia marcescens, enterobacteria, Proteus, Salmonella and Shigella, and fungi such as Candida and Aspergillus fumigatus are also found. Mixed infections are common. Viruses (e.g. hepatitis B) can also be acquired and transmitted in hospital. Table 70 summarises the occurrence, mode of transmission, clinical picture and the use of antibiotics in such cases.

The **spread** of these organisms in hospital may be encouraged by the indiscriminate use of antibiotics. Antibiotics which exert a strong selective pressure can, given excessively to patients undergoing operations or at high risk in intensive care units, lead to infections with klebsiellae and other gram-negative bacilli. The main reason for such infections is immunological impairment, particularly when the patient is receiving immunosuppressive drugs such as

Table 70. Main causes of hospital infection.

Organism	Reservoir	Mode of transmission	Important clinical infections	Usual antibiotic susceptibilities
Staphylococcus aureus	Respiratory tract, nasal mucosa and skin of patients and staff, infected wounds and venous catheters	Droplets, contact, hands, contaminated objects, e.g. beds, hand towels, autoinfection, infected food	Post-operative wound infection, pneumonia, suppurative parotitis, mastitis, sepsis, osteomyelitis, post-antibiotic enterocolitis, foreign-body infection	Penicillinase-stable penicillins, cephalosporins, fusidic acid, clindamycin, erythromycin, vancomycin
Pseudomonas aeruginosa	Dirt, waste water, infected wounds, sometimes faeces	Contact, contaminated hands, fluids, disinfectants, catheter lubricant, infected milk, ventilators	Wound infections, particularly burns, septicaemia, urinary infections after urological operations, foreign-body infections, otitis externa	Tobramycin, amikacin, azlocillin, piperacillin, cefsulodin, ceftazidime, norfloxacin
Multi-resistant gram-negative bacilli (Klebsiella, Enterobacter, Proteus, Serratia etc.)	Varies according to organism and hospital, intestinal tract	Contact, contaminated objects, autoinfection, ventilators	Urinary infections, wound infections, pneumonia, septicaemia	Gentamicin, amikacin, cefoxitin, cefuroxime, cefotaxime, norfloxacin
Candida, especially C. albicans	Mouth and intestinal tract of patients and staff, air	Autoinfection, contact (genitalia, birth canal), fomites (dummies, milk bottle, teats etc.)	Thrush, napkin dermatitis, post-antibiotic stomatitis, vaginitis, burns, septicaemia (mainly from infected venous catheters), pneumonia	Local nystatin etc. and, in severe generalised infections, amphotericin B and/or flucytosine, miconazole or ketoconazole

cytotoxic agents and corticosteroids. Some secondary infection (e.g. of the respiratory tract during long-term ventilation) is often unavoidable in an intensive care unit. The organisms may be endogenous bacteria or fungi from the patient's own skin or mucous membranes (autoinfection). On the other hand, patients debilitated by their underlying disease can become infected from other patients or from carriers among the hospital staff (cross-infection). Hospital infections are more common in surgical and gynaecological patients than in medical and paediatric wards. Portals of entry can be provided by infected venous catheters, urethral catheters, feeding tubes, aerosol and breathing equipment, air conditioners and the incorrect use of disinfectants. Contaminated intravenous infusion solutions are particularly dangerous. Food from hospital kitchens has on occasion been contaminated with salmonellae, pseudomonas etc., which can be a danger to patients with serious underlying disease.

The **prevention** of hospital infection is difficult since the patients themselves are usually the reservoir of potentially pathogenic organisms. The introduction of single unproven measures (e.g. UV lamps) is of no value. Good general hospital design and nursing practice are much more important, and careful hand-washing and hand-disinfection by all staff after every contact with a patient is essential.

Certain categories of infected patients should be isolated and nursed with special procedures. In other areas of the hospital, however, the routine use of disinfectants for walls, floors, furniture, sinks etc., is very expensive and of no value. Accommodation where infected patients have been isolated should be terminally disinfected. Any equipment (including beds, mattresses, linen), which comes into close contact with patients and then has to be re-used, such as baby incubators, ventilators etc., should be thoroughly cleaned, dried and decontaminated.

The environmental hygiene of operating theatres requires stricter control and the details of air changes and filtration, sterilisation of instruments, the pre-operative "scrub-up" and sterile gowning for the surgeon and his assistants, and general operating theatre discipline are beyond the scope of this book.

A key role can be played by infection control staff in advising on safe procedures and policies in all areas of the hospital, including nursing, medical services, catering, the collection and transmission of pathology specimens, and the disposal of clinical waste. The correct function of hospital plant, e.g. autoclaves, air conditioning, incinerators should be regularly tested by engineering staff. The routine screening of hospital staff for bacterial carriage is not worthwhile unless carried out so frequently that the expense would be prohibitive. Kitchen and nursing staff should, however, have a faecal examination after a diarrhoeal illness and possibly after returning from abroad. Ward and operating staff may be required to submit specimens, e.g. nose or throat swabs, when outbreaks of infection are investigated.

The judicious use of antibiotics should reduce the selection of multi-resistant hospital bacteria and in many hospitals general antibiotic policies which allow antibiotic use to be controlled are now accepted. Good general principles, such as the avoidance of systemic antibiotics for topical use, should also be applied. Antibiotics are seldom the direct cause of hospital infection, even when the selection of resistant strains is involved. Antibiotics should, therefore, never be withheld from a patient in whom there is a clear clinical indication for their use, purely because of the fear of spreading resistant bacteria.

There is no general answer to the **control of hospital infection.** Some surveillance is useful, whether general or selective, so that clusters of infection can be identified and control measures instigated where appropriate. Indiscriminate bacteriological sampling of the environment is of little value, though occasional, planned surveys using surface or contact swabs, settle plates and measured air sampling may be useful in commissioning a new ward or operating theatre, investigating a specific incident or outbreak, or for general educational purposes. Such exercises should only be carried out after consultation and agreement with the microbiologist or hospital hygienist. Typing methods (e.g. phage typing of staphylococci and salmonellae, M and T typing of streptococci, serotyping of gram-negative bacilli) can be useful in clarifying the source and modes of spread of bacteria, and can form a basis for the introduction of control measures.

Good standards of hygiene, discipline and education are essential if hospital infection is to be controlled. Those responsible for hospital hygiene should, with any others involved, formulate policies for the limited use of disinfectants in the hospital, the standardisation of nursing and domestic procedures, the safe functioning of support departments (catering, laundry, sterile supply) and the management of infected patients. All of these can be embodied in a hospital control of infection policy. The organisation of the control of infection is best carried out by a full-time interdisciplinary clinician or medical microbiologist with the support of a representative committee, and who can also advise physicians on the rational use of antibiotics.

References

DASCHNER, F.: Hygiene auf Intensivstationen. Springer, Berlin 1981.

KIOSZ, D., CHR. STOFFREGEN, C. SIMON: Über den Luftkeimgehalt in Inkubatoren und auf neonatologischen Intensivstationen. Mschr. Kinderheilk. 132: 274 (1984).

KONOLD, P., U. ULLMANN, C.-P. SCHRADER, G. KIENIGER: Klinische und bakteriologische Beobachtungen bei intravenös eingeführten Kathetern. Dtsch. med. Wschr. 99: 1009 (1974).

MARSHALL, B. R., J. K. HEPLER, W. S. JINGUJI: Fatal streptococcus pyogenes septicemia associated with an intrauterine device. Obstet. Gynecol. *41:* 83 (1973).

MERTZ, J. J., L. SCHARER, J. H. McCLEMENT: A hospital outbreak of Klebsiella pneumoniae from inhalation therapy with contaminated aerosol solutions. Amer. Rev. resp. Dis. *95:* 454 (1976).

PICHLER, H., G. KRYSTOF, F. CORAIM, W. KOLLER, G. WEWALKA: Einfluß der Antibiotika-prophylaxe auf die Infektionserreger von Intensivpatienten und die Flora der Intensiv-behandlungsstation. Mschr. Kinderheilk. *125:* 284 (1977).

SMITH, P. W., R. M. MASSANARI: Room humidifiers as the source of Acinetobacter infections. JAMA *237:* 795 (1977).

WEWALKA, G., W. KOLLER, M. ROTTER, F. LACKNER, F. CORAIM, H. PICHLER: Der Patient als Keimquelle in der Intensivpflegestation. Einfluß von Antibiotika und trachealer Intuba-tion. Infection *4:* 204 (1976).

9. Antibiotics in the Elderly

Frequency of infection: Infections which require antibiotics are commoner in patients over 65 years than in young adults, largely because of the increased incidence of diseases which lower the resistance to infection such as malignancies, diabetes and cirrhosis. Deaths from pneumonia in Europe are mainly in the over 65 age group (80–85%) whereas deaths from pneumonia in those aged between 5 and 40 are uncommon. The frequency of newly detected tuberculosis in adult males increases steadily with age and reaches its peak above the age of 60. The relative frequency of tuberculosis in the elderly comes from post-mortem statistics; active tuberculosis is often not detected in life. Elderly patients often suffer from chronic respiratory and urinary disease, mainly due to anatomical changes (e. g. pulmonary emphysema, prostatism, vaginal prolapse etc.). Fungal skin infections and organ mycoses are apparantly commoner in the elderly. Infected gangrene in arteriosclerosis and recurrent erysipelas mainly occur in later years.

Susceptibility to infection: Increased susceptibility with age is only found for certain diseases (pneumonia, septicaemia, urinary infections etc.) which are generally related to factors such as the ageing of organs or systems, or a severe underlying disease such as malignancy. The humoral and cellular immunities normally remain intact with age and the secondary immune response is not reduced. Evidence exists, however, that defects in the T-cell system become commoner in the elderly and can considerably influence the course of infections.

Special clinical and diagnostic features: Typical symptoms of localised infection or septicaemia, such as fever or leucocytosis, are often absent in the elderly. Pneumonia can be present without clear signs in the chest. Bacteriological sputum results are often difficult to interpret since gram-negative bacilli can colonise the mouth as a result of frequent courses of antibiotics (e.g. ampicillin) and mix with the bronchial secretions. More useful results may be obtained of bronchial secretion by bronchoscopy for other indications, or by transtracheal aspiration. A sudden hypotension may be the only sign of gram-negative septicaemia with shock. Pulmonary tuberculosis can be present in the elderly even though the tuberculin reaction is weak (positive at 10 or 100 U only). Urinary infections are often silent. The examination of a mid-stream urine in elderly females is often unreliable because of difficulties of collection, and bladder puncture or catheterisation may be necessary. The presence of several diseases, such as arteriosclerosis, cardiac insufficiency, diabetes, cirrhosis, renal insufficiency can obscure the symptoms of infectious diseases.

Tolerance to antibiotics: Underlying diseases sometimes reduce the tolerance to drugs. When the patient has liver disease, potentially hepatotoxic agents such as the tetracyclines, rifampicin, isoniazid etc. should only be used with caution. The dosage must be considerably modified in cases of renal insufficiency (p. 510). In severe cardiac failure, the renal function is affected and the excretion of certain antibiotics (e.g. amikacin) is delayed, often giving rise to side effects. Potentially nephrotoxic antibiotics should be avoided in patients with acute or impending impaired renal function. The combination of cephalothin and gentamicin can cause kidney function in the elderly to deteriorate. Nalidixic acid, carindacillin and pivampicillin are badly tolerated in patients with gastric disorders. If several drugs are given they can interfere with one another; anticoagulants are particularly susceptible. By competition for plasma albumin binding sites, the concentration of free coumarin anticoagulants can be increased by sulphonamide therapy, thus potentiating this anticoagulant effect.

Pharmacokinetics: Pharmacokinetic studies comparing the elderly with young adults have only been carried out with a few antibiotics, e.g. benzyl penicillin, propicillin, ampicillin, cefazolin, cephradine and doxycycline. With the exception of doxycycline the mean serum concentrations in subjects over 60 years of age were significantly higher than in those aged between 20 and 30. The biological *half-life* of the penicillins and cephalosporins was prolonged in the elderly and the total clearance and renal clearance were reduced in the presence of normal serum urea and creatinine values. The higher serum concentrations in the elderly can only be partially explained by physiological renal impairment. The *volume of distribution* and tissue diffusion of certain drugs are obviously reduced in the elderly. The lipophilic doxycycline with a half-life of about 15 hours behaves, on the other hand, as in young adults. The elimination of penicillins such as carbenicillin and ampicillin is delayed in severe cardiac failure. The *plasma protein* *binding* of penicillins (benzyl penicillin, cloxacillin) is not reduced in persons over 70, although hypoalbuminaemia which occurs in certain diseases can increase the concentrations of free antibiotic in the blood. The *absorption* of propicillin, for example, is not reduced on oral administration; relevant studies are missing for many other antibiotics. The simultaneous administration of antacids can reduce the absorption of tetracyclines by chelate formation. Oral pivampicillin was only slightly less absorbed after partial or total gastrectomy than in healthy subjects.

Practical therapeutic recommendations: *Early diagnosis* (including laboratory and x-ray examination) and *prompt initiation of treatment* are very important in the treatment of many serious infections in the elderly. Bacteriological cultures of blood, sputum or urine should be taken before starting any treatment so that if the patient fails to respond, a change can be made on the basis of culture and sensitivities. When choosing an antibiotic, one should remember that multiresistant gram-negative bacilli (Klebsiella, Enterobacter, Pseudomonas, Serratia etc.) are commoner in chronic respiratory or urinary infections than in acute bacterial infections; a β-lactamase-stable cephalosporin or an aminoglycoside should therefore be given. Wherever possible, treatment should be based on sensitivity testing. Less sensitive organisms or life-threatening infections should be treated with a combination to achieve synergy or broaden the spectrum of action. The bacteriological investigations should be repeated during therapy in case the infecting organism changes, and to monitor the effectiveness of therapy.

Treatment in hospital often has advantages, including better facilities for investigation, the possibility of parenteral administration and control of the drug administration and clinical effectiveness. The elderly often take oral drugs irregularly. Long-acting preparations can be useful at home, such as depot penicillins, doxycycline or rolitetracycline which can be given parenterally at a daily visit.

Oral antibiotics can conveniently be given to the elderly in calendar packs so that the patient or his physician can check whether the drug has been taken (control of compliance). If the patient is receiving a large number of drugs, some may be better omitted temporarily to ensure that the antibiotic is reliably taken and absorbed.

The patient should only be kept in bed during the acute phase of the infection. *Early mobilisation* is beneficial and the careful treatment of symptoms can be lifesaving.

Pneumonia in the elderly is usually bronchopneumonia. Aspiration, a previous viral infection (influenza) or alcoholism often play a role. Carcinoma of the bronchus should always be considered in recurrent or abscess-forming pneumonia. The causative organism is unlikely to be cultured without a transtracheal aspiration. Pneumococci, streptococci, staphylococci, Haemophilus and Bacteroides should be considered in pneumonias which originate at home. Cefoxitin is a suitable antibiotic treatment, as are a combination of doxycycline + clindamycin, erythromycin or amoxycillin plus metronidazole. Pneumonias originating in hospital may also be due to gram-negative bacilli, when a combination such as gentamicin + piperacillin or cefotaxime + azlocillin should be used, since gram-negative pneumonia has poor prognosis in the elderly.

Infected arteriosclerotic gangrene: This nearly always involves mixed infections of aerobic and anaerobic streptococci, Bacteroides sp., staphylococci, clostridia (gas gangrene) and resistant gram-negative bacilli. Narrow-spectrum therapy is not advisable. The antibiotics used should have as wide a range of activity as possible and also penetrate the ischaemic tissue adequately. Initial treatment with 20–30 megaunits of benzyl penicillin i. v. a day does not cover the full range of possible pathogens and a combination with a β-lactamase-stable cephalosporin, clindamycin or metronidazole is recommended. The chances of success of such antibiotic therapy should not be overestimated. If amputation becomes necessary, antibiotic cover must be given to prevent postoperative gas gangrene.

Recurrent erysipelas: The portals of entry are often small skin erosions; if they occur on the legs, there is a particular risk of relapse through postthrombotic changes or lymphoedema. Acute erysipelas is best treated with high doses of benzyl penicillin, and relapses may be prevented with long-term benzathine penicillin, 1.2 megaunits i. m. once a month.

Geriatric urinary infections: Disorders of micturition (e. g. by prostatic adenoma or vaginal prolapse) are often present. The range of organisms may depend on the number of previous urological operations; an indwelling catheter or a prostatectomy often lead to infections with multiresistant bacteria. Treatment should if possible be based on culture and sensitivities.

References

Brühl, P.: Zur Therapie der Harnwegsinfektion bei alten Menschen. Z. Geront. *4:* 258 (1971).
Coper, H.: Pharmakologische Grundlagen der Therapie beim alten Menschen. Acta geront. *6:* 207 (1976).
Estler, C. J.: Wirkungsveränderungen von Pharmaka im Alter. Med. Welt *26:* 795 (1975).
Falck, I.: Das Tuberkuloseproblem in der Geriatrie. Z. Geront. *8:* 12 (1975).
Freeman, J. T.: Some principles of medications in geriatrics. J. Amer. Geriat. Soc. *22:* 289 (1974).
Götz, H.: Immunologische Besonderheiten im Alter. In: Falck, J. et al. (ed.): Infektionen beim alten Menschen. Roche, Basel, 1977.

GSELL, O.: Besonderheiten der Pharmakotherapie in der Geriatrie. Z. präklin. Geriatrie *5:* 1 (1975).
HALL, M. R. P.: Use of drugs in elderly patients. N. Y. St. J. Med. *24:* 67 (1975).
SIMON, C., V. MALERCZYK, U. MÜLLER, G. MÜLLER: Zur Pharmakokinetik von Propicillin bei geriatrischen Patienten im Vergleich zu jüngeren Erwachsenen. Dtsch. med. Wschr. *97:* 1999 (1972).
SIMON, C., V. MALERCZYK, G. ZIEROTT, K. LEHMANN, U. THIESEN: Blut-, Harn- und Gallespiegel von Ampicillin bei intravenöser Dauerinfusion. Arzneimittel-Forsch. *25:* 654 (1975).
SIMON, C., V. MALERCZYK, H. ENGELKE, I. PREUSS, H. GRAHMANN, K. SCHMIDT: Die Pharmakokinetik von Doxycyclin bei Niereninsuffizienz und geriatrischen Patienten im Vergleich zu jüngeren Erwachsenen. Schweiz. med. Wschr. *105:* 1615 (1975).
SIMON, C., V. MALERCZYK, B. TENSCHERT, F. MÖHLENBECK: Die geriatrische Pharmakologie von Cefazolin, Cefradin und Sulfisomidin. Arzneimittel-Forsch. *26:* 1377 (1976).
WEINSTEIN, L.: Whatever happened to the "old-time" infections? J.A.M.A. *229:* 196 (1974).
WILLEROTH, C., H. GEISSMEYER: Die Tuberkulose in einem großen Obduktionsgut der Jahre 1962 bis 1971. I. Inaktive und aktive Lungentuberkulosen und Miliartuberkulosen. Zbl. allg. Path. path. Anat. *118:* 37 (1974).

10. Failure of Chemotherapy

Reasons: The failure of fever to resolve, clinical improvement to occur or bacterial cultures to become sterile can have various causes. The wrong choice of antibiotic, an inappropriate dose or route of administration, or the omission of bacteriological investigations are avoidable. Other reasons for failure are the virulence of the pathogen, impaired host resistance because of severe underlying disease in the patient, delay in starting treatment, secondary infections, development of antibiotic resistance in the pathogen, or a change in infecting agent. Treatment may appear to be ineffective if assessed too early in a severe general infection such as typhoid fever, septicaemia, osteomyelitis or meningitis, when resolution may be slower, perhaps not until 5–8 days after beginning treatment. Fever can also persist despite antibiotic treatment in viral infections, intracranial complications, development of an empyema, malignant disease and drug allergy; it should not, therefore, necessarily be blamed on the antibiotic.

Discrepancy between clinical and bacteriological results: Considering the large number of factors which affect the course of an infection, it is not surprising that sensitivity testing does not always correlate with the results of treatment. Facultative pathogens present as contaminants in blood cultures, pus swabs etc. can be misinterpreted as the causative organisms. Bacteriological specimens should therefore be taken wherever possible by the doctor himself using aseptic precautions, and sent to the bacteriology laboratory promptly, if possible within

1–2 hours. Infections with organisms which are difficult to culture may need to be inoculated at the bedside on fresh media (e. g. blood cultures, or pernasal swabs on special media for whooping-cough). If there is no local bacteriological laboratory, transport media should be used, or kits (e. g. dip-slides for urine) should be inoculated on collection. Transport media are essential if fragile organisms such as anaerobes are to survive.

Treatment occasionally fails even though the organism has been shown to be sensitive in vitro; conversely, infections sometimes resolve despite apparent resistance of the organisms cultured. Antibiotic sensitivities are usually tested by disc-diffusion using average concentrations. Discrepancies from clinical results may occur because the tissue concentrations in the body are lower than the test concentrations used in vitro. Sometimes, however, higher concentrations occur in vivo, e. g. in urine, than are tested in the laboratory. Moreover, the standard in vitro tests do not apply to antibiotics for local use, where large concentrations can occur. The value of antibiotic sensitivity testing is mainly to enable the clinician to choose, from a range of antibiotics with activity in vitro, that agent which is pharmacokinetically the most suitable, gives the best results according to clinical experience and has the least danger of side effects.

If antibiotics fail when given before the bacterial cause has been isolated, the likeliest reason is that the *pathogen is resistant* and has been treated with an inappropriate antibiotic. After 2–3 days treatment should then be changed to an agent or combination with a broader spectrum.

Supplementary measures: Other forms of treatment such as operation, aspiration of pus, treatment of shock, and parenteral nutrition should not be overlooked. This is especially true of empyema, cerebral abscess, subphrenic abscess and chronic osteomyelitis, where surgical measures are often required for antibiotic therapy to be successful.

11. Chemotherapy of Viral Diseases

Most viral infections do not require chemotherapy, resolve spontaneously and should be managed symptomatically. Potentially fatal diseases, however, such as herpes simplex encephalitis and herpes neonatorum should be treated with antiviral agents. Otherwise mild viral infections (e. g. chicken-pox, herpes zoster or cytomegalovirus infection) can be severe or prolonged in patients with immunosuppression from treatment with cytotoxic agents, radiotherapy, or malignancy. Persistent viral infections, e. g. chronic aggressive hepatitis or

Table 71. Mode and spectrum of action of clinically tested antiviral agents. VZV = varicella zoster virus, EBV = Epstein-Barr virus, CMV = cytomegalovirus.

Process affected	Drug	Virus inhibited
Penetration, uncoating	Amantadine, rimantadine	Influenza A, influenza B
Replication	Idoxuridine Adenine arabinoside	Herpes simplex DNA-viruses, VZV, EBV, herpes simplex, CMV, pox viruses
	Acyclovir	DNA-viruses, VZV, EBV, herpes simplex, CMV
Viral protein synthesis	Methisazone, interferon	Vaccinia, variola, DNA and RNA viruses
Assembly, release	Interferon	RNA-tumour viruses

subacute sclerosing panencephalitis, have a poor prognosis and rapid elimination of the pathogen is important. Unfortunately, few selective antiviral agents are yet available. Only acyclovir and adenine arabinoside (Table 71) are now licensed for systemic use. Other agents are still undergoing clinical trials. Idoxuridine and adenine arabinoside are available for local use. Unproven drugs propagated for the treatment of viral diseases should be avoided.

Only two preparations, methisazone and amantadine, are currently useful for the *prevention of viral infections*. Some viral infections may be prevented or suppressed with pooled normal human immunoglobulin or in some cases with human hyperimmune immunoglobulin containing more specific virus antibodies. Immunoglobulins are only prophylactic as long as the viruses are extracellular. The value of immunostimulants, such as isoprinosine (dimethylamino-2-propranol-4-acetamidobenzoate) is not established.

Methisazone (N-methylisatin-β-thiosemicarbazone) affects viral maturation at a later stage by inhibiting the incorporation of nucleic acid in the viral capsid; it was formerly used for smallpox prophylaxis, when prompt administration during the early stages of the disease (3 g twice a day at 12 h intervals in adults, and 1.5 g twice a day in children aged 3–10 years) reduced the number of cases and fatalities. This drug has the disadvantage of poor tolerance (vomiting and alcohol tolerance). It has been successfully used to treat post-vaccinial complications such as eczema vaccinatum, vaccinia gangrenosum and generalised vaccinia. Children should be given 200 mg/kg/day in 2–3 single doses for 2–3 days. After the eradication of smallpox, this agent may be useful in cases of African monkey pox.

Proprietary name: Marboran.

Amantadine (1-adamantane hydrochloride) inhibits viral penetration into the cell and, when given early, acts against influenza A_2 infection but not against influenza B virus. *Well absorbed* by mouth. *Urinary recovery:* >90% (unchanged). There are considerable side effects such as restlessness, tremor, ataxia, lack of concentration, lassitude, depression, dryness of the mouth, rashes etc.; the drug is mainly used in the treatment of Parkinson's disease. *Contra-indications:* pregnancy. Use with caution in patients with epilepsy, cerebral arteriosclerosis and

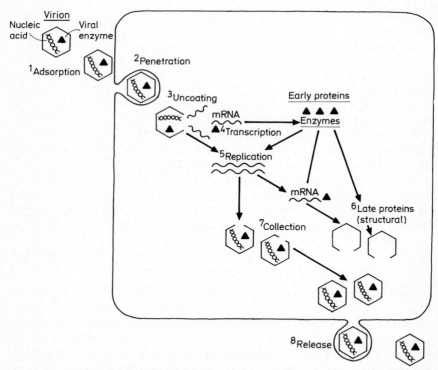

Fig. 35. Stages of viral reproduction within the cell. (After Y. J. BRYSON: Antiviral Agents. In: R. D. FEIGIN, M. D. CHERRY [eds.]: Textbook of Pediatric Infectious Diseases. Saunders, Philadelphia 1981.)

kidney disease. When used for the prophylaxis of influenza, it should only be given with simultaneous immunisation under certain circumstances. The *dose* is 200 mg a day by mouth for adults, 150 mg for children from 5–9 years, 50–100 mg for children from 1–5 years, all for at least 10 days after infection.

Proprietary name: Symmetrel.

Idoxuridine (5-iodo-2'-desoxyuridine) is a halogenated thymidine analogue which inhibits viral synthesis by competitive antagonism with thymidine (5-methyl-desoxyuridine) through the incorporation of altered nucleotide bases. Since it has a similar function in uninfected cells and is rapidly degraded in the body, it cannot be used in general therapy. Systemic use in generalised herpes or herpes encephalitis is no longer justified on account of its unreliable action and considerable side effects. A skin ointment containing 0.2% idoxuridine is available for the treatment of *herpes simplex infections of skin and mucous membranes;* but because of the poor solubility of idoxuridine, its effectiveness is limited and of little value in this largely self-limiting condition. A solution with 0.11% idoxuridine should be applied to areas of skin affected by herpes simplex several times a day. A 5% solution of idoxuridine in dimethyl sulphoxide may be painted on affected areas of *cutaneous herpes zoster* 4 times a day, but has the side effect of severe burning. Idoxuridine drops are used as local treatment of *herpes simplex keratitis,* applying 1–2 drops to the infected cornea, firstly every hour during the day and every 2 hours at night, then every 2 hours by day and every 4 hours at night (for 3–5 days) once improvement sets in. The eye ointment is applied every 4 hours into the conjunctival sac, that is, about 5 times a day. When used too frequently, signs of irritation can appear (pain, itching, oedema, photophobia, and even small areas of surface ulceration).

Proprietary names: Aedurid, Herpid, Iduridin, IDU, Synmiol.

Commercial forms: Eye drops (0.1%; 0.15%), eye ointment (0.1%; 0.2%; 0.5%), gel (0.3%) and a solution for subconjunctival injection (0.5%).

Trifluorothymidine is a halogenated pyrimidine structurally similar to idoxuridine and thymidine. Its action on herpetic corneal ulcers is greater and more rapid than idoxuridine but it can only be used locally because of its toxicity. Trifluorothymidine is available as eye drops and ointment.

Adenine arabinoside is a purine nucleoside analogue which blocks intracellular viral reproduction by inhibition of DNA polymerase. The *action* on herpes simplex virus (types 1 and 2), varicella zoster and vaccinia viruses is much stronger than that on cytomegalovirus. It is better tolerated and less immunosuppressive than cytosine arabinoside which should no longer be used to treat viral infections. After i.v. infusion, preferably over 12 hours, adenine arabinoside is mainly *metabolised* in the liver to hypoxanthine arabinoside which has a weaker antiviral action than the original substance. The *half-life* of adenine arabinoside is 4 hours and elimination is mainly urinary (unchanged and as a metabolite). Adenine arabinoside has proved in clinical trials to be an effective treatment of progressive mucocutaneous herpes simplex in patients with malignant disease, as well as in herpetic uveitis and herpes simplex infections of the newborn. *Systemic use* in cancer patients with progressive zoster can heal the skin lesions rapidly. Adenine arabinoside has now been largely superceded by acyclovir, which is more reliable and has fewer side effects. Adenine arabinoside is still useful for the *local treatment* of herpes simplex keratitis and is better tolerated than idoxuridine. The 3% ointment may be used to treat herpes simplex and zoster of both the eye and the skin. The effectiveness in cytomegalovirus infection of the newborn is very unreliable. *Side effects* including nausea, vomiting and mild diarrhoea have been observed in 5–10% of cases given i. v. infusions of 5–15 mg/kg a day for 5–15 days. Tremor, EEG changes, bone marrow suppression and loss of weight have been reported at higher doses.

Acyclovir (acycloguanosin) is a guanine derivative with an acyclic side-chain:

9–(2-hydroxyethoxymethyl) guanin

Mode of action: Acyclovir inhibits viral replication in infected cells in the body without interfering with the function of non-infected cells. After uptake into the infected cell, acyclovir is first transformed to acycloguanosine monophosphate by a viral thymidine kinase. The triphosphate is then derived from the monophosphate using the cell's own kinases. This triphosphate is the active substance which inhibits the virus-specific DNA polymerase, hence interrupting the chain of viral DNA synthesis. The body's own cellular DNA polymerase, on the other hand, is only inactivated 1/10th to 1/30th as much. Acyclovir is effective against herpes simplex virus (types 1 and 2) and varicella zoster virus. The activity against cytomegalievirus, hepatitis B virus and Epstein-Barr virus is questionable. Only 1/3000th of the concentration needed to inhibit the body's cells will completely inhibit herpes simplex virus. Resistance of varicella zoster virus to acyclovir has not yet been reported, although 5–10% of herpes simplex infections are now resistant. Because of its selectivity and low toxicity, acyclovir is now the agent of choice in the treatment of herpes simplex and varicella zoster infections in oncological patients and after organ transplantation.

The *dosage* in herpes simplex is 5 mg/kg 3 times a day as an i.v. infusion for 5 days; in chicken pox, zoster and herpes encephalitis, 10 mg/kg should be given 3 times a day for 10 days. The dose-interval should be extended in renal failure to 12 hours when the creatinine clearance is 25–50 ml/min/1.73 m^2 and to 24 hours when the creatinine clearance is 10–25 ml/min/1.73 m^2. When the clearance is 0–10 ml/min/1.73 m^2, *half* the normal dose is given every 24 hours.

Side effects include a slight increase in serum creatinine and urea. There is a danger of crystalluria so the solution must always be diluted according to instructions, and adequate diuresis must be achieved during administration. Cutaneous zoster may be treated locally with acyclovir eye ointment but this is not sufficient in oncological patients. The eye ointment has proved effective in herpes simplex keratitis and in ocular zoster.

Prophylaxis of herpes simplex infections with intravenous acyclovir is recommended in the first 4 weeks after bone marrow transplantation. Acyclovir tablets (200 mg 4 times a day) also appear to be suitable for this purpose. The bioavailability with oral administration is only 20%, so high dosage is necessary. Intravenous acyclovir may prevent chicken pox when given in therapeutic dosage to children with malignant disease after exposure.

Interferons are formed in the body's cells during viral infections. They are species-specific proteins which inhibit the early stages of viral reproduction. The interferons act against many viruses and are part of the body's defences.

All interferons have (among other properties) antiviral activity, but they are distinguishable biochemically according to their cellular origin and the type of inducer used. Thus, diploid cells from human fibroblasts produce a different interferon than that from human leucocytes which has been induced by stimulation of viral or double-stranded RNA.

Immune interferon is obtained from lymphocytes by treatment with mitogens (e.g. phytohaemagglutinin) or specific antigens (e.g. herpes simplex virus). Gene technology will lead to a sufficient supply with different interferons in future. Interferons inhibit the synthesis of viral proteins in cells, which thereby become resistant to the viruses. Interferon given parenterally is rapidly removed from the blood (half-life 2–4 hours) but its antiviral activity is maintained for longer in the tissues. Clinical trials of purified human leucocyte interferon in immunosuppressed oncological patients with *herpes zoster* showed the primary lesions to heal more rapidly and generalised spread to be less likely after the i.m. injection of a highly concentrated preparation (5×10^5 units/kg/day). The frequency of severe *varicella* in children with malignant disease was reduced by interferon, and the

Table 72. Passive prophylaxis of viral infections with normal pooled human (polyvalent) immunoglobulin of specific high titre hyperimmune globulin.

Passive protection against	Dose (ml/kg) of	
	polyvalent immuno-globulin (intramuscular)	specific hyperimmune globulin (intramuscular)
Measles	0.2–0.4	0.2–0.4
Varicella	0.2–1.0	0.2–0.4
Rubella in pregnancy	0.2–0.8* (at least 40 ml in total)	0.2
Mumps	0.2–0.5	0.3
Hepatitis A	2–5 ml (total)	–
Hepatitis B	–	0.06 (−0.1)
Non-A, non-B hepatitis	10 ml (total)	–

*When rubella exposure was more than 7 days previously, give 50 ml in total including at least 15 ml of rubella hyperimmune globulin simultaneously.

viraemia and viral excretion were reduced in renal transplant patients with cytomegalovirus infection. Patients with *aggressive hepatitis* given interferon showed a decrease in DNA polymerase in the Dane particles and a reversal of the hepatitis B core antigenaemia. The incidence of *side effects* depends on the dosage and partially on the purity of the preparation used. A severe flu-like syndrome is associated with the action of interferon itself. Fever was not uncommon, occasionally with nausea, vomiting, myalgia, an increase in transaminases and a reversible decrease in the peripheral leucocyte, platelet and reticulocytes counts.

Immunoglobulins for the treatment and prophylaxis of viral disease should be used only in especial indications. The former use of i. v. immunoglobulin for treatment of herpes zoster in immunocompromised patients is now largely replaced by acyclovir. Immunoglobulins should also be considered when a pregnant mother is exposed to *chicken pox* in the last 5 days before delivery, never having had the disease before. She should be given 0.1 ml/kg of zoster immuno-globulin i. m. forthwith. When the mother is infected earlier (in the last 3 weeks before delivery), the newborn baby can be treated with acyclovir, which is usually effective in preventing fatal neonatal varicella. When infection occurs after birth, the danger to the baby is no longer so great, and 0.6 ml/kg of normal pooled human (polyvalent) immunoglobulin should then be given. The use of immuno-globulins in the prophylaxis of *other viral diseases* is summarised in Table 72.

References

ADAMS, H. G., E. A. BENSON, E. R. ALEXANDER: Genital herpetic infection in men and women: Clinical course and effect of topical application of adenine arabinoside. J. infect. Dis. *133* (Suppl.): A151 (1976).

ARVIN, A. M., S. FELDMAN, T. C. MERIGAN: Human leukocyte interferon in the treatment of varicella in children with cancer: A preliminary controlled trial. Antimicrob. Ag. Chemother. *13:* 605 (1978).

BARON, S., P. A. BRUNELL, S. E. GROSSBERG: Mechanisms of action and pharmacology: The immune and interferon systems. In: GALASSO, G. J. et al. (eds.): Antiviral Agents and Viral Diseases of Man, pp. 131. Raven Press, New York 1979.

BRYSON, Y. J., C. MONAHAN, M. POLLACK: A prospective, double-blind study of side effects associated with the administration of amantadine hydrochloride or influenza A prophylaxis. Side effects of amantadine. J. infect. Dis. *141:* 545 (1980).

CANTELL, K., L. PYHALA: Pharmacokinetics of human leukocyte interferon. J. infect. Dis. *133* (Suppl.): A6 (1976).

CHEESEMAN, S. H., R. H. RUBIN, J. STEWART: Controlled clinical trial of prophylactic human-leukocyte interferon in renal transplantation. Effects on cytomegalovirus and herpes simplex virus infections. New Engl. J. Med. *300:* 1345 (1979).

GOLDMAN, J. M., P. M. CHIPPING, G. AGNARSDOTTIR: Acycloguanosine for viral pneumonia. Lancet *1:* 820 (1979).

GREENBERG, H. B., R. B. POLLARD, L. I. LUTWICK: Effect of human leukocyte interferon on hepatitis B virus infection in patients with chronic active hepatitis. New Engl. J. Med. *295:* 517 (1976).

MERIGAN, T. C., K. H. RAND, R. B. POLLARD: Human leukocyte interferon for the treatment of herpes zoster in patients with cancer. New Engl. J. Med. *298:* 981 (1978).

MONTO, A. S., R. A. GUNN, M. G. BANDYK: Prevention of Russian influenza by amantadine. J.A.M.A. *241:* 1003 (1979).

POLLARD, R. B., J. L. SMITH, A. E. NEAL: The effect of adenine arabinoside on chronic hepatitis B virus infection. J.A.M.A. *21:* 1648 (1977).

RYTEL, M. W., H. M. KAUFFMAN: Clinical efficacy of adenine arabinoside in therapy of cytomegalovirus infections in renal allograft recipients. J. infect. Dis. *133:* 202 (1976).

12. Evaluation of New Antibiotics

The introduction of a new antibiotic is not necessarily a therapeutic advance. The ideal agent would have good solubility and stability, strong antibacterial activity, no bacterial resistance, favourable pharmacokinetic properties (high blood *and* tissue concentrations with little metabolism in the body), convincing therapeutic results and very good tolerance. Whenever a new antibiotic is introduced, sometimes with exaggerated commercial publicity, the clinician should examine the accompanying literature critically according to the following criteria:

The **chemical structure** of the antibiotic and its membership of a particular class of substances will show whether it is a completely new drug or a variation of an existing compound. It is not sufficient for the manufacturer only to provide an incomprehensible chemical description which obscures the correct classification.

The **antibacterial activity** of a new antibiotic must be tested against a large number of different organisms of clinical significance. The results are best summarised as the *minimal inhibitory concentrations* as measured in serial dilution tests. *Disc diffusion* is not suitable for comparison with other antibiotics since the results are much more susceptible to variations in method than those of serial dilution. Bactericidal function in vivo should only be claimed for a new antibiotic if bactericidal concentrations are rapidly achieved at the site of action. The frequency of primary or secondary bacterial **resistance** should be stated as far as known. *Cross-resistance* with other antibiotics gives information about the relationship to existing agents.

The **pharmacokinetics** of a new antibiotic must be investigated in a large number of healthy subjects. Analysis of the results gives important information about the *amount and rate of absorption,* the *rate of elimination,* the *necessary dose interval* and the relationship of blood concentrations with the dose. The presentation of maximum (peak) blood concentrations alone is not enough for an assessment because it is dependent on a number of factors such as absorption and elimination rates, tissue diffusion and metabolism. The *urinary recovery* or the detection of metabolites in the urine allows the rate of metabolism to be calculated for substances whose elimination after parenteral administration is predominantly renal. The water and lipid solubility, molecular size and CSF concentrations of the new drug give information about its distribution in the body. These indices should be compared with the corresponding properties of other antibiotics.

New antibiotics are normally only approved after relatively extensive clinical trials (500–1000 cases) in which the most common **side effects** will normally be detected. With completely new drugs, however, there are still some unknown factors such as rare side effects or unexpected interactions which have not yet been tested. There are good reasons why a new antibiotic should be given with caution during the first 2 years after being licensed. Some countries (e. g. Britain) have a scheme by which possible side effects experienced in clinical use can be reported by clinicians to the drug licensing body. The immediate widespread use of a new compound is only justified when it is a major innovation (e. g. a well-tolerated antibiotic against Candida albicans). Many new compounds are only minor improvements on existing agents which require a controlled and critical introduction but do not justify replacement antibiotics of proven value.

The **indications** for the rational use of new antibiotics are based on the properties of the agent and the published results of large clinical trials of the drug's effectiveness in various diseases. It is wrong when a manufacturer declares a series of indications based only on in vitro activity but without clinical trials or for which other existing antibiotics are more suitable. New antibiotics are normally only licensed for certain indications. An antibiotic which has been approved for special indications should not, therefore, be used for "blind" therapy, and should not be used for certain potentially fatal conditions such as meningitis or endocarditis until these indications have been approved for that antibiotic.

The **dosage** should be decided on the basis of measured blood levels, tolerance and clinical experience. The dosage recommended when an antibiotic is introduced may on occasion be too low in order to make the treatment appear cheaper.

Illogical fixed **antibiotic combinations** or combinations of an antibiotic with other drugs (e. g. expectorants or spasmolytics) are not recommended because the clinician must be able to decide individually at each stage of the disease whether a combination is required.

The manufacturer has to provide evidence of bioavailability for every presentation of the drug, since the right **galenic formulation** is important for adequate uptake in the body (bioavailability). Any solvents or additives should be stated on the label. Studies have shown that similar preparations from different firms can show considerable variation in their absorption because of different galenic properties. As a rule, regular careful quality control is needed to ensure that a product has reliable activity.

The **clinical examination** of a new antibiotic can be an important scientific work. The requirements for clinical trials of new drugs are normally controlled by legislation which may be applied by official licensing bodies such as the Committee for Safety of Medicines (CSM) in Great Britain or the Food and Drug Administration (FDA) in the United States of America. Clinical trials should follow the Declaration of Helsinki. The qualifications of the examiner, informed consent of the patient, insurance of the patient (in some countries) and proper study design are the main general requirements. Double-blind studies in comparison with a placebo are only ethically justifiable in trivial infections such as interdigital fungal infections; comparative studies generally compare current standard therapy with the new treatment. The use of licensed preparations for approved indications is usually not a clinical trial but a clinical study. Such studies can deliver valuable additional information, especially when two different forms of a compound are compared. The value of non-comparative clinical studies is limited. As a general principle, drugs for clinical trials and studies are provided free of charge by the manufacturer, usually in special containers under their own control.

Very occasionally, **antimicrobials** may need to be used which are **not licensed** in that country, for example in the treatment of imported tropical diseases. Such use is legally acceptable in many countries but the manufacturer may not be liable. If this is the case, the patient should be clearly informed and legal consent obtained.

Index